ENCYCLOPEDIA OF
Sport and Exercise Psychology

Editorial Board

ENCYCLOPEDIA OF
Sport and
Exercise
Psychology

Editors

Robert C. Eklund
University of Stirling

Gershon Tenenbaum
Florida State University

⑤SAGE reference

Los Angeles | London | New Delhi
Singapore | Washington DC

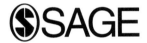

Los Angeles | London | New Delhi
Singapore | Washington DC

FOR INFORMATION:

SAGE Publications, Inc.
2455 Teller Road
Thousand Oaks, California 91320
E-mail: order@sagepub.com

SAGE Publications Ltd.
1 Oliver's Yard
55 City Road
London, EC1Y 1SP
United Kingdom

SAGE Publications India Pvt. Ltd.
B 1/I 1 Mohan Cooperative Industrial Area
Mathura Road, New Delhi 110 044
India

SAGE Publications Asia-Pacific Pte. Ltd.
3 Church Street
#10–04 Samsung Hub
Singapore 049483

Acquisitions Editor: Jim Brace-Thompson
Developmental Editor: Sanford J. Robinson
Reference Systems Manager: Leticia M. Gutierrez
Reference Systems Coordinators: Anna Villasenor,
                                           Laura Notton
Production Editor: Tracy Buyan
Copy Editors: Diane DiMura, Megan Markanich
Typesetter: Hurix Systems (P) Ltd.
Proofreaders: Sally Jaskold, Kate Peterson
Indexer: Sheila Bodell
Cover Designer: Candice Harman
Marketing Manager: Carmel Schrire

Printed in the United States of America.

Library of Congress Cataloging-in-Publication Data

Encyclopedia of sport and exercise psychology / edited by Robert C. Eklund, Gershon Tenenbaum.

pages cm
Includes bibliographical references and index.

ISBN 978-1-4522-0383-6 (hardcover)

1. Sports—Psychological aspects—Encyclopedias.
2. Exercise—Psychological aspects—Encyclopedias. I. Eklund, Robert C. (Robert Charles), 1958– II. Tenenbaum, Gershon.

GV706.4.E5 2014
796.03—dc23   2013021776

MIX
Paper from
responsible sources
FSC® C014174

14 15 16 17 18 10 9 8 7 6 5 4 3 2 1

DISCLAIMER: All information contained in the *Encyclopedia of Sport and Exercise Psychology* is intended only for informational and educational purposes. The information is not intended to diagnose medical problems, prescribe remedies for illness, or treat disease. We recommend that you always seek the advice of a health care professional with respect to any medical condition, illness, or disease.

Contents

List of Entries

Reader's Guide

Psychological Skills and Interventions

Affirmations
Attention Training
Breathing Exercises
Centering
Cognitive Restructuring
Concentration Skills
Coping
Energizing (Activation) Strategies
Goal Setting
Humor
Hypnosis
Imagery
Mental Blocks
Mental Rehearsal
Mentoring
Mindfulness
Multimodal Mental Training
Music-Based Interventions
Positive Thinking
Preperformance Routines
Psychological Skills
Psychological Skills Training
Relaxation
Rest
Self-Regulation
Self-Talk
Simulation Training
Stress Management
Support Group
Thought Stopping

Psychosociocultural Considerations

Adaptation
Assimilation
Collectivism/Individualism
Cultural Competence
Cultural Safety
Diversity
Ethnicity
Feminism
Gender
Heterosexism, Homonegativism, and
    Transprejudice
Multiculturalism
Race
Racism/Whiteness
Stereotyping, Cultural/Ethnic/Racial

Self-Concept, Self-Perceptions, and Identity

Body Awareness
Body Dissatisfaction
Body Dysmorphic Disorder, Muscle Dysmorphia
Body Image
Body Self-Esteem
Hierarchical Self
Identity
Possible Selves
Self-Acceptance
Self-Appraisal/Assessment/Perception
Self-Awareness
Self-Compassion
Self-Construal
Self-Criticism
Self-Discrepancy
Self-Doubt
Self-Efficacy
Self-Fulfilling Prophecy
Self-Handicapping
Self-Monitoring
Self-Objectification
Self-Presentation
Self-Schema
Social Comparison

Youth Sport

Coach–Athlete Relations
Friendships/Peer Relations
Parenting
Participation Motives
Talent Development
Youth Sport, Participation Trends in

About the Editors

Robert C. Eklund, PhD, is currently professor and chair in physical activity and health in the School of Sport at the University of Stirling in Scotland. Previously, and while working on this encyclopedia, he served as distinguished professor of sport psychology in the Department of Educational Psychology and Learning Systems at Florida State University. His doctoral degree was earned at the University of North Carolina at Greensboro in exercise and sport science with a specialization in sport and exercise psychology. He is a fellow of both the American College of Sports Medicine (ACSM) and the National Academy of Kinesiology (NAK).

Dr. Eklund has published more than 75 peer-reviewed articles, coedited (with Gershon Tenenbaum) the prestigious *Handbook of Sport Psychology* (3rd ed.), *Measurement in Sport and Exercise Psychology, Critical Readings in Sport Psychology,* and *Critical Readings in Exercise Psychology,* in addition to having coauthored two measurement manuals on flow, and authored or coauthored 12 book chapters in edited sport and exercise psychology compendia. Eklund has presented his research and participated as a keynote lecturer and invited colloquia speaker at numerous conferences worldwide.

With regard to professional service to the field, Dr. Eklund is the current editor-in-chief of the *Journal of Sport & Exercise Psychology,* the premier journal in the field, and has served in that capacity since January 2003. He has also served as associate editor for the *Journal of Applied Sport Psychology* and section editor (Psychology) for *Research Quarterly for Exercise and Sport.* In addition to providing editorial review services for a range of scholarly journals, Eklund presently serves as an editorial and advisory board member for *The Sport Psychologist; Sport, Exercise, and Performance Psychology; Pamukkale Journal of Sport Sciences;* and *Hacettepe Journal of Sport Sciences.* In the past, he has also served on the editorial boards for the *Journal of Sport & Exercise Psychology* and the *Journal of Applied Sport Psychology.*

Dr. Eklund resides in Stirling, Scotland, with his wife, Colleen, and their two sons Garth (12 years of age) and Kieran (10 years of age). He immensely enjoys their sport involvements and intense interest in being physically active.

Gershon Tenenbaum, PhD, is Benjamin S. Bloom Professor of Educational Psychology and professor of sport and exercise psychology at Florida State University. He is a former director of the Ribstein Center for Research and Sport Medicine at the Wingate Institute in Israel, and coordinator of the graduate program in sport psychology at the University of Southern Queensland, Australia. From 1997 to 2001 he was president of the International Society of Sport Psychology, and from 1996 to 2008 served as editor of the *International Journal of Sport and Exercise Psychology.* He has published extensively in psychology and sport psychology in the areas of expertise and decision making; linking emotions, cognitions, and motor systems; psychometrics; and coping with physical effort experiences. Dr. Tenenbaum has written and edited several books. In 2012, he edited *Measurement in Sport and Exercise Psychology* (with Robert C. Eklund and Akihito Kamata); *Case Studies in Applied Psychophysiology: Neurofeedback and Biofeedback Treatments for Advances in Human Performance* (with William A. Edmonds); and the *Handbook of Sport Psychology* (3rd ed., with Robert C. Eklund).

Dr. Tenenbaum has received several awards for his academic and scientific achievements, such as the Distinguished Scientific and Research Contributions to Exercise and Sport Psychology Award from the American Psychological Association, Division 47–Exercise and Sport Psychology, the International Society of Sport Psychology (ISSP) Presidential Award, the ISSP Honor Award, the ISSP Distinguished International Scholar Award, and the Journal of Educational Research's Harold E. Mitzel Award for Meritorious Contribution to Educational Practice through Research. He is a member of several professional organizations and a fellow of the American Psychological Association (Division 47), Association for the Advancement of Applied Sport Psychology, and the American Academy of Kinesiology. Dr. Tenenbaum is a scientific advisor to the Israeli Olympic Committee and has been invited to lecture in many conferences and for organizations worldwide.

Contributors

Bruce Abernethy
University of Queensland

Edmund O. Acevedo
Virginia Commonwealth University

Brandon L. Alderman
Rutgers University

Dorothee Alfermann
University of Leipzig

Sebastian Altfeld
Ruhr-University Bochum

Mark B. Andersen
Victoria University

Mark H. Anshel
Middle Tennessee State University

Renee N. Appaneal
Australian Institute of Sport

Shawn M. Arent
Rutgers University

Calum Alexander Arthur
Stirling University

Kelly J. Ashford
Brunel University

Joseph Baker
York University

Michael Bar-Eli
Ben-Gurion University of the Negev

Jamie Barker
Staffordshire University

Vassilis Barkoukis
Aristotle University of Thessaloniki

Itay Basevitch
Florida State University

Mark R. Beauchamp
University of British Columbia

Peter J. Beek
VU University Amsterdam

James Bell
Bangor University

Tanya R. Berry
University of Alberta

Robyn Bertram
Wilfrid Laurier University

Natalia Bessette
McGill University

Stuart J. H. Biddle
Loughborough University

Bettina Bläsing
Bielefeld University

Boris Blumenstein
Wingate Institute

Ian D. Boardley
University of Birmingham

Brenda Light Bredemeier
University of Missouri–St. Louis

Britton W. Brewer
Springfield College

Cameron Brick
University of California, Santa Barbara

Mark W. Bruner
Nipissing University

Jennifer Brunet
CHUM Research Centre, University of Montreal

Kevin L. Burke
Queens University of Charlotte

Ted M. Butryn
San Jose State University

Winston D. Byblow
University of Auckland

Martin Camiré
University of Ottawa

Albert V. Carron
University of Western Ontario

Andree Castonguay
McGill University

Derwin K.-C. Chan
University of Nottingham

Yu-Kai Chang
National Taiwan Sport University

Melissa A. Chase
Miami University

Nikos L. D. Chatzisarantis
Curtin University

Packianathan Chelladurai
Professor emeritus, Ohio State University

Graig M. Chow
University of Nevada, Las Vegas

Pete Coffee
University of Stirling

David E. Conroy
Pennsylvania State University

Brian Cook
Neuropsychiatric Research Institute

Kelly A. Cotter
Sacramento State University

Cathy Craig
Queen's University Belfast

Peter R. E. Crocker
University of British Columbia

Jennifer Cumming
University of Birmingham

Andreas Daffertshofer
VU University Amsterdam

Keith Davids
Queensland University of Technology

Matt S. Dicks
University of Portsmouth

James Dimmock
University of Western Australia

Shawna E. Doerksen
Pennsylvania State University

Rachel L. Duckham
Loughborough University

William L. Dunlop
University of British Columbia

David A. Dzewaltowski
Kansas State University

Peter R. Eastwood
University of Western Australia

David W. Eccles
Durham University

Jacquelynne S. Eccles
University of Michigan

Alfred Effenberg
University of Hanover

Panteleimon Ekkekakis
Iowa State University

Robert C. Eklund
University of Stirling

Steriani Elavsky
Pennsylvania State University

Lydia Emm
University of Bath

Paul A. Estabrooks
Virginia Polytechnic Institute and State University

Roger Eston
University of South Australia

Jennifer L. Etnier
University of North Carolina at Greensboro

Mark Eys
Wilfrid Laurier University

Damian Farrow
Victoria University and Australian Institute of Sport

Guy Faulkner
University of Toronto

Bradley Fawver
University of Florida

Luke Felton
Loughborough University

Leah J. Ferguson
University of Saskatchewan

Edson Filho
University of Chieti-Pescara

Lucie Finez
Laboratoire SPMS

Leslee A. Fisher
University of Tennessee

Brian Focht
Ohio State University

Emily Galvin
Miami University

Kimberley L. Gammage
Brock University

Jennifer I. Gapin
Southern Illinois University, Edwardsville

Frank L. Gardner
Kean University

Lael Gershgoren
Wingate Institute

Diane L. Gill
University of North Carolina at Greensboro

Fiona B. Gillison
University of Bath

Todd A. Gilson
Northern Illinois University

Adam D. Gorman
Australian Institute of Sport

Daniel Gould
Michigan State University

Rob Gray
University of Birmingham

Christy Greenleaf
University of Wisconsin–Milwaukee

Iain Greenlees
University of Chichester

J. Robert Grove
University of Western Australia

Daniel F. Gucciardi
Curtin University

Katie E. Gunnell
University of British Columbia

Oscar Gutierrez
Florida State University

Martin S. Hagger
Curtin University

G. M. Hancock
University of Central Florida

P. A. Hancock
University of Central Florida

Yuri L. Hanin
Research Institute for Olympic Sports, Jyväskylä University

James Hardy
Bangor University

Heather Hausenblas
Jacksonville University

Kate F. Hays
The Performing Edge

Kathleen Haywood
University of Missouri–St. Louis

Herbert Heuer
*IfADo–Leibniz Research Centre
for Working Environment
and Human Factors*

Nicola Jane Hodges
University of British Columbia

Nicholas L. Holt
University of Alberta

Thelma S. Horn
Miami University, Ohio

Amanda L. Hyde
Pennsylvania State University

Ben Jackson
University of Western Australia

Robin C. Jackson
Brunel University

Susan Jackson
*www.bodyandmindflow.com.au
and Queensland University of
Technology*

Brittany K. Jakubiak
Villanova University

Christopher M. Janelle
University of Florida

Marc V. Jones
Staffordshire University

Sophia Jowett
Loughborough University

Svetlana Kamarova
Curtin University

Cindra S. Kamphoff
*Minnesota State University,
Mankato*

Costas I. Karageorghis
Brunel University

Maria Kavussanu
University of Birmingham

Masato Kawabata
*Nanyang Technological
University*

David A. Keatley
University of Nottingham

Michael Kellmann
Ruhr-University Bochum

J. A. Scott Kelso
*Center for Complex Systems
and Brain Sciences, Florida
Atlantic University*

Deborah Kendzierski
Villanova University

Kieran Kingston
Cardiff Metropolitan University

Camilla J. Knight
University of Alberta

Dirk Koester
Bielefeld University

Anthony P. Kontos
*University of Pittsburgh School
of Medicine*

Kent C. Kowalski
University of Saskatchewan

Vikki Krane
Bowling Green State University

Daniel R. Lalande
*Université du Québéc à
Chicoutimi*

William Land
University of Texas, San Antonio

Edel Langan
University College Dublin

Amy E. Latimer-Cheung
Queen's University

Hedda Lausberg
German Sport University

Domagoj Lausic
*U.S. Professional Tennis
Association*

David Lavallee
University of Stirling

Lambros Lazuras
*South-East European Research
Centre*

Ronnie Lidor
Wingate Institute

Sonia Lippke
Jacobs University Bremen

Keith R. Lohse
University of British Columbia

Chris Lonsdale
University of Western Sydney

Britta Lorey
*Neuromotor Behavior Lab,
Justus-Liebig-Universität
Gießen*

Andrew MacIntosh
Michigan State University

Katherine M. Maciulewicz
University of Saskatchewan

Diane Mack
Brock University

Clare MacMahon
Victoria University

Leilani Madrigal
*University of North Carolina at
Greensboro*

Neha Malhotra
University of Hong Kong

George Mammen
University of Toronto

David L. Mann
*Faculty of Human Movement
Sciences*

Mallory Mann
Bowling Green State University

Matthew P. Martens
University of Missouri

Caoimhe Martin
Bangor University

Eric Martin
*Michigan State University
Institute for the Study of
Youth Sports*

Jeffrey J. Martin
Wayne State University

Luc J. Martin
*University of British
Columbia*

Rich Masters
University of Hong Kong

Lauren Mawn
Bangor University

Carolyn McEwen
*University of British
Columbia*

Kerry R. McGannon
Laurentian University

Tara-Leigh McHugh
University of Alberta

Colin McLaren
Wilfrid Laurier University

Eva V. Monsma
University of South Carolina

Zella E. Moore
Manhattan College

Aidan Moran
University College Dublin

Katie L. Morton
University of Cambridge

Amber D. Mosewich
University of British Columbia

Robert Motl
University of Illinois

Jörn Munzert
*Neuromotor Behavior Lab,
Justus-Liebig-Universität*

Nanette Mutrie
University of Strathclyde

Nicholas D. Myers
University of Miami

Richard Neil
Cardiff Metropolitan University

Maria Newton
University of Utah

Nikos Ntoumanis
University of Birmingham

Emily J. Oliver
Aberystwyth University

Iris Orbach
Wingate Institute

Michael W. Otto
Boston University

Derek Panchuk
Victoria University

Kyle F. Paradis
University of Western Ontario

Gaynor Parfitt
University of South Australia

William D. Parham
Loyola Marymount University

Sunghee Park
University of Stirling

Cassandra D. Pasquariello
*Virginia Commonwealth
University*

Frank M. Perna
National Cancer Institute

Melanie Perreault
University of South Carolina

Marie-Josee Perrier
Queen's University

Trent Petrie
University of North Texas

Steven J. Petruzzello
*University of Illinois at Urbana-
Champaign*

Aaron T. Piepmeier
*University of North Carolina
at Greensboro*

Eva Pila
University of Toronto

Artur Poczwardowski
University of Denver

Leslie Podlog
University of Utah

Jamie Poolton
University of Hong Kong

Timothy W. Puetz
Emory University

Anke Raabe-Oetker
German Sport University

Thomas D. Raedeke
East Carolina University

Selen Razon
Ball State University

Claudia L. Reardon
University of Wisconsin

Justy Reed
Chicago State University

Tim Rees
University of Exeter

Erin J. Reifsteck
*University of North Carolina
at Greensboro*

Anke Reints
Vrije Universiteit Brussel

Ian Renshaw
*Queensland University of
Technology*

Ryan E. Rhodes
University of Victoria

Stephan Riek
University of Queensland

Kaitlin Riley
Arizona State University

Elisa Robey
*University of Western
Australia*

Emily A. Roper
Sam Houston State University

Catherine M. Sabiston
University of Toronto

Michael L. Sachs
Temple University

Geert J. P. Savelsbergh
VU University Amsterdam

Lawrence A. Scanlan
University of California, Los Angeles

Tara K. Scanlan
University of California, Los Angeles

Thomas Schack
Bielefeld University

Robert J. Schinke
Laurentian University

Richard A. Schmidt
Human Performance Research, Marina Del Rey, California

Ralf Schwarzer
Freie Universität Berlin

Ludovic Seifert
University of Rouen

Brian Seiler
University of South Carolina

Charles H. Shea
Texas A&M University

David K. Sherman
University of California, Santa Barbara

David Light Shields
St. Louis Community College–Meramec

Sandra Short
University of North Dakota

Jeffery P. Simons
California State University East Bay

Brett Smith
Loughborough University

Erin M. Smith
Virginia Tech

J. Carson Smith
University of Maryland

Jasper A. J. Smits
Southern Methodist University

John C. Spence
University of Alberta

Kevin S. Spink
University of Saskatchewan

Christopher M. Spray
Loughborough University

Natalia Stambulova
Halmstad University

Martyn Standage
University of Bath

Tino Stöckel
University of Rostock

Joachim Stoeber
University of Kent

Sharon Kay Stoll
University of Idaho

Jeff Stone
University of Arizona

Shaelyn M. Strachan
University of Manitoba

Cheryl Stuntz
St. Lawrence University

Danielle Symons Downs
Pennsylvania State University

Katherine Tamminen
University of British Columbia

Adrian H. Taylor
University of Exeter

Gershon Tenenbaum
Florida State University

Owen Thomas
Cardiff Metropolitan University

Katy Tran Turner
U.S. Army Comprehensive Soldier and Family Fitness Program

Martin J. Turner
Staffordshire University

Sarah Ullrich-French
Washington State University

M. Renée Umstattd Meyer
Baylor University

Robert J. Vallerand
Université du Québec à Montréal

John van der Kamp
VU University Amsterdam

Judy L. Van Raalte
Springfield College

Jérémie Verner-Filion
Université du Québec à Montréal

Bas Verplanken
University of Bath

Joan N. Vickers
University of Calgary

Francesca Vitali
University of Verona

Dana K. Voelker
State University of New York College at Brockport

Michelle W. Voss
University of Iowa

Paul Ward
University of Greenwich

Jack C. Watson
West Virginia University

Matthias Weigelt
University of Paderborn

Laurel Whalen
Wayne State University

Diane E. Whaley
University of Virginia

David M. Williams
Brown University

Sarah E. Williams
University of Birmingham

Gabriele Wulf
University of Nevada, Las Vegas

Frank Zhu
University of Hong Kong

Tim Woodman
Bangor University

Paul Wylleman
Vrije Universiteit Brussel

Sam J. Zizzi
West Virginia University

Craig A. Wrisberg
University of Tennessee

Howard Zelaznik
Purdue University

Introduction

Sport psychology and exercise psychology are two closely interrelated fields of scientific study and professional practice. Human movement is central in both instances. In general, competitive physical activities characterized by athleticism and/or physical skill are typically categorized as sport, particularly when governed by rules and conventions to ensure fair competition and reasonably clear and consistent determinations of competitive outcomes. Exercise, again speaking broadly, involves planned and regular engagement in physical activity for the purpose of improving or maintaining physical fitness. The categories of "sport" and "exercise," however, do not encompass the entirety of possibilities available in physical activity. This is a matter that is fairly obvious given that not all physical activity inherently, or necessarily, involves competing or efforts to improve or maintain fitness. Research on both sport psychology and exercise psychology has tended to be inclusive and definitely elastic on this account as long as the participants are engaged in physical activity. Nonetheless, as noted in Diane Gill and Erin Reifsteck's entry on the history of exercise psychology, sport psychology and exercise psychology have essentially always been deeply interconnected despite the relatively recent interest in making more emphatic subdisciplinary distinctions. The ambiguities involved in making these distinctions have generally been addressed by acknowledging that the psychological aspects of particular subcategories of physical activity warrant recognition—that the uniquenesses are not entirely trivial even if the commonalities are very substantial.

Psychological factors have long been implicated as influencing, and being influenced by, involvement in sport and exercise. As discussed in entries on the histories of sport psychology and exercise psychology, and as is evident in the timeline included in the encyclopedia's appendix, commentary connecting engagement in human movement activity and psychological factors can be identified across millennia. The emergence of systematic scientific study of the psychology of human movement endeavors, however, is relatively recent. In the last half century, the acceleration, accumulation, and span of quality research-based knowledge on human behavior in the area has been impressive. The research knowledge conveyed in the encyclopedia stems from the many areas and traditions of psychological inquiry pursued in sport and exercise psychology. Findings from investigations involving participants relevant for the given research questions being examined in experimental, quasi-experimental, and descriptive correlational designs as well as findings from qualitative, naturalistic, and observational inquiry are featured across entries in this compendium.

Although sport and exercise psychology is fundamentally grounded in scientific study of human behavior in physical activity settings, it is also inherently an area of applied practice. Simply seeking to acquire knowledge and understanding on psychological influences and consequences of sport and exercise involvement without any applied application would be an incredibly sterile endeavor. In fact, the growth and acceptance of the practice of applied sport and exercise psychology has been no less impressive than the accelerating growth of research-based knowledge. Importantly, the developments in sport and exercise psychology research and applied practice have been synergistic in nature with both research informing practice and practice informing research in some meaningful degree. Clearly there is variation in opinions on whether or not the science of sport and exercise psychology is too distant from (and hence of limited relevance to) applied practice in the area, as well as whether or not applied practice in sport and exercise psychology is too distant from, and insufficiently grounded in, research in the area. It is, nonetheless, reasonable to suggest that the applied and research spheres within sport and exercise psychology are not entirely disconnected. Certainly, however, the days when athletes and coaches shunned the presence of applied sport psychologists are now largely in the past. Applied sport psychologists now enjoy more generalized acceptance and valuing of their potential contributions. There is now broader recognition than in past decades that individuals with relevant sport psychology expertise can offer avenues for optimizing both on-field performance and athlete health and well-being. Although not everyone would agree, we suggest that this recognition has also opened doors for more extensive and intensive research in applied settings, and the fruits of that applied research have increasingly provided credibility and greater trust in the applied practice of sport psychology. Certainly parallel developments and gains in professional acceptance can be observed for applied exercise psychologists as well, and for the vibrancy brought by healthy synergies across research and applied endeavors.

Rationale for the *Encyclopedia of Sport and Exercise Psychology*

Given the previously mentioned rapid growth and acceptance of research and applied practice during the relatively short history of formal recognition of these subdisciplinary areas, it is not surprising that a variety of substantial scientific journals and a cavalcade of books and scholarly resources have also come into existence. Nonetheless, a single authoritative, comprehensive resource explicating and supporting exploration of topics, constructs, issues and theories in the field had not yet been compiled at the time that we started contemplating the possibilities and challenges involved in undertaking such a tantalizing project. This two-volume *Encyclopedia of Sport and Exercise Psychology* is the result of our contemplations and the input received from the membership of the stellar advisory board assembled to guide our efforts in this daunting task. Of course, the real substance of the compendium lies in the 300+ authoritative entries written by researchers with expertise particular to the topics of focal

interest in each instance—researchers and practitioners who are typically among the world leaders in their areas of expertise. The notable enthusiasm of these authors for this project was gratifying. We believe that readers will find the results of the authors' efforts to be edifying in their utility for answering questions of interest and in expanding understanding of the state of knowledge in the area.

Questions on sport and exercise participation relating to psychological matters are myriad. For examples: How do athletes overcome fears, mental blocks, or injuries and how do they deal with stress and anxiety? Does engaging in exercise really make people feel good? What influence do competitors, teammates, audiences, parents, and coaches have on athletic performance? How do I get my spouse, children, friends, patients, or colleagues to be more physically active? What specific psychological techniques have proven effective in mental training for peak performance, maintaining concentration, motivation, and competitive drive? How can an athlete enhance his or her commitment to a training regimen, or how might the average person better adhere to a regime of exercise intended to advance health and well-being? What are the psychological risks and consequences associated with serious competition, training "too much," using performance-enhancing drugs, or training under aversive conditions? Does exercise really build self- and body-esteem? How does emotional experience in sport and exercise play into the behaviors exhibited by physical activity participants? Does sport involvement build character or does it really undermine moral development? How do coaches provide effective leadership for their athletes? Though final and complete answers to such questions may never be entirely at hand, the existing knowledge base is substantial and hence answers—some tentative, others more maturely concrete—are available in many areas. The *Encyclopedia of Sport and Exercise Psychology* was assembled to provide readers with a single authoritative, comprehensive resource to explore state-of-the-art scientific knowledge in seeking answers to the array of possible questions that might be asked, as well as to spur interest in areas beyond the specifics of any particular question that someone might have initially turned to the encyclopedia for an answer. The entries contained in this two-volume compendium explore the theory, research, and application of psychology as they relate to sport and exercise behavior.

The Audience of the Encyclopedia

The entries in this compendium convey information in a manner that is open, accessible, and relatively jargon-free. This stands in stark contrast with other available primary and secondary resources reporting scientific findings in the field where intimate knowledge of the specific topic is required to fully understand the issues and findings being addressed. In the encyclopedia, effort has been invested by the authors, advisory board members, and editors to ensure that the information is accessible to any reasonably well-educated reader having an inquiring mind regardless of the topical focus of that education. Readers with backgrounds in psychology (particularly health, exercise, and sport psychology), physical education, kinesiology, athletic training, and related fields will likely find the information more accessible than readers having little or no topical exposure to the area, but overall the entries have been shaped to convey information to as broad an audience as possible. The intent in having authors convey information in this manner was to help a wide array of interested readers to better understand human behavior in sport and exercise settings while avoiding the pitfalls engendered by an overly ponderous reliance on scientific jargon or area-specific terminology.

Content of the Encyclopedia

The entries in the encyclopedia span the spectrum of topics in the scientific study and applied practice of sport and exercise psychology, as well as on matters of foundational importance. The content of the encyclopedia can reasonably be captured within the 18 topical categories identified below.

- Career Transition
- Certification, Credentialing, and Roles of Sport and Exercise Psychologists
- Disability
- Emotion
- Exercise Health
- Group Dynamics
- History and Foundation
- Leadership
- Morality, Aggression, and Ethics in Sport
- Motivation
- Motor Control
- Perception and Cognition in Sport
- Personality and Psychological Characteristics in Sport
- Psychobiology
- Psychological Skills and Interventions
- Psychosociocultural Considerations
- Self-Concept, Self-Perceptions, and Identity
- Youth Sport

It is important to note that these categories are not mutually exclusive. Many individual entries cut across more than one topical area and some cut across many. Emotional experiences in sport and exercise, for example, have motivational implications, but motivation and emotion are not topically one and the same thing. Moreover, both also impact upon and are shaped by self-concept, self-perceptions, identity, and so on but not necessarily in the same ways. Identification of topical categories that were entirely independent of one another would have been impossible simply because of the nature and complexity of the human psyche. It should also be intuitively obvious that some categories are much broader than others. Motivation, for example, is fundamental to all human behavior, but commentary on, for example, disability or youth sport, is inherently focused more specifically.

Entries relating to these topics range from approximately 1,000 to 3,000 words in length. Some are very broadly focused and theoretical in nature (e.g., entries describing key psychological theories employed in sport and exercise psychology) while others are much narrower and more concrete in focus (e.g., use of humor in sport or on the nature of preperformance routines). Specific entry lengths were largely dictated by topical breadth and/or extent of available scientific or professional practice evidence.

Organization of the Encyclopedia

The 300-plus signed entries appearing in the encyclopedia are organized alphabetically for easy location of specific entries. A thematic Reader's Guide is provided in the front matter so that the specific entries can be identified relative to the primary topics they were associated with during development of the encyclopedia's content. Cross-references within the encyclopedia are provided with all entries to ensure topically related entries are brought to the reader's attention. Moreover, suggestions for further readings are provided with every entry so that avenues for deeper topical exploration are readily identifiable to satisfy the interested reader. Finally, a representative timeline on the History of Sport and Exercise Psychology is provided in the Volume 2's appendix.

How the Encyclopedia Was Created

This two-volume encyclopedia is the manifestation of a multistep process. Our initial considerations were focused upon developing a suitable keyword "skeleton" to serve as the roadmap for our efforts to create the encyclopedia. The first step in creating this skeleton involved collation of subject index entries from prominent textbooks in sport and exercise psychology, motor learning, and motor control, as well as article keywords appearing in prominent journals in sport and exercise psychology. This list of candidate keywords relating to constructs, theories, effects, and so on was subsequently reduced to a more manageable length by the removal of obvious redundancies, and through omission of potential keywords deemed too idiosyncratic or obscure for inclusion. We completed this initial phase of the process by conducting an "intuitive factor analysis," subjectively lumping potential keywords together that seemed to have topical coherence. Armed with this array of potential keywords and a potential topical organization to guide our invitations, a seventeen-member advisory board was recruited. As an aside, recruitment of the advisory board was far easier than expected given the amount of work involved in the project. Seventeen of 18 scholars on our list of candidates accepted our invitations—most were accepted immediately and the balance, a small minority, were accepted following relatively brief periods of contemplation.

The keyword lists generated by the editors for each potential topical area were first forwarded to the advisory board member recruited for his or her expertise in that area. The feedback obtained in this process was used to refine each of the area listings as well as the foci of identified topical areas themselves. Not surprisingly, suggestions for some keyword additions were common across several topical areas. Subsequent to making adjustments to these sublists, a single overall list of keywords was forwarded to all advisory board members so that they could comment on the totality of potential entries as well as the placement of keywords within topical areas. More excellent feedback was obtained in the course of a couple of iterations of this process, after which the final working "skeleton" keyword list was settled upon. Adjustments to the overall list after that point were relatively rare and minor and occurred only as terms, concepts, constructs, and so on were tripped across, or identified by contributing authors as really "needing" to be added. From that point forward, the process of creating the encyclopedia involved "putting meat" on the 300-plus keyword "skeleton" by securing authors to write the entries. This process was greatly facilitated by the stature and "connectedness" of our advisory board members.

Acknowledgments

The *Encyclopedia of Sport and Exercise Psychology* came to fruition only as a result of the committed involvement of many people. Completion of a project of this magnitude and complexity cannot occur in a timely manner otherwise. We acknowledge this fact and extend our sincerest and deepest appreciation to everyone who contributed to this project. We particularly thank the advisory board members identified in the front matter of the encyclopedia because their input and efforts were crucial at every stage of the process. They contributed to identification of topics and entry keywords in the developmental process, facilitated the identification and securing of authors of suitable expertise and stature, and subsequently provided feedback to those authors on entries submitted within their topical areas. They all have our gratitude for their Herculean efforts. The many authors who invested their time and expertise in this project also have our gratitude. They are all identified by name in conjunction with their entries. Their willingness to join us in this project was both bracing and satisfying. We also deeply appreciate the terrific support we received from "our" team on this project at SAGE: Jim Brace-Thompson,

Sanford Robinson, Leticia Gutierrez, Anna Villaseñor, Laura Notton, Tracy Buyan, Diane DiMura, Megan Markanich, Candice Harman, and Carmel Schrire. Their willingness to respond to questions, offer advice and guidance to ease our labors, and improve the product facilitated our efforts greatly. Surely the process would have been greatly more difficult without their cheerful, constructive, and proactive support. Finally, we thank Vista Beasley, our managing editor (and stellar doctoral student), for her contributions and assistance in making this effort run smoothly, effectively, and on time. She went above and beyond the call of duty and was amazing throughout.

Robert C. Eklund
Gershon Tenenbaum

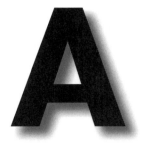

ACHIEVEMENT GOAL THEORY

Achievement goals refer to the aim, purpose, or focus of a person's achievement behavior. These goals are dynamic cognitive entities representing future-based possibilities that respond to changes in the person as well as the situation. They do not refer strictly to the level of aspired performance (as in the goal-setting literature) but, rather, to how people evaluate their competence or incompetence and orient their behavior accordingly. Achievement goal theory has emphasized the role of achievement goals in regulating a wide variety of affective, behavioral, and cognitive outcomes during people's competence pursuits. More recently, research on achievement goal theory has developed the hierarchical model of achievement motivation, which integrates a variety of achievement motivation theories. This entry defines key constructs in achievement goal theory, reviews major models of achievement goals, reviews the consequences of different achievement goals, and explains how achievement goals have been integrated with other theoretical approaches in the hierarchical model of achievement motivation.

Key Constructs in Achievement Goal Theory

Achievement goal theory posits three major explanatory constructs: *states of goal involvement, goal orientations,* and *goal climates.* A person's state of achievement goal involvement reflects the aim, purpose, or focus of the achievement behavior in a specific context at a particular moment in time. States of goal involvement can change over time, so it is very important to understand their contextual and temporal frame of reference. The narrower and more specific the frame of reference, the closer the construct will be to the theoretical conception of a goal as a dynamic cognitive entity. The predictive power of states of involvement varies based on the correspondence between the frame of reference for the goal and the outcome. For example, goals for today's practice session will be more effective at predicting outcomes in today's practice than in predicting outcomes over the course of the 6 months ahead. Unfortunately, research on states of achievement goal involvement is limited, in part because of the challenges associated with assessing goals in relevant performance contexts repeatedly over time.

An individual's achievement *goal orientation* reflects one's typical state of achievement goal involvement over time within a particular context. Goal orientations can be thought of as the central tendency of a distribution representing a person's states of involvement for an activity sampled repeatedly over time. Goal orientations are thought to be more stable than states of goal involvement because they are contextually—but not temporally—specific. Goal orientations emerged as a preferred level of analysis in achievement goal research because they can be assessed via self-reports on a single occasion and do not require repeated assessment to capture a process.

Despite the relative ease of assessing goal orientations, a noteworthy limitation of this construct is that it cannot distinguish goal-based variability from variability associated with other stable individual differences (e.g., motives). For example, a person who has a strong fear of failure will tend to adopt some achievement goals more than others, and the difference between fear of failure-based variability and variation due to the actual aim, purpose, or focus of that person's achievement behavior is blurred. Likewise, goal orientation ratings may be tainted by situational factors at the time the measure is completed. Notwithstanding these limitations, the achievement goal orientation construct has provided a very accessible entry point for testing the propositions of achievement goal theory, and the vast majority of the research on achievement goals has focused on goal orientations.

Finally, achievement *goal climates* represent the situational cues that lead people to adopt different states of involvement. Joyce Epstein proposed a set of TARGET structures within achievement contexts, which influence the goals that people adopt. This model is derived from research on academic achievement motivation but also provides a rich conceptual framework for dissecting the motivational climate in physical activity settings.

The TARGET acronym stands for the *task, authority, recognition, grouping, evaluation,* and *timing structures* in a particular situation. *Task structures* refer to the type of task that people are working on. Tasks that are perceived as challenging will evoke different goals than tasks that are perceived as repetitive and boring. *Authority* refers to how decisions were made about the task. Activities that are perceived as more autonomously selected by participants evoke different goals than those that are selected by leaders such as coaches or teachers. *Recognition* refers to the procedures used to recognize performers' accomplishments. Praise and criticism that are provided privately evoke different goals than similar feedback that is provided publicly. *Grouping* refers to whether participants are assigned to groups of similar or diverse ability levels. Groups formed with the intention of having a diverse range of abilities evoke different goals than groups formed with the intention of creating status differences between groups. *Evaluation* describes how participants' competence is evaluated and recognized. Evaluations that emphasize improvement evoke different goals than evaluations that emphasize normative comparisons. *Timing* refers to whether

the time demands promote a focus on learning or immediate performance. It is worth noting that the perceived motivational climate (i.e., TARGET structures) may differ from an objective assessment of the motivational climate. As in other social cognitive approaches, it is the perceived climate that is held to influence states of goal involvement.

Structure of Achievement Goals

The structure of and terminology for describing achievement goals have evolved considerably over the past 3 decades. Goals were originally proposed to account for differences between mastery and helpless responses to failure. People who exhibited a mastery response to failure (i.e., attributions to low effort, increased persistence, greater enjoyment, and enhanced problem solving) were thought to exhibit this response because they focused on learning and improving. In contrast, people who exhibited a helpless response to failure (i.e., attributions to low ability, decreased persistence, less enjoyment, and reduced problem solving) were thought to exhibit this response because they focused on protecting themselves from undesirable social comparisons. These goals became the focus of the dichotomous model of achievement goals.

Dichotomous Achievement Goals

The dichotomous model of achievement goals emphasizes two primary definitions of competence. *Task goals* emphasize learning and improving, whereas *ego goals* emphasize outperforming others. Task and ego goals have also been referred to as mastery–learning and performance–competitive goals, respectively.

Based on research in sport and physical education contexts, task goal orientations are associated with greater enjoyment, interest, pleasant emotional experiences, prosocial behavior, commitment, perceived improvement, intrinsic motivation, moral functioning, life satisfaction, and satisfaction with coaching and competitive results. Ego goals are associated with consequences such as anxiety, worry, competitiveness, public self-consciousness, motivation for social status and recognition, extrinsic motivation, hypercompetitive attitudes, and antisocial behavior. Relations between dichotomous goal orientations and perceived competence are more equivocal in the literature and require further attention. Both task and ego goal orientations positively predict perceptions of task and ego goal climates, respectively.

Goal climates have also been linked with a number of affective, behavioral, and cognitive outcomes. This literature has emphasized the distinction between mastery (i.e., task) and performance (i.e., ego) motivational climates without attending much to the *approach–avoidance* distinction that became the focus in subsequent extensions of the goals model. It has also focused on physical education settings. Compared with control groups and groups exposed to performance goal climates, interventions that created mastery goal climates in physical education classes have been associated with more positive attitudes toward the activity, greater enjoyment, increased health and fitness, improved skill, lower anxiety, and greater use of effective learning strategies compared with performance goal climates.

Trichotomous Achievement Goals

The trichotomous model of achievement goals was noted as a possibility in early writing on the dichotomous model of goals but only received empirical attention in the 1990s when it was used to explain an inconsistent finding in the literature. Specifically, relations between performance (or ego) goals and intrinsic motivation varied considerably, from negative to nil, across studies. Scholars posited that these goals had no influence on intrinsic motivation when they were approach oriented but reduced intrinsic motivation when they were avoidance oriented. This hypothesis was supported by a meta-analysis of existing studies and a series of experiments. Subsequent research has identified a number of other variables with different relations to performance goals depending on whether those goals are approach or avoidance oriented. Thus, the trichotomous model of achievement goals includes *mastery goals, performance–approach goals,* and *performance–avoidance goals.* These goals reflect aims of learning and improving, outperforming others, and not being outperformed by others, respectively.

In the physical domain, the added value of distinguishing performance–approach from performance–avoidance goals in physical activity was established in experimental research. These studies manipulated the instructions given to participants to induce particular goals. Participants who received mastery or performance–approach goals exhibited greater intrinsic motivation than participants who received performance–avoidance goals, and these relations were not due to differences in perceived competence. The latter finding was particularly important because early critics of expanding the dichotomous model of achievement goals speculated that the approach–avoidance distinction was simply a reflection of differences in perceived competence—a hypothesis that was clearly refuted by these studies. These findings were instrumental for introducing the approach–avoidance dimension to achievement goal theory in physical activity.

2x2 Model of Achievement Goals

Shortly after the introduction of the trichotomous model of achievement goals, the model was expanded to a fully symmetric 2x2 model of achievement goals. This model outlined four possible achievement goals based on (a) the *definition of competence* and (b) the *valence of the competence-based incentive.* The two levels for definitions of competence were consistent with the dichotomous and trichotomous models. Mastery goals defined competence in reference to the self or absolute standards, and performance goals defined competence in reference to normative standards. The two competence-based possibilities that orient people's behavior in achievement situations are success (which people typically approach) and failure (which people typically avoid).

A 2x2 taxonomy emerges from the combination of the definition of competence with the valence of the incentive. The *performance–approach* and *performance–avoidance* goals in this model mirror those goals in the trichotomous model. Mastery goals from the trichotomous model are specified as *mastery–approach goals* in the 2x2 model. These goals involve striving to improve or execute a skill as it should be executed (i.e., self- and absolutely referenced competence, respectively, with a focus on being successful). The new addition to the 2x2 model involves *mastery–avoidance goals,* which describe strivings not to have one's skills deteriorate or not to make mistakes (i.e., self- and absolutely referenced competence, respectively, with a focus on not failing). One of the major objectives for researchers interested in the 2x2 model over the past decade has involved evaluating whether the added complexity of this model is warranted in relation to increases in predictive power. Following is a summary of bivariate relations between each goal and a variety of affect, behavioral, and cognitive consequences in physical activity; this summary does not account for any overlap between goals due to a shared definition of competence or valence.

Mastery–approach goals have been linked with affective consequences such as heightened enjoyment and positive affect, and reduced boredom. Behaviorally, these goals are associated with increased fitness, perceived exercise intensity, physical activity participation and, in some studies, even performance (typically in timed races or similar tasks). They have also been linked with reduced self-handicapping. From a cognitive standpoint, mastery–approach goals have been linked with (a) greater meta-cognitive regulation, relative autonomy, intrinsic motivation, perceived usefulness and importance of the activity, effort, tolerance, help-seeking, situational interest, satisfaction, intentions to continue in sport, preferences for the activity, and utility value, and (b) reduced amotivation.

Mastery–avoidance goals have been linked with mixed affective consequences such as increased enjoyment and increased negative affect. Behaviorally, these goals are associated with increased fitness, shuttle run performance, and self-reported intensity of activity. From a cognitive standpoint, mastery–avoidance goals have been linked with stronger preference for the activity, tolerance, effort, physical activity participation, and intentions to participate in sport.

Performance–approach goals have been linked with affective consequences, such as increased enjoyment and positive affect, and decreased boredom. Behaviorally, these goals are associated with physical activity and performance (typically in timed races or similar tasks). From a cognitive standpoint, performance–approach goals have been linked with greater meta-cognitive regulation, effort, introjected and external regulation, intentions to participate in sport, value (intrinsic and utility), and satisfaction.

Performance–avoidance goals have been linked with affective consequences such as increased enjoyment and negative affect as well as decreased boredom. Behaviorally, these goals are associated with fitness, self-handicapping, and physical activity participation. From a cognitive standpoint, performance–avoidance goals are associated with interest; identified, introjected, or external

regulation; and intentions to continue in sport as well as decreased satisfaction with sport.

Even a cursory review of this list reveals that some outcomes (e.g., enjoyment) are associated with all four goals in the same way. This finding reflects, at least in part, the overlap between goals. It also suggests that a general achievement goal profile elevation may be contaminating some of these results, that is, people may be high or low in all goals because of some other factor such as the importance of the domain to them. Shifting the focus of future research from achievement goal orientations to states of involvement will help to resolve this issue. Notwithstanding this limitation, clear nomological networks for each goal are emerging. Taken as a whole, these findings indicate that mastery–approach goals have unequivocally desirable consequences, and the other goals have mixed profiles, with performance–approach goals appearing preferable to mastery–avoidance goals, which seem preferable to performance–avoidance goals.

Although the 2x2 model of achievement goals is fairly comprehensive, there may be reasons to make further distinctions between goals. For example, scholars have debated the merits of differentiating between mastery goals based on a self-referenced definition of competence and mastery goals based on a task-referenced definition of competence. Any such expansions of the 2x2 model of achievement goals must ensure that the new goals are grounded in competence-based incentives and must demonstrate that the explanatory or predictive power of the new goals is sufficient to offset the added complexity of the model.

Hierarchical Model of Achievement Motivation

The hierarchical model of achievement goals was proposed at the beginning of the 21st century to integrate the classic, motive-based approaches and contemporary, goal-based approaches to studying achievement motivation. This model posits goals as the proximal regulators of affect, behavior, and cognition during competence pursuits. It also proposes that many established achievement motivation constructs in other approaches predispose people to adopt certain goals. These goal antecedents include achievement motives, self-related constructs (e.g., perceived competence, self-theories of ability), neurophysiological predispositions, and the motivational climate in a given situation.

For example, mastery–approach goals are more likely to be adopted by people with high need for achievement, perfectionistic strivings, perceived competence, incremental theories of ability, and approach motivational temperaments and in situations that create a mastery motivational climate. In contrast, performance–avoidance goals are more likely to be adopted by people with high fear of failure, perfectionistic concerns, entity theories of ability, avoidance motivational temperaments, and low perceived competence and in situations that create a performance motivational climate.

One benefit of this hierarchical, antecedent–consequence model of achievement goals is that it has increased conceptual precision in research on achievement goal theory. Researchers now tend to differentiate between factors that lead to goal adoption and those that are produced by goal adoption. Although the vast majority of this literature is nonexperimental and does not provide a strong basis for causal claims, coherent and logical conceptual articulations of relations within the antecedent–consequence framework are contributing to theoretical clarity. Another trend worth noting in recent literature is a slight increase in the number of longitudinal research studies that investigate how goals fluctuate within people over time. This approach is valuable because it shifts the focus from goal orientations to states of involvement and removes threats from confounding third variables that may be antecedents of goals (e.g., fear of failure). Finally, as evidenced by the preceding review, the majority of the research on achievement goal theory as it relates to physical activity has been conducted in the context of sport and physical education. Exercise and rehabilitation contexts have received considerably less attention but also involve competence pursuits and therefore may be useful contexts for understanding the role of achievement goals in regulating affect, behavior, and cognition.

Conclusion

In sum, achievement goal theory has developed considerably since it was first proposed over 3 decades ago. Extensions of the theory have met with resistance in some quarters, but the associated debates have clarified differences in assumptions and contributed to a more precise articulation of the theory. The hierarchical model of achievement motivation represents the current state of the science. It is a significant development because it (a) links multiple levels of analysis in motivation from the neurophysiological to the social; (b) integrates diverse theories of achievement motivation; (c) differentiates the causes of goals from their effects, at least conceptually; and (d) specifically addresses the factors that energize and orient achievement strivings.

David E. Conroy and Amanda L. Hyde

See also Achievement Motive Theory; Attribution Theory

Further Readings

Braithwaite, R., Spray, C. M., & Warburton, V. E. (2011). Motivational climate interventions in physical education: A meta-analysis. *Psychology of Sport and Exercise, 12,* 628–638.

Conroy, D. E., & Hyde, A. L. (2012). Measurement of achievement motivation processes. In G. Tenenbaum, R. C. Eklund, & A. Kamata (Eds.), *Handbook of measurement in sport & exercise psychology* (pp. 303–317). Champaign, IL: Human Kinetics.

Cury, F., Elliot, A., Sarrazin, P., Da Fonseca, D., & Rufo, M. (2002). The trichotomous achievement goal model and intrinsic motivation: A sequential meditational analysis. *Journal of Experimental Social Psychology, 38,* 473–481.

Dweck, C. S. (1986). Motivational processes affecting learning. *American Psychologist, 41,* 1040–1048.

Dweck, C. S., & Leggett, E. (1988). A social-cognitive approach to motivation & personality. *Psychological Review, 95,* 256–273.

Elliot, A. J. (1997). Integrating "classic" and "contemporary" approaches to achievement motivation: A hierarchical model of approach and avoidance achievement motivation. In P. Pintrich & M. Maehr (Eds.), *Advances in motivation and achievement* (Vol. 10, pp. 143–179). Greenwich, CT: JAI Press.

Elliot, A. J. (1999). Approach and avoidance motivation and achievement goals. *Educational Psychologist, 34,* 169–189.

Elliot, A. J., Conroy, D. E., Barron, K. E., & Murayama, K. (2010). Achievement motives and goals: A developmental analysis. In R. Lerner, M. Lamb, & A. Freund (Eds.), *Handbook of lifespan development, Vol. 2: Social and emotional development* (pp. 474–510). New York: Wiley.

Epstein, J. L. (1989). Family structures and student motivation: A developmental perspective. In C. Ames & R. Ames (Eds.), *Research on motivation in education* (Vol. 3, pp. 259–295). New York: Academic Press.

Nicholls, J. G. (1984). Achievement motivation: conceptions of ability, subjective experience, task choice, and performance. *Psychological Review, 91,* 328–346.

Papaioannou, A. G., Zourbanos, N., Krommidas, C., & Ampatzoglou, G. (2012). The place of achievement goals in the social context of sport: A comparison of Nicholls' and Elliot's models. In G. C. Roberts & D. C. Treasure (Eds.), *Advances in motivation in sport and exercise* (3rd ed., pp. 59–90). Champaign, IL: Human Kinetics.

Roberts, G. C., Treasure, D. C., & Conroy, D. E. (2007). The dynamics of motivation in sport: The influence of achievement goals on motivation processes. In G. Tenenbaum & R. C. Eklund (Eds.), *Handbook of sport psychology* (3rd ed., pp. 3–30). New York: Wiley.

ACHIEVEMENT MOTIVE THEORY

Competence is a recurring theme in human movement whether the setting is sport, exercise, or rehabilitation. From the earliest days of life, people strive to feel effective in their unfolding interactions with the environment and, throughout the lifespan, people's well-being is compromised when this need is thwarted. Despite the apparent universality of competence motivation, there are clear differences in the ways that people pursue competence. Achievement motivation theories strive to explain the processes that initiate, direct, and maintain achievement behavior. Achievement motives are relatively stable individual differences that influence people's motivation during competence pursuits. This entry defines achievement motives, provides an overview of how they develop, reviews implicit and explicit measures of motives, and summarizes documented outcomes of achievement motives.

Achievement Motives

The earliest achievement motivation theories focused on people's aspired level of behavior and the perceived utility of different behaviors as indicated by the expectancies and values that people associated with those behaviors. A key assumption underlying these approaches was that people make conscious and rational choices about their achievement behavior. Around the same time that the expectancy-value theories were emerging,

personality psychologist Henry Murray proposed a system of psychological needs that included *achievement* (a need for efficiency and effectiveness) and *infavoidance* (a need to avoid humiliation and to refrain from action due to fear of failure). These needs were proposed to explain individual differences in behavior. David McClelland and colleagues in several works subsequently introduced the construct of achievement motives to account for individual differences in people's achievement behavior under similar conditions. Motives represented the strength of associations between environmental cues (e.g., competence pursuits where success or failure are possible) and learned affective responses to those cues. Given the importance of competence to the self, self-evaluative emotions such as pride and shame provided logical affective bases for these motives.

Two motives were proposed based on people's orientation toward or away from competence-based incentives during competence pursuits. The *motive to approach success* (sometimes referred to as hope for success) described individual differences in people's tendency to experience anticipatory pride while engaged in a competence pursuit. The *motive to avoid failure* described individual differences in people's tendency to experience anticipatory shame while engaged in a competence pursuit. Over time, these motives have been referred to as the need for achievement and fear of failure, respectively.

The anticipatory pride and shame involved in motives are instrumental in energizing and orienting achievement behavior. For example, pride fosters persistence and heightened engagement in goal pursuit, promotes long-term achievement, stimulates interpersonal expressiveness, engages flexible social behavior, and contributes to the development of social capital over time. Shame, on the other hand, motivates withdrawal. It can promote appeasement or aggressive behaviors depending on how people regulate their shame. From an achievement motivation perspective, shame will undermine persistence and create difficulties in achieving long-term goals.

In their achievement motivation theory, McClelland et al. posited that a person's motivation is influenced by a tendency toward success and a tendency away from failure. Each of these tendencies was represented as the product of the person's perceived probability of succeeding (or failing), the value of the reward for succeeding (or the punishment for failing), and the person's motives. Thus, motives were proposed to refine basic expectancy-value predictions and elaborate on interindividual variation in behavior. Over time, the independence of *approach* and *avoidance* motivation became apparent, and the idea that approach and avoidance tendencies produced a single resultant motivation orientation was abandoned. In contemporary research, the approach- and avoidance-based achievement motives are typically treated as independent predictors of motivational outcomes, and their direct effects on motivational outcomes receive more attention than their interactions with expectancies and values.

Development of Achievement Motives

Research on the development of self-evaluative emotions informs our understanding of how the two achievement motives develop. Self-evaluative emotions are a unique class of emotions because they are not present at birth and require some cognitive development before they appear. The necessary cognitive milestones include (a) the development of a sense of self (typically 15–24 months of age); (b) the internalization of rules, standards, or goals for desired behavior (typically 24–41 months of age); and (c) the evaluation of oneself in relation to those internalized rules, standards, or goals (as early as 30 months of age). If children appraise that they are complying with the rules, standards, or goals that they internalized through socialization, they should feel proud. On the other hand, if they appraise that they are not complying with those rules, standards, or goals, and attribute that deviance to a personal flaw (as opposed to a simple behavioral error), they should feel shame. As children develop a history of experiencing pride and shame in their competence pursuits, those competence pursuits increasingly become cues for anticipatory pride and shame. This association and anticipatory affective response is the basis for achievement motives. With roots in such foundational self-evaluative processes, these motives are likely to generalize across achievement contexts and should not be domain specific.

Measuring Implicit and Explicit Motives

One major controversy in the achievement motives literature concerned the measurement operations used to assess these motives.

Originally, McClelland and his colleagues adapted the Thematic Apperception Test and asked participants to view ambiguous images of people involved in competence pursuits, and to write a story about the image (e.g., What is happening? What happened previously? What will happen next?). Content from the ensuing narratives can be coded using different schemes for the need for achievement or fear of failure, which was called *hostile press* in an early scoring system. This procedure has been refined in the contemporary picture story exercise. This fantasy-based assessment procedure is relatively time-consuming and requires extensive training, so a number of researchers attempted to develop parallel self-report measures that could be administered quickly and easily without sacrificing (and possibly even enhancing) validity. When scores from self-reported achievement motives were compared with scores from projective tests, the correlations were unexpectedly small.

After extensive debate over which score was the more valid measure of achievement motives, researchers concluded that both scores were valid and that the difference reflected differences in the motivational systems that were assessed. This discovery contributed to the distinction between implicit and explicit motivation. *Implicit achievement motives* are rooted in affective arousal and are reflected in scores from the projective, fantasy-based measures. *Explicit achievement motives* involve cognitive elaboration and are reflected in scores from the self-report measures. Implicit motives are posited to predict spontaneous, nondeclarative outcomes that may be regulated outside of a person's conscious awareness (e.g., procedural learning), whereas explicit motives are posited to predict declarative outcomes of which people are self-consciously aware (e.g., enjoyment). Although the implicit or explicit distinction is still common in the achievement motivation literature, other models refer to these dual processes as *impulsive or automatic* and *reflective or controlled* processes, respectively.

Overall, the motivational taxonomy at the heart of motive-based approaches can be summarized as a 2x2 taxonomy. Both approach- and avoidance-based achievement motives exist at implicit, impulsive, or automatic levels and explicit, reflective, or controlled levels of analysis. The vast majority of research on achievement motives in physical activity contexts has employed explicit motivation measures so relatively little is known about implicit measures of motivation in these contexts.

Within the context of sport, most of the research on achievement motives has focused on fear of failure. This research often equated fear of failure with performance anxiety although it is now clear that athletes may experience anxiety over threats other than failure (e.g., injury, success). This distinction is important because contemporary models of emotion hold that emotions reflect people's ongoing adaptational struggles. Thus, the possibility of failure by itself is insufficient as a stimulus for activating a person's fear of failure because the meaning of failure can vary considerably from one person to the next.

The cognitive–motivational–relational theory of emotion has been applied to understand the meaning of failure. In a series of studies, five major aversive consequences of failing have been identified. These include *shame and embarrassment, devaluing one's self-estimate, having an uncertain future, upsetting important others*, and *having important others lose interest*. Beliefs in each of these consequences are strongly correlated so there appears to be a general fear of failure that underlies beliefs in each of these specific consequences. Beliefs that failure leads to shame and embarrassment are most closely related to the original definition of fear of failure. Perhaps not surprisingly, this belief was also the most strongly associated with the general fear of failure and seems to be the most relevant for achievement motivation. It is clear that all five of the beliefs are strongly associated, and collectively they provide a better representation of the universe of the fear of failure domain than does any single belief by itself.

Consequences of Achievement Motives

Achievement motives influence people's lives in a variety of ways, although more attention has focused on the impact of fear of failure than on need for achievement. In academic contexts, fear of failure has been linked with decreased moral functioning and increased attention-seeking behavior. From a health perspective, fear of failure is positively associated with anorexia, anxiety, depression, and headache disorders. College students who present for counseling services frequently cite fear of failure as a problem that interferes with their lives and academic performance.

Research within the context of sport has documented that young athletes report fear of failure as a salient source of stress and a reason for dropping out of sport. Athletes have also attributed their use of ergogenic drugs to their fear of failure. Officials, such as umpires and referees, cite fear of failure as a common reason for burnout and turnover in their work.

The most well-established consequences of achievement motives involve achievement goals. People with a strong need for achievement tend to adopt *approach–valenced achievement goals* such as *mastery–approach* (focused on learning and improving) and *performance–approach goals* (focused on outperforming others). People with a strong fear of failure tend to adopt avoidance–valenced achievement goals such as mastery-avoidance (focused on not making mistakes or getting worse) and performance–avoidance goals (focused on not being outperformed others). People who fear failing may also adopt an approach-to-avoid strategy whereby they adopt performance-approach goals because demonstrating normative competence provides immediate, albeit short-lived, evidence that one is not incompetent. Each of these achievement goals has important consequences for achievement behavior. Over time, consistent patterns of achievement goal involvement contribute to the achievement differences between people with different motive profiles.

Conclusion

Achievement motives are useful theoretical constructs for explaining factors that energize and initially orient achievement behavior. These motives emphasize fundamental differences between people in their approach and avoidance tendencies during competence pursuits. They remain a relevant component of contemporary achievement motivation theories by virtue of their role in predisposing people toward characteristic achievement goals during their competence pursuits. These constructs will remain useful as motivation theories develop more nuanced explanations of how people respond in the different psychological contexts of their competence pursuits.

David E. Conroy

See also Achievement Goal Theory; Automaticity: Implicit Attitudes; Dual Process Theory; Expectancy-Value Theory

Further Readings

Conroy, D. E., Elliot, A. J., & Thrash, T. M. (2009). Achievement motivation. In M. R. Leary & R. H. Hoyle (Eds.), *Handbook of individual differences in social behavior* (pp. 382–399). New York: Guilford Press.

Conroy, D. E., & Hyde, A. L. (2012). Measurement of achievement motivation processes. In G. Tenenbaum, R. C. Eklund, & A. Kamata (Eds.), *Handbook of measurement in sport & exercise psychology* (pp. 303–317). Champaign, IL: Human Kinetics.

Elliot, A. J., Conroy, D. E., Barron, K. E., & Murayama, K. (2010). Achievement motives and goals: A developmental analysis. In R. Lerner, M. Lamb, & A. Freund (Eds.), *Handbook of lifespan development, Vol. 2: Social and emotional development* (pp. 474–510). New York: Wiley.

McClelland, D. C., Atkinson, J. W., Clark, R. A., & Lowell, E. L. (1953). *The achievement motive.* New York: Appleton Century Crofts.

McClelland, D. C., Koestner, R., & Weinberger, J. (1989). How do self-attributed and implicit motives differ? *Psychological Review, 96,* 690–702.

Schultheiss, O. C. (2008). Implicit motives. In O. P. John, R. W. Robins, & L. A. Pervin (Eds.), *Handbook of personality* (pp. 603–633). New York: Guilford Press.

ADAPTATION

The term *adaptation* has been integrated within the sport psychology literature, from as early as 1986. Initially mentioned in relation to elite athlete retirement, adaptation is a broad term associated with monumental change in the athlete's life. People experience stress in their lives, and at certain times stress reaches a threshold, after which one must make decisions to alleviate that stress and reestablish psychological balance. When the performer integrates the necessary information about a significant stressor or the accumulation of several smaller stressors, that person can begin to establish or reestablish control, ideally culminating in adaptation.

Adaptation has been discussed in relation to contributive pathways, comprised of *understanding, control, self-enhancement, belonging,* and *trust.* Understanding facilitates adaptation when one gains an accurate appreciation of the stress episode, in advance of action. Control is sought through either direct or indirect means. Self-enhancement encompasses decisions that lead to

better performance via purposive effort and learning. Trust delineates the performer's belief that social support within the performance context holds the performer's best interests in mind, that supporters are creditable, and that they will act when assistance is needed. Belonging, like trust, is a social pathway. However, through belonging one facilitates social affiliations that in turn make trust more likely. Any of these five adaptation pathways can segue to a larger adaptation process, and so to the outcome of adaptation.

Adaptation interventions are temporal in nature, with at least a search for understanding preceding all other pathways. However, understanding is not necessarily acquired in its totality before the performer begins an adaptation process. The rule of thumb, however, is for the performer to seek as much detail about the stress episode and how one might engage in the process when the information is most needed. For example, the elite junior athlete who is drafted to a professional ice hockey, baseball, or football team will encounter several stressors that catalyze an adaptation process. The performer's understanding of the previously unfamiliar in such circumstances would include the coach's performance expectations, social norms that build relations with one's teammates, relocation to a new city and a new sport environment, media demands, fan expectations, and a significant change in financial status. Learning of these new contextual changes and beginning to engage in effective responses that lead to restored ease, the athlete can perform at the optimum. Hence, the process can generally be regarded as the move into, the move through, and the move onward from stress, with adaptation.

There are cases when performers maladapt, meaning they engage in an incorrect psychological process that manifests in rumination, apathy, or ego-protective thinking. It is human tendency to seek understanding throughout the adaptation process. However, how one chooses to view the stressor, via personal reflections and social support resources, will help determine whether the stress episode is resolved and the performer reestablishes psychological balance. There are, indeed, cases where an athlete's best performances are early in the career, with results waning at the juncture when the athlete should be performing at potential. When athletes encounter barriers during formative points in their athletic careers and there is incomplete or inaccurate understanding as a pattern, the athletes engage in negative contemplation and impede their own career development. The objective is for athletes and those who work with them to identify the barriers to performance in advance of the challenge, take only as much time and effort as is necessary to resolve the stress episode, and then reengage with correctly chosen personal and social support strategies. With the process of adaptation accomplished, the athlete gains (or regains) efficacy in personal abilities to resolve stress episodes in advance of further—inevitable—challenges.

In a similar vein, people who engage in exercise and move toward healthier choices can also experience adaptation processes when life changes are required, be these changes foreseen or unforeseen. The process would pertain to cardiac patients and people suffering from obesity who are seeking to begin a targeted exercise program. The identification of what is expected of oneself in relation to the program, and also of one's barriers in advance of the required behavior change, would increase the likelihood that personal and social support strategies are correctly chosen and implemented, leading to good change.

Up to the present day, formal adaptation research in sport and exercise psychology has included investigations into the adaptation processes of National Hockey League athletes during various stages of a professional sport career; immigrant athletes performing in major league baseball; Olympians; elite amateur cyclists; and indigenous developmental, elite amateur and professional athletes. These investigations have been for the most part qualitative, with several projects positioned as atheoretical, and others reflecting various adaptation, career, or life transition frameworks. This author proposes that adaptation research, reflecting its reality in application, should include cross-cultural investigations, community sport contexts, developmental sport, youth sport, sport for the elderly, and interventions in exercise and health settings with at-risk cohorts. Indeed, every performer experiences adaptation processes, though not all adaptation attempts are successful. Through a more systematic approach to research and practice, the sought after outcome of adaptation can become the performer's effective resolution to stress episodes in sport and exercise contexts.

Robert J. Schinke

See also Anticipation; Burnout; Career Transitions; Choking; Competition; Coping; Decision Making; Effort; Injury, Psychological Susceptibility to; Resilience

Further Readings

Magnusson, K. C., & Redekopp, D. E. (1992). Adaptability for transitions: Components and implications for intervention. *Canadian Journal of Counselling, 26,* 134–143.

Pummell, B., Harwood, C., & Lavallee, D. (2008). Jumping to the next level: A qualitative examination of within-career transition in adolescent event riders. *Psychology of Sport and Exercise, 9,* 427–447. doi: 10.1016/j.psychsport.2007.07.004

Schinke, R. J., Tenenbaum, G., Lidor, R., & Battochio, R. C. (2010). Adaptation in action: The transition from research to intervention. *The Sport Psychologist, 24,* 542–557.

Sinclair, D., & Orlick, T. (1993). Positive transitions from high-performance sport. *The Sport Psychologist, 7,* 138–150.

Tenenbaum, G., Jones, C. M., Kitsantis, A., Sachs, D. N., & Berwick, J. P. (2003). Failure adaptation: An investigation of the stress response process in sport. *International Journal of Sport Psychology, 34,* 27–62.

ADAPTED PHYSICAL EDUCATION

Physical education (PE) is considered an important vehicle for the promotion of physical activity, psychosocial development, and teaching dance, games, and sports skills. Unfortunately, children with disabilities are often inactive and socially isolated during PE despite laws requiring children with disabilities to be included in general educational schools, PE not excepted. This entry centers on the psychosocial and educational research in four related areas: PE teachers, peer tutors, able-bodied classmates of children with disabilities in PE, and children with disabilities.

Most teachers find that including children with disabilities in PE is challenging because of the need to change activities and adapt how they are implemented and evaluated. Many PE teachers report that they lack knowledge on disability conditions and have limited experiences in teaching children with disabilities. Because many school districts do not hire adapted physical education specialists, general PE teachers are required to teach children with disabilities. Hence, PE teachers' lack of knowledge and experience is likely grounded in the limited to nonexistent adapted PE training they receive while in teacher preparation programs. In turn, their limited experiences lead to feelings of low perceived competence. In addition to a lack of perceived competence, researchers have also documented that teachers often have negative attitudes toward including children with disabilities into their general PE classes, although other reports suggest teachers tend to have more mixed attitudes. Teachers also tend to grade children with disabilities differently by emphasizing participation and effort versus fitness and skill development. Whether such grading differences reflect reasonable accommodations of children's limitations versus lowered expectations of their abilities is unclear from the literature.

In brief, most of the research on PE teachers of children with disabilities indicates they feel their professional preparation is inadequate. Hence, they lack the ability to effectively accommodate children with disabilities into their general PE classes. It would seem reasonable that providing support for PE teachers in the form of adapted physical education (APE) specialists who have received extensive training in adapted physical activity would be helpful. Unfortunately, very little research has been done in this area, and the limited research often involves case studies or very small samples. For instance, many physical education classes might have only two or three students with disabilities in them. Nonetheless, researchers conducting studies in this area have suggested that APE teachers can enhance student outcomes.

In addition to research on support offered by trained APE specialists, PE teachers are also helped by trained peer tutors and teacher aides. Although only a handful of researchers have examined the effectiveness of peer tutors, the results have consistently established that peer tutors are effective. Children with disabilities working with peer tutors have increased their physical activity engagement and in some cases enhanced motor skill development. Added benefits also include increased social interaction and subsequent feelings of belonging. Based on limited research, teacher aides, while lacking training in PE, appear to be beneficial, especially if they are paired up with peer tutors.

Although it might be assumed that APE specialists may lack the same concerns as general PE teachers, APE specialists have noted they often lose access to the gymnasium or have to share it, which limits the space they have to work with. Lack of adequate functional equipment is also a complaint of APE teachers. Many APE teachers travel from school to school and may teach students ranging from preschool to high school at 4 to 14 different schools. To ensure they have adequate equipment, they often buy their own and transport it back and forth between schools. The constant travel while carrying equipment is often quite tiring. Similar to general physical education (GPE) teachers, APE specialists also receive support from teacher aides. Unfortunately, they have sometimes reported aides as apathetic and as exhibiting negative behaviors. Some APE specialists have also reported that they perceive themselves as disrespected and do not feel valued or part of the *family* of teachers at the schools where they teach. It should be noted, however, that the above concerns were not universally shared by all study participants. For instance, some APE teachers felt quite respected by colleagues and have very dedicated and competent teacher aides.

When GPE teachers are provided with teaching support from peers, teacher aides, or APE specialists, it is thought that any negative impact on children without disabilities as a result of inclusion is negated or minimized. Historically, a major concern arising from the inclusion of children with disabilities in general PE is that the educational experiences of children without disabilities may suffer. Accordingly, many scientists have examined how children without disabilities are affected by inclusion. In situations where children do not have significant disabilities, such as mild developmental delays, the experiences of both able-bodied and disabled children are similar; they experience comparable levels of physical activity and on-task behavior. In another study, researchers examined 15 students with disabilities and 20 students without as they participated in a regular game of volleyball and an adapted game of volleyball. All students enjoyed success, expressed fun and interest, and were physically active. The one caveat to these findings was that some of the older students (i.e., 12 years old) were not particularly keen on the adapted version of volleyball that included a smaller court and net. Despite the portrayal of a successful adapted PE class where all students do well, there is a less optimistic line of research examining the social dynamics of adapted PE classes.

In contrast to the reported results, more mixed findings have been reported on the experiences of nine elementary-age children who participated in inclusive PE classes. The scientists reporting the study categorized the children's experiences into *good* and *bad* days. Children reported having bad days if they experienced being teased. While teasing was seen as an example of being rejected, the children were also ignored and neglected. Finally when able-bodied classmates seemed to focus on children's disabilities, those children felt objectified and seen as curiosities. Being seen as objects of curiosity or rejected and neglected were all classified as forms of social isolation. A second major theme was represented by instances where the children perceived that their abilities were questioned and devalued. It was not uncommon for their mental as well as their physical abilities to be questioned. Finally, in the third theme, there were situations where the children were inactive or had minimal levels of participation. Common reasons were environmental barriers like a grass field that inhibited wheelchair access, lack of teacher and classmate support, as well as outright neglect. In summary, when children could not be active, had their capabilities questioned, or were socially marginalized, they experienced these situations as constituting a bad day in PE.

Fortunately, the same participants also described how they had good days in PE. There were times when classmates were quite encouraging and helpful. For example, during relay races children with disabilities remarked on how they were cheered on. Moments like those described above were categorized as promoting a sense of belonging. When participants were engaged in PE, they recognized they were reaping the intended benefits of PE, such as developing skills, enhancing their health, and learning fitness and health concepts. The recognition that they were obtaining benefits just like the able-bodied children represented having a good day in PE. One final theme indicative of having a good day was the intrinsic (pride) and extrinsic (compliments) rewards they experienced from being successful and demonstrating their skills.

In a research effort similar to the above study, Donna Goodwin sought to understand if all children with disabilities perceived offers of assistance positively. She found that children with disabilities viewed some forms of help as supportive and other types of help as threatening. There were a number of key differences between the types of support seen as threatening versus supporting. First, support that was pragmatic or functional and helped the children engage in a game was seen as supportive—being pushed in the wheelchair across a grass field to reduce travel time when the alternative was wheeling all the way around the field. When children without disabilities did not ignore children with disabilities and encouraged their sport participation, this was perceived as being done to secure control over their moves.

In contrast, threatening help was that which was provided unilaterally, where the helper refrained from asking if the help was needed. If help was offered when it was not needed, it was seen as interfering and threatening to children's sense of independence. Furthermore, some enactments of help were dangerous, such as pushing a child's wheelchair too fast and causing the child to fall. Finally, when children viewed offers of help as tantamount to an indictment of their capabilities, it was seen as a threat to their self-worth and interpreted negatively. Individuals with disabilities have to weigh the short-term task-oriented benefits, such as being helped across a grass field quickly, against the more long-term self-oriented costs, such as a missed opportunity to experience pride in independently wheeling around the entire field.

The authors of this research suggested that their findings have some bearing on the findings presented earlier on peer tutors. Given the various interpretations that children with disabilities might make about whether help is beneficial or harmful, it would be of value if PE teachers understood these complexities. Peer tutors and teacher aides could then be informed about the various ways their help might be interpreted and act accordingly.

In summary, researchers of inclusive PE have documented a mixed and complex picture of teachers, support personnel, and children's experiences. Teachers often feel unprepared and hence are reticent about engaging with and teaching children with disabilities. While support personnel, such as peer tutors, teachers' aides, and adapted PE specialists, have the potential to enrich the experiences of children with disabilities, their own lack of training and challenges can compromise their ability to deliver quality education. Finally, children with disabilities have mixed experiences in PE resulting from reliance on the quality of instruction they obtain from educators and the quality of the peer interactions they experience with their classmates. Clearly, adapted PE can be improved.

Jeffrey J. Martin

See also Disability; Disability and Exercise; Disability and Sport

Further Readings

Block, M. E., & Obrusnikova, I. (2007). Inclusion in physical education: A review of the literature from 1995–2005. *Adapted Physical Activity Quarterly, 24,* 103–124.

Goodwin, D. L., & Watkinson, E. J. (2000). Inclusive physical education from the perspective of students with physical disabilities. *Adapted Physical Activity Quarterly, 17,* 144–160.

Hodge, S. R., & Akuffo, P. B. (2007). Adapted physical education teachers' concerns in teaching students with disabilities in an urban public school district. *International Journal of Disability, Development and Education, 54,* 399–416.

Klavina, A. (2008). Using peer-mediated instructions for students with severe and multiple disabilities in inclusive physical education: A multiple case study. *European Journal of Adapted Physical Activity, 1*(2), 7–19.

Martin, M. R., & Speer, L. (2011). Leveling the playing field: Strategies for inclusion. *Strategies: A Journal for Physical and Sport Educators, 24*(5), 24–27.

ADDICTION, EFFECTS OF EXERCISE ON

Exercise has been proposed as a potential treatment to help people quit smoking and, more recently, to treat addictions to alcohol and other drugs of abuse. This entry discusses the rationale and empirical support for the use of exercise as a treatment for addiction.

Rationale

Exercise has been proposed as a stand-alone or supplementary treatment for addiction. The focus has been on exercise as a potential treatment to assist with successful quitting and prevention of relapse among those who are initially motivated to discontinue use of the addictive substance, rather than to produce intentions to quit among those who are not initially motivated. The rationale for exercise as a potential treatment for addictive substances is predicated on a number of potential mechanisms, including potential effects of exercise on (a) affective states, (b) cravings or urges to use the addictive substance, and (c) reduced concerns about postcessation weight gain.

Affective States

Withdrawal from addictive substances typically results in chronic negative shifts in affective valence (i.e., negative mood states). It has been proposed that exercise might help to prevent relapse by attenuating chronic negative mood states or providing a substitute means for producing an acute positive shift in affective valence. This proposed pathway was predicated on early research findings supporting the general notion that "exercise feels good." More recent research has shown that the effect of exercise on affective states (e.g., emotion, mood, pleasure or displeasure) is more complex. It now appears that affective response *during* exercise varies greatly based on a number of variables, including personal factors, such as exercise history, fitness, health status; exercise setting and mode; and, perhaps most importantly, exercise intensity. Nonetheless, across populations, settings, and exercise modes and intensities, people generally tend to have a positive shift in affective valence (feel more pleasure or less displeasure) immediately *after* an acute session of exercise. Additionally, there is accumulating evidence that engaging in a program of regular exercise for at least 8 weeks results in reduced depressive symptoms among clinically depressed adults. Thus, given these caveats, there is reason to believe that exercise might serve as a treatment for addictive substances through its influence on affective states.

Craving

A second potential pathway through which exercise may serve as a treatment for addictive substances involves the effects of exercise on acute cravings or urges for the addictive substance. It has been posited that acute exercise may serve as a substitute or distraction for use of the addictive substance during a craving or urge, particularly to the extent that it is difficult—if not impossible—to use the addictive substance while exercising.

Concerns About Weight Gain

Another potential pathway through which exercise might serve as a treatment for smoking cessation is through its effects on concerns about postcessation weight gain—a common barrier to smoking cessation, especially among women. Indeed, women who are concerned about post-cessation weight gain are less likely to attempt smoking cessation, less likely to successfully quit smoking, more likely to relapse postpartum, and more likely to drop out of smoking cessation programs. Exercise plays a major role in preventing weight gain, as a moderate increase in one's level of exercise can minimize weight gain in women who have quit smoking. The ability for exercise to combat weight gain in the general population and particularly during smoking cessation is likely to make it especially attractive for women smokers who are concerned about gaining weight during their smoking cessation attempt.

Evidence

Exercise as a Smoking Cessation Treatment

Numerous research studies have shown that a single exercise session has favorable effects on immediate changes in affective states and cigarette cravings. However, the optimal mode, intensity, and duration of the exercise stimulus remain unclear. Moreover, the duration of the effects of a single session of exercise on affect and cravings remains uncertain.

While outcomes of studies examining a single session of exercise on affect and cravings have been generally positive, results from the first 14 randomized controlled trials conducted have been equivocal, with only a single study showing positive effects of exercise on rates of successful smoking cessation at the end of the trial. Some problems with these studies are (a) a lack of adherence to the exercise treatments; (b) an inability to objectively verify adherence to the exercise program; (c) lack of data on who continues to exercise during the study follow-up period, following the initial exercise treatment (usually about three months); (d) high drop-out among study participants; and (e) lack of data on the potential mechanisms of treatment (see above). Thus, more research is needed to determine whether exercise is an effective treatment for smoking cessation, and if so, the optimal dose.

Exercise as a Treatment for Addiction to Alcohol and Other Drugs of Abuse

Research on exercise as a treatment for alcohol and other drugs has thus far been limited to studies conducted on animals and a few small-scale studies among humans. While the existing research shows promise, no large-scale clinical trials have been conducted in humans. Thus, it remains unclear as to whether exercise will serve as an effective treatment for addiction to alcohol and other drugs

Conclusion

There is a strong rationale for exercise as treatment for addiction to various substances. Findings from research on animals and small-scale studies with humans are supportive of the rationale. However, outcomes of randomized control trials have been equivocal for smoking cessation and are yet to be conducted for alcohol and other drugs of abuse.

David M. Williams

See also Alcohol Abuse; Affective Responses to Exercise; Drug Use and Control; Multiple Behavior Change; Obesity; Stress Management

Further Readings

Brown, R. A., Abrantes, A. M., Read, J. P., Marcus, B. H., Jakicic, J., Strong, D. R., et al. (2009). Aerobic exercise for alcohol recovery: Rationale, program description, and preliminary findings. *Behavior Modification, 33,* 220–249.

Roberts, V., Maddison, R., Simpson, C., Bullen, C., & Prapavessis, H. (2012). The acute effects of exercise on cigarette cravings, withdrawal symptoms, affect, and smoking behaviour: Systematic review update and meta-analysis. *Psychopharmacology, 222,* 1–15.

Ussher, M. H., Taylor, A., & Faulkner, G. (2012). Exercise interventions for smoking cessation. *Cochrane Database of Systematic Reviews, 1,* CD002295.

ADHERENCE

Many of the benefits of exercise come through sustained participation. Unfortunately, it is difficult for sedentary individuals to start an exercise program, and of those that do approximately 50% on average will drop out in the first 3 to 6 months. Furthermore, after 12 months most people who started a new exercise program will be sedentary again. As a result, a large body of literature is available on the degree to which different factors contribute to *exercise adherence*, defined as the degree to which an individual is able to sustain an exercise program. Among the many psychological factors that may contribute to exercise adherence, three broad categories that have received extensive research attention are outcome expectations, social influences, and perceptions of control.

Outcome Expectations

Outcome expectations include the value that an individual puts on the outcomes associated with regular exercise as well as the likelihood that the person believes the outcome will occur. Outcome expectations can be positive (reduce the risk of cardiovascular disease) or negative (sore muscles or injury). The literature is mixed on the relationship between outcome expectations and exercise adherence. Still, most literature supports the notion that having positive outcome expectations is a necessary, though potentially insufficient, characteristic of exercise adherence. Further, when evaluating what value a person places on an outcome, one must take into account age and other demographics. Values vary significantly depending on the person involved. For example, older adults may place a higher value on perceived health and longevity than do younger adults. Older women may place more importance on the social aspects of exercise, while younger women may find physical activity as an important way to control weight. Value expectations may also differ between demographic groups. For example, Caucasian women generally may value physical activity as a method to lose weight, while Latina women may positively associate overweight with a healthy ideal and, therefore, not value physical activity from a weight-loss perspective. Finally, there is some evidence that the expected timing of the outcome is important. Specifically, if someone expects to lose 10 pounds in 1 week because of a new exercise program, it will be demotivating when that outcome does not happen when one wants it to happen.

Social Influences

Like outcome expectations, social influences are included in most theoretical models developed to predict exercise adherence. Social influences can include social support from a family member or friend, group norms or cohesion in an exercise class, or social environmental factors related to economic status or culture. The way people perceive social support can have positive and negative influences on exercise adherence. Positive social

support from family members, friends, and others can include opportunities to exercise with the person, planning activities around exercise, and giving encouragement for the person to continue exercising. However, even these kinds of activities can negatively influence exercise adherence if the person receiving the support feels pressured. Social norms can also have a positive or negative impact on exercise adherence. Within an exercise class, norms and a sense of cohesion result in increased adherence. Similarly, normative beliefs related to people who are important to us or have expertise can influence adherence. Normative beliefs are formed when a person's perception that other people who are personally important think the individual should engage in a specific behavior. For example, if a son believes that his mother is convinced track is the safest form of exercise for him, this belief will influence the subjective norm of the son, who may be apt to run instead of playing baseball, football, or another team sport. Alternatively, an individual who lives in a house full of other sedentary people may have a hard time initiating and sustaining an exercise regimen if the following is taking place: (1) subtle teasing ("Look at you wanting to be Mr. Universe"), (2) complaints about the time spent exercising, and (3) instances of sabotage.

Perception of Control

When people feel they have control over a situation, they are more likely to participate in a given behavior. Perceptions of control can be thought of as expectations related to one's ability to complete a task. Self-efficacy is the most commonly studied control belief—the belief that one has the ability or the competency to complete a certain action. It is predictive of attendance of exercise classes, and like value expectancy, can be influenced by demographics or age. Older adults who may be afraid of injury could have lower self-efficacy than younger adults; however, researchers have hypothesized that methods to increase self-efficacy and exercise adherence include (1) having participants experience personal successes with their exercise regimen; (2) providing vicarious experiences, or modeling exercise behaviors; (3) integrating social and verbal persuasion; and (4) monitoring physiological states (soreness, sickness, etc.).

Although many people are likely to not stick with exercise programs and regimens, these factors may improve exercise adherence. Outcome expectations, social influences, and perceptions of control are closely related to the intentions and goals of a person. Indeed, these broad categories are interrelated. Outcome expectations are typically lower when participants do not value the outcomes of regular exercise. Also, when one's self-efficacy is low, the likelihood of valued outcomes also decreases. Conversely, when social influences are supportive of exercise, then perceptions of control increase. All of these factors interact within the broader ecological milieu. Laws and policies related to ensuring safe biking, opportunities for children to walk to school, and traffic calming all contribute to exercise adherence, sometimes acting through outcome expectations, social influences, and perceptions of control and other times directly impacting an individual's opportunities for exercise.

Paul A. Estabrooks and Erin M. Smith

See also Control Theory; Enjoyment; Expectancy-Value Theory; Health Promotion; Satisfaction; Self-Efficacy

Further Readings

Anderson, E. S., Wojcik, J. R., Winett, R. A., & Williams, D. M. (2006). Social-cognitive determinants of physical activity: The influence of social support, self-efficacy, outcome expectations, and self-regulation among participants in a church-based health promotion study. *Health Psychology, 25*(4), 510–520.

Carron, A. V., Hausenblas, H. A., & Mack, D. (1996). Social influence and exercise: A meta-analysis. *Journal of Sport & Exercise Psychology, 18*(1), 1–16.

Dishman, R. K. (1994). *Advances in exercise adherence.* Champaign, IL: Human Kinetics.

Hagger, M. S., Chatzisarantis, N. L. D., & Biddle, S. J. H. (2002). A meta-analytic review of the theories of reasoned action and planned behavior in physical activity: Predictive validity and the contribution of additional variables. *Journal of Sport & Exercise Psychology, 24*(1), 3–32.

AFFECT

Affect, also referred to as *core affect,* is the basic substrate of consciousness, its most elementary constituent. It is the constant readout of human feeling. Affect has a distinctive experiential quality that does not consist of nor require cognition or reflection. It is an inherent and necessary ingredient of emotions and moods; it is what gives these states affective *color.* However, affect is not only present during emotions and moods. Rather, it is always accessible to conscious awareness, although its experiential nature and intensity constantly fluctuate in response to internal and external stimuli.

Emotions and moods are considerably more complex and multifaceted constructs than affect. For example, the emotion of anxiety includes, besides unpleasant affect, a redirection of attentional and cognitive resources, attribution to the eliciting stimulus (a remark by a supervisor alluding to possible layoffs); a cognitive appraisal of threat (to one's life, social status, or self-image); a pattern of physiological changes (activation of the autonomic nervous system and the main neuroendocrine stress axes); observable changes in behavior (nervousness; altered voice modulation, facial expressions, muscular tics; exaggerated mannerisms); characteristic cognitions (distractability, thoughts of failure and negative consequences); and coping efforts (a search for solutions or sources of support). Similarly, moods also include multiple components besides affect. Although this may not always be immediately apparent, moods like emotions are also *about something.* They follow an eliciting stimulus, although the stimulus might have occurred long before the mood. They also require a cognitive appraisal, although what is appraised might be something as unspecific as one's life overall or one's place in the universe. In contrast, affect is not about something—it is not directed at anything; it is noncognitive, and it does not require an antecedent cognitive appraisal.

Examples of affect include pleasure, displeasure, energy or vigor, tiredness or fatigue, tension or distress, and calmness or relaxation. It is important to recognize that these affective states may occur by themselves or embedded as essential ingredients within emotions or moods. For example, when one is injured, the displeasure of pain is an affective reaction. It occurs instantaneously and automatically, without any need for cognitive recognition, evaluation, and interpretation. When one feels exhausted, drained of energy after a strenuous run on a hot and humid day, the sense of exhaustion is an affective state that stems directly from the physiological condition of the body, without any need for cognitive mediation. Similarly, the feelings of energy, invigoration, and revitalization that a physically fit individual may experience after a great workout are also affective states.

On the other hand, the fear that a patient in cardiac rehabilitation feels during the first exercise session after a heart attack is an emotion; it includes affect at its core (fear is unpleasant) but it is more than that. There are memories of the heart attack, a fixation on the somatic sensations elicited by exercise in search for anything suspicious, an appraisal of threat due to the severity and the unpredictability of the situation, an accentuation of the physiological stress response to exercise, and avoidance tendencies. Likewise, the pride experienced by a formerly sedentary individual after being able to walk continuously for 30 minutes is also an emotion; there is again affect at the core (pride is pleasant), but there are several additional components. These include, for example, a cognitive appraisal of achievement (one has succeeded in attaining an important and challenging personal milestone) and characteristic behavioral manifestations (smiles, happy vocal expressions, arms raised in celebration). Put differently, when one says "I feel great that I was able to finish my first marathon," the "I feel great" part is a reference to affect. The "that I was able to finish . . ." part is a reference to a cognitive appraisal that qualifies this state as an emotion.

Conceptualization and Measurement of Affect

As an object of scientific study, affect has been approached from two perspectives. Some investigators have considered each affective state as a separate entity, independent of all others. Examples of this *distinct–states* or *discrete–states* approach are questionnaires that assess various assortments of states (tension, fatigue, vigor, energy, revitalization). Such questionnaires are developed on the basis of factor analyses followed by orthogonal rotations, based on the assumption that the resultant factors are statistically independent of one another.

A different perspective considers affective states as systematically interrelated; some states are similar to others, some are unrelated, and some are antithetical. So, since the early twentieth century, investigators have been searching for a core set of dimensions that could explain these differences and similarities among affective states. Although various such dimensional models have been proposed, the first two dimensions are usually the same. The first dimension, and the one that accounts for a larger portion of the variance, is pleasure-versus-displeasure (also termed *affective valence* or *hedonic tone*). The second dimension is low-versus-high perceived activation (also termed *arousal*). These two dimensions are bipolar and orthogonal to each other. So, when used in combination, they can be thought of as a Cartesian coordinate system in which one can place the various affective states, depending on the degree of pleasure or displeasure and perceived activation they entail. For example, there are states that combine pleasure and high activation (energy, vigor), displeasure and high activation (tension, distress), pleasure and low activation (calmness, relaxation), and displeasure and low activation (tiredness, boredom). In psychology, this two-dimensional model of affect is known as the *affect circumplex*. Alternatively, researchers have also used a version of this coordinate system rotated by 45°. In that case, the dimensions extend from pleasant high activation (termed high *positive activation*) to unpleasant low activation (termed low *positive activation*) and from unpleasant high activation (termed high *negative activation*) to pleasant low activation (termed low *negative activation*).

Regardless of which rotational variant is used, these dimensional models of affect can serve as encompassing maps of affective space. By gathering information about each respondent's position on only two dimensions, investigators can get a meaningful representation of the respondent's affective state and, with repeated assessments, track the individual's movement in response to experimental manipulations, including sport- and exercise-related stimuli.

Panteleimon Ekkekakis

See also Affective Disorders; Affective Responses to Exercise; Emotional Reactivity; Emotional Responses; Energy, Effects of Exercise on; Hedonic Theory

Further Readings

Ekkekakis, P. (2013). *The measurement of affect, mood, and emotion: A guide for health-behavioral research.* New York: Cambridge University Press.

Larsen, R. J., & Diener, E. (1992). Promises and problems with the circumplex model of emotion. In M. S. Clark (Ed.), *Review of personality and social psychology: Emotion* (Vol. 13, pp. 25–59). Newbury Park, CA: Sage.

Russell, J. A. (2005). Emotion in human consciousness is built on core affect. *Journal of Consciousness Studies, 12*(8–10), 26–42.

Russell, J. A., & Feldman Barrett, L. (1999). Core affect, prototypical emotional episodes, and other things called emotion: Dissecting the elephant. *Journal of Personality and Social Psychology, 76,* 805–819.

AFFECTIVE DISORDERS

Affective disorders, also known as mood disorders, are clinical psychological disorders. The most common affective disorders are major depressive disorder, dysthymic disorder, bipolar disorder, and cyclothymic disorder. A core feature of these disorders is dysfunction in emotion processing and neurohormonal regulation leading to subjective feelings of sadness, depressed mood, and loss of pleasure in things normally pleasurable (anhedonia) for 2 weeks or more. These symptoms must also subjectively impair the fulfillment of social or occupational responsibilities. Additional possible symptoms include cycling episodes of mania in bipolar disorder; insomnia or hypersomnia; feelings of worthlessness, guilt, suicidal thoughts; and psychomotor agitation (restlessness, pacing) or psychomotor retardation (fatigue, tiredness). Affective disorders often co-occur with anxiety disorders, such as panic disorder, generalized anxiety disorder, posttraumatic stress disorder, and social phobia. Women are at greater risk than men for the development of both affective and anxiety disorders.

Diagnosis of an affective disorder, mood disorder, or anxiety disorder requires an extensive in-person interview with a licensed clinical psychologist or psychiatrist to establish whether criteria for the diagnosis are met. A score on a self-report survey of depression or anxiety symptoms, even when administered by a licensed clinician, is not sufficient for diagnosis. The primary diagnostic criteria have been set forth by the American Psychiatric Association (APA) in the *Diagnostic and Statistical Manual for Mental Disorders, 4th Edition, Text Revision (DSM-IV-TR)* and by the World Health Organization in the *International Statistical Classification of Diseases and Related Health Problems,* 10th revision (*ICD-10*). Adherence to these diagnostic standards have been difficult in the fields of sport and exercise psychology, as few in the field have the necessary credentials or lack the financial or collegial resources.

Nevertheless, it is critical to understand the effects of leisure-time physical activity and acute and chronic exercise on affective and anxiety disorders. The focus here will be on the use of exercise as a treatment intervention among individuals diagnosed with affective or anxiety disorders. However, it is also important to understand how these disorders may affect physical activity behavior in general. Symptoms of depression are associated with lower levels of physical activity and inhibition of behavioral activation. For example, feelings of hopelessness and fatigue are difficult to overcome, and, as such, these patients experience difficulty in engaging in effortful tasks. In addition, among athletes, there is evidence that a core feature of the staleness syndrome (as a result of overtraining) is depressed mood, and the symptoms of staleness map directly onto the diagnostic criteria for a major depressive episode. Monitoring depressed mood in athletes may be a method to help avoid staleness during an overtraining period.

Major Depressive Disorder

Epidemiological studies consistently indicate that greater levels of physical activity or cardiorespiratory fitness are related to reduced risk for the future development of major depression in both men and women. Engaging in regular physical activity provides protection against symptoms of depression, compared with being sedentary. However, there is not strong evidence for a dose response effect, so greater levels of physical activity are not necessarily more protective. Exercise training has been shown to be an effective treatment for major depression. Both aerobic exercise (walking, jogging) and resistance exercise, compared with a wait list or non-exercise control condition, have been shown to effectively reduce symptoms of depression and result in a remission in symptoms of depression. Walking or jogging exercise interventions, 4 to 6 months in duration (but longer is better), have been shown to be as effective as antidepressant drug therapy and cognitive behavioral therapy compared with a placebo. Exercise is a good treatment option or adjuvant to treatment for major depression; however, adding exercise training to pharmacologic or cognitive behavioral therapy does not produce synergistic effects. The behavioral deactivation and extreme feelings of hopelessness and fatigue present clear challenges to the initiation of and adherence to a physical activity or exercise training program, although one possible advantage of exercise training over pharmacotherapy is that remission of symptoms may persist for a longer time after the exercise and drug treatments have ended.

Bipolar Disorder

Although there is increasing interest in using exercise as a treatment in bipolar disorder, and high-functioning bipolar disorder patients report exercise as one of many methods they use to help maintain emotional stability, very little empirical research and no clinical trials for exercise have been conducted in patients with bipolar disorder. One study has shown that markers of cardiovascular disease risk can be improved with exercise in patients diagnosed with bipolar disorder, but it is unknown if exercise can improve the core symptoms of bipolar disorder.

Panic Disorder

Patients diagnosed with panic disorder tend to be less physically active than their healthy counterparts. This may be due, in part, to feelings of discomfort experienced during exercise. The physiological arousal due to exercise (increased heart rate and respiration) is similar to the core symptoms of a panic attack, and thus may be avoided. Another reason may be due to false beliefs that exercise will cause a panic attack. The evidence, however, clearly indicates that exercise is safe for people diagnosed with panic disorder and exercise, even at maximal capacity, does not cause panic attacks. The very few documented instances of panic attack during exercise can be viewed as chance occurrences relative to the number of documented exercise and physical activity sessions that did not involve a panic attack. Exercise training is known to be a very useful treatment for panic disorder and can be useful as a cognitive restructuring tool ("I can sweat and breathe hard and my heart can beat very fast, and it does not mean I am about to die or that I am going crazy"). Exercise is comparable to pharmacological treatments for reducing clinician rated symptoms of panic disorder. However, the combination of drug treatment with exercise training does not produce a synergistic effect.

Generalized Anxiety Disorder

There is epidemiological evidence that greater levels of physical activity or cardiorespiratory fitness are related to reduced risk for the future development of anxiety disorders. However, very few studies have tested the effects of exercise as a treatment for generalized anxiety disorder (GAD). In two clinical trials, both aerobic exercise and resistance exercise resulted in significant symptom reductions compared with a wait-list control condition. Exercise has not currently been compared with drug treatments or other treatment methods. Additionally, the affective experience during or immediately after exercise in GAD patients has not been examined. There is very little information about how a single session of exercise affects symptoms in people clinically diagnosed with affective or anxiety disorders.

J. Carson Smith

See also Affect; Emotional Reactivity; Emotional Responses; Mental Health; Psychological Well-Being; Stress Reactivity

Further Readings

Babyak, M. A., Blumenthal, J. A., Herman, S., Khatri, P., Doraiswamy, M., Moore, K. A., et al. (2000). Exercise treatment for major depression: Maintenance of therapeutic benefit at 10 months. *Psychosomatic Medicine, 62*(5), 633–638.

Blumenthal, J. A., Babyak, M. A., Moore, K. A., Craighead, W. E., Herman, S., Khatri, P., et al. (1999). Effects of exercise training on older patients with major depression. *Archives of Internal Medicine, 159*(19), 2349–2356.

Dishman, R. K., Berthoud, H. R., Booth, F. W., Cotman, C. W., Edgerton, V. R., Fleshner, M. R., et al. (2006). Neurobiology of exercise. *Obesity (Silver Spring), 14*(3), 345–356.

Herring, M. P., O'Connor, P. J., & Dishman, R. K. (2010). The effect of exercise training on anxiety symptoms among patients: A systematic review. *Archives of Internal Medicine, 170*(4), 321–331.

Hoffman, B. M., Babyak, M. A., Craighead, W. E., Sherwood, A., Doraiswamy, M., Coons, M. J., et al. (2011). Exercise and pharmacotherapy in patients with major depression: One-year follow-up of the SMILE study. *Psychosomatic Medicine, 73*(2), 127–133.

AFFECTIVE RESPONSES TO EXERCISE

Exercise can influence how people feel. This observation has attracted considerable research attention in the last 50 years. There are several reasons for this. First, if exercise can improve how people feel, this could have significant implications for mental health. Disorders impacting mood (depression, dysthymia, bipolar disorder) and anxiety (generalized anxiety, phobia, posttraumatic stress) are prevalent and can have a devastating effect on quality of life for sufferers and their families. Moreover, standard therapies such as pharmacotherapy and psychotherapy are costly and not always effective. Psychoactive drugs in particular can have several undesirable side effects. Against this backdrop, exercise offers the promise of an intervention that can be effective (by some estimates, at least as effective as the standard forms of therapy), inexpensive, free of undesirable side effects, and associated with many additional benefits for the body (e.g., reduced cardiovascular risk) and mind (e.g., reduced risk for dementia).

Second, people engage in various unhealthy lifestyle behaviors to regulate how they feel. For example, they consume caffeine and sugary snacks to feel more energized and they smoke cigarettes or drink alcohol to calm the nerves and relax. In pursuit of a feel-better effect, some people even engage in illicit and dangerous activities, such as abusing psychotropic drugs. Over time, these behaviors may lead to serious problems, from obesity and diabetes to chronic cardiorespiratory conditions to life-endangering addictions. Therefore, it would be desirable to replace these behaviors with an alternative that has the same affect-enhancing properties without a negative impact on health. Exercise engages some of the same brain mechanisms targeted by widely abused chemical affect regulators, such as dopamine, endogenous opioids, and endocannabinoids; can increase perceived energy and calmness; and has positive, rather than negative, effects on overall health.

Third, the low adherence to exercise represents a major public health problem. Most people who become physically active either do not exercise regularly or quit. Although most contemporary theories assume that nonadherence and drop-out are the result of a rational decision-making process, these phenomena may also be driven by affective processes. Affect is a powerful motive in human behavior. People may adhere to exercise if their affective responses are positive and may drop out if their affective responses are consistently negative. This possibility, which has received empirical support, offers researchers new insight into the mechanisms underlying exercise behavior.

History

The first studies on affective responses to exercise appeared in the late 1960s. The typical methodological approach consisted of administering a questionnaire of mood (such as the Profile of Mood States) or anxiety (such as the State-Trait Anxiety Inventory) shortly before and after an exercise bout. At the time, very few questionnaires were designed to assess nonclinical forms of how people feel. Therefore, the limited availability of measures dictated the dependent variables being studied. Consequently, those variables might or might not have been the most relevant, raising the possibility that changes also occurred in variables other than those being measured. The samples of respondents typically consisted of conveniently accessible groups, such as young, healthy, physically active, and fit university students. The intensity of exercise was rarely monitored via objective means (electrocardiography or expired gases) and, when it was standardized across participants, the method was often based on estimated, rather than directly measured, maximal exercise capacity (typically, age-predicted maximal heart rate, known to result in considerable errors). Despite these methodological limitations, which were consistent with a nascent line of research, early studies provided voluminous evidence of an exercise-associated anxiolytic and mood-enhancing effect.

Mechanisms

In the 1980s and 1990s, along with numerous replications of the anxiolytic and mood-enhancing effects across different settings, samples, and types of exercise, research attention turned to mechanistic hypotheses. These included proposals that exercise makes people feel better because (a) they perceive that they are doing something challenging and, at the same time, beneficial (the mastery hypothesis); (b) it provides an opportunity to temporarily escape the stresses and hassles of daily life (the distraction or time-out hypothesis); (c) it provides an opportunity for enjoyable social interaction (the social interaction hypothesis); (d) it corrects imbalances in monoaminergic neurotransmission that are associated with negative affectivity (the monoamine hypothesis); (e) it promotes the release of peripheral and central endogenous opioids (the endorphin hypothesis); and (f) it raises core temperature, which creates a sense of relaxation or exhilaration (the thermogenic hypothesis).

The conclusions from these investigations have been mixed. What seems clear is that no single explanation can provide an exclusive account of the reasons why exercise can make people feel better. Studies on the mastery hypothesis have demonstrated that participants whose physical confidence is strengthened report feeling better than those whose physical confidence is weakened. On the other hand, the thermogenic hypothesis has been largely discredited, with studies demonstrating that elevations in core temperature during exercise are associated with feeling worse, not better. The endorphin hypothesis continues to hold promise. However, interest in this idea has declined following a string of studies that produced conflicting results and, thus, confusion and frustration among researchers. However, upon closer analysis, the inconsistencies can be attributed to methodological weaknesses, which, in turn, could be due to the lack of interdisciplinary expertise on the physiology and pharmacology of the endogenous opioid system. The distraction and social-interaction hypotheses may provide partial explanations, but there are caveats for both. Specifically, while other distracting activities may also produce a feel-better effect, exercise often produces changes that are qualitatively different. For example, while a session of meditation or a period of quiet rest may primarily induce relaxation, a typical response to a bout of moderate-intensity exercise consists of an increase in perceived energy during and immediately following the bout and, only later, an increase in relaxation compared to baseline. Furthermore, while an enthusiastic and supportive social group can enhance the positive affective response to exercise, an indifferent group may experience no effect and a group or an exercise leader perceived as critical can have a negative effect. Moreover, studies have shown that people can feel better even when they exercise in an empty room while staring at a barren wall. The monoamine hypothesis remains viable, with findings showing that monoamines (serotonin, dopamine) may be implicated in the

feel-better effect. However, at least for now, this research is limited to experimental animals, with all the interpretational challenges that this entails, that is, inability to directly extrapolate from observable animal behavior to subjective human feelings.

Mechanistic research has now moved in some notable new directions. First, studies have begun exploring associations between affective responses to exercise and neurotransmitter dynamics. Advances in positron emission tomography have made it possible to quantify exercise-associated changes in receptor occupancy in the human brain. Second, research is emerging on the role of endocannabinoids, a class of substances discovered relatively recently, that are extensively involved in reward. Both experimental studies with animals and preliminary correlational studies of peripherally circulating endocannabinoids in humans suggest that these substances may add one more piece to the mechanistic puzzle. Third, research is examining the role of exercise-upregulated neurotrophic factors in anatomical adaptations in the human brain that may be associated with how people feel. While chronic psychological stress is associated with reduced synthesis of neurotrophic factors and reduced volumes of brain structures involved in emotion and mood regulation, exercise is among the most potent known stimuli for the upregulation of these neurotrophic factors.

Beyond the Feel-Better Effect

Critics express skepticism about the ability of exercise to make people feel better based on a simple but intriguing argument: If exercise could, in fact, make people feel better, would most people be sedentary? Research based on a new methodological platform is beginning to show that the feel-better effect, while feasible, is neither automatic nor guaranteed for everyone. It should more accurately be described as conditional.

One of the methodological innovations was the introduction of measures that tap the main dimensions of affect, as opposed to a few discrete affective states. Theoretically, the advantage is no major variant of affective experience resulting from exercise (including negative variants) can go undetected. A second aspect of the revised methodology is the timing of affect assessments. It became clear that, by measuring only before and after the exercise bout, the shape of the affective response could be misrepresented. For example, depending on the intensity of exercise, pleasure could be reduced during exercise but rebound postexercise. However, if affect is assessed only before and after the bout, one could conclude that the only change was a pre-to-post increase in pleasure. Thus, newer studies have employed repeated assessments of affect, both during and after the bout. Thirdly, newer studies use more accurate methods for standardizing exercise intensity, reducing error variance and increasing statistical power. The measurement of expired gases has become common practice. Furthermore, several laboratories base the standardization of intensity on the more laborious but more meaningful practice of identifying physiological markers, such as the ventilatory or lactate threshold and the respiratory compensation point. These markers differ among individuals, even of the same sex, age, health status, activity habits, and aerobic capacity. Research suggests that exercising at intensities slightly above and below these markers may be associated with considerable differences across several physiological systems as well as differences in affective responses. Finally, once it became clear that affective responses varied between individuals, even in response to the same, well-standardized, exercise stimulus, it also became apparent that analyses of change restricted to the level of entire groups could be misleading. This is because subgroups within the same sample may respond in different directions (e.g., increased versus decreased pleasure). Thus, it is possible for two subgroups to exhibit changes of equal magnitude but in opposite directions, resulting in a group mean that appears unchanged over time. In such cases, the sample mean fails to reflect the actual response of individuals, becoming merely a statistical abstraction. To address this problem, in newer studies, change is examined both at the level of the entire sample and at the level of individuals and subgroups.

The conclusion from studies based on this revised methodology is that the feel-better effect represents only one aspect of the multifaceted exercise–affect relationship. Interindividual differences are prevalent and reductions in pleasure are common. For example, obese and inactive middle-age women report declines in pleasure across the entire range of exercise intensity.

Affective Responses and Exercise Prescription

The optimization of affective responses to exercise is gradually being adopted as one of the pillars of exercise prescription guidelines, alongside the maximization of biological adaptations like gains in fitness and health and the minimization of risk. Exercise practitioners are advised to systematically monitor the affective responses of participants and to regulate exercise intensity to ensure that affective responses remain positive or at least nonnegative. This can be achieved by (a) allowing participants to self-select their intensity, in order to engender a sense of perceived autonomy and self-efficacy; and (b) ensuring that intensity does not greatly exceed the ventilatory threshold (which can be estimated without instruments as the level of intensity that brings about a perceptible increase in the frequency and depth of ventilation and a subjective characterization of perceived exertion as "somewhat hard" or "hard"). Maintaining proper hydration and comfortable ambient temperature and humidity levels is also important.

Furthermore, it is crucial to recognize that the relationship between exercise intensity and affective responses is influenced by individual differences. Because of a combination of genetic and epigenetic factors, people develop varied preferences for levels of exercise intensity and different degrees of tolerance to intense exercise. These differences influence the affective responses that individuals experience at different intensities. Although a standard method of tailoring exercise intensity to individual levels of preference and tolerance has yet to be developed, practitioners should keep in mind that what was pleasant for one participant may not be pleasant for another.

Finally, it is advisable to maintain a social environment in which participants can feel confident and secure. The presence of other exercisers who appear to be of superior fitness or an exercise leader who emphasizes skill, appearance, or interpersonal comparisons could induce social-evaluative and self-presentational concerns.

Panteleimon Ekkekakis

See also Addiction, Effects of Exercise on; Affect; Emotional Responses; Energy, Effects of Exercise on; Hedonic Theory; Runner's High

Further Readings

Chaouloff, F., Dubreucq, S., Matias, I., & Marsicano, G. (2013). Physical activity feel-good effect: The role of endocannabinoids. In P. Ekkekakis (Ed.), *Routledge handbook of physical activity and mental health* (chap. 3). London: Routledge.

Ekkekakis, P., Parfitt, G., & Petruzzello, S. J. (2011). The pleasure and displeasure people feel when they exercise at different intensities: Decennial update and progress towards a tripartite rationale for exercise intensity prescription. *Sports Medicine, 41,* 641–671.

Henning, B., & Dishman, R. K. (2013). Physical activity and reward: The role of endogenous opioids. In P. Ekkekakis (Ed.), *Routledge handbook of physical activity and mental health* (chap. 2). London: Routledge.

Rhodes, J. S., & Majdak, P. (2013). Physical activity and reward: The role of dopamine. In P. Ekkekakis (Ed.), *Routledge handbook of physical activity and mental health* (chap. 4). London: Routledge.

AFFIRMATIONS

Affirmation is the act of reflecting on core aspects of the self, such as important values, relationships, and personal characteristics like religion, music, or sports. Previous research shows that self-affirmation interventions can reduce psychological and physiological stress and defensiveness, while boosting personal responsibility and performance. Self-affirmation interventions and theory have promising applications in sports and exercise, including facilitating achievement and helping individuals respond adaptively to setbacks.

Self-Affirmation Theory

The social psychologist Claude Steele proposed self-affirmation theory in 1988. It holds that individuals are motivated to maintain self-integrity: a sense that one is a person of worth, morally adequate and effective at making changes in one's life. There are many routes to self-integrity, and affirmations of the self in one part of life (e.g., reflecting on being a good father) can buffer threats in other parts of life (e.g., poor performance). Affirmations in the context of threat can protect the self and allow people to respond with reduced stress and defensiveness because they are reassured that they possess integrity and worth.

When an event such as a sports loss or failure to complete a workout regimen threatens a valued self-image (e.g., being a good athlete or motivated exerciser), people are at risk of responding defensively by rejecting responsibility or giving up. If, however, the person affirms an important personal value before the threat, their sense of moral adequacy and efficacy can be reinforced and protected. Within social psychology, interventions involving values affirmations often take the form of having individuals reflect and write briefly about an important personal value such as relationships with friends and family. Writing about important personal values can fulfill the global need for self-integrity and enable people to constructively respond to threatening events.

Reduction of Defensive Strategies

Sport and exercise present psychological threats like the fear of low performance that can impact one's personal and public image. There is empirical evidence that people can respond to these threats by construing situations as less threatening to personal worth and well-being. For example, athletes may use defensive strategies such as attributing more internal causes for success than for failure (e.g. "I won because of my ability," but "I lost because of the weather": self-serving biases); denying their team's responsibility for a negative outcome or exaggerating their role in victory (group-serving biases); or claiming handicaps (e.g., claiming back pain before a competition to have an excuse for failure or to enhance credit for success: claimed self-handicapping). These defensive strategies help maintain self-integrity by reducing threats but can limit achievement when personal responsibility is denied and failure is attributed to external causes. Self-affirmation can reduce engagement in these maladaptive strategies.

For instance, a field study demonstrated how self-affirmation can lower athletes' engagement in self-handicapping strategies. Claimed self-handicapping was assessed before and after an affirmation intervention. First, coaches asked their athletes to report to what extent handicaps such as physical pain or stress could disrupt their training. Using a classic self-affirmation study design, athletes assigned to an affirmation condition ranked a list of values (e.g., relationships with friends) from the most important to the least important, and then wrote an essay about their most important value. Athletes in a no-affirmation control condition ranked the same values but wrote an essay on why their least important value might be important to someone else. Athletes in the affirmation condition claimed fewer handicaps after the intervention (no difference in the control condition).

Field studies with athletes immediately after competition examined their attributional patterns for victories and defeats. The studies demonstrated that an affirmation manipulation reduced self-serving and group-serving attributional biases. Without affirmation, winning team members claimed that their efforts and their team's efforts were more responsible for the outcome of the game than losing team members'. These findings were observed for players as well as nonplayer fans, such that collegiate fans were less defensive in their attributions about their team's outcomes when they affirmed a value central to their university. In health psychology, affirmed individuals are less defensive and more open to learning about their health risks, and more likely to take behavioral steps to address drinking, diabetes, or excessive weight. One study found that overweight women who completed a self-affirmation lost more weight than women in a control condition, suggesting that the threat and stress stemming from their appearance may have hindered their attempts to diet and exercise.

Reduced Stress

Self-affirmation can reduce physiological and psychological stress responses. Compared to a control group, participants who affirmed personal values by reporting their thoughts and feelings about an important value had lower salivary cortisol responses, a marker of stress, in a stressful laboratory task. In a longitudinal study, compared to control students who had a marked increase, students who affirmed personal values 2 weeks prior to an academic evaluation did not have increased cumulative epinephrine levels from baseline (an indicator of stress measured in urine).

Increased Performance

Whereas threat depresses performance, affirming core values could alleviate threat and improve performance. In both laboratory and field studies, self-affirmations have improved academic performance among people confronting a negative stereotype about their ability; for example, it improved the academic performance of African American and Latino American, but not White, students in mixed middle schools in the United States. These effects persist for years by changing the narrative students tell themselves about their

ongoing experience, thereby instigating recursive processes and positive feedback loops.

Conclusion

In sum, sports research demonstrates that self-affirmation reduces athletes' defensiveness, whereas other research shows that it helps address health problems, reduces stress responses, and boosts academic performance. Future research should address the specific effect of self-affirmation on the stress, performance, and commitment to a training regimen among both athletes and exercisers.

Lucie Finez, David K. Sherman,
and Cameron Brick

See also Attribution Theory; Identity; Self-Appraisal/ Assessment/Perception; Self-Handicapping; Self-Presentation; Stereotype Threat; Team Attributions

Further Readings

Finez, L., & Sherman, D. K. (2012). Train in vain: The role of the self in claimed self-handicapping strategies. *Journal of Sport & Exercise Psychology, 34,* 600–620.

Logel, C., & Cohen, G. L. (2012). The role of the self in physical health: Testing the effect of a values-affirmation intervention on weight loss. *Psychological Science, 23,* 53–55.

Sherman, D. K., & Cohen, G. L. (2006). The psychology of self-defense: Self-affirmation theory. In M. P. Zanna (Ed.), *Advances in experimental social psychology* (Vol. 38, pp. 183–242). San Diego, CA: Academic Press.

Sherman, D. K., & Kim, H. S. (2005). Is there an "I" in "team"? The role of the self in group-serving judgments. *Journal of Personality and Social Psychology, 88,* 108–120.

AGGRESSION

Aggression has a long history in both sport and nonsport contexts. There is some variation in the definitions of aggression employed by different people. However, it is commonly agreed that *aggression* is a verbal or physical behavior that is directed intentionally toward another individual and has the potential to cause psychological or physical harm. In addition, the target of the behavior should be motivated to avoid such treatment. Typically, definitions of aggression incorporate the notion of *intent to cause harm;* that is, for behavior to be classified as aggressive, the perpetrator must have the intent to harm the victim. However, strict behavioral definitions of aggression exclude the term *intent* because it refers to an internal state, which cannot be observed.

Aggression has been distinguished between *instrumental* and *hostile.* Instrumental aggression is a behavior directed at the target as a means to an end, for example, injuring a player to gain a competitive advantage, or late tackling to stop an opponent from scoring. Thus, instrumental aggression is motivated by some other goal. In contrast, hostile aggression is a behavior aimed toward another person who has angered or provoked the individual and is an end in itself. Its purpose is to harm for its own sake, for example, hitting an opponent who has just been aggressive against the player. Hostile aggression is typically preceded by anger. Instrumental aggression, in pursuit of a goal, is not normally associated with anger and, in sport, is far more frequent than hostile aggression. In both types of aggression, a target person is harmed, and the harm can be physical or psychological.

In this entry, the construct of aggression is presented. First, the distinction is made between aggression and assertion, and difficulties with the notion of intent in the definition of aggression are discussed. Then measures of aggression are outlined followed by factors associated with aggression in sport.

Aggression, Assertion, and Intent

In sport, the word *aggressive* is often used when *assertive* is more appropriate. For example, coaches describe strong physical play as aggressive, when this type of play is actually assertive; it is within the rules of the game and there is no intention to cause harm. The difference between aggression and assertion lies in the intention to harm. If there is no intent to harm the opponent, and the athlete is using legitimate means to achieve goals, the behavior is assertive, not aggressive. When one is being assertive, the intention is to establish dominance rather than to harm the opponent. Behaviors such as tackling in rugby, checking in ice hockey, and breaking up a double play in baseball may be seen as assertive as long as these are performed as legal components of the contest and without malice. However, these same actions would represent aggression if the athlete's intention was to cause injury.

It is often difficult to distinguish aggression from assertion in sport. Although assertive behaviors are forceful behaviors that are not intended to injure the victim, by their nature, they may result in unintended harm to the athlete's opponent. In addition, some sports involve forceful physical contact, which *has the capacity* to harm another person, but this contact is within the rules of sport. Assertive behaviors have also been labeled *sanctioned aggression.* Thus, sanctioned aggression is any behavior that falls within a particular sport's rules or is widely accepted as such: for example, using the shoulder to force a player off the ball in soccer and tackling below the shoulders in rugby. Examples are combat sports, such as judo, karate, and wrestling, and team contact sports, such as rugby, ice hockey, American football, and lacrosse. Perhaps the confusion between assertion and aggression arises because both have the capacity to harm the target, although, as noted earlier, only aggression involves intention to harm.

Incorporating the notion of intent in definitions of aggression has the difficulty of establishing which behavior is aggressive. This is because the only person knowing whether there is intent to cause harm is the person who carries out the action. Two features of definitions of aggression that have not been questioned are the capacity of behavior to cause harm and the intentional (nonaccidental) nature of the behavior.

The Measurement of Aggression

The notion of *intent,* which is part of most definitions of aggression, has created difficulties in the measurement of aggression. Therefore, many studies have operationally defined and measured aggression without considering intent, or the reasons for the behavior. A very common aggression measure in the laboratory context is administering electric shocks, which is known to hurt the participant. Thus, aggression is reflected in the intensity of the shock administered. Other studies used delivering an aversive stimulus, for example a loud noise, as their measure of aggression.

In the sport context, aggression has been measured in a variety of ways, such as number of fouls, coach ratings, penalty records, as well as using self-reports and behavioral observation. In studies of behavioral observation, instrumental and hostile aggression have been measured. *Instrumental aggression* has been operationally defined as aggression occurring during game play and involves opponent-directed physical interactions that contribute to accomplishing a task. In contrast, *hostile aggression* has been operationally defined as physical or verbal interactions aimed at various targets but not directly connected to task accomplishment; these behaviors are directed at opponents, teammates, or referees. For example, in handball, repelling, hitting, and cheating have been coded as instrumental aggression, and insulting, threatening, making obscene gestures, and shoving against opponents, referees, teammates, and others have been coded as hostile aggression. Aggressive behaviors (e.g., late tackle, hitting, elbowing) have also been measured as part of the construct of *antisocial behavior*, which has been defined as behavior intended to harm or disadvantage another individual and has considerable overlap with aggression.

Other studies have used athlete self-reports to measure aggression, either by presenting them with a scenario that describes an aggressive behavior and asking about their intentions or likelihood to aggress, or by asking them to respond to a number of items measuring aggressive or antisocial behavior. Self-described likelihood to aggress has been used as a proxy for aggression. In these studies, participants are presented with a scenario in which the protagonist is faced with a decision to harm the opponent to prevent scoring and they are asked to indicate the likelihood they would engage in this behavior if they were in this situation. Finally, aggression (e.g., trying to injure another player) has been measured as part of antisocial behavior in sport.

Why Aggression Occurs

Aggression has a long history in both mainstream psychology and sport psychology. One view is that aggression results from *frustration*. In sport, frustration can occur for a variety of reasons: because of losing, not playing well, being hurt, and perceiving unfairness in the competition. Frustration heightens one's predisposition toward aggression. Contextual factors come into play so that the manner in which an individual interprets the situational cues at hand best predicts whether this athlete, or spectator, will exhibit aggression.

Some theorists view aggression as a learned behavior, which is the result of an individual's interactions with personal social environment over time. Aggression occurs in sport where an athlete's expectancies for reinforcement for aggressive behavior are high (receiving praise from parents, coaches, peers), and where the reward value outweighs punishment value (gaining a tactical or psychological advantage with a personal foul). Situation-related expectancies, such as the time of game, score opposition, or the encouragement of the crowd, also influence the athlete in terms of whether this is deemed an appropriate time to exhibit aggression.

A number of individual difference factors have been associated with aggression. Three of them are *legitimacy judgments, moral disengagement,* and *ego orientation*. When athletes judge aggressive and rule-violating behaviors as legitimate or acceptable, they are more likely to be aggressive. Moral disengagement refers to a set of psychosocial mechanisms that people use to justify aggression. Through these justifications, athletes manage to engage in aggression without experiencing negative feelings like guilt that normally control this behavior. For example, players may displace responsibility for their actions to their coach, blame their victim for their own behavior, claim that they cheated to help their team, or downplay the consequences of their actions for others. Finally, individuals who are high in ego orientation feel successful when they do better than others; they are preoccupied with winning and showing that they are the best. These players are more likely to be aggressive in sport.

Social environmental variables are also associated with aggression. One of them is the performance motivational climate, which refers to the criteria of success that are dominant in the athletes' environment. Through the feedback they provide, the rewards they give, and, in general, the way they interact with the players, coaches make clear the criteria of success in that achievement context. As an example, when coaches provide feedback about how good a player is relative to others and reward only the best players, they create a performance motivational climate, sending a clear message to athletes that only high ability matters. Players who perceive a performance climate in their team are more likely to become aggressive.

Conclusion

Aggression is a construct with a long history and considerable debate around its definition, primarily due to the difficulties of determining whether the perpetrator has the intention to harm the victim when acting in a certain way. Aggression can be instrumental or hostile. Many sports involve forceful play, which could result in an injury. However, if players do not intend to harm the opponent, this play is considered as an assertive act, not an aggressive one. Finally, several individual difference and social environmental factors have been associated with aggression in sport.

Maria Kavussanu and Gershon Tenenbaum

See also Moral Behavior; Moral Disengagement

Further Readings

Anderson, C. A., & Bushman, B. J. (2002). Human aggression. *Annual Review of Psychology, 53,* 27–51.

Baron, R. A., & Richardson, D. R. (1994). *Human aggression* (2nd ed.). New York: Plenum Press.

Coulomb-Cabagno, G., & Rascle, O. (2006). Team sports players' observed aggression as a function of gender, competitive level, and sport type. *Journal of Applied Social Psychology, 36,* 1980–2000.

Kavussanu, M. (2008). Moral behaviour in sport: A critical review of the literature. *International Review of Sport and Exercise Psychology, 1,* 124–138.

Stephens, D. (1998). Aggression. In J. L. Duda (Ed.), *Advances in sport and exercise psychology measurement* (pp. 277–292). Morgantown, WV: Fitness Information Technology.

ALCOHOL ABUSE

Hazardous alcohol use is a significant health problem that affects many people. In the United States, almost 10% of the population will meet past-year diagnostic criteria for either alcohol abuse or alcohol dependence, with the highest rates occurring among college students and other young adults. Alcohol use disorders co-occur with mental health problems like depression, anxiety, and other substance use disorders, and can cause a variety of physical ailments. According to Bouchery, Harwood, Sacks, Simon, and Brewer (2011), the economic cost of alcohol use disorders in the United States is approximately $223.5 billion each year.

Despite the fact that alcohol use is known to be harmful toward athletic performance, rates of alcohol use are relatively high among some groups of athletes. This entry compares rates of alcohol use between athletes and nonathletes, discusses sport-related factors that might impact alcohol use among athletes, and highlights effective intervention and prevention strategies.

Rates of Alcohol Use Among Athletes

A number of studies across several countries have shown adolescent athletes consume alcohol at rates similar to or higher than peers. Findings from several recent studies, though, suggest the relationship between sport participation and alcohol use among adolescents is impacted by other factors. One national study of U.S. adolescents found self-reported rates of heavy drinking and drinking and driving in the past 30 days were higher for male athletes versus male nonathletes. In contrast, female athletes reported lower rates of ever using alcohol or use within the past 30 days versus female nonathletes. Another national, longitudinal study found that adolescents within the United States whose extracurricular activities included only sports display accelerated rates of alcohol use and alcohol-related problems. In contrast, involvement in sports and extracurricular academic activities was associated with a deceleration in alcohol use and related problems. Additionally, a national study of Norwegian high school students found participation in collaborative team sports like soccer was associated with an increase in alcohol intoxication over time, but participation in endurance sports like running was associated with a decrease in alcohol intoxication over time. Thus, the answer to the degree to which sports participation among adolescents is a risk or protective factor for alcohol use is not a simple one, but is instead often contingent upon a variety of factors.

Research examining the relationship between sport participation and alcohol use among college athletes in the United States has provided clear evidence that athletes tend to consume more alcohol than nonathletes. For example, in three national studies with sample sizes ranging from 12,777 to 51,483, the researchers reported past 2-week binge drinking rates of 57% to 62% and 48% to 50% among male and female college athletes, respectively. These percentages were approximately 15 points higher than corresponding rates for nonathletes. Similar patterns emerged for other measures of alcohol use, such as frequent binge drinking and average number of drinks per week. As one might expect given these differences in heavy drinking rates, college athletes were also more likely than other students to experience problems from alcohol like impaired academics, trouble with the authorities, and participation in behaviors later regretted. There is also evidence to suggest that college students who engage in recreational sports like club teams and intramurals are more at risk for excessive alcohol use than other students.

Relatively few studies have examined rates of alcohol consumption among professional or other elite athletes, particularly in terms of comparing them with relevant nonathlete groups. Those that have been conducted suggest rates of alcohol use among adult elite athletes are higher than general population rates. Research is also lacking on rates of alcohol use disorders among athletes. However, it is likely that rates of alcohol abuse and dependence are particularly high among some groups of athletes, especially those where evidence suggests they experience more alcohol-related problems than others (e.g., college athletes).

Sport-Related Factors and Alcohol Use

Researchers have identified numerous factors that increase the likelihood of hazardous alcohol use in the general population, including demographic characteristics, genetic factors, personality variables, environmental factors, and a host of other individual, interpersonal, and contextual variables. The impact of such factors is presumably consistent between athletes and nonathletes, but researchers have also identified several sport-related factors that may increase the likelihood of heavy drinking among athletes.

There is a clear cultural link between athletics and alcohol use in many countries. Alcohol beverage companies advertise heavily during televised sporting events and provide key sponsorship for many sporting leagues. In some countries, alcohol companies even provide direct sponsorship for individual teams and players. Research has shown that athletes receiving alcohol industry sponsorship report higher rates of hazardous drinking than those who do not receive such sponsorship. Other research has documented an association between exposure to alcohol advertising and subsequent alcohol consumption. It is therefore possible that athletes are more likely than others to be influenced by the advertising or sponsorship efforts of alcohol beverage companies.

A second set of factors that may be associated with heavy alcohol use among athletes is a particular susceptibility to the positive and negative reinforcing aspects of alcohol. For example, the personality trait of sensation seeking has been shown to be positively associated with alcohol consumption, and several studies have shown that athletes are more likely than others to report high levels of this trait. Similarly, a number of writers have suggested that some groups of athletes experience especially high levels of stress and other pressures, such as college athletes attempting to balance the demands of athletics and academics. Such individuals are thought to be particularly prone to using alcohol as a negative reinforcing coping strategy (e.g., reducing stress, distracting from life's problems), although research studies have not provided convincing support that this is in fact the case. There may be other factors that are associated with both the likelihood of participating in athletics and the likelihood of engaging in at-risk alcohol use.

Increased access to alcohol may also account for heavier drinking rates among athletes in comparison with the general population. Athletes at many competitive levels often have more social opportunities involving alcohol than others. For example, college athletes are usually among the most popular students on campus, and therefore have ample opportunities to attend parties or other gatherings where they will be provided alcohol. Similarly, many athletes socializing in public establishments, particularly those who are recognizable in their communities, will experience the phenomenon of others wishing to buy them drinks or otherwise supply them with alcohol. Thus, heavy drinking among some athletes may be partially explained by relatively easy access to a supply of free or low-cost alcoholic beverages, which would be consistent with basic behavioral economics theories.

A final factor that may impact at-risk drinking among athletes involves their seasonal calendar cycle. Research suggests athletes tend to limit alcohol use during their competitive seasons, but drinking rates increase in the off-season. Some athletes may engage in particularly heavy drinking during the off-season believing (a) they are not harming their athletic performance since they are not in-season; and (b) they have to take advantage of a limited timeframe that does not involve regular practices, games, and accountability to coaches. Such a spike in heavy drinking can lead to increased likelihood of a host of severe alcohol-related consequences.

Interventions for Hazardous Drinking Among Athletes

Unlike both recreational and performance enhancing drugs, regular testing for the presence of a substance is not a logistically feasible deterrent for alcohol use among athletes. Thus, it is particularly important to explore alternative strategies for preventing harmful alcohol use among athletes. Several effective treatments have been identified for individuals experiencing alcohol use disorders, including cognitive behavioral therapy, twelve-step facilitation therapy, and behavioral family therapy. Athletes experiencing significant problems with alcohol should be referred to settings where intensive treatment could be provided.

It is also important to provide interventions to those who may be at risk for experiencing alcohol-related problems but whose current alcohol use habits do not necessarily warrant extensive treatments. Over the past 10 to 15 years, clinical researchers have examined the efficacy of brief interventions in reducing harmful alcohol use. One of the most popular and efficacious approaches involves a single-session model where the clinician uses a motivational interviewing-based style and provides personalized feedback about one's drinking habits. Motivational interviewing is designed to increase an individual's motivation to change behavior by exploring and resolving ambivalence regarding change, and this process can be facilitated by receiving personalized information on one's drinking habits. Commonly included pieces of personalized feedback include social norms information (how one's own alcohol use and perceived typical alcohol use among others compares to actual population norms), a summary of alcohol-related risks or problems experienced, and possible genetic risk for an alcohol use disorder. More recently, researchers have explored the efficacy of personalized feedback-only interventions where the feedback is provided without one-on-one clinician contact. Three studies have examined the effects of these interventions specifically among athletes, all of which showed positive effects in terms of reducing alcohol consumption relative to control conditions. One of the studies included feedback that was targeted specifically for athletes (e.g., the impact of alcohol use on one's athletic performance), which was shown to be more effective than personalized feedback that did not include the athlete-targeted information. Other studies have provided promising support for interventions focusing exclusively on correcting misperceptions of drinking norms, although they have been limited by the lack of proper control conditions.

An important gap in the literature on the efficacy of alcohol-related interventions among athletes is that the effectiveness of interventions delivered via sporting organizations themselves has not been examined. There are, though, potentially promising avenues that could be explored in this area. For example, research has supported the efficacy of brief advice interventions delivered by physicians and parent-based interventions, both of which could be modified to be delivered by athletic organization personnel like coaches and team doctors. It may also be possible to integrate alcohol interventions into the context of a team's sports medicine staff, which would be advantageous given the degree to which athletic trainers and other sports medicine staff are often the ones working most closely with athletes on a variety of health-related issues.

Conclusion

Some groups of athletes are particularly at risk for excessive alcohol use that can lead to a variety of negative or harmful outcomes, including impaired athletic performance. Researchers and theorists have explored several sport-related factors that might serve to heighten the risk of heavy drinking among athletes, although the specific ways in which many of these factors impact alcohol use are not well understood. Fortunately, a number of interventions exist that can either reduce or prevent problematic alcohol use, including brief models that have been shown to be efficacious specifically among athletes.

Matthew P. Martens

See also Moral Behavior; Performance-Enhancing Drugs; Recreational Drugs

Further Readings

Bouchery, E. E., Harwood, H. J., Sacks, J. J., Simon, C. J., & Brewer, R. D. (2011, November). Economic costs of excessive alcohol consumption in the U.S., 2006. *American Journal of Preventive Medicine, 41,* 516–524.

Dimeff, L. A., Baer, J. S., Kivlahan, D. R., & Marlatt, G. A. (1999). *Brief alcohol screening and intervention for college students: A harm reduction approach.* New York: Guilford Press.

Grant, B. F., Dawson, D. A., Stinson, F. S., Chou, S. P., Dufour, M. C., & Pickering, R. P. (2004). The 12-month prevalence and trends in DSM-IV alcohol abuse and dependence: United States, 1991–1992 and 2001–2002. *Drug and Alcohol Dependence, 74,* 223–234.

Lisha, N. E., & Sussman, S. (2010). Relationship of high school and college sports participation with alcohol, tobacco, and illicit drug use: A review. *Addictive Behaviors, 35,* 399–407.

Martens, M. P., Kilmer, J. R., Beck, N. C., & Zamboanga, B. L. (2010). The efficacy of a targeted personalized drinking feedback intervention among intercollegiate athletes: A randomized controlled trial. *Psychology of Addictive Behaviors, 24,* 660–669.

Mays, D., DePadilla, L., Thompson, N. J., Kushner, H. I., & Windle, M. (2010). Sports participation and problem alcohol use. A multi-wave national sample of adolescents. *American Journal of Preventive Medicine, 38,* 491–498.

Nelson, T. F., & Wechsler, H. (2001). Alcohol and college athletes. *Medicine and Science in Sports and Exercise, 33,* 43–47.

O'Brien, K. S., & Kypri, K. (2008). Alcohol industry sponsorship of sport and drinking levels in New Zealand sportspeople. *Addiction, 103,* 1961–1966.

Anticipation

In sport and exercise psychology, *anticipation* usually refers to the ability to quickly and accurately predict the outcome of an opponent's action before that action is completed. Skilled athletes can use bodily cues to anticipate outcomes at earlier moments in an action sequence than can unskilled athletes, allowing them more time to perform an appropriate response in time-stressed tasks. A basic understanding of anticipation requires a comprehension of how skilled athletes anticipate actions, how anticipation is best tested, and what the practical implications are for training anticipation.

How Skilled Athletes Anticipate Actions

Anticipation is most commonly tested by occluding vision at a critical point in an action sequence, after which the observer must predict the action outcome. For instance, a tennis player may observe an opposing player performing a serve, but at the moment of racquetball contact, vision is occluded, and the receiver must predict the direction of the serve. Skilled athletes in a wide range of sports do better than lesser skilled performers in these tests, including in tennis, soccer goalkeeping, squash, and batting in baseball and cricket. Occlusion is achieved in the laboratory using edited video footage or in the field by using liquid crystal glasses that quickly and selectively occlude vision.

Skilled athletes anticipate action outcomes based on events presented earlier in a movement sequence, providing a distinct advantage for sports skill that must be performed under severe time constraints. The selective occlusion of different body segments (e.g., the arms or legs) in video displays has shown that experts—when compared with novices—rely on the movement of body segments that are more remote from the end effector. For example, novice badminton players typically anticipate based on the movement of the opponent's racquet, whereas skilled players use the movement of the opponent's racquet *and* arm. Attention toward the arm provides a temporal advantage, as movement of the arm precedes the movement of the racquet. The expert advantage in anticipation is based on sensitivity to kinematic movement patterns, rather than to figural or contextual cues. Point-light displays replace video footage of an opponent with a series of isolated points of light located at critical joint centers; expert–novice differences in anticipation are replicated when athletes view these displays. Evidently, skilled athletes have developed the ability to understand the consequences of the underlying kinematic movement pattern of their opponents. It is likely that this skill has developed not only as a consequence of *observing* these movements but also by skilled athletes *performing* the same actions. Perception may share a mutual form of neural programming with the production of action; recent work has shown that anticipation of an action relies on the same brain region that is used when generating the same action.

Testing Anticipation

Anticipation can be tested using a range of different display stimuli and responses. While it is most favorable to use conditions that accurately reflect those found in the natural environment, the need for consistency and control in testing conditions means that this is not always possible. Skilled athletes outperform lesser skilled players in simulated conditions; however, the degree of superiority will be an underrepresentation of the true ability that would be found in the natural environment.

Display Stimuli

Video simulations allow anticipation to be tested in a very reliable and repeatable manner, though they often lack the size, contrast, or depth information available in real life. Liquid crystal occlusion goggles allow anticipation to be tested in the performance setting; this improvement in display fidelity usually leads to a commensurate increase in the size of the expert–novice difference.

Perception-Action Coupling

Athletes make perceptual predictions in most tests of anticipation (e.g., verbal or pen-and-paper); however, the separation of perception from action may miss an important element of sporting expertise. It is likely that perceptual responses test only the vision-for-perception neurological pathway; in contrast, skilled athletes rely on a specific vision-for-action pathway to produce real-time movements in the natural setting. Accordingly, it has been found that movement-based responses provide a better assessment of skilled anticipation than purely perceptual responses do.

Practical Implications

Facilitation of Performance

Skilled athletes use prerelease information to facilitate early and appropriate body positioning, rather than to stipulate the exact location the ball or target will arrive. This allows for better use of postrelease information to engender successful interception. The kinematic movement pattern of the opponent is also used to coordinate the timing and movement of an athlete's response. The importance of anticipatory skill suggests the need for advance information to be present in the training environment to optimize learning; for example, this principle has been used to argue against the use of ball projection machines, as they remove the kinematic movement information essential for anticipation.

Training Anticipatory Skill

Perceptual training programs are used to improve the anticipatory skill of developing athletes. These programs expose learners to a high volume of action sequences (usually occluded), observed either using video displays or in the field setting and often accompanied by some form of guiding information to accelerate skill acquisition. Perceptual training generally leads to an improvement in anticipatory skill, though there is conjecture about the most effective forms of training. Intuitively, practitioners have sought to provide learners with explicit information about how they should search for and interpret kinematic cues. More recent work suggests that implicit means of training, which guide attention without the provision of explicit rules, may enhance the likelihood that a skill is retained and may render the skill more robust under stress.

David L. Mann

See also Cue Utilization; Decision Making; Expertise; Perception; Skill Acquisition

Further Readings

Abernethy, B., & Russell, D. G. (1987). Expert-novice differences in an applied selective attention task. *Journal of Sport Psychology, 9*, 326–345.

van der Kamp, J., Rivas, F., van Doorn, H., & Savelsbergh, G. J. P. (2008). Ventral and dorsal contributions in visual anticipation in fast ball sports. *International Journal of Sport Psychology, 39*(2), 100–130.

Williams, A. M., Ward, P., Knowles, J. M., & Smeeton, N. J. (2002). Anticipation skill in a real-world task: Measurement, training, and transfer in tennis. *Journal of Experimental Psychology: Applied, 8*, 259–270.

Antisocial/Prosocial Behavior

See Moral Behavior

Assimilation

Assimilation refers to the integration of one culture into another. This integration may include changes in cultural characteristics such as language, appearance, food, music, and religion among other customs. Cultural values and beliefs also influence this integration of cultures. Assimilation is relevant to sport performance in that sports occur in the context of culture, society, and politics. In addition, each sport has its own culture and characteristics that may reflect or be in contrast with the values and beliefs of society and the individual athletes that play a particular sport. As such, an athlete's cultural milieu may interact with that of the sport and society in which the sport occurs to influence performance. For instance, a sport that focuses on individual performance and recognition may not fit well for an athlete from a culture that emphasizes teamwork and humility.

Assimilation may influence the type of sport an athlete selects and the roles assumed within sports and may also manifest in interactions and relationships with teammates and coaches. Typically, cultural assimilation involves an underrepresented (minority) group integrating into a dominant group's culture. An athlete from rural American Samoa playing American football at an urban college in the United States, for example, might integrate into the dominant cultural group of the city in which he plays by adopting the cultural practices of that region. However, the preceding example and description represent a unidirectional and oversimplified version of the concept of assimilation, as they suggest that assimilation necessarily occurs in the direction of the dominant group and that it is a linear process of change. Assimilation can also occur from the direction of the dominant to the underrepresented group, though this is less common. For example, a White athlete playing American football at a predominantly Black college may assimilate toward the culture of his fellow students, campus, and teammates, which may not reflect the dominant culture per se. Moreover, assimilation is not a process that is linear with a finite endpoint of *being assimilated*; rather it is a process that is constantly evolving. Individual athletes may assimilate to varying degrees based on situational, historical, and other factors. Thus, a Cuban immigrant playing professional baseball may be less assimilated around other Cuban or Latin American teammates or coaches, whereas he may be more assimilated around teammates and coaches from other cultures. In other words, assimilation is an evolving process that may be state dependent and also reflect the evolution of an athlete's assimilation.

The way in which assimilation is initiated may also affect how it is perceived, thereby influencing the athlete in negative or positive aspects or both. Assimilation may occur voluntarily or involuntarily: A soccer player from North Africa may be traded to a team in Russia, with little control over the decision. In contrast, another athlete may decide to immerse himself or herself in a culturally different environment to expand life experience. The perceived level of control over assimilation may affect how an athlete responds to it.

Enculturation and Acculturation

Regardless of the mechanism for assimilation, there are two primary components to assimilation: (1) *enculturation*, or the level to which someone adheres to primary cultural beliefs, values, and customs, and (2) *acculturation*, or the level to which someone adopts dominant or other cultural beliefs, values, and customs. One might think of complete enculturation and acculturation as extreme endpoints on a balancing continuum (see Figure 1). Most athletes' assimilation will balance between some percentage of acculturation and enculturation that together equals 100%; for example, 75% enculturated, 25% acculturated. This percentage is based on which side the cultural characteristics discussed earlier reside. An athlete's assimilation balance may shift based on the situation and may change over time to reflect life experiences.

Effects of Assimilation

Assimilation can sometimes result in acculturative stress (stress related to adapting to another culture) and may adversely affect performance in sport. In

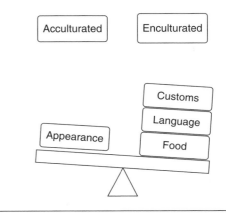

Figure 1   Balancing the Assimilation Continuum
Source: Anthony P. Kontos.

extreme cases, if not addressed, acculturative stress may develop into depression, anxiety, or hostility. These negative effects of assimilation may be more salient for athletes who are highly acculturated and then return to their own culture. When athletes return to their own culture, they may be perceived as having sold out their own culture for the dominant culture. In contrast, a recently immigrated athlete or one who is highly enculturated may struggle to adapt to a new culture and the athletes from that culture. As a result, such an athlete may be isolated in the new cultural environment. However, for some athletes assimilation may not play any role at all in creating stress or adversely affecting sport performance. For these athletes, assimilation may even help alleviate stress and anxiety by allowing them to fit in better and feel more comfortable in an unfamiliar culture.

Conclusion

Assimilation is nonlinear and constantly evolving through both direct and indirect experiences with one's own and other cultures. An athlete's level of enculturation and acculturation occurs on a balanced continuum that may shift back and forth based on the situation and cultural context, as well as the evolution of the athlete's assimilation process. It is important to point out that assimilation does not typically involve a purposeful integration of another culture. In fact, assimilation may simply occur as a product of direct or indirect exposure to and familiarity with another culture over time. As such, many athletes are unaware of how assimilated they are or of assimilation's potential role on performance and sport. Therefore, assimilation should be viewed as neither positive nor negative but rather as an evolving process that is highly individualized for each athlete.

Anthony P. Kontos

See also Cultural Competence; Cultural Safety; Diversity; Ethnicity; Multiculturalism; Racism/Whiteness; Stereotyping, Cultural/Ethnic/Racial

Further Readings

Kontos, A. P., & Arguello, E. (2009). Sport psychology consulting with Latin American athletes. In R. Schinke (Ed.), *Contemporary sport psychology* (pp. 181–196). Hauppauge, NY: Nova Science.

Kontos, A. P., & Breland-Noble, A. (2002). Racial/ethnic diversity in applied sport psychology: A multicultural introduction to working with athletes of color. *The Sport Psychologist, 16,* 296–315.

Ryba, T. V., Schinke, R. J., & Tenenbaum, G. (2010). *The cultural turn in sport psychology.* Morgantown, WV: Fitness Information Technology.

Schinke, R. J., & Hanrahan, S. J. (2009). *Cultural sport psychology.* Champaign, IL: Human Kinetics.

ATHLETE LEADERSHIP

An *athlete leader* in sport is defined as an individual who holds a formal or informal leadership role within a team and influences other group members in the pursuit of common objectives. Researchers suggest that approximately one quarter of athletes occupy some form of leadership role within a team, and highlight the potential importance of athlete leadership toward positive group functioning as well as the need for a more thorough understanding of the topic. The following entry briefly highlights the characteristics, types, and functions of athlete leaders, as well as other important variables associated with the presence of these individuals on sport teams.

Characteristics of an Athlete Leader

Research generally demonstrates that individuals possessing athlete leadership roles within a group have similar characteristics. Maureen Weiss and colleagues Molly Moran and Melissa Price revealed that athlete leaders self-report greater friendship quality and peer acceptance, while Joseph Bucci, Gordon Bloom, Todd Loughead, and Jeffrey Caron found that these individuals have a stronger work ethic, desire for high performance, and respect from teammates. The latter researchers also noted that possessing these characteristics leads to positive relationships with both coaches and teammates, helping foster effective levels of communication within the overall group structure. However, despite the importance and prevalence of the social psychological characteristics noted above, the most consistent characteristic of athlete leaders found in previous research pertains to sport-related competence; in other words, athletic ability is positively associated with ratings of athlete leadership.

Types of Athlete Leadership

To garner an understanding of how athlete leadership manifests itself in the sport context, it is important to understand the emergence of the leadership role, as well as the extent to which leadership behaviors influence group members.

Formal and Informal Athlete Leadership

The formal athlete leader represents a role that is prescribed by another individual within the group or sport organization, usually a member of the coaching staff. This type of leader is highly visible within the group and is assigned specific responsibilities. A common example of a formal athlete leader in sport is the team captain. In many instances, the coach selects the captain of the team and, within certain sports, the occupant of this role may even be formally designated by such things as a C on the uniform or an armband to wear during competitive matches.

Conversely, an informal athlete leader emerges as a function of (a) group interaction, (b) distinct group needs, and (c) the personality traits of individual athletes. This type of athlete leader acts in a way that often complements the style of an established leader within the group (the formal athlete leader). However, the informal leader emerges naturally, without designation by another group member or the organization. For example, an athlete may assume the role of an emotional leader to help rally a team around its goals. This potential informal athlete leader may exist on teams in which the formal leader is more task driven (less expressive in nature); however, in other teams this informal role may be redundant if the formal leader possesses high interpersonal attraction and engages in socially supportive behaviors.

Team- and Peer-Level Athlete Leaders

In addition to the level of formality, athlete-to-athlete leadership is categorized in terms of the scope of influence held by each individual. Todd Loughead, James Hardy, and Mark Eys discussed the presence of both team- and peer-level leaders. First, a team-level leader is more influential and is identified as an athlete leader by the majority of the team (over 50% of the membership). Examples include veteran players who provide valuable advice to all members of a group at different times or who are highly vocal (in a productive manner) during team meetings. It is also worthwhile to note that the team-level athlete leader likely emerges through the formal leadership process discussed previously.

In contrast, peer-level leaders represent those who are identified by a lower percentage of the team (less than 50%). Equally important in a team setting, peer-level leaders exert individualized influence on a small number of athletes. An example of this type of leader is an individual within the team who acts as a mentor to two or three less-experienced teammates. Although other team members may never be influenced by this specific individual, the inexperienced athletes may view the mentor as a very important leader.

Functions of Athlete Leadership

Athlete leadership roles are often differentiated by their specific functions within the group. These functions revolve around both internal and external activities. Athlete leaders who attend to the internal functions focus on the (a) task or (b) social related activities of the group.

- *Internal task functions.* Task-related functions represent the behaviors executed by a leader surrounding a group's instrumental objectives, such as the performance of the sport team. The behaviors oriented toward this function, for example, influence group members to perform to the best of their abilities and to coordinate effectively with their teammates.

- *Internal social functions.* Social-related functions represent the behaviors executed by a leader surrounding interpersonal relations and optimal team unity. An example of an athlete leader concerned with the social activities of the group would be someone who works to resolve conflict or plans events aimed at bonding the members of a team together.

- *External functions.* Athletes can also serve the function of leading their team in external activities. Todd Loughead et al. described the external athlete leader as one who leads and represents the group outside of the competitive setting. Specifically, an external athlete leader helps a team cope and adapt to the surrounding environment. As examples, individuals who represent the team at different community-driven events or speak to the media on behalf of the group undertake external functions.

It is important to note that the various functions of an athlete leadership role, although distinct from one another, are not necessarily performed by different people. One individual may have the ability to occupy a leadership role that is solely task-related, whereas another individual may occupy a leadership role that executes all three functions.

Correlates of Athlete Leadership

Interesting insights have been yielded with respect to the presence of athlete leadership in sport. The following sections briefly highlight both individual (satisfaction) and team level (group cohesion and collective efficacy) correlates of athlete leader behavior.

Athlete Satisfaction

Following research that linked leadership behaviors of the coach with athlete satisfaction, Mark Eys, Todd Loughead, and James Hardy demonstrated that athletes who perceived a balanced dispersion of athlete leaders across the aforementioned functions (approximately equal number of leaders focusing on task, social, and external objectives) had higher satisfaction with their sport experiences. Specifically, these athletes were more satisfied with team performance and the degree of integration of team members than those who perceived a relative imbalance with respect to the focus of athlete leaders on their team, as with a high number of task leaders but low numbers of social and external leaders.

Group Cohesion

Athlete leadership is also related to the perceptions of cohesion experienced by group members. Two studies provide different perspectives on the relationship between these variables. First, Price and Weiss found that adolescent female soccer players who self-reported higher leadership abilities with respect to instrumental and prosocial behaviors perceived greater task and social cohesion on their teams. Furthermore, those who were rated higher by their teammates in the same leadership abilities perceived greater social cohesion.

In a second study, Hardy, Eys, and Loughead were interested in the links between the percentage of athlete leaders on sport teams (i.e., dispersion) and group members' perceptions of cohesion. Their findings indicated that the dispersion of leaders focused on task functions was negatively related to perceptions of task cohesion. In other words, a more constrained number of task-focused

leaders was associated with increased group unity. Furthermore, these researchers found that intrateam communication mediated this relationship. The interpretation of these results was that a lower number of task leaders leads to better quality communication in terms of consistency, clarity, and overall effectiveness that, in turn, is associated with more positive perceptions of task cohesion.

Collective Efficacy

Finally, athlete leadership is linked to members' beliefs regarding the group's ability to carry out required tasks, as well as its general ability to perform at a high level. Price and Weiss revealed that the self-reported instrumental and prosocial leadership behaviors of athletes were positively related to their indications of efficacy related to the team's ability, unity, effort, preparation, and persistence.

Conclusion

Overall, athlete leadership represents an important aspect of group functioning. This entry has briefly highlighted the characteristics, types, and functions of athlete leadership. Future research, however, must continue to build upon the current breadth of knowledge regarding the influence of athlete leaders within sport. In doing so, sport psychology researchers can continue moving toward unearthing different individual and group level variables that are related to both effective and ineffective cases of athlete leadership. Furthermore, another future step can involve translating this knowledge into the group exercise setting to test similar relationships to those found in sport like individual satisfaction and group cohesion and determine if exerciser-to-exerciser leadership influences important outcomes such as physical activity adherence.

Mark Eys, Colin McLaren, and Robyn Bertram

See also Cohesion; Friendships/Peer Relations; Leadership in Sport: Multidimensional Model; Leadership in Sport: Transactional and Transformational; Mentoring; Roles

Further Readings

Bucci, J., Bloom, G. A., Loughead, T. M., & Caron, J. G. (2012). Ice hockey coaches' perceptions of athlete leadership. *Journal of Applied Sport Psychology, 24,* 243–259.

Eys, M., Loughead, T. M., & Hardy, J. (2007). Athlete leadership dispersion and satisfaction in interactive sport teams. *Psychology of Sport and Exercise, 8,* 281–296.

Hardy, J., Eys, M., & Loughead, T. M. (2008). Does communication mediate the athlete leadership to cohesion relationship? *International Journal of Sport Psychology, 39,* 329–345.

Loughead, T. M., Hardy, J., & Eys, M. (2006). The nature of athlete leadership. *Journal of Sport Behavior, 29,* 142–158.

Moran, M. M., & Weiss, M. R. (2006). Peer leadership in sport: Links with friendship, peer acceptance, psychological characteristics, and athletic ability. *Journal of Applied Sport Psychology, 18,* 97–113.

Price, M. S., & Weiss, M. R. (2011). Peer leadership in sport: Relationships among personal characteristics, leader behaviors, and team outcomes. *Journal of Applied Sport Psychology, 23,* 49–64.

ATTACHMENT THEORY AND COACHING

The aim of attachment theory has largely been to explain how relationships with parents in childhood have such a persistent effect on personality development. The focus of attachment theory has subsequently been extended from child to adolescent and adult development and social relationships within the context of both contemporary personality and social psychology. Attachment has been viewed as a natural phenomenon sought by all human beings. Subsequently, the theory postulates that, whereas successful bids for proximity and connectedness with warm, kind, dependable, and encouraging attachment figures are important for optimal functioning, the loss of such proximity and connection can be a natural source of distress and psychosocial dysfunction.

In sport and exercise psychology, attachment theory has recently been used to understand (a) how athletes and coaches perceive and cope with fears and anxieties, injuries, and performance slumps; and (b) how personal relationships (parent–athlete or parent–child) and social relationships (coach–athlete, athlete–athlete) help their members to either flourish or diminish. The appeal of attachment theory to explain a whole host of research questions has sparked research within sport and exercise psychology that has the potential to advance theory, measurement, and practice,

as seen in work by Sam Carr and Neil Fitzpatrick and by Louise Davis and Sophia Jowett.

Attachment Figures, Interactions, and Relationships

Attachment figures are not just any close relationship member. Attachment figures are special individuals to whom, for example, an athlete turns when assistance, encouragement, and cooperation are needed. In the context of sport, coaches serve as attachment figures when they allow their athletes to act independently. Athletes, in these cases, are encouraged to explore and discover new techniques, skills, or competition in the knowledge that their coaches are near and they can reliably provide protection, comfort, encouragement, or relief should the athletes need it (failing to execute the technique or the skill, failing to qualify, losing a major championship, getting injured during a task). While there are numerous interpersonal behaviors that cannot be characterized as *attachment interactions,* such as organizing a training session or providing feedback and criticism, there are other interpersonal behaviors that can be characterized as attachment interactions. In such interactions, the expectation is that the athlete would feel a degree of threat or distress, thus compelling that athlete to seek comfort and support from the coach. In competitive sport especially where the stakes are high, athletes undergo numerous stressful situations, including dealing with complicated technical routines, serious injuries, team selections, career transitions, or personal circumstances such as the loss of a loved one, financial problems, and social pressures—all of which could require them to seek comfort and support from people they trust. The *attachment bond* becomes apparent when coaches are shown to be available, sensitive to the needs of their athletes, and responsive to the athletes' feelings of threat, worries, distress, hurt, or bids for proximity when in need.

Attachment Working Models

According to attachment theory, variations in attachment figure responses to an attached individual's bids for proximity, connectedness, and protection are capable of progressively producing lasting changes in how attached individuals function personally and interpersonally. For example, over time, athletes (attached individuals) have a host of interactions with their coaches (attachment figures) and the quality and type of responses of these interactions are stored in athletes' long-term memories. This stored knowledge takes the form of *internal working models* (IWMs) and allows, for example, athletes to predict future interactions with their coaches and guide their behavior, cognitions, and feelings. Specifically, IWMs are capable of orienting individuals in specific ways toward their own self and toward their close others. On one hand, *IWM of the self* reflects how worthy one feels in obtaining assistance when in need (I am a valued member), and on the other hand, *IWM of others* refer to whether an individual can expect assistance, including responsive and caring behavior, from an attachment figure in times of stress (I expect or don't doubt coaches' understanding and help). According to attachment theory, IWMs are thought to account for the long-term effects on individuals' personality functioning as this relates to attachment interactions during infancy, childhood, adolescence, and adulthood. An individual's *attachment style* reflects the most constantly accessible IWM, and thus how typically an individual functions within one's attachment system at a local level and within a specific relationship like the coach–athlete relationship or at a global level and across a number of relationships in general attachment style.

Attachment Styles

There are three most commonly referred to attachment styles: *secure, anxious,* and *avoidant.* Individuals with a secure attachment style display confidence in the availability of close others like a coach for comfort and support in times of need. Those who display an anxious attachment style have a desire for proximity and intimacy to an attachment figure even in nondistressing conditions. Under stressful situations, they can display excessive distress and may withdraw in anger even if support is offered from the close other on the basis that the support offered is not good enough. Finally, individuals with an avoidant attachment style display little distress during stressful events and few attempts at maintaining contact with an attachment figure. As mentioned earlier, attachment styles are thought to be determined by an individual's IWM of both the self and others. Individuals with a secure attachment style typically have an expectation that assistance should be available in times of need and that they

are worthy of such assistance; this helps them develop and maintain a positive IWM of themselves and others. Conversely, individuals with insecure attachment styles typically expect either inconsistent assistance (anxious), or no assistance at all (avoidant), in times of need; this results in the development and maintenance of feelings of unworthiness regarding others' care and affection while also becoming suspicious of any affection they may receive. This leads individuals with anxious attachment to display a negative IWM of themselves, and for those with an avoidant attachment style to display negative IWMs of others.

Lifespan Perspective of Attachment

It is important to note that although an individual's attachment style could remain stable over time, this can be dependent on the caregiving environment or attachment figure. If, for example, an individual's attachment bond with the coach supports and reinforces one's dominant or currently most active IWM, the stability of an attachment style would be expected. However, if an individual develops an attachment bond (e.g., with the coach) that is substantially different from attachment bonds formed in the past (predominantly by the primary caregiver, such as a parent or indeed a previous coach), then there is a chance of altering IWMs (tendencies to anticipate, attend to, interpret, and recall behavior) and, in turn, attachment style. For example, an athlete who has constantly received inconsistent support and responsiveness from previous attachment figures, such as parents, teachers, or coaches, is likely to develop a negative IWM of self and thereby bring about an anxious attachment style. However, the intense and enduring support, responsiveness, and encouragement demonstrated by a new coach over a period of time can foster a much more positive intrapersonal outlook, which can potentially lead to an alteration of the athlete's IWM and consequently the adoption of a secure attachment style within the coach–athlete relationship.

Attachment Theory in Sport

Research within the broader discipline of social psychology on adult attachment has demonstrated the importance of secure attachments for relationship quality and functioning as well as psychological well-being (for a comprehensive review, see Mikulincer & Shaver, 2007). In sport and exercise psychology, research is gathering momentum in this area. At present, the findings suggest that athletes displaying insecure attachment (anxious or avoidant attachment) are likely to report poor relationship quality with the coach, less sport satisfaction, greater risk of developing an eating disorder, low perceptions of basic psychological need satisfaction, and ill-being (e.g., lack of vitality, negative affect, depression) when compared to more securely attached athletes. Moreover, findings highlight that the satisfaction of basic psychological needs, such as connectedness, competence, and autonomy, can potentially explain the association between insecure attachment and well- or ill-being. It would appear that while security attachment can satisfy basic needs and thus lead to athletes' well-being, insecure attachment can thwart basic needs and lead to athletes' ill-being. These studies started to underline the significance of attachment theory in understanding important research questions of practical significance for effective coaching and successful athletic performance.

Coaching Practice

Given that coaching is an interpersonal affair revolving primarily around the coach and the athlete, it is important that both coach and athlete have an appreciation of the potential impact that their attachment styles can have on their own and the other's behaviors, thoughts, and feelings. As described earlier, an avoidant attachment style is reflected in an individual's being heavily self-reliant and uninterested and unwilling to connect with others. If an athlete appears to be distant to the coach when interacting in training or competitions, it does not mean that that athlete is being indifferent toward sport or dislikes the coach; it may simply be a reflection of the athlete's personality. Athletes with insecure attachment styles may be misunderstood by their coaches, and thus coaches may decide to write them off or not give them the time and attention they require to progress. Coaches who recognize their athletes as insecure can, instead of adopting a similar pattern of behavior (e.g., less connection, responsiveness) that only serves to strengthen the athlete's IWM and further reinforces the athlete's negative IWM, try creating a positive, caring, and nurturing environment that is consistently unambiguous. Ultimately, coaches' persistent positive interpersonal behaviors are more likely to help athletes satisfy basic

psychological needs and promote their well-being. Happy and satisfied athletes are more likely to persist and achieve in their chosen sports. Thus, coaches who (a) behave in an autonomy-supportive manner, while avoiding controlling behaviors, allow the athlete to take on a more integral role in their training and competition; and (b) develop positive relationships characterized by trust, respect, appreciation, commitment, readiness, reassurance, and security are more likely to help their athletes recognize that they are being valued and cared for. Such enduring, supportive, responsive, and encouraging interactions may begin to lay the foundations for a substantial change in the insecure athletes' IWMs, leading to a more secure attachment style for that athlete within the coaching context. Theory and research suggest that secure attachment styles are more advantageous for optimal functioning at both intrapersonal and interpersonal levels. Given that sporting success is the product of the combined interrelation between the coach and the athlete, as typically neither of them can do it alone, understanding their personalities can make the journey to achieving performance success much happier, easier, and rewarding.

Sophia Jowett and Luke Felton

See also Caring Climate; Coach–Athlete Relations; Coaching Efficacy; Friendships/Peer Relations; Interdependence Theory and the Coach–Athlete Relationship

Further Readings

Ainsworth, M. D. S., Blehar, M. C., Waters, E., & Wall, S. (1978). *Patterns of attachment: Assessed in the strange situation and at home*. Hillsdale, NJ: Lawrence Erlbaum.

Bowlby, J. (1969/1982). *Attachment and loss: Vol. 1. Attachment* (2nd ed.). New York: Basic Books.

Carr, S., & Fitzpatrick, N. (2011). Experiences of dyadic sport friendships as a function of self and partner attachment characteristics. *Psychology of Sport and Exercise, 12*, 383–391.

Davis, L., & Jowett, S. (2010). Investigating the interpersonal dynamics between coaches and athletes based on fundamental principles of attachment. *Journal of Clinical Sport Psychology, 4*, 112–132.

Felton, L., & Jowett, S. (2013). Attachment and well-being: The mediating effects of psychological needs satisfaction within the coach-athlete and parent-athlete relational contexts. *Psychology of Sport and Exercise, 14*, 57–65.

Mikulincer, M., & Shaver, P. R. (2007). *Attachment in adulthood: Structure, dynamics, and change.* New York: Guilford Press.

Shanmugam, V., Jowett, S., & Meyer, C. (2011). Application of the transdiagnostic cognitive-behavioral model of eating disorders to the athletic population. *Journal of Clinical Sport Psychology, 5,* 166–191.

ATTENTION THEORY

Every waking moment we face an important selection problem. How do we pick some information for further processing while ignoring almost everything else? This problem is not easy to solve given the brevity and fragility of our *working memory* (the mental system that regulates our conscious awareness) and the all but unlimited array of information available to us—not only from the external world but also from the internal domain of our own memory and imagination. So, the mind has developed a system that helps us select some information for further processing while blocking out other information. This system is called *attention*—a term that denotes the process of exerting mental effort on specific features of the world around us or on our own thoughts and feelings. For example, in sport, making a conscious effort to listen carefully to a coach's instructions before a match involves attention. Similarly, a soccer goalkeeper who is preparing to defend against a corner kick from the opposing team must pay attention to the flight of the incoming ball while disregarding the movements of the players in the penalty area. These two examples show that the ability to focus on what is most important in any situation while ignoring distractions is vital for success in sport. But when we delve deeper into the psychology of attention, a number of questions arise. Are there different types of attention? If so, how can these different attentional processes be measured? Finally, what theories best explain how the attention system works? The purpose of this entry is to answer these and other relevant questions.

Describing Attention: Nature and Types

For well over a century, cognitive psychologists (researchers who study how the mind works in seeking, storing, and using knowledge) have investigated attentional processes. From this research, three different types of attention have been identified.

First, *concentration* refers to a person's decision to invest mental effort in what is most important in any situation (as in the example above of listening to a coach's instructions). Next, *selective attention* is the perceptual ability to zoom in on task-relevant information (the flight of the ball) while ignoring distractions (the movement of players). Finally, *divided attention* refers to a form of mental time-sharing ability whereby people can learn, as a result of extensive practice, to execute two or more concurrent skills equally well. To illustrate, a skilled basketball player can dribble the ball while simultaneously looking around for a teammate who is in a good position to receive a pass. In summary, *attention* is a multidimensional term that refers to at least three different cognitive processes—concentration or effortful awareness, selectivity of perception, or the ability to coordinate two or more skills at the same time. Having explained what attention involves, let us now consider how attentional processes can be measured.

Measuring Attention

In general, cognitive sport psychology researchers have developed three main strategies for the measurement of attentional processes. These strategies include the *psychometric approach* (the use of psychological tests to measure individual differences in people's attentional skills), the *neuroscientific approach* (measurement of the brain processes underlying attention), and the *experimental approach* (which involves testing people's ability to perform two or more tasks at the same time in laboratory settings).

The Psychometric Approach

The psychometric approach involves the use of standardized paper-and-pencil tests in an effort to measure individual differences in attentional processes in athletes. Such tests are both administratively convenient, as they are usually quick and easy to use, and amenable to empirical validation. To illustrate this approach, Robert Nideffer developed the Test of Attentional and Interpersonal Style (TAIS), which is based on a model that postulates that people's attentional focus varies simultaneously along two independent dimensions—width and direction. With regard to width, Nideffer proposed that attention can range along a continuum from a broad focus (where one is aware of many stimulus features at the same time) to a narrow one (where irrelevant information is excluded effectively). Attentional direction refers to the target of one's focus: whether it is external or internal (see also the "Attentional Focus" entry). These dimensions of width and direction may be combined to yield four hypothetical attentional foci: (1) broad external, (2) broad internal, (3) narrow external, and (4) narrow internal. These various types of attentional focus can be illustrated as follows. First, a broad external focus is required for sport skills that involve the ability to read a game and quickly assess a situation for relevant information. For example, a good midfield player in soccer must be able to quickly size up the best passing options available having gained possession of the ball. Second, a narrow external focus is necessary when an athlete locks on to a specific target in the environment. To illustrate, a golfer needs this type of focus when looking at the hole before putting. Third, a broad internal focus is necessary when a tennis player develops a general tactical game plan for a forthcoming match. Last, by contrast, a narrow internal focus is demanded when a gymnast mentally rehearses a skill such as a backflip while waiting to compete.

Nideffer speculated that optimal athletic performance is possible only if performers manage to ensure that their attentional focus matches the specific requirements of the sport skill that they are required to execute. Some evidence to support this idea comes from a study of the attentional strategies used by former Olympic cyclists to cope with the pain of physical exertion in their sport. Briefly, these cyclists reported that they had regularly used all four types of focus when competing. For example, they used a broad external focus when concentrating on getting to the finish line and a broad internal focus when concentrating on their body movements. Similarly, they used a narrow external focus when trying to keep up with the riders ahead of them and a narrow internal focus when concentrating on maintaining a smooth pedaling stroke. Unfortunately, despite their intuitive plausibility, Nideffer's theory and his Test of Attentional and Interpersonal Style have been criticized on a number of grounds. His theory does not distinguish between task-relevant and task-irrelevant information in sport settings. Similarly, the Test of Attentional and Interpersonal Style is questionable because it assesses people's *perceived* rather than their actual attentional skills. Despite its limitations, however, the psychometric approach

has made progress recently with the development of self-report tests that purport to measure athletes' susceptibility to *internal* distractions or thoughts and feelings that divert focus away from its intended target (see also the "Concentration Skills" entry). In sport psychology, for example, researchers have devised psychometric measures of *cognitive interference* (task-irrelevant, self-preoccupied thinking) in athletes. Although these measures seem promising, however, they require comprehensive evidence of validity before they can be recommended for use in applied settings.

The Neuroscientific Approach

The second approach to measuring attentional processes in athletes comes from cognitive neuroscience—a field that is concerned broadly with the identification of the neural substrates of mental processes. Typically, this approach involves a range of neuroscientific techniques in an effort to reveal which parts of the brain are activated when an athlete is paying attention to a sport-related task. Among the most popular of these techniques are electroencephalography (EEG), a method that records electrical activity in the brain using special electrodes placed on the scalp; functional magnetic resonance imaging (fMRI), a method that detects changes in the activity of the brain by measuring the amount of oxygen brought to a particular location within it; and transcranial magnetic stimulation (TMS), a method in which the functioning of a specific area of the brain is temporarily disrupted through the application of pulsating magnetic fields to the skull using a stimulating coil. Using EEG measures, sport psychology researchers have discovered cerebral asymmetry effects (differences between the activities of the two hemispheres of the brain) in athletes involved in target shooting. Specifically, it seems that just before expert archers and pistol performers execute their shots, their EEG profiles tend to reveal a distinctive shift from left-hemisphere to right-hemisphere activation. This shift may indicate a deliberate suppression of self-talk (what one says to oneself silently) on the part of the shooters in an effort to achieve a truly focused state of mind. Another finding—this time from fMRI research—is that compared to expert players, novice golfers have difficulty in filtering out irrelevant information when imagining the appropriate shot to play in a golf simulation task. More recently, TMS studies have shown that expert basketball players have developed finely tuned *resonance* mechanisms that enable them to simulate and predict other players' actions.

Taken together, neuroscientific techniques have a major advantage over their psychometric counterparts in yielding objective data on biological processes that can be recorded *while* the athlete is performing skills. Unfortunately, key drawbacks associated with such neuroscientific measures are excessive cost and impracticality of use in everyday sport settings.

The Experimental Approach

The third approach to measuring attentional processes comes from experimental psychology and is called the *dual-task paradigm*. This method is based on the capacity theory of attention (explained below) and investigates how well people can divide their attention between two concurrent tasks like reading and listening to music. More precisely, it compares people's performance when executing the tasks separately with that when executing the tasks simultaneously. The logic of this method is as follows. If people's performance on one or both tasks is *worse* when the tasks are executed *simultaneously* as compared with when they are performed separately, then these two tasks must be interfering with each other—suggesting that they are competing for the same limited pool of attentional resources in the brain. However, if the two tasks can be performed as well simultaneously as individually, then at least one of these tasks must be automatic, hence making minimal demands on available attentional resources.

When the dual-task paradigm is used in sport psychology, the primary task usually consists of a self-paced skill (one that can be performed without interference from others such as target shooting in archery), whereas the secondary task tends to involve monitoring the environment for a signal such as an auditory tone. To illustrate this approach, a study was designed to investigate the effects of anxiety on skilled performance. The researchers used a dual-task design to examine the effects of manipulating people's focus of attention on performance on a driving simulator under low- or high-anxiety experimental conditions. Attention was directed explicitly to either the participants' own driving performance or to a distracting secondary task. In this study, participants were required to perform a primary task

(simulated rally driving) as fast as possible while responding as accurately as possible to one of two theoretically-derived secondary tasks. The skill-focused secondary task required participants to respond to an auditory tone by indicating at that moment whether their left hand on the steering wheel was higher, lower, or at the same height as their right hand. The distraction secondary task required participants to remember the pitch of an auditory tone presented while they were driving. Results showed that racing performance effectiveness (as measured by lap times) was maintained under anxiety-provoking conditions—although occurred at the expense of reducing processing efficiency. Unfortunately, despite its ingenuity, the dual-task paradigm has not been used widely to measure attentional processes in athletes—mainly because of the difficulty in locating pairs of attentional tasks that engage athletes' interest in laboratory settings.

Explaining Attention: Theories and Issues

Cognitive psychologists have developed three main theories of attention: *filter theory, capacity theory,* and *spotlight theory.*

Filter Theory

The first modern theory of attention, proposed by Donald Broadbent in the 1950s, was based on a series of laboratory experiments on selective listening tasks. Two key assumptions of this theory were that people are limited in their ability to process information, and there must be a mechanism that facilitates the selection of some information while inhibiting the selection of competing information. To explain this mechanism, Broadbent drew an analogy between attention and a filtering device or bottleneck that restricts the flow of information into the mind in accordance with a set of criteria. He proposed that just as the neck of a bottle restricts the flow of liquid, a hypothetical filter in the mind limits the quantity of information to which we can pay attention at any given time. In addition, Broadbent suggested that although multiple channels of information reach the filter, only one channel is permitted to pass through for further information processing. Unfortunately, Broadbent's filter model of attention soon ran into difficulty. Attentional researchers failed to agree on either the location or timing of the filter. Also, this model could not explain the *cocktail party phenomenon.* Imagine that you are at a noisy party and trying to pay attention to a conversation. Suddenly, you hear your name being mentioned in another conversation somewhere else in the room. How can Broadbent's theory explain the fact that you recognized your name? Clearly, if you heard your name being mentioned, then it could not have been blocked by the hypothetical filter in the first place. Problems like these hastened the demise of filter theory.

Capacity Theory

Capacity or resource theory was developed by Daniel Kahneman in an effort to explain the mechanisms underlying divided attention (explained earlier in this entry). This theory postulates that attention is analogous to a pool of mental energy that can be allocated to tackle various processing demands according to certain strategic principles—such as the influence of the performer's arousal level. For example, people usually have a greater amount of attentional capacity available to them when they are fully alert than when they are sleepy. Also, the notion of automaticity suggests that the more practiced a task is, the more automatic (or unconscious) it becomes and the fewer attentional resources it requires. One implication of this latter notion is the prediction that expert athletes are especially vulnerable to distractions because they have considerable spare attentional capacity due to the largely automated nature of their highly practiced skills.

A recurrent weakness of resource models of attention, however, stems from the possible circularity of some of their terminology. For example, there is a logical flaw in the explanation offered by resource theorists for people's inability to divide their attention successfully between two concurrent tasks. Specifically, the assumption in such cases that the resources of some central attentional capacity system have been exceeded by the joint demands of these concurrent tasks is circular in the absence of an independent measure of attentional resources.

Spotlight Theory

According to spotlight theory, as developed by researchers such as Michael Posner, selective attention or our ability to zoom in on some aspects of a stimulus while ignoring other features of it, resembles an adjustable mental beam that we shine at things that are important to us at any given moment. These targets of our concentration beam can be external (in the world around us) or internal (in the private domain of our own thoughts and feelings). Aiming one's golf drive at a specific target on the fairway, for example, involves an external focus of attention, whereas concentrating on the rhythm or feeling of one's golf swing involves an internal focus of attention. This idea of attention as a mental spotlight appeals to athletes and coaches for two main reasons. First, it shows us that our concentration can never be really lost because our mental spotlight is always shining *somewhere*—either at external or internal targets. But lapses of attention can occur whenever we focus on the *wrong* target (something that is irrelevant to the task at hand or that lies outside our control). In such cases, our performance is likely to deteriorate (see also the "Concentration Skills" entry). Second, the spotlight theory of attention suggests that athletes can exert voluntary control over where they shine their mental beam. In other words, athletes have choice over their attentional focus (see earlier discussion of Robert Nideffer's theory).

Unfortunately, although the spotlight metaphor of attention is intuitively appealing, it has three main weaknesses. First, spotlight theorists have largely neglected the issue of what lies *outside* the beam of one's conscious attention; they have tended to ignore the possibility that *unconscious* factors, such as ironic or counterintentional effects, can affect people's attentional processes in certain situations, as when they are cognitively overloaded (see the "Concentration Skills" entry). Second, spotlight theory has historically been concerned with external targets (stimuli in the external world) rather than the internal distractions that often afflict athletes. Finally, spotlight theory has little to say about the influence of emotional factors like anxiety on attentional processes (but see the "Choking" entry).

Aidan Moran

See also Attention Training; Attentional Association and Dissociation; Attentional Focus; Automaticity; Choking; Concentration; Concentration Skills

Further Readings

Baddeley, A. (2012). Working memory: Theories, models, and controversies. *Annual Review of Psychology, 63,* 1–29.

Chun, M. M., Golomb, J. D., & Turk-Browne, N. B. (2011). A taxonomy of external and internal attention. *Annual Review of Psychology, 62*, 73–101.

Kremer, J., Moran, A. P., Walker, G., & Craig, C. (2012). *Key concepts in sport psychology.* London: Sage.

Moran, A. P. (1996). *The psychology of concentration in sport performers: A cognitive analysis.* Hove, East Sussex, UK: Psychology Press.

Moran, A. P. (2012). Concentration: Attention and performance. In S. Murphy (Ed.), *The Oxford handbook of sport and performance psychology* (pp. 117–130). New York: Oxford University Press.

Moran, A. P. (2012). *Sport and exercise psychology: A critical introduction* (2nd ed.). London: Routledge.

ATTENTION TRAINING

The term *attention* denotes the process by which we exert mental effort in focusing either on specific features of the world around us or on our own thoughts and feelings. An example would be a soccer goalkeeper who is preparing to defend against a corner kick from the opposing team must pay attention to the flight of the incoming ball while disregarding a variety of distractions arising from the movements of players in the penalty area and from any irrelevant thoughts he or she might have at that time. Clearly, the ability to focus on what is most important in any situation while ignoring a multitude of distractions is vital for successful performance in sport. Accordingly, researchers in sport and exercise psychology have developed a variety of practical strategies that purport to improve attentional skills in athletes. Although these strategies differ in the extent to which they have been validated by empirical evidence, they share a common purpose—namely, to help sports performers to achieve a focused state of mind in which there is no difference between what they are thinking about and what they are doing.

Specifying Performance Goals

Psychologists commonly distinguish between result goals, such as the outcome of a sporting encounter, and performance goals, or specific actions that lie within the athlete's control, such as attempting to achieve 100% accuracy in one's first serve in tennis. Some evidence has accumulated to suggest that athletes who specify performance goals while competing can improve their concentration skills. To illustrate a practical implication of this finding, a golfer could strive to improve concentration during a round by focusing on maintaining a slow, rhythmic swing on every shot rather than worrying about the score. Theoretically, performance goals should enhance athletes' concentration because they encourage them to focus only on task-relevant information and controllable actions. Support for this conjecture comes from studies that have contrasted psychological variables associated with sports performers' best and worst competitive performances. One finding from these studies is that collegiate athletes reported performing worst when they were preoccupied by result goals but best when they focused on performance goals.

Adhering to Preperformance Routines

Sport is a highly ritualized activity. To illustrate, most top-class athletes display characteristic sequences of preparatory actions before they perform key skills: Golfers tend to waggle their clubs a consistent number of times before striking the ball and tennis players tend to bounce the ball a standard number of times before serving. These preferred action sequences or repetitive forms of behavior are called *preperformance* routines and are typically followed prior to the execution of self-paced skills—actions that are carried out largely at the performer's own speed and without interference from other people.

As in the case of performance goals, preperformance routines should facilitate concentration because they encourage athletes to stay in the present moment, focusing only on specific, controllable actions. Implementing this theory, many soccer goalkeepers go through identifiable prekick routines in an effort to block out external distractions such as hostile noise that is directed at them by supporters of opposing teams. Unfortunately, despite their potential value as attentional strategies, preperformance routines often overlap with superstitious rituals in the minds of athletes. So, what exactly is a superstition?

In psychology, a *superstition* can be defined as the belief that, despite evidence to the contrary, certain behavior is causally related to certain outcomes. Research shows that athletes are notoriously superstitious—perhaps because of the capricious nature of success in their field. For example, in competitive matches, the tennis star Rafael Nadal appears to believe that he must have two water bottles beside the court, perfectly aligned and with the labels facing the baseline. Psychologically, routines and superstitious behavior differ on two key criteria—control and purpose. The essence of superstitious behavior is the belief that one's fate is governed by factors that lie *outside* one's control. But the virtue of a routine is that it allows the player to exert complete control over preparation. Indeed, players often shorten their preperformance routines in adverse circumstances—as happens, for example, when a competitive event is delayed unexpectedly. Unfortunately, the converse is true for superstitions. They tend to grow *longer* over time as performers chain together more and more illogical links between behavior and outcome. The second criterion that may be used to distinguish between routines and rituals concerns the technical role of each behavioral step followed. To explain, whereas each part of a routine should have a rational basis, the components of a superstitious ritual may not be justifiable objectively.

Returning to routines, at least three psychological factors have been postulated to explain their apparent efficacy in enhancing athletic performance. First, some theorists believe that routines are effective because they encourage athletes to prioritise task-relevant information over other available stimuli, such as penalty takers in soccer who may follow prekick routines to remind themselves to focus only on the target that they are aiming at rather than on distractions such as the movements of the goalkeeper. Second, routines may be useful because their sequential nature helps athletes concentrate on the present moment rather than on past events or on possible future outcomes. Finally, paying attention to each step of a routine involves conscious mental effort and consumes short-term or working memory resources. Therefore, adhering to a preperformance routine may prevent athletes from devoting too much attention to the mechanics of well-learned skills—a habit that can unravel automaticity and precipitate skill failure in certain circumstances. In short, routines may work by helping athletes to suppress the type of inappropriate conscious control that often occurs in pressure situations.

Some empirical evidence to support the attentional benefits of preperformance routines has emerged in recent years. Research has shown that amateur international golfers reported using routines explicitly for focusing purposes such as

attempting to *switch on and off* when required and trying to stay in the present while playing.

Using Trigger Words as Cues to Concentrate

Many athletes talk to themselves covertly as they train or compete—usually in an effort to improve their concentration and performance. Such self-talk, or what athletes say to themselves silently, may involve praise, criticism or instruction. An example of the instruction type of self-talk is the use of *trigger words*, which are short, vivid, and positively phrased verbal reminders to cue athletes to focus on a specific target or to perform a given action. An example would be gymnasts may say the word *forward* silently to themselves as a reminder to push their bodies upward when executing a floor routine. A graphic example of athletes' use of trigger words occurred during the 2002 Wimbledon ladies' singles tennis final between the Williams sisters, Serena and Venus. During this match, Serena (who defeated Venus 7–6, 6–3) was observed by millions of television viewers reading hand-written notes as she sat down beside the court during the change-overs between games. Afterwards, she explained that she had written these notes to herself as instructional reminders to *hit in front* or *stay low* during the match. Another example of trigger words in action occurred recently when Paula Radcliffe, who holds the current women's world record time for the marathon, advocated a trigger word strategy involving silently counting her steps in an effort to maintain her concentration in a race.

Does empirical research support the claim that trigger words can improve attentional skills? Unfortunately, although studies have shown that instructional self-talk is one of the strongest predictors of successful performance among U.S. Olympic athletes, there is a dearth of empirical evidence on the efficacy of trigger words as concentration cues. However, it seems plausible that instructional self-talk could enhance attentional skills by reminding athletes about what to focus on in a given situation. For example, novice golfers may miss the ball completely on the fairway in the early stages of learning to swing the club properly. So, in an effort to overcome this problem, golf instructors may advise learners to concentrate on *sweeping the grass* rather than hitting the ball. This evocative trigger phrase ensures that learners focus down on the ball instead of looking up to see where it went after they had struck it. Research suggests that for optimal effectiveness, trigger words should be short, vivid, and positively phrased. They should also emphasize positive targets (what to aim for) rather than negative ones (what to avoid).

Mental Practice

In psychology, the term *mental imagery* refers to the cognitive simulation process by which we can represent perceptual information in our minds in the absence of appropriate sensory input. If you close your eyes, you should be able to *see* yourself in your mind's eye throwing a bright yellow tennis ball up in the air (a visual mental image), *feel* yourself catching it (a kinesthetic mental image) and then bouncing it (a motor mental image). In sport, many athletes use motor imagery or *mental practice* to cognitively rehearse their skills. This technique involves seeing and feeling a skill in one's imagination before actually executing it. Jenson Button, the Formula One star who won the 2009 World Drivers' Championship, regularly rehearses his gear shifts by sitting on a Swiss ball with a steering wheel in his hands—imagining himself navigating the course. Although there is considerable empirical evidence that such mental practice can facilitate skill learning and competitive performance, their value specifically as a concentration tool remains unproven. Anecdotally, however, mental imagery is used widely by performers to improve their focusing skills. Swimmer Michael Phelps, who has won more Olympic gold medals than any other athlete in history, uses imagery to see and feel his strokes and turns before a race. Such use of imagery helps sports performers to prepare for various hypothetical scenarios, thereby ensuring that they will not be distracted by unexpected events. However, this hypothesis has not been tested empirically to date. Therefore, despite the fact that mental imagery is known to improve athletic performance, its status as a concentration technique is uncertain.

Simulation Training

The term *simulation training* refers to the idea of practicing under conditions that replicate key aspects of an impending competition. Certain football teams have tried to simulate the noisy conditions that they expect to encounter in opposing teams' stadia by training on their home grounds using giant screens playing loud music and recordings of rival fans cheering. Intuitively, it seems plausible that simulation training could help skilled performers concentrate because research suggests that people's recall of information is facilitated by conditions that resemble those in which the original encoding occurred. Based on this principle, the simulation of competitive situations in practice should lead to positive transfer effects to the competition itself. Another advantage of adversity training is that it may counteract the tendency for novel or unexpected stimuli to distract athletes in competition. Interestingly, simulation training was used by the renowned swimming coach Bob Bowman, who admitted deliberately breaking the goggles of Michael Phelps during practice so that he could learn to swim calmly without them, if necessary, in a competition. Remarkably, this situation actually arose in the 2008 Olympics when Phelps won the 200-meter butterfly event even though his goggles had been broken for the last 100m of the race.

To summarize, the ability to pay attention to what is most important in any situation while ignoring distractions is vital for successful performance in sport. We have reviewed five attentional strategies that are intended to help athletes achieve a focused state of mind in which there is no difference between what they are thinking about and what they are doing. Empirical research evidence is available to support the efficacy of four of these strategies—setting performance goals (or actions that lie under the control of the athlete), adhering to preperformance routines, using trigger words (or covert verbal cues), and engaging in mental practice (or seeing and feeling a skill in one's imagination before executing it). The fifth attentional strategy—simulation training—has a plausible theoretical rationale but currently lacks relevant empirical validation.

Aidan Moran

See also Attention Theory; Automaticity; Choking; Concentration; Concentration Skills

Further Readings

Cotterill, S. T. (2010). Pre-performance routines in sport: Current understanding and future directions. *International Review of Sport and Exercise Psychology, 3*, 132–153.

Hatzigeorgiadis, A., Zourbanos, N., Galanis, E., & Theodorakis, Y. (2011). Self-talk and sports performance: A meta-analysis. *Perspectives on Psychological Science, 6,* 348–356.

Kremer, J., & Moran, A. P. (2013). *Pure sport: Practical sport psychology* (2nd ed.). London: Routledge.

Kremer, J., Moran, A. P., Walker, G., & Craig, C. (2012). *Key concepts in sport psychology.* London: Sage.

Moran, A. P. (2012). *Sport and exercise psychology: A critical introduction* (2nd ed.). London: Routledge.

ATTENTIONAL ASSOCIATION AND DISSOCIATION

Coping with acute exertional sensations during physical effort expenditure requires optimal use of attentional resources. *Association* and *dissociation* are two broad attentional strategies for coping with exertional stimuli during effort expenditure. Association represents the shift of the attentional focus inward (to somatic sensations), and dissociation represents the shift of the attentional focus outward (away from somatic sensations). Association and dissociation, therefore, correspond to internal and external foci, respectively.

Comparative research findings indicate that both association and dissociation can be effective and ineffective. Specifically, depending on several characteristics inherent in task and effort conditions either strategy was shown to be more or less potent. There is a general consensus that associative strategies may help performance in competitive events such as long-distance running, while dissociative strategies may help adherence in noncompetitive physical activity settings such as a routine treadmill walk.

Associative Versus Dissociative Strategies

Associative strategies increase awareness of physiological cues, such as breathing, heart pounding, and muscle pain, leading to increased negative affective responses during physical activity. Nevertheless, association also enables better effort monitoring and self-regulation, thereby allowing increased time on task as well as greater performance efficiency, performance outcome, and injury prevention. Dissociative strategies, on the other hand, are closely linked to a number of task-related variables, including task-related pleasure, confidence, feelings of ease, and motivation. Moreover, dissociating helps lower perception of fatigue and exertion, thereby allowing reduced sense of task difficulty.

In sum, because associative strategies correspond to an inward focus of attention, their use increases awareness of somatic cues during effort expenditure. In contrast, the use of dissociative strategies decreases awareness of somatic cues, helps curb the physiological stress posed by the effort, and overall results in a greater potential for enhancing the physical activity experience.

It is evident that, while an associative attentional focus is more beneficial for performance enhancement during competitive events, a dissociative attentional focus is of greater value for relatively untrained individuals or during noncompetitive events. Distraction from aversive sensations via the use of dissociative strategies is, however, limited and closely depends on the effort intensity (workload).

Attention Inflexibility and Attention Threshold

As a limited capacity, attention is compromised in its flexibility to cope with physiological sensations as the effort expenditure increases. Specifically, at the onset of effort expenditure or at submaximal workloads, attentional focus is flexible: It can be switched back and forth effortlessly between associative and dissociative foci. Increase in physiological stress, however, leads the system to be challenged and compromised in its attentional flexibility. Specifically, as the workload gets harder or time on task increases, attention shifts inwards, preventing the system from distracting. The point at which attention loses its flexibility to shift between dissociation and association is termed the *dissociative/associative* (D/A) *attention threshold*. The concept entails that, once a subjective perceptual threshold relative to perceived physiological cues is exceeded, attention shifts from a dissociative focus to an associative one. Thus, as this perceptual threshold is attained, dissociative strategies are compromised in their capacity to distract from aversive cues of fatigue. The latter results in a final tuning into an associative focus, hence a growing concentration on the acute stress of exertion. The attention threshold occurs in parallel to the aerobic–anaerobic transition. Thus, when the physical effort expenditure is maintained below the attention threshold, effort can be sustained significantly longer than when the effort expenditure is at or above the aerobic–anaerobic transition levels. Specifically, a shift from dissociative to associative focus of attention takes place as the workload intensity begins exceeding approximately 50% of the individual's maximal capacity. In fact, when individuals report equal employment of associative and dissociative strategies, associative strategies gradually take over rendering the cessation of the effort imminent. The issue of attention inflexibility and interventions to address it are the subject of a growing number of studies.

Methods for Extending the D/A Threshold

Distractive capabilities of dissociative strategies are compromised once the D/A attention threshold is exceeded, that is, as marked by the final tune into the associative attention focus. Successful attempts to delay the occurrence of the D/A threshold may aid in extending effort expenditure. To that aim, exposure to polysensory feedback including the use of auditory stimuli such as music, use of olfactory stimuli such as differential odorants, and use of mental imagery and virtual reality, have been shown to help postpone the final tune into the associative focus—but at low to moderate workload intensities only. Because the optimal use of attentional resources is central to sport and exercise performance and adherence, testing the effectiveness of further modalities designed to address the issue of attentional inflexibility remains important.

Gershon Tenenbaum and Selen Razon

See also Adherence; Attention Theory; Attention Training; Attentional Focus; Attention–Performance Relationships; Choking; Concentration

Further Readings

Lind, E., Welch, A. S., & Ekkekakis, P. (2009). Do "mind over muscle" strategies work? Examining the effects of attentional association and dissociation on exertional, affective, and physiological responses to exercise. *Sports Medicine, 39*(9), 743–764.

Morgan, W. P. (1978). The mind of the marathoner. *Psychology Today, 11*, 38–49.

Morgan, W. P., & Pollock, M. L. (1977). Psychological characterization of the elite distance runner. *Annals of New York Academy of Sciences, 301*, 382–403.

Noble, B. J., & Robertson, R. J. (1996). *Perceived exertion*. Champaign, IL: Human Kinetics.

Tenenbaum, G. (2001). A social-cognitive perspective of perceived exertion and exertion tolerance. In R. N. Singer, H. A. Hausenblas, & C. M. Janelle (Eds.), *Handbook of sport psychology* (pp. 810–822). New York: Wiley.

Tenenbaum, G. (2005). The study of perceived and sustained effort: Concepts, research findings, and future directions. In D. Hackfort, J. L. Duda, & R. Lidor (Eds.), *Handbook of research on applied sport psychology* (pp. 335–349). Morgantown, WV: Fitness Information Technology.

ATTENTIONAL FOCUS

The effect of an individual's focus of attention on motor performance and learning has long intrigued both researchers and practitioners. Numerous studies have shown that what a performer focuses or concentrates on while executing a motor skill has an impact how well that person performs the skill. An important distinction is that between an *external focus* of attention on the intended movement effect, as on an implement versus an *internal focus* on body movements. These foci have differential effects on motor performance—sometimes seen almost immediately—as well as more long-term effects on motor learning. There is considerable evidence for the superiority of an external focus of attention with respect to both the effectiveness and efficiency of movements.

Movement Effectiveness

Numerous studies have assessed movement effectiveness as a function of attentional focus using outcome measures such as deviations from a balanced position, the accuracy in hitting a target or producing forces, or movement speed. The first study, by Gabriele Wulf and Rebecca Lewthwaite, demonstrated learning advantages of instructions inducing an external relative to an internal focus of attention using dynamic balance tasks. The results showed that the learning of those tasks was enhanced when participants' attention was directed to the movements of the platform on which they were standing as compared to the movements of their feet. Since then, numerous researchers have replicated the benefits of an external focus for other tasks.

Learning advantages of an external focus have also been shown for many sport skills, such as hitting golf balls, shooting basketball free throws, throwing darts, serving in volleyball or kicking in soccer, kayaking, swimming, and running. For example, the accuracy in hitting golf balls is greater when performers focus on the swing of the club or on the intended ball trajectory (external focus), rather than on the swing of their arms or on their wrists (internal focus). Similarly, in dart throwing, accuracy is increased with an external focus on the flight of the dart or bull's eye. In swimming or running, performance (speed) is enhanced when performers focus on the force they are exerting against the water or ground as opposed to the movement of their arms or legs exerting the force, respectively. When the goal is to produce a certain amount of force, concentrating on the device, such as a weight bar or force platform, against which the force is exerted generally results in greater accuracy than focusing on the effector, such as the arms or legs.

Interestingly, when the effectiveness of external and internal focus conditions is compared to that of control conditions without focus instructions, performance in the control condition is typically similar to that with internal focus instructions, and external focus instructions result in more effective outcomes than both. One possible reason for this result is that people spontaneously focus on their body movements if they are not specifically asked to adopt an external focus. The only exception to this pattern of results is sometimes seen with highly skilled athletes who show similar performances in external focus and control conditions but degraded performance with an internal focus. This pattern of results suggests that—aside from relatively rare cases in which performance is already highly automatized (see below)—an external focus *enhances* performance or learning.

An intriguing finding is the so-called *distance effect*. Some studies have compared the effectiveness of external foci that differed with respect to the distance of the intended movement effect from the body. For example, a task may involve a balance platform that has markers attached to it, and learners are asked to concentrate on the markers while keeping the platform horizontal. Performers whose markers are placed at a greater distance from their feet show more effective balance learning than performers who are asked to focus on markers that are closer to their feet. Greater benefits of more distal relative to more proximal external foci have also been found for kayaking, golf, dart throwing, and long jump. Thus, concentrating on a movement effect that is more remote from one's body movements seems to be even

more advantageous than a focus on an effect that is closer to the body.

Overall, the benefits of an external compared to an internal focus have been shown not only for a variety of skills but also levels of expertise and age groups, as well as healthy individuals and those with motor impairments (for a review, see Wulf, 2012).

Movement Efficiency

If the same movement outcome is achieved with less energy, the movement is considered more efficient. While some studies have used direct measures of efficiency, such as muscular activity or oxygen consumption, others have used more indirect measures such as maximum force production, movement speed, or endurance to examine the effects of attentional focus. If more effective outcomes (e.g., greater forces) are achieved with the same (physical) resources, they reflect greater movement efficiency as well. There is converging evidence that an external relative to an internal focus optimizes movement efficiency.

Muscular Activity

For weight lifting tasks, electromyographic (EMG) activity has been found to be reduced when performers concentrate on the weight they are lifting (external focus) as compared to their arms or legs that are lifting the weight (internal focus), or compared to lifting without an instructed focus (control conditions). An external focus has been shown to be associated with greater efficiency *within* muscles, as only the necessary motor units are recruited, whereas superfluous recruitment of larger motor units is seen when performers adopt an internal focus. In addition, fewer cocontractions between the agonist and antagonist muscles occur with an external focus, indicating a more efficient coordination *between* muscle groups. As a result, performers are able to execute more repetitions with the same weight or produce greater maximum force (see below) with an external focus.

Reduced EMG activity has also been found for tasks requiring accuracy such as free-throw shooting in basketball or dart throwing, when performers concentrate on the target as opposed to their arm. Interestingly, with an internal focus, increased EMG activity is seen not only in those muscles on which the performer focuses but also in other muscle groups—indicating that a focus on one part of the body *spreads* to other muscle groups. Thus, movement inefficiency is increased at a more general level, presumably contributing to the greater observed inaccuracies in the movement outcome with an internal focus.

Oxygen Consumption and Heart Rate

If the same (or more effective) movement outcome is achieved with less muscular activity, cardiovascular responses should be lowered as well. Indeed, studies confirm this assumption. In experienced runners who ran on a treadmill at a certain speed, oxygen uptake was reduced with an external focus (on the surrounding environment) relative to internal foci (on running technique or breathing). Furthermore, lower heart rates have been found when exercisers adopted an external relative to an internal focus while performing sit-ups.

Maximum Force Production

Producing maximum forces requires optimal muscle fiber recruitment within muscles and optimal activation patterns among muscles. Studies examining maximum force production demonstrate differences in muscular coordination as a function of attentional focus. Greater maximum forces with an external focus have been found for isokinetic contractions (e.g., biceps contractions on a dynamometer) and for dynamic tasks such as vertical jumps and standing long jumps. Also, complex tasks such as discus throwing benefit from an external focus (discus) as opposed to an internal focus (throwing arm or hand).

Speed and Endurance

Movement speed has been found to be increased for an external focus compared with an internal one, presumably due to the greater movement efficiency associated with an external focus. The tasks used to demonstrate this advantage have ranged from functional reach tasks in persons following cerebrovascular accident (stroke) where a focus on the manipulated object resulted on more fluid and faster motions than a focus on the grasping hand, to riding a paddle boat powered by pedals (Pedalo) in young healthy adults, where focusing on the boards under their feet led to higher speeds than focusing on the feet themselves.

In longer duration tasks in which fatigue is a limiting factor, the adoption of an external focus can enhance performance as well. In tasks that require the production of submaximal or maximal forces over a longer period of time, an external focus enables performers to maintain those forces longer or to produce greater force in a given period of time (e.g., 10 secs). Performance on sprinting and agility tasks involving running and turning components has been shown to be enhanced by external focus instructions, relative to internal focus or no instructions. Similarly, (intermediate) swimmers swim faster when they focus on pushing the water back as opposed to pulling their hands back.

Also, the attentional focus of exercisers has an influence on muscular endurance. Trained individuals performing various exercises like bench press or squat lift were able to complete a greater number of repetitions to failure with a given weight when instructed to focus on the weight as opposed to the movements of the limbs involved or without focus instructions. In a study using an isometric force production task (wall-sit), participants' ability to hold the posture increased with an external focus (imaginary horizontal lines between their hips and knees), relative to an internal focus on the horizontal position of their thighs.

Mechanisms Underlying the Attentional Focus Effect

An internal focus induces a conscious type of control, causing individuals to constrain their motor system (*constrained action hypothesis*) and interfere with automatic control processes that have the capacity to control movements effectively and efficiently. In contrast, an external focus promotes an automatic mode of control. Adopting an external focus allows unconscious, fast, and reflexive processes to control the movement, with the result that the desired outcome is achieved effectively and relatively effortlessly. Several converging lines of evidence support the notion that an external focus facilitates automaticity relative to a focus on body movements. For example, attentional-capacity demands have been shown to be reduced with an external focus. High-frequency movement adjustments while balancing with an external focus indicate the use of reflex-based feedback loops, while slower and more conscious feedback loops seem to be utilized with an internal focus. Other findings, such as the reduced EMG activity seen with an external focus, also indicate that an external focus allows individuals to perform at the higher, more advanced level—essentially reflecting a speeded learning process.

Conclusion

The benefits of an external compared with an internal focus have been shown for a variety of skills, ranging from pressing keys to driving golf balls. They have also been found for different levels of expertise, ranging from novice to skilled performance; for people of various age groups, ranging from children to older adults; and for healthy people as well as those with injuries or with motor impairments (stroke, Parkinson's disease, intellectual disabilities). Performance-enhancing effects of an external focus are often seen immediately, but practice with an external focus also has more permanent effects on motor skill learning. These effects are seen in movement effectiveness like accuracy, consistency, and balance as well as movement efficiency like EMG, heart rate, force production, speed, and endurance. Adopting an external focus during practice promotes movement automaticity and accelerates the learning process. In practical settings, coaches, trainers, and physical therapists often use less-than-optimal instructions and feedback by referring to body movements, thus inducing an internal focus. Rewording instructions to direct performers' attention to the intended movement outcome, and away from body movements, has the potential to significantly enhance performance and learning.

Gabriele Wulf

See also Attention Theory; Attention Training; Attentional Focus; Attention–Performance Relationships; Feedback

Further Readings

Lohse, K. R., Wulf, G., & Lewthwaite, R. (2012). Attentional focus affects movement efficiency. In N. J. Hodges & A. M. Williams (Eds.), *Skill acquisition in sport: Research, theory & practice* (2nd ed., pp. 40–58). London: Routledge.

Marchant, D. C. (2011). Attentional focusing instructions and force production. *Frontiers in Psychology, 1*, 210. doi: 10.3389/fpsyg.2010.00210

Wulf, G. (2012). Attentional focus and motor learning: A review of 15 years. *International Review of Sport and Exercise Psychology, 6*(1), 77–104. doi: 10.1080/1750984X.2012.723728

Wulf, G., & Lewthwaite, R. (2010). Effortless motor learning? An external focus of attention enhances movement effectiveness and efficiency. In B. Bruya (Ed.), *Effortless attention: A new perspective in attention and action* (pp. 75–101). Cambridge: MIT Press.

ATTENTION–PERFORMANCE RELATIONSHIPS

The desire to perform as well as possible in situations with a high degree of (personally felt) importance is thought to create *performance pressure*. Paradoxically, despite the fact that performance pressure often results from aspirations to function at one's best, pressure-packed situations are where major performance failures may be most visible. The term *choking under pressure* has been used to describe this phenomenon. *Choking* is defined as performing more poorly than expected given one's skill level and is thought to occur across many diverse task domains where incentives for optimal performance are at a maximum. Two of the most common examples of situations in which choking under pressure can occur are sport competitions and exams or tests.

Many different theories have been put forth to explain how and why choking under pressure occurs with the ultimate goal of developing interventions and training methods to prevent it. These theories can be roughly divided into three categories: drive theories, biomechanical theories, and attentional theories. *Drive theories*, which are primarily descriptive in nature, propose that there is an optimal level of physiological arousal for each skill that we perform. *Biomechanical theories* provide hypotheses about how the kinematics and motor control strategies involved in skill execution (e.g., control of the velocity of the racquet head in a tennis serve) change in response to pressure. Finally, *attentional theories* seek to describe the cognitive processes governing pressure-induced failure—how pressure changes the attentional mechanisms and memory structures supporting performance.

The remainder of this entry focuses on the major attentional theories.

Distraction Theory

Distraction theory is one of the primary attentional theories of choking under pressure. This theory assumes that every performer has a limited amount of information processing capacity that can be devoted to the execution of one's skill. Information processing involves multiple resources, including perception, working memory, and attention. Successful skill execution requires accurate perception of objects in environment such as judging the speed at which a ball is approaching or discriminating between opponents and teammates on a basketball court. Working memory is a short-term memory system that maintains, in an active state, a limited amount of information with immediate relevance to the task at hand (e.g., a phone number you are about to dial) while preventing distractions from the environment and irrelevant thoughts. Attention is a resource that allows us to enhance the processing of relevant objects or locations in our environment (analogous to the way in which a spotlight allows one to see more clearly in small areas). Resource allocation models of human performance typically assume that each of these resources is capacity limited.

As an example of these information processing capacity limits in sport, consider an attacker in soccer processing the locations of opponents and teammates on a pitch. In this situation, there are only a limited number of players that the attacker can focus attention on in a given instant and there are only limited number of player locations that can be held in working memory. Therefore, anything else in the performer's environment that uses processing resources, such as a fan drawing the player's attention by yelling an insult, may require that resources are taken away from skill execution, which can lead to degraded performance (e.g., the attacker passes the ball to an opponent). In this example, player locations are an example of task-relevant information, an information source needed for successful skill execution, while the words spoken by the fan are an example of task-irrelevant information, a source that does not aid skill execution.

According to distraction theory, the introduction of performance pressure creates additional sources of task-irrelevant information that could potentially draw processing resources away from skill execution. These information sources primarily come in the form of negative thoughts or worries about the outcome of the action being performed and its potential consequences. Examples of such worries could include losing a large monetary prize, being booed by fans, letting down

one's teammates, or failing a class in school. These negative thoughts are hypothesized to sap both working memory (as the performer plays out the disastrous outcomes in their mind) and attentional resources (as the performer's attention is shifted from the external environments to these internal thoughts). Another way to conceptualize this effect is that pressure serves to change a single task situation where the performer is only required to execute one particular skill into a multitasking situation in which the performer must do two things at once. In sum, in distraction theory, performance pressure serves to distract the performer and draw processing resources away from the task at hand. As described below, this account is the polar opposite to explicit monitoring theory, which proposes that pressure serves to increase the amount of attention and working memory resources devoted to skill execution.

Processing Efficiency Theory

Does the distraction created by the negative thoughts and worries always lead to performance failure? A related theory, called *processing efficiency theory*, suggests this might not always be the case. Similar to distraction theory, processing efficiency theory proposes that pressure serves to draw processing resources away from task-relevant information; however, it further proposes that decreases in resources available to support skill execution can be partially or fully compensated for by an increase in the effort devoted to the task. Therefore, the main outcome predicted by processing efficiency theory is that *skill efficiency* (defined as the ratio of performance to the amount of effort exerted) will decrease under pressure. The extent to which associated declines in performance also occur will depend on how much additional effort is exerted by the performer. In any case, both theories propose the same mechanism for the effects of pressure with the difference between them being the degree to which performance is affected in the end.

Because it is based on the assumption that information processing capacity is limited, a strong prediction made by distraction theory is that pressure-induced performance failures will be greatest for skills that normally in nonpressure situations require a large amount of working memory and attentional resources. When a task has very low processing demands, it follows that a performer will have more available capacity, that is, will have more working memory and attention resources available for handling task-irrelevant information, as compared to a skill with high processing demands. Therefore, when a low demand skill is performed under pressure, it is less likely that the additional resources required to process distracting thoughts and worries will cause an overloading of processing capacity. Instead, it is possible that the performer will be able to successfully process both task-relevant and task-irrelevant information. This prediction has received strong support from research involving academic test anxiety. For example, it has been demonstrated that individuals who become highly anxious during test situations, and consequently perform at a suboptimal level, often divide their attention between task-relevant and task-irrelevant thoughts more so than those who do not become overly anxious in high pressure situations. However, suboptimal performance only appears to occur for test problems with high working memory demands like a difficult math problem, while performance for low-demand problems is relatively unaffected.

Thus, there is evidence that pressure can compromise working memory resources, causing failure in tasks that rely heavily on this system. But, not all tasks *do* rely heavily on working memory. Specifically, the types of high-level motor skills that have been the subject of the majority of choking research in sport (well-learned golf putting, baseball batting, soccer dribbling) are thought to become proceduralized (unconscious, automatic) with practice. Proceduralized skills do not require constant online attentional control and are in fact thought to run largely outside of working memory. Such skills, then, should be relatively robust to conditions that consume working memory resources as distraction theory proposes. However, these types of skills may be sensitive to other attention-induced disruptions under pressure. A second class of theories, generally known as explicit monitoring theories, has been used to explain such failures.

Explicit Monitoring Theories

Explicit monitoring theories suggest that pressure situations raise self-consciousness and anxiety about performing correctly. This focus on the self is thought to prompt individuals to turn their attention inward on the specific processes of performance in an attempt to exert more explicit monitoring and control than would be applied in a nonpressure situation. Explicit attention to step-by-step skill processes and procedures is thought to disrupt well-learned or proceduralized performance processes that normally run largely outside of conscious awareness. This proposal is based on the assumption that the processing demands for complex motor skills change systematically during skill acquisition.

For example, consider a golfer attempting to make a putt. A performer relatively new to the sport is likely to have been given a lot of explicit instructions about how to putt effectively (e.g., keep head down, use a smooth backstroke, keep your eye on the ball, etc.). Executing a skill based on these types of instructions is assumed to require a large amount of working memory (the golfer must actively hold in working memory all these instructions and the order they should be executed) and attentional resources (the golfer must focus attention on the position of the head, hands, etc. to determine consistency with the instructions). Through extensive practice, it is assumed these instructions become internalized (or *proceduralized*) so that expert performance is guided by a set of motor programs, and procedures, once initiated, can run without the need for working memory or attention. How to perform the skill is no longer held actively in working memory but rather it is stored in *muscle memory*. And the performer no longer needs to consciously monitor the position of the body by focusing attention because the execution of movement is now controlled by unconscious, automatic processes. Instead, more attentional and working memory capacity can be devoted to processing external or strategic information.

In explicit monitoring theory, it is assumed that not only is attention to the execution of a complex motor skill not required, but also that it can be harmful for performance if it does occur. It is argued that directing one's attention to a well-learned skill effectively serves to disrupt the highly efficient and automatic motor procedures developed through practice. Instead, if skill execution is controlled consciously in a step-by-step manner using a large amount of attentional and working memory resources, performance becomes slow, nonfluent and error prone, outcomes typical of novice performance. Evidence for explicit monitoring theory is provided by dual-task experiments, which require a performer to execute a skill—such as putting or batting—while simultaneously performing a secondary task designed to reorient attention toward skill execution (judging the angle of the putter head or direction of bat movement) or away from skill execution (judging the pitch of an irrelevant sound). Consistent with explicit monitoring theory, it is typically found that expert performance suffers for tasks that direct attention to skill execution and is relatively unaffected by tasks that direct attention away from it. Also consistent with the theory, novice performers typically show the reverse pattern where performance is harmed by irrelevant dual tasks and relatively unaffected (or in some cases actually improved) by skill-focused dual tasks.

Reinvestment Theory

One type of explicit monitoring theory, called *reinvestment theory,* suggests that the specific mechanism governing explicit monitoring is *dechunking.* Pressure-induced attention to execution causes an integrated or proceduralized control structure that normally runs off without interruptions to be broken back down into a sequence of smaller, independent units—similar to how the performance was organized early in learning. Once dechunked, each unit must be activated and run separately. Not only does this process slow performance, it creates an opportunity for error at each transition between units that was not present in the integrated control structure.

Explicit Monitoring and Distraction Theories Compared

Explicit monitoring and distraction theories essentially make opposite predictions regarding how pressure exerts its impact. While distraction theories suggest that pressure shifts needed attention away from execution, explicit monitoring theories suggest that pressure shifts too much attention to skill execution processes. Can both theories be correct? One possibility is that performance pressure creates two effects that alter how attention is allocated to execution: (1) Pressure induces worries about the situation and its consequences, thereby reducing working memory capacity available for performance—as distraction theories would propose; and (2) at the same time, pressure prompts individuals to attempt to control execution in order to ensure optimal performance—in line with explicit monitoring theories. This suggests that how a skill fails is dependent on performance

representation and implementation. That is, skills that demand working memory will fail when pressure consumes the resources necessary for performance, while proceduralized skills that run largely outside of working memory will fail when pressure-induced attention brings such processes back into conscious awareness. Therefore, it is perhaps better to think of these two theories of pressure-induced failures of performance as complementary rather than competing.

It is important to note that it does not seem to be merely a cognitive versus motor distinction that predicts how a skill will fail under pressure. That is, just because one is performing an academically based, cognitive task does not mean this task will show signs of failure via pressure-induced distraction. And, likewise, sports skills do not necessarily fail via pressure-induced explicit monitoring. Rather, it appears to be the manner in which skills utilize on-line attentional resources that dictates how they will fail (though often, this is related to skill domain). Thus, sports skills that make heavy demands on working memory, such as strategizing, problem solving, and decision making (skills that involve considering multiple options simultaneously and updating information in real time), will likely fail as a result of pressure-induced working memory consumption—similar to a working-memory-dependent academic task. In contrast, motor skills that run largely outside of working memory—for instance, a highly practiced golf putt or baseball swing—will fail when pressure-induced attention disrupts automated control processes.

Explicit monitoring and distraction theories have very different implications for how to prevent choking under pressure. According to explicit monitoring theory, choking is best prevented by not allowing a performer to turn attention inward and explicitly control movements. Two promising interventions for achieving this end have been identified. First, it has been shown that allowing a performer to become accustomed to the desire to turn attention inward during practice (through the use of videotaping or some other means of evaluation that tends to induce self-consciousness) can help prevent choking from occurring during a subsequent competition. A more radical solution, based on the reinvestment theory described above, is to change the way a performer acquires a skill: If the performer acquires less knowledge about how to explicitly control a skill (e.g., a golfer is not given instructions about where to place the feet, hands, etc.), it is less likely he or she will switch to this control mode under pressure. Indeed, research evidence suggests that skills acquired implicitly, as in learning by doing as opposed to following instructions, are less prone to choking under pressure.

The primary means for remedying pressure-induced failure, according to distraction theory, is to increase the amount of processing resources devoted to task-relevant information when a performer is placed in a high pressure situation. This could be achieved in different ways. First, as discussed above with reference to processing efficiency theory, it is theoretically possible to reduce (or eliminate) the effects of pressure on performance by increasing effort. Studies that incorporated effort measurement under pressure have shown that this does indeed occur for many performers, suggesting that learning to put more effort into one's skill can be an effective means of handling pressure. An alternative remedy is to reduce the level of processing demands required for the task-irrelevant worries and negative thoughts that can occur under pressure. Research has shown that this can be achieved by having the performer explicitly verbalize (or write down) the negative thoughts immediately prior to performing the high-pressure skill.

Rob Gray

See also Attention Theory; Attentional Focus; Automaticity; Choking; Chunking/Dechunking; Concentration; Information Processing; Memory; Motor Control

Further Readings

Baumeister, R. F. (1984). Choking under pressure: Self-consciousness and paradoxical effects of incentives on skillful performance. *Journal of Personality and Social Psychology, 46,* 610–620.

Beilock, S. L., & Gray, R. (2007). Why do athletes "choke" under pressure? In G. Tenenbaum & R. C. Eklund (Eds.), *Handbook of sport psychology* (3rd ed., pp. 425–444). Hoboken, NJ: Wiley.

Eysenck, M. W., & Calvo, M. G. (1992). Anxiety and performance: The processing efficiency theory. *Cognition and Emotion, 6,* 409–434.

Masters, R. S. W. (1992). Knowledge, knerves and know-how—The role of explicit versus implicit knowledge in the breakdown of a complex motor skill under pressure. *British Journal of Psychology, 83,* 343–358.

Wine, J. (1971). Test anxiety and direction of attention. *Psychological Bulletin, 76,* 92–104.

Wulf, G., & Prinz, W. (2001). Directing attention to movement effects enhances learning: A review. *Psychonomic Bulletin & Review, 8,* 648–660.

ATTRIBUTION THEORY

Attributions are explanations about why particular performances or behaviors have occurred. When faced with important, negative, novel, or unexpected events, individuals search for meaningful explanations for the causes of those events. In this regard, it is widely acknowledged that attributions are an area of importance in the field of applied psychology because of their implications for motivation and emotion. This entry discusses the historical theories that have provided the framework for research into, and application of, attribution theory in sport and exercise settings, then moves on to highlight recent theoretical advances, assessments of attributions, empirical evidence for attribution theory, and the application of attribution theory.

Historical Theories

If a particular individual were to be singled out as the founder of the scientific study of attributions, it would be Fritz Heider. He proposed that people explore explanations for events or behaviors to increase their control over the environment and to satisfy a desire to understand and gain knowledge about the world. His insights provided the impetus for numerous theories and investigations. Three of the most well known are Edward Jones and Keith Davis's correspondent inference theory, Harold Kelley's covariation model, and Bernard Weiner's attributional theory of achievement motivation and emotion.

Correspondent inference theory proposes that people infer dispositions and intentions of others, as a result of observing their behavior. That is, behavior is seen as corresponding to or reflecting an underlying disposition of the actor. In general, correspondence is high when behavior is atypical and has clear implications. In other words, behavior is informative to the extent that it is seen to involve choice among alternatives. Whereas correspondent inference theory focused mainly on person perception (or attributing to others), the covariation model made contributions to our understanding of self-perception. The covariation model suggests that people arrive at a cause for an event by processing information about whether accompanying conditions and circumstances vary or not as the event changes. According to the model, people use three types of information—consistency, distinctiveness, and consensus—to verify whether they have correctly linked causes and effects.

The approach that has had most influence on attribution research in sport and exercise psychology is the attributional theory of achievement motivation and emotion. A central premise of this theory is that there is a dimensional structure underpinning the explanations people give for events. Building on previous works in this field, Bernard Weiner, a key figure in conceptualizing the attributional categories into dimensions, initially identified four main attributions (or attribution elements), namely, ability, effort, task difficulty, and luck; these were then classified into two dimensions, locus of causality and stability. *Locus of causality* refers to whether the cause is inside (internal) or outside (external) the person; *stability* refers to whether the cause will (unstable) or will not (stable) change over time. Later deductive theorizing led to the identification of a third dimension, *controllability*, referring to whether the cause could be viewed as controllable or uncontrollable.

Recent Theoretical Advances

Despite warnings by a number of researchers that the three dimensions of locus of causality, stability, and controllability may not be appropriate for all types of situations (e.g., sport and exercise), until recently, there has been little effort to examine alternative approaches. In 2005, Tim Rees, David Ingledew, and Lew Hardy published an article that examined the congruence between theory, research, and practice of attributions in sport. On the basis of their observations, they proposed a broader conceptual approach to our understanding of attributions. They encouraged (a) a focus on the controllability dimension, (b) an expanded conceptualization of generalizability attributions (in addition to stability, examining globality and universality attributions), and (c) exploring interactive effects of controllability and generalizability attributions upon performances or behaviors.

The focus on controllability is based on empirical and theoretical grounds. Empirically, studies

in a wide array of domains have shown that perceived personal control is an important psychological predictor. For example, within general social psychology, perceived personal control has been shown to affect a person's level of depression, loneliness, and shyness, and in sport an athlete's level of subsequent self-efficacy. Theoretically, the need to exert control over future events was foundational to early attribution theorizing, with Harold Kelley commenting that the purpose of causal analysis is effective control. Further, drawing upon attribution theory, the expectancy of future uncontrollability is at the heart of Lyn Abramson, Martin Seligman, and John Teasdale's reformulation of the learned helplessness model: The *expectancy of future uncontrollability* is the most direct determinant of helplessness.

The second proposal is that, in addition to the stability dimension, attribution research in sport and exercise should examine the dimensions of globality and universality. The addition of globality refers to whether the cause affects a wide range of situations with which the person is faced (a global attribution) or a narrow range of situations (a specific attribution); universality refers to whether the cause is common to all people (a universal attribution) or unique to the individual (a personal attribution). This leads to an expanded conceptualization of generalizability: In addition to whether causes generalize across time (stability), attribution research should examine whether causes generalize across situations (globality) or all people (universality).

The final proposal is that researchers need to move beyond testing solely main effects of attributions to exploring interactive effects of controllability and generalizability attributions upon performances or behaviors. Until recently, the focus of much attribution research had been upon main or independent effects of attribution dimensions. To model *generalizability,* however, implies the need to consider *interactive* effects. Interactions of attribution dimensions may well be important because attributing, for example, less successful performances to uncontrollable causes may only lead to negative effects when causes are also considered to be stable (unlikely to change over time), global (likely to affect a wide range of situations), or personal (unique to the individual). For example, an athlete attributing poor performance to poor concentration might say, "There was nothing I could do about it" (an uncontrollable attribution), together with "and this will never change" (a stable attribution), or "and this affects a lot of situations I find myself in" (a global attribution), or "and this only happens to me" (a personal attribution). In this instance, the athlete might well be expected to experience poorer subsequent performance. Conversely, higher levels of performance would be expected if the athlete were to combine this uncontrollable attribution with "but this will change" (an unstable attribution), or "however, this only affects a few situations I find myself in" (a specific attribution), or "but this affects everyone, not just me" (a universal attribution).

Assessing Attributions

Various methods have been employed in the measurement and categorization of attributions. *Open-ended methods* involve the researcher categorizing the oral replies of participants to open-ended questions. *Derived score methods* require the participant to rate reasons for a success or failure on five-point scales for different elements (e.g., ability, effort, task difficulty) related to the attribution dimensions. Problems can arise, however, when researchers try to summarize attributions along dimensions or otherwise assume the dimensional categories of attributions. Recent attribution measures, such as the Causal Dimension Scale (CDS), the Causal Dimension Scale II (CDSII), and the Measure of Controllability, Stability, Globality, and Universality Attributions (CSGU), have used *direct rating methods*. These methods require the participants to state their reasons for the event and then map those reasons onto items referring to attribution dimensions.

The CDS was developed to reflect Weiner's three-dimensional model of attributions. A number of methodological criticisms have been leveled at the CDS, in particular concerns over the nature of the controllability subscale, which contains items referring to *controllability, responsibility,* and *intentionality*. The revision of the CDS (the CDSII) focused on changes to the controllability items, with all six of the items from the locus of causality and stability subscales left unaltered. In the CDSII, the controllability dimension was subdivided into personal control (control by the actor) and external control (control by others). Based upon recent proposals in the sport and exercise psychology literature, measures of attributions should include four scales for controllability and the generalizability dimensions of stability, globality, and universality. Following this, researchers developed the CSGU, a 16-item, 4-factor measure of attributions that assesses the four dimensions of controllability, stability, globality, and universality.

Empirical Evidence for Attribution Theory

A number of research articles have been published, exploring the following key propositions of the attributional theory of achievement motivation and emotion: (a) the locus-of-causality dimension affects intrapersonal emotions including pride and shame; (b) the stability dimension affects expectations of future success and feelings of hopefulness; and (c) the controllability dimension affects interpersonal emotions including blame, anger, and pity. Despite empirical support, these propositions are limited to the extent they explore the effects of attribution dimensions in isolation. In other words, the proposals focus solely upon main effects of attribution dimensions upon outcomes.

Recent research has reported the interactive effects of attribution dimensions upon outcomes. Collectively, the research demonstrates that the independent effects of attribution dimensions upon outcomes—such as emotions, self-efficacy, and performance—may be conditioned by interactive effects. For example, research has demonstrated that, following failure, higher levels of perceptions of controllability may only lead to beneficial effects if causes are also considered to generalize, such as across time (interaction of controllability and stability).

Application of Attribution Theory

Attributional retraining involves attempts to change maladaptive explanations for outcomes (attributing failure to uncontrollable or stable causes) toward more adaptive explanations (attributing failure to controllable or unstable causes). Although there is discrepancy in the literature regarding whether negative behaviors or outcomes should be perceived as inside the individual (internal locus of causality) or outside the individual (external locus of causality), there is agreement in regard to the need to perceive such causes as controllable. For example, following failure like a loss in sport or a relapse from a positive behavior like smoking a cigarette following a period of abstinence, an individual is encouraged to attribute the negative outcome or behavior to causes that are within one's control. In situations where such causes are perceived as outside one's control (i.e., a maladaptive attribution), the procedure of attributional retraining involves practitioners manipulating causes toward aspects that are within one's control.

Conclusion

Attribution theory has a rich history in general (social) psychology, and has significantly influenced applied practice in sport and exercise settings. Recent theoretical advances, supported by empirical evidence, suggest a promising future for attribution theory to continue as a principal theory in sport and exercise psychology.

Pete Coffee

See also Cognitive Restructuring; Feedback; Positive Thinking; Psychological Skills Training; Self-Fulfilling Prophecy; Team Attributions

Further Readings

Abramson, L. Y., Seligman, M. E. P., & Teasdale, J. D. (1978). Learned helplessness in humans: Critique and reformulation. *Journal of Abnormal Psychology, 87,* 49–74.

Biddle, S. J. H., Hanrahan, S. J., & Sellars, C. N. (2001). Attributions: Past, present, and future. In R. N. Singer, H. A. Hausenblas, & C. M. Janelle (Eds.), *Handbook of sport psychology* (2nd ed., pp. 444–471). New York: Wiley.

Heider, F. (1958). *The psychology of interpersonal relations.* New York: Wiley.

Jones, E. E., & Davis, K. E. (1965). From acts to dispositions: The attribution process in person perception. In L. Berkowitz (Ed.), *Advances in experimental social psychology* (Vol. 2, pp. 219–266). New York: Academic Press.

Kelley, H. H. (1967). Attribution theory in social psychology. In D. Levine, *Nebraska symposium on motivation* (Vol. 15, pp. 192–240). Lincoln: University of Nebraska Press.

Rees, T., Ingledew, D. K., & Hardy, L. (2005). Attribution in sport psychology: Seeking congruence between theory, research and practice. *Psychology of Sport and Exercise, 6,* 189–204.

Weiner, B. (1986). *An attributional theory of achievement motivation and emotion.* New York: Springer.

AUDIENCE EFFECT

See Social Processing Effects

AUTOMATICITY

Automaticity is the ability to execute a skill using no (or very few) information processing resources: attention and working memory. When a skill can be executed in this fashion, the performer has resources available to process other sources of information not directly required for the task. Automaticity is thought to be a hallmark of expert performance that is acquired through learning and extensive practice. A breakdown of automaticity resulting from a performer turning attention inward toward skill execution is thought to be one of the primary causes of choking under pressure (see also the "Attentional Focus" entry).

When one performs a skill, there are different modes of control that can be used. At one extreme, commonly called *controlled processing mode,* a performer executes an action by following a series of explicit steps that are held in working memory and by focusing attention on each part of the action. Each stage during skill execution is consciously controlled and monitored. For example, when executing a complex movement in sports, the performer must remember the instructions to position different body parts and focus attention on these parts to determine if positioning is correct. In this performance mode, the information-processing demands of the skill are very high and there are few, if any, leftover resources available for processing task-irrelevant information. At the other extreme, commonly called *automatic processing* mode, skill execution relies on motor programs or procedures that, once initiated, run without the use of attentional or working-memory resources. The skill is executed unconsciously as it is thought to involve *muscle memory* (well-developed internal commands for how the different body parts should be moved) rather than high-level cognitive control. In this performance mode, the performer has information processing resources available for handling task-irrelevant information. Planning a play to be executed on the next possession in basketball is an example of a highly controlled task, whereas running down the court is thought to be a highly automatic one.

As first proposed by Paul Fitts, the controlled and automatic processing modes are thought to be characteristics of the early and late stages of skill acquisition, respectively. For novice performers, it has been proposed that skill execution requires that attention be paid to each component stage of the motor act (in golf, back-swing, down-swing, club-head angle in putting). At this level of performance, referred to as the *cognitive* or *declarative* stage, it is assumed that skill execution depends on a set of unintegrated control structures that must be held in working memory and attended in a step-by-step fashion. The attentional and memory requirements result in the slow, nonfluent, and error-prone movement execution that is characteristic of a novice performer. As expertise develops through practice and the performer reaches the highest stage of skill execution (the *autonomous* or procedural stage), it has been proposed that the role of attention and working memory in performance changes dramatically. As procedural knowledge develops, the conscious step-by-step control of execution is no longer required. Instead, skill execution is assumed to operate by fast, efficient control procedures that function largely without the assistance of working memory or attention. At this final stage, it is proposed that skill automaticity has been achieved. It is frequently also proposed that automatic skills are encapsulated such that, once they are initiated, it is difficult for the performer to inhibit or disrupt them.

A key advantage that automaticity is thought to give an athlete is the availability of attentional and working-memory resources to process information in the environment not directly related to movement control. First, the performer is more likely to detect situational or contextual information that is not required for movement control but may serve to improve performance success. If an expert footballer does not need to actively monitor the position of the body when taking a penalty kick, that player will have processing capacity available to attend to the movements of the goalkeeper. Second, the performer is less likely to be affected by the introduction of stimuli completely irrelevant to the task like a fan yelling an insult or waving hands in the background.

Theories of skill acquisition and automaticity make several predictions about the nature of performance (and the supporting attentional mechanisms and memory structures) as a function of skill level. For example, if it involves the automatic processing mode, expert performance should be (a) unaffected by the introduction of an irrelevant secondary task that requires attentional or working memory resources, and (b) associated with a poorer ability to verbalize the stages involved in skill execution (*expertise-induced amnesia*) since these stages are not attended or held actively in memory. For the most part, research evidence is consistent with these predictions; however, for most tasks, it has also been shown there is some decrement in performance when a highly demanding secondary task is introduced. Therefore, it may not be the case that automatic processes are completely resource free; rather, automaticity may be best characterized by a reduction in the processing resources required.

Another important prediction of skill acquisition and automaticity theories concerns pressure-induced failures of performance (choking under pressure). One of the dominant theories of choking, called *explicit monitoring theory*, proposes that pressure can cause the deautomization of well-learned skills. This occurs because an increase in self-consciousness and anxiety about performing well causes an athlete to turn attention inward on the specific processes of performance in an attempt to exert more explicit monitoring and control. This increase in skill-focused attention is thought to disrupt the automatic motor procedures.

Rob Gray

See also Attention Theory; Attentional Focus; Attention–Performance Relationships; Choking; Information Processing; Memory; Motor Control

Further Readings

Anderson, J. R. (1983). *The architecture of cognition.* Cambridge, MA: Harvard University Press.

Beilock, S. L., & Gray, R. (2007). Why do athletes "choke" under pressure? In G. Tenenbaum & R. C. Eklund (Eds.), *Handbook of sport psychology* (3rd ed., pp. 425–444). Hoboken, NJ: Wiley.

Fitts, P. M., & Posner, M. I. (1967). *Human performance.* Belmont, CA: Brooks/Cole.

AUTOMATICITY: EVALUATIVE PRIMING

Priming effects occur when the processing of a target stimulus is influenced by a preceding stimulus on the basis of a relationship between prime and target. Processing of the target word *surgeon*, for example, may be facilitated by the prime word *injury*. The priming effect in this example is based on associative and nonevaluative semantic relationships between prime and target, and is called *semantic priming*. Evaluative priming, on the other hand, focuses on evaluative (positive or negative) relationships between primes and targets. In an evaluative priming paradigm, a positive or negative target (delight) is preceded by a prime of the same valence (healthy) or of the opposite valence (failure).

Usually, participants in these reaction-time tasks are asked to decide whether the target denotes something positive or negative. Responses are typically faster and more accurate when the prime and target share the same valence (healthy delight). Thus, presentation of *healthy* as the prime is likely to automatically activate a positive evaluation. If the target word that is subsequently presented is also positive (delight), then the individual is likely to respond quickly and accurately to the adjective. If the target word is negative, however, response accuracy and speed are likely to be compromised. Consequently, evaluative priming effects are based on a significant interaction between the valence of the prime and the valence of the target.

Automatic Evaluation: A Consistent Finding

By using a short timeframe (called *stimulus onset asynchrony*) between the presentation of primes and targets, research on evaluative priming has found that evaluative information about stimuli is activated very quickly (automatically) upon presentation of the prime. Also, the evaluative priming effect has been replicated numerous times using a variety of experimental stimuli. The effect has emerged, for instance, when the primes consist of words, pictures, or odors. Moreover, the effects have been evidenced when the response task given to participants is to evaluate the target ("Is the target word positive or negative?"), when they are asked to pronounce the targets, or when they are required to generate a motor response task to the primes.

Compatibility Between Automatic Evaluation and Self-Report Evaluation

Traditionally, to gauge people's evaluation of an object or concept, researchers have utilized self-report measures that invite conscious introspection among participants. One of the most significant benefits of evaluative priming studies, however, is that they allow researchers to tap fast evaluative processes that often occur without, and sometimes against, the respondents' intentions. For research on socially sensitive topics, such as exercise and body image, significant differences might emerge between these automatic evaluations and self-report evaluations. Therefore, social stigmatization acts as a possible moderator to the relationship between self-report and automatic evaluations. Another possible moderator to this relationship is evaluation strength. In other words, people who possess strong automatic evaluations of concepts are also likely to report strong, compatible evaluations in self-report questions. If one has a strong passion for basketball, for example, the individual is likely to report congruent positive evaluations of the sport on both self-report measures and implicit measures.

Research on Consequences of Automatic Evaluation

There are two streams of literature on the consequences of automatic evaluation. One of these streams relates to the question of whether primed evaluations are predictive of approach or avoidance behaviors toward that stimulus. In other words, do automatic evaluations increase one's tendency to behave in particular ways toward the priming stimulus? Research is now emerging to suggest that these evaluations can significantly influence one's reactions toward the stimulus itself. Another stream of research focuses on the implications of a primed evaluation for the subsequent processing of unrelated stimuli. There is a possibility that interpretation of ambiguous stimuli can be guided by previous exposure to positively or negatively evaluated primes. In fact, past work has established that interpretation of words such as *beat* can be guided by strongly valenced primes, such that people are more likely to interpret the word as meaning *rhythm* after a positive prime and *hit* after a negative prime. Collectively, these findings suggest that one's automatic evaluations of sport or exercise are likely to predict the individual's approach or avoidance of these activities, as well as influence the interpretation of information about them. Someone who possesses a negative automatic evaluation of exercise, for instance, is likely to reject an offer to join an exercise class without giving much thought to the offer. Also, that person will be likely to bias any ambiguous information in an exercise advertisement (or other communication) in a negative manner.

Mechanisms

Evaluative priming effects are most often discussed in terms of a spreading activation within a participant's semantic network. According to the spreading activation hypothesis, priming *success*, for example, would make the concept of all positively valenced representations more accessible. These salient representations are then more readily used to encode subsequent information. Although the spreading activation account to evaluative priming has conceptual appeal, it has also been criticized by some scholars. One of the key criticisms has been that the spreading activation account is based on the *fan effect*. If a prime stimulus activates many concepts in memory (as it would in the context of evaluative priming), the amount of activation should disperse over many pathways, making the activation of any one representation quite minimal. Other mechanisms for evaluative priming have been forwarded, but more research is needed to establish which of them offer the best explanation for these effects.

James Dimmock

See also Affect; Automaticity; Automaticity: Implicit Attitudes; Priming

Further Readings

Bluemke, M., Brand, R., Schweizer, G., & Kahlert, D. (2010). Exercise might be good for me, but I don't feel good about it: Do automatic associations predict exercise behavior? *Journal of Sport & Exercise Psychology, 32,* 137–153.

Ferguson, M. J., & Bargh, J. A. (2003). The constructive nature of automatic evaluation. In J. Musch & K. C. Klauer (Eds.), *The psychology of evaluation: Affective processes in cognition and emotion* (pp. 173–193). Mahwah, NJ: Lawrence Erlbaum.

Ferguson, M. J., Bargh, J. A., & Nayak, D. A. (2005). After-affects: How automatic evaluations influence the interpretation of subsequent, unrelated stimuli. *Journal of Experimental Social Psychology, 41,* 182–191.

Automaticity: Implicit Attitudes

Implicit attitudes, also referred to as automatic evaluations, are immediate and spontaneous evaluations of objects, groups, or behaviors as being pleasant or unpleasant. They occur unintentionally within a fraction of a second after exposure to the stimulus, preceding any reflective deliberation. Typically, these attitudes are inferred from systematic variations of performance on indirect priming or categorization tasks. Implicit attitudes can collaborate or conflict with more controlled and deliberated explicit attitudes to influence decisions and behaviors. It has been shown that implicit attitudes predict physical activity behavior, but little research has been conducted on implicit attitudes in the context of sport. This entry briefly overviews (a) measurement, (b) attitudinal concordance with explicit attitudes, (c) proposed origins, and (d) proposed consequences of implicit attitudes. Special emphasis is placed on implicit attitudes in the context of physical activity and sport.

Measurement

Implicit attitudes are typically measured indirectly via performance tasks because self-assessment (self-report) is susceptible to inaccuracy due to people's lack of awareness or willingness to report their implicit attitudes. The most common methods for implicit attitude assessments are priming procedures or categorization tasks, such as the Implicit Association Tests (IAT). Given the nature of response latency tests, error variability can be easily introduced (e.g., distraction, sneeze, fatigue). This, among other concerns about validity and reliability of the measures, remains an important issue in the field.

Attitudinal Concordance With Explicit Attitudes

Research suggests implicit attitudes are related, but distinct, from explicit attitudes. *Implicit attitudes* are automatic, efficient, rapid, and goal-independent evaluations that involve the neural circuits of the amygdala and right insula; *explicit attitudes* are effortful, deliberative, and controlled evaluations that involve areas of the frontal cortex. Explicit attitudes may serve to override or validate implicit attitudes through reflective cost–benefit analyses, especially when ample motivation and opportunity to deliberate is present. Implicit and explicit attitudes typically show weak positive correlations within studies, although the magnitude of the relation differs as a function of the attitude being assessed. For example, implicit and explicit attitudes are largely divergent for socially sensitive topics where impression management may occur, as with racial prejudices, but less divergent for topics toward which people have little motivation to disguise their attitudes, as with preference for flowers. The magnitude of the relation between implicit and explicit attitudes also is a function of study design. Correlations are strongest when there is strong convergence of the conceptual and format structure of the implicit and explicit measures, for example. Implicit and explicit attitudes toward physical activity have been shown to be independent of one another, but little is known about concordance of implicit and explicit attitudes in the context of sport.

Proposed Origins

The origins of implicit attitudes are not fully understood; however, there is research connecting implicit attitudes to early emotional responses to the stimuli, such as averseness of the first cigarette smoked and to more recently learned affective associations, such as priming associations between valence and object. Implicit attitudes tend to show low or moderate stability across time, supporting the notion that they comprise both trait- and state-like components. Although some aspect of implicit attitudes may be resistant to change, it seems that appropriate environmental pairings have potential to counter these learned associations. Most theories propose that implicit attitudes are some manifestation of both early and recent experiences, but it has also been proposed that implicit attitudes represent knowledge of cultural biases, rather than personal attitudes. Very little is understood about the origins of implicit attitudes in the context of physical activity and sport.

Consequences

Implicit attitudes have been shown to have physiological consequences, such as an elevated heart rate response to stimuli; cognitive consequences, such as phobias and judgments; and behavioral consequences, such as prejudice and consumer and voting behavior. Within an evolutionary context, implicit attitudes have been proposed as a survival strategy to quickly differentiate hostile from friendly stimuli. Favorable implicit attitudes elicit immediate approach behavior, whereas unfavorable implicit attitudes elicit immediate avoidance behavior. Implicit attitudes seem to guide behavior without people's conscious awareness. Implicit and explicit attitudes have been shown to predict unique portions of variance of the same behavior and to interact to predict behavior. Additionally, a double-dissociative connection between attitudes and behavior has been supported in which implicit and explicit attitudes predict behaviors under different circumstances. Whereas explicit attitudes tend to direct volitional behavior or behavior when people have ample time and resources to deliberate, implicit attitudes tend to direct spontaneous behaviors or behaviors when people are under time pressure, distracted, or unmotivated for reflective deliberation. Physical activity and fitness level have also been shown to be related to implicit attitudes above and beyond explicit motivational constructs. Again, little is known about how implicit attitudes may impact outcomes in the competitive or training contexts of sport.

Conclusion

Implicit attitudes have been shown to influence peoples' physiology, judgments, and behavior independently of explicit attitudes. It has been established that implicit and explicit attitudes toward physical activity are distinct, and that implicit attitudes predict physical activity behavior; however, little is known about the origins or malleability of these attitudes. Implicit attitudes within the context of sport remain largely uninvestigated. The potential for implicit attitudes to serve as an avenue for physical activity and sport interventions needs to be clarified with future research.

David E. Conroy and Amanda L. Hyde

See also Automaticity: Evaluative Priming; Dual-Process Theory; Habit

Further Readings

Conroy, D. E., Hyde, A. L., Doerksen, S. E., & Ribeiro, N. F. (2010). Implicit attitudes and explicit motivation prospectively predict physical activity. *Annals of Behavioral Medicine, 39,* 112–118.

De Houwer, J., Teige-Mocigemba, S., Spruyt, A., & Moors, A. (2009). Implicit measures: A normative analysis and review. *Psychological Bulletin, 135,* 347–368.

Evans, J. S. B. T. (2008). Dual-processing accounts of reasoning, judgment, and social cognition. *Annual Review of Psychology, 59,* 255–278.

Greenwald, A. G., Banaji, M. R., Rudman, L. A., Farnham, S. D., Nosek, B. A., & Mellott, D. S. (2002). A unified theory of implicit attitudes, stereotypes, self-esteem, and self-concept. *Psychological Review, 109,* 3–25.

Nosek, B. A., Greenwald, A. G., & Banaji, M. R. (2006). The Implicit Association Test at age 7: A methodological and conceptual review. In J. A. Bargh (Ed.), *Automatic processes in social thinking and behavior* (pp. 265–292). New York: Psychology Press.

Perugini, M. (2005). Predictive models of implicit and explicit attitudes. *British Journal of Social Psychology, 44,* 29–45.

Rudman, L. A. (2004). Sources of implicit attitudes. *Current Directions in Psychological Science, 13,* 79–82.

AUTONOMIC NERVOUS SYSTEM

The central nervous system (CNS) is composed of the brain and spinal cord. The CNS receives sensory information from the peripheral nervous system and controls the body's responses. The peripheral nervous system involves all of the nerves outside of the brain and spinal cord that carry messages to and from the CNS. The peripheral nervous system has two branches: the somatic nervous system and the autonomic nervous system. The somatic nervous system controls skeletal muscle as well as external sensory organs such as the skin. This system is described as voluntary because the responses can be controlled consciously, although reflex reactions of skeletal muscles are an exception.

The autonomic nervous system is the branch of the peripheral nervous system that controls involuntary actions, such as pulmonary respiration (breathing), heart rate and the force of contraction of the heart, and vasoconstriction and dilation (widening and narrowing of blood vessels) that impact blood pressure. This system is further divided into two systems: the sympathetic system and the parasympathetic system. The sympathetic division of the autonomic nervous system regulates flight-or-fight responses. This division is responsible for tasks such as relaxing the bladder, increasing heart rate, and dilating eye pupils. The parasympathetic division of the autonomic nervous system supports homeostasis and conserves physical resources. This division performs tasks such as controlling the bladder, slowing down heart rate, and constricting eye pupils.

Like other nerves, those of the autonomic nervous system convey their messages to the appropriate end organs (blood vessels, viscera, etc.) by releasing transmitter substances to which the receptors of the target cells are responsive. The most important of these transmitters in the autonomic nervous system are acetylcholine and norepinephrine. In the parasympathetic system, acetylcholine is responsible for most of these transmissions between the afferent (leading toward the CNS) and efferent nerves (leading away from the CNS) and between the efferent nerve endings that innervate cells or organs. Acetylcholine also serves to transmit nerve-to-nerve messages in the afferent nerves and the brain centers of the sympathetic nervous system. Norepinephrine is released from sympathetic nerve endings to end organs or cells, except at the sweat glands where acetylcholine is released. Epinephrine is also released from the adrenal medulla in response to sympathetic activation.

The rate and strength of cardiac contractions is under the predominant control of the sympathetic nervous system. Sympathetic stimuli from cardiac nerves cause acceleration of the heart rate. Increases in heart rate are also complemented by simultaneous reduction in the parasympathetic stimuli via the vagus nerve, which is responsible for slowing the heart rate. Thus, heart rate responses are often used as indirect measures of sympathetic and parasympathetic activity (autonomic nervous system activation).

Situations such as emotional excitement, fear, apprehension, psychological distress, panic reactions, and fight-or-flight stimuli activate the sympathetic nervous system. In addition, the activation of the autonomic nervous system, often demonstrated in preparation for and during activity, has been an area of investigation in sport and exercise physiology. Noninvasive measures of autonomic function (heart rate, blood pressure, galvanic skin response, etc.) have been used to investigate the role of the peripheral nervous system in human performance, infer affect and infer changes in affect during and following physical activity, understand the effects of overtraining, and explain potential positive adaptations that occur in parallel with improvements in fitness. In summary, biofeedback studies have demonstrated a relationship between effective control of autonomic function and human performance, a number of affective states have been shown to correlate with autonomic responses, overtraining seems to be associated with parasympathetic dysfunction, and improvements in fitness are associated with enhanced parasympathetic tone and diminished sympathetic activity. More specifically, the changes in response to aerobic training seem to occur primarily due to an alteration in the balance of sympathetic and parasympathetic activity. With training, several adaptations, including enhanced parasympathetic tone and increased stroke volume, explain the reduction in resting heart rate. At rest the enhanced parasympathetic activity seen in trained individuals leads to a reduction in heart rate; however, when presented with a mental challenge, trained individuals demonstrate greater vagal withdrawal and possibly an enhanced sympathetic response compared with untrained individuals. This adaptation seems to be beneficial for cardiovascular health.

Edmund O. Acevedo

See also Biofeedback, Neurofeedback; Cardiac Function; Electromyography (EMG); Eye Movements/Gaze; Neuroscience, Exercise, and Cognitive Function; Overtraining Syndrome; Psychophysiology; Stress Reactivity

Further Readings

Acevedo, E. O., Webb, H. E., & Huang, C. J. (2012). Cardiovascular health implications of combined mental and physical challenge. In E. O. Acevedo (Ed.), *The Oxford handbook of exercise psychology* (pp. 169–191). New York: Oxford University Press.

Boutcher, S. H., & Hamer, M. (2006). Psychobiological reactivity, physical activity, and cardiovascular health. In E. O. Acevedo & P. Ekkekakis (Eds.), *Psychobiology of physical activity* (pp. 161–175). Champaign, IL: Human Kinetics.

AUTONOMY-SUPPORTIVE COACHING

Motivation is one of the foundations of successful sport performance, and coaches play a critical role in developing or undermining this attribute in their athletes. The techniques coaches use to instruct and motivate their athletes can influence whether athletes learn and achieve at a high level, develop a strong sense of confidence, enjoy their experience, and persist in their sport over a long period of time.

Self-Determination Theory

In 1985, Edward Deci and Richard Ryan wrote their influential book, *Intrinsic Motivation and Self-Determination in Human Behavior*. In this text, and numerous subsequent publications, Deci and Ryan outlined their theory of human motivation, *self-determination theory*. This theory, often known as SDT, has guided much research examining the influence that coaches can have on their athletes' motivation and subsequent outcomes in sport.

Deci and Ryan suggested that motivation is multidimensional, meaning that a person can be simultaneously motivated by multiple factors. Central to SDT is the distinction between self-determined and controlled forms of motivation. To be *self-determined* means to act with a sense of self-direction and choice. An athlete who is self-determined participates because that athlete finds sport enjoyable or interesting (intrinsic motivation) or values the benefits of sport participation. In contrast, motivation that is fueled by pressure from others or pressure from within (guilt) is referred to as *controlled motivation*. A growing body of research has provided evidence regarding the benefits of being involved in sport for more self-determined reasons. For example, athletes whose participation is driven largely by self-determined factors as opposed to controlled forces perform at a higher level; experience more positive emotions; use positive coping strategies in stressful situations; and invest higher levels of concentration, persistence, and effort than athletes with lower self-determined motivation and stronger controlled motivation. In comparison, athletes with high levels of controlled motivation tend to experience a variety of negative outcomes such as drop-out from sport, burnout, antisocial behavior, anxiety, and negative affect.

Given our understanding of the effects of controlled and self-determined types of motivation on the athlete sport experience, a natural question that arises is: How do athletes' self-determined and controlled motivations develop? According to SDT, self-determined motivation is most likely to develop when three basic psychological needs, known as autonomy, competence, and relatedness, are fulfilled. Autonomy represents the need to feel personal control over one's actions. Competence reflects the need to feel effective. Relatedness represents the need to feel connected with others and a secure sense of belonging. There is evidence that athletes require all three psychological needs to be satisfied in order for optimal motivation and well-being to develop. However, there is also research that suggests that some needs may be more important in certain circumstances. For example, competence may have a greater impact than relatedness on elite athletes' motivation.

Coaching Behaviors and Athlete Motivation

When coaches' actions support their athletes' needs, self-determined motivation will develop. When coaches' behavior undermines these needs, athletes are likely to experience increased controlled motivation. Therefore, it is important to understand the specific aspects of coaching behaviors that are positively or negatively related to athlete motivation.

Coaches' behavior can be classified in a variety of ways. When exploring motivation from a SDT perspective, coaches' provision of psychological needs support is often examined. Specifically, support that pertains to each of the three psychological needs has been investigated: autonomy support, competence support, and relatedness support. When a coach acts in an autonomy supportive way, the coach considers the athletes' perspective, provides appropriate and meaningful feedback, and offers opportunities for choice, while at the same time minimizing the use of pressures and demands to control the athletes. The process of creating an autonomy-supportive climate requires considerable skill, particularly considering the authoritarian role that coaches have often been expected to play in the past. Even within the somewhat rigid structure of many organized sports, coaches can take steps to create an autonomy-supportive climate for their athletes. Specifically, researchers suggest a number of key practices that would help a coach become autonomy supportive:

1. Provide choice—athletes making decisions about some aspects of a training session.

2. Provide a rationale for tasks, limits, and rules—explaining the reasons behind key coaching decisions.

3. Inquire about and acknowledge athletes' feelings—getting to know athletes as people first and athletes second; acknowledging that some training drills may be repetitive or tedious.

4. Promote athlete responsibility—allowing athletes to create and deliver a training drill.

5. Provide noncontrolling competence feedback—having constructive feedback that is *solution* focused rather than *problem* focused.

6. Avoid guilt inducing criticisms and controlling statements—providing critiques that focus on the behavior, not the athletes' character.

7. Limit ego involvement—encouraging athletes to improve their own performance, avoiding intrateam rivalries and social comparisons.

Studies exploring the relationship between coach autonomy support and athlete outcomes suggest a positive relationship exists. For example, various studies report that athletes who perceived their coach to be autonomy supportive displayed greater levels of psychological and physical well-being, self-determined motivation, sport persistence and adherence, enjoyment, and positive appraisal for their sports participation.

Coaching research based on SDT has largely focused on autonomy support. However, competence and relatedness support have also received some attention. A coach who supports the athletes' sense of competence by helping his athletes set clear and realistic performance targets, for example, ensures those athletes have the necessary information and experience to develop and progress. Additionally, a coach who displays high levels of involvement with relatedness support ensures the athletes feel a sense of belonging and connection. Research suggests all three types of coach support (autonomy, competence, and relatedness support) create a favorable environment for the satisfaction of athletes' needs.

Unfortunately, the very nature of organized sport can lend itself to the development of a controlling climate that undermines athletes' needs for autonomy, competence, and relatedness. Offering rewards with a condition attached, such as an activity if athletes satisfy the coach's expectations, is a common practice. Also, athletes' schedules are often planned well in advance, thus creating rigid deadlines for training and performance. Additionally, athletes' choice is often limited, particularly in youth sport, as coaches take ownership for developing strategies that they believe will provide their athletes with a competitive advantage. Hence, it is unsurprising that many coaches tend to favor a controlling style, whereby their athletes feel pressured to think, feel, or behave in a set way. As a result, athletes will often comply with, but may not fully support, requests from the coach, which contributes to the development of controlled motivation (non-self-determined). Coaching behaviors that are viewed as controlling include the following:

- offering rewards such as guaranteed selection to motivate athletes if they put all their effort into training;
- using feedback that pressures athletes to continue with their behavior;
- making demands concerning aspects of an athlete's life not associated with sport participation;
- intimidating athletes by using verbal abuse or threats;
- promoting rivalry among athletes; and
- withholding affection and attention if athletes don't perform to an expected standard.

Unfortunately, little is known about the impact of these controlling coach strategies. A number of studies suggest that athletes who viewed their coach to predominantly display autocratic and controlling behaviors reported less self-determined motivation and greater levels of controlled motivation. Recent research indicates that athletes who view their coach as using controlling strategies report low levels of psychological needs satisfaction. In turn, these low levels of psychological needs satisfaction have been associated with negative athlete outcomes, such as disordered eating behaviors, depression, burnout, and negative affect. These findings suggest that although controlling behaviors may sometimes appear to be adaptive in that they prompt desired behaviors and performance outcomes in the short term, these behaviors may contribute to negative outcomes in the long term.

It is important to note that a coach can display elements of controlling and needs-supportive behavior. A coach may frequently issue additional physical exercises to the athletes as a discipline strategy (controlling behavior) but may often provide opportunities for player input about other aspects of training (autonomy-supportive behavior). It is also important to note that the lack of needs-supportive behaviors does not automatically necessitate the presence of controlling coach behaviors. The lack of needs support might, for instance, simply be a sign of a more neutral rather than a controlling style. Nonetheless, in terms of the impact of these different coaching styles, needs support versus controlling behavior, the majority of studies indicate that needs-supportive behaviors are associated with self-determined motivation and positive athlete outcomes.

Autonomy-Supportive Approaches

These research findings provoke an important question as to whether it is possible for a sports coach to learn *how* to become more needs supportive and less controlling. While a needs-supportive coach training program has yet to be experimentally tested, preliminary evidence demonstrates that needs-supportive practices can be employed by coaches working with elite athletes. Clifford Mallet described an autonomy-supportive approach when coaching two Australian relay teams competing at the 2004 Athens Olympic Games. Some of his autonomy supportive strategies included (1) providing choice to the athletes in a number of management and performance areas; (2) providing a rationale for executive decisions; (3) actively seeking suggestions, opinions, and feedback from athletes and their personal coaches; and (4) encouraging athletes to take personal responsibility for their learning. Mallet concluded that by adopting this autonomy supportive approach he promoted their levels of self-determined motivation. This preliminary evidence suggests that needs-supportive coaching is feasible, even in elite sport settings.

Additional evidence supporting the potential efficacy of needs-supportive coach training programs comes from intervention studies designed to improve coaches' interpersonal skills. Although not focused specifically on needs support, these studies provide evidence that coaches can learn to alter their interpersonal behaviors when working with athletes. For example, coaches can learn to (a) provide instruction and encouragement, (b) avoid sarcasm or degrading comments, (c) establish clear expectations, and (d) avoid nagging or threatening athletes. Promisingly, coaches who participated in these training programs were evaluated more positively by their athletes compared with athletes whose coaches did not take part. Additionally, a variety of positive athlete outcomes were reported. For example, compared with controls, athletes of the trained coaches displayed lower levels of anxiety and drop-out, higher levels of healthy motivation and fun, and a greater liking for their teammates.

Finally, research outside of the sport setting indicates that authority figures like teachers, managers, and health care professionals can successfully alter their interactions to become more needs supportive after attending a training program and this increased support had positive effects on subordinates' motivational outcomes. Coach education research has taken this evidence on board and preliminary guidelines are now available and can help coaches learn how to be needs supportive in their interactions with their athletes.

Conclusion

There is a great deal of evidence that needs-supportive coaching is associated with more positive forms of motivation and better experiences for athletes. Preliminary data suggests that sport coaches can learn to effectively apply needs-supportive coaching principles. Further research is required to test the effects of coach training programs specifically designed to promote needs support and lessen controlling coaching.

Chris Lonsdale and Edel Langan

See also Coach–Athlete Relations; Coaching Efficacy; Leadership in Sport: Multidimensional Model; Relational Efficacy Beliefs in Coach–Athlete Relations; Self-Determination Theory

Further Readings

Amorose. A. J. (2007). Coaching effectiveness: Exploring the relationship between coaching behavior and self-determined motivation. In M. S. Hagger & N. L. D. Chatzisarantis (Eds.), *Intrinsic motivation and self-determination in exercise and sport* (pp. 209–227). Champaign, IL: Human Kinetics.

Mageau, G. A., & Vallerand, R. J. (2003). The coach-athlete relationship: A motivational model. *Journal of Sports Sciences, 21*, 883–904.

Mallett, C. J. (2005). Self-determination theory: A case study of evidence-based coaching. *The Sport Psychologist, 19*(4), 417–429.

Treasure, D. C., Lemyre, P., Kuczka, K. K., & Standage, M. (2007). Motivation in elite-level sport. In M. S. Hagger & N. L. D. Chatzisarantis (Eds.), *Intrinsic motivation and self-determination in exercise and sport* (pp. 153–164). Champaign, IL: Human Kinetics.

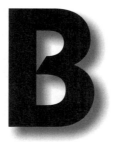

BASIC EMOTIONS IN SPORT

Emotion is a central feature of many sporting events. Athletes, as well as supporters, can experience many emotions, including joy, sadness, anger, fear, anxiety, shame or guilt, and pride. Most emotion theorists argue that emotions have the power to motivate and regulate cognitions and behaviors in sport. To understand the antecedents, experience, and consequences of emotions, theorists have attempted to classify emotions into various categories. One central question is whether some emotions should be considered basic. That is, are some emotions fundamental to human experience? To answer this question, it is important to consider the criteria to identify such basic emotions, the functions of basic emotions, and whether basic emotions be modified by social learning.

The discussion about basic emotions is challenging because there is much disagreement among emotion theorists on many critical issues. Some theorists believe basic emotions are linked to evolutionary development (phylogeny), whereas others hold that emotions are social constructions and reflect only social learning through shared experiences across cultures and the past history of the person (ontogeny). These views, of course, influence the criteria used to identify basic emotions. There are others, however, who reject the notion of basic emotions all together. Rather than address all these competing perspectives, this entry will attempt to capture the key features of basic emotions that are common to several prominent theorists, such as Paul Ekman, Robert Levenson, Robert Plutchik, and Carroll Izard. For alternative views, the reader is directed to publications by Andrew Ortony and Terence Turner, and by Jesse Prinz.

Criteria for Basic Emotions

Basic emotion theorists tend to agree on a number of central criteria for basic emotions: They have been shaped by evolutionary history; they are associated with subcortical brain structures; they are triggered by prototypical evolutionary meaningful stimuli; they have a rapid onset with limited higher order cognitive involvement; they have potentially adaptive functions based on evolutionary needs; and they have specific neural, expressive, and physiological mechanisms. For example, Robert Levenson has argued that for emotions to be considered basic, they must meet three general criteria. First, basic emotions have distinct behavioral, expressive, and physiological responses. Second, basic emotions are hardwired in the brain, although the emotion systems are plastic, such that learning over the lifespan may modify and enhance the emotional response. Third, basic emotions have specific functionality, in that each emotion is triggered by an affect program that rapidly recognizes a survival-critical situation and produces an action to enhance survival. Paul Ekman, a leading figure on basic emotion theory and research, has identified numerous criteria that are generally consistent with Levenson's three general criteria. The criteria for basic emotions according to Ekman include distinctive universal signals, distinctive physiology, automatic appraisals, distinctive universals in antecedent events, presence in other primates, capable of quick onset, brief duration, unbidden occurrence, distinctive thought memories and images, and distinctive subjective experiences.

Identifying which specific emotions are basic is challenging because not all the criteria are readily testable in humans; nor do theorists agree on all criteria. Thus, it is not surprising the number of emotions and specific emotions identified by various theorists ranges greatly, and theorists may even add or delete emotions from their lists over time. Carroll Izard identified seven basic or primary emotions, for example, whereas Paul Ekman identified six basic emotions in 1972 (but expanded his list to 15 emotions in 1999). Overall, there seem to be five discrete emotions—fear, happiness and joy, sadness, anger, and disgust—that most theorists agree upon and include on their lists of basic emotions. Other commonly identified basic emotions are contempt, surprise, and interest. Ekman makes the argument that each basic emotion term should be viewed as being part of a basic emotion family; thus there are many emotions that could be considered basic in his view. For example, sadness would include terms such as *distress* and *anguish* within its emotion family.

Do Basic Emotions Have Adaptive Motivational Features in Sport?

To determine whether basic emotions have adaptive motivational features in sport, we need to consider if the behavioral and physiological responses associated with each emotion can be regulated by higher order cognitions and whether social learning can modify the antecedent triggers and behavioral responses. Most emotion theorists believe that the emotion process can be modified by social learning and can be regulated by higher order cognitive functioning. Carroll Izard suggests that basic or primary emotions are only present in infants and that most emotional experience in youth and adults is governed by emotional schema involving an interface between emotion and cognitive brain structures. Others such as Ekman believe that basic emotions exist across the lifespan but are modified by the life experiences of the person. He believes that learning can change aspects of the emotion process like antecedent triggers and behavioral expression, and that cognition helps regulate the emotion response. Ekman, however, believes that

such learning would be biologically primed by the basic emotions. Fear, for example, should be triggered by prototypical stimuli that result in rapid automatic appraisal and trigger an evolutionary response—specific facial expression, high physiological arousal, blood shunting away from hand and toward legs, urge to flee. Through experience and observations, athletes can learn that certain situations, such as falling off a gymnastic beam, facing large and powerful opponents, skiing icy steep slopes with surrounding cliffs, or trying to hit a 95 mph fastball are dangerous. These stimuli can become incorporated into the evolutionary affect program as prototypical events for fear, although the way in which this occurs is not clear. Thus, these stimuli can rapidly trigger a fear response. The interface of the basic emotion system with higher level cognitive systems, however, can either enhance or inhibit the emotion response. The fear emotion can activate fear-related memories and learned behaviors, thus increasing the strength of the fear response. Conversely, higher order cognitions can also activate a number of potential coping strategies that help regulate the fear response as well as formulate solutions to manage the situation. It should be noted that the fear response may not be maladaptive, especially if it causes athletes to flee or avoid a situation that exceeds their resources and endangers their lives.

Basic emotions may have constructive and destructive functions in sport. Emotions can influence short-term individual performance, as well as persistence and engagement over time. Basic emotions can be rapidly triggered with minimal awareness, so specific emotional responses might interfere with effective performance through disruptive effects on physiological, motoric, and cognitive functioning. Moreover, the basic emotion response may overwhelm higher order cognitive functioning when a situation is extreme. The inability to override or reduce the responses to specific basic emotions may even cause the athlete to attack opponents, coaches, officials, or even fans. The news is replete with many examples of athletes losing emotional control. On the other hand, basic emotion responses may facilitate performance under some conditions when the behavioral and physiological responses augment the necessary resources needed for success. Motivational research also suggests that participation in sport is facilitated by positive emotions, such as happiness, joy, and enjoyment. Many motivational models used in sport consider the impact of basic emotions, such as happiness and sadness, along with related emotional states, such as enjoyment and interest.

Basic emotions are also important in social functioning in sport because they can signal significant information to others. Repeated expression of basic emotions, such as happiness, joy, and anger, in specific sport situations, allows others to understand what sport situations are important. Social functioning in sport also depends on the ability to recognize basic emotions in others such as teammates, opponents, coaches, and fans. For example, when an athlete is angry, with corresponding facial and bodily (and maybe voice) expression signals, others are alerted to not only the potential reasons for the anger but also to potential consequences. Others begin to regulate their behavior in response to the anger. Athletes can, however, learn to inhibit signals, as the demonstration of specific emotions may not be socially appropriate or may interfere with sport performance. Athletes can also learn to send false signals. German sport researcher Dieter Hackfort has written about how athletes show, hide, or fake emotions for multiple reasons, such as to influence officials and fans, deceive or irritate opponents, and motivate teammates.

Research, as well as anecdotal evidence in sport, generally supports the basic tenets associated with basic emotions. Happiness and joy are associated with the attainment of important goals and the demonstration of competence. When happy, athletes are more likely to smile and embrace significant others. Loss is more likely to lead to sadness, with tell-tale facial expressions, occasional crying, initial behavioral isolation, and the urge to seek comfort from others. Anger is generated by the frustration of important goals. Expressions include flushed face, furled brow, lips curled back to expose teeth, increased heart rate and blood pressure, and the urge to attack. Fear is triggered by the appraisal of impending danger related to physical or psychological harm. Athletes are more likely to behaviorally freeze and tremble or engage in disengagement (flight) behaviors. Obvious physical reactions also can include increased respiration and perspiration, combined with facial expressions of eyes open, eyebrows raised, and mouth slightly open. In extreme cases of fear, bowel and bladder emptying may occur. For the last of the commonly agreed upon basic emotions (i.e., disgust), there is neither much empirical research nor much anecdotal evidence in sport.

Although basic emotions are likely to be hard-wired, there is no doubt that social learning and culture (and sporting culture) has a large impact on the appraisal and expression of basic emotions. Anger is a classic example. Anger is not always triggered by goal frustration that threatens the self either psychologically or physically but can also involve rapid evaluation of whether the offending other is violating normative rules and has control over the offending behavior. For example, an athlete may feel anger toward an opponent who appears to be cheating and violating the normative rules of the game. Even if the initial neural or physiological components of anger are initiated, the expression can also be modulated by higher cognitive processes. These cognitions can include evaluation of who was to blame (self: internalized anger; other: externalized anger), coping potential (what actions are possible?), and acceptable actions (determined by general and sport culture). The influence of higher order cognitions in the basic emotion process helps to explain individual differences as well as differences across sports. These higher order cognitions explain why an athlete may try to ignore the cheating opponent's behavior, or may instead tell the coach or the referee about the opponent's apparent cheating, resisting the urge to directly attack the opponent.

Conclusion

The study of basic emotions is full of controversy. For those who support the existence of basic emotions, there is a general consensus that they are rooted in evolutionary history, are associated with subcortical brain structures, and have important motivational functions. Basic emotional processes are influenced over the lifespan by social learning, with higher order cognitions influencing emotional response and emotional regulation. Basic emotions can facilitate or hinder performance and social functioning in sport. Athletes can learn to regulate the expression of basic emotions, but such regulation can be overwhelmed in extreme situations. Understanding how social learning is integrated into the brain mechanisms regulating basic emotion has critical implication for emotional regulation interventions.

Peter R. E. Crocker

See also Affect; Choking; Coping; Emotional Schemas; Self-Conscious Emotions; Stress Management

Further Readings

Crocker, P. R. E., Kowalski, K., Hoar, S., & McDonough, M. (2004). Emotions in sport across adulthood. In M. Weiss (Ed.), *Developmental sport and exercise psychology: A lifespan perspective* (pp. 333–356). Morgantown, WV: Fitness Information Technology.

Ekman, P. (1999). Basic emotions. In T. Dalgleish & M. Power (Eds.), *Handbook of cognition and emotion* (pp. 45–60). West Sussex, UK: Wiley.

Ekman, P., & Cordaro, D. (2011). What is meant by calling emotions basic. *Emotion Review, 3,* 364–371.

Hackfort, D. (1993). Functional attributions to emotions in sport. In J. R. Nitsch & R. Seiler (Eds.), *Movement in sport: Psychological foundations and effects. Proceedings of the VIIIth European Congress of Sport Psychology* (Vol. 1, pp. 143–149). Sandt Augustin, Germany: Academic Verlag.

Hanin, Y. L. (2000). *Emotions in sport.* Champaign, IL: Human Kinetics.

Izard, C. E. (2011). Forms and functions of emotions: Matters of emotion-cognition interactions. *Emotion Review, 3,* 371–378.

Levenson, R. W. (2011). Basic emotion questions. *Emotion Review, 3,* 379–386.

Ortony, A., & Turner, T. J. (1990). What's basic about basic emotions? *Psychological Review, 97,* 315–331.

Prinz, J. (2004). Which emotions are basic? In P. Cruise & D. Evans (Eds.), *Emotion, evolution and rationality* (pp. 69–87). Oxford, UK: Oxford University Press.

BIOFEEDBACK, NEUROFEEDBACK

In recent years, there has been an increase in research and practical applications concerning the use of biofeedback training for athletic performance enhancement. It is important to be aware that the terms *biofeedback* and *biofeedback training* are not identical, and therefore need to be defined separately. Biofeedback (BFB) is the output from an electronic device with sensors and electrodes, which allows immediate and objective measurements of personal biological functions. This information is monitored on a computer screen and is transformed into auditory and visual signals, helping in learning to regulate body–mind activity in line with a basic psychophysiological principle. The main idea of this principle is that for every physiological change there is a parallel change in an emotional or mental component of human behavior, and vice versa. Biofeedback training (BFBT) is a process of learning psychophysiological self-regulation skills using information from a feedback device. Possible models of BFBT are as follows:

- *One-to-one model:* Sport psychologist or consultant and athlete work together throughout the sessions.
- *Group model:* Sport psychologist or consultant and several athletes with BFB equipment for each athlete work in one laboratory.
- *Home practice:* Athlete trains with portable BFB equipment at home, following sport psychologist or consultant's written instructions.

Biofeedback Modalities

Biofeedback modalities refer to the types of physiological indicators used for feedback during BFBT:

1. *Cardiovascular* or *heart rate* (HR) feedback measures heart activity using beats per minute (bpm) by electrocardiography. In addition, practitioners use measurements of interbeat interval (IBI), the time between heart beat and msec-heart rate variability (HRV). HR generally increases with an increase in stress, and vice versa.

2. *Muscle* or surface *electromyographic* feedback measures muscle activity in microvolts (μV). In cases of an increase in stress, electromyography (EMG) usually increases, as does muscle tension, and vice versa.

3. *Temperature* or *thermal* (T) feedback is a measurement of skin temperature as an indication of peripheral blood flow. Temperature feedback is measured in Fahrenheit (F) or Celsius (C) degrees. During an increase in stress, skin temperature decreases, and vice versa.

4. *Blood pressure* (BP) feedback is the measurement of the force exerted by circulating blood on the walls of blood vessels. BP is measured in terms of the systolic pressure over diastolic pressure (mmHg), and it usually increases with increases in stress.

5. *Electrodermal activity* (EDA) feedback is a measurement of changes in the electrical activity of the skin surface. It can be measured by skin resistance (historically known as *galvanic skin response* [GSR], units of kohms, kΩ), by skin conductance (SC, units of microsiemens, μS), and by skin potential (SP, units of millivolts,

mV). SC is the preferred method in psychophysiology research. SC increases with higher arousal, and vice versa.

6. *Respiration* (R) feedback is a measurement of the respiration rate, which is the number of breaths taken within a set amount of time (breaths per minute). Respiration rate can be recorded using a tensometric sensor inserted into a cuff that is fixed around the individual's chest. R increases with increased stress, and vice versa.

7. *Electroencephalograph* (EEG) feedback, more recently known as *neurofeedback* (NFB), is a measurement of brain wave activity. EEG frequency groups are: Delta (1–4 Hz), Theta (4–7 Hz), Alpha (8–12 Hz), Beta (13–36 Hz), and Gamma (36–44 Hz). The response range under stress increases from sleep states (Theta waves) to excitement (Beta waves).

Research and Applications

Biofeedback research and applications can be dated back to the 1960s, when the focus was on the medical and clinical field. The primary modalities used in research in health care and cases of trauma and injury were EMG, EEG, and HR, especially in the laboratory setting.

The main goals of the BFB studies in this period were to demonstrate self-regulation skills and symptom reduction. Moreover, researchers attempted to describe an optimal model of BFBT and its applications in clinical practice. Later, in 1975, Leonard Zaichkowsky, the pioneer of biofeedback application in sport, described the positive effect biofeedback had on athletic performance. Research on BFB (usually EMG) efficiency in sport focused on reducing anxiety, increasing muscle strength, and decreasing muscle fatigue and pain in different kinds of sports. The EEG BFB (neurofeedback) studies focused on psychomotor efficiency and skilled motor performance; for example, enhanced performance in golf, shooting, and archery was shown to be associated with an increase in alpha (decreased cortical activation) activity in the left hemisphere. An additional trend in research and application of BFBT in sport was to include BFBT as part of a larger package of psychological interventions. A major limitation of this period was the inability to transfer the results from sterile laboratory conditions to a field setting and integrating BFBT into the training process.

The Wingate Five-Step Approach (W5SA) was developed to overcome this limitation.

The Wingate Five-Step Approach (W5SA)

The W5SA consists of five steps and a self-regulation test (SRT). Three of the steps are provided in a laboratory setting and the last two under field and training conditions. The steps are as follows:

1. *Introduction:* The main goal is to teach the athlete basic self-regulation techniques, such as relaxation, imagery, self-talk, and concentration. At the end of this step, EMG, HR, and GSR BFB are used as part of the athlete's mental training, especially the use of auditory or visual signals. The duration of this step can last up to 10 to 15 sessions, while each session can last approximately 45 to 50 minutes.

2. *Identification:* In this step, most of the work that is done focuses on identifying and strengthening the most suitable biofeedback modality. Different sports require different biofeedback modalities. For example, in combat sports, EMG and GSR BFB are the most efficient modalities for measuring and practice. In contrast, EEG and HR are more suitable for sports such as golf, archery, and shooting. Additionally in this step, personal characteristics and the specific demands of the sport discipline should be taken into account. The duration of this step is approximately 15 sessions, each lasting 45 to 50 minutes.

3. *Simulation:* The main goal of this step is to practice self-regulation and concentration skills in the laboratory setting using BFB in the natural environment, such as watching video scenes under competitive situations. In addition, the basic self-regulation techniques are modified according to the sport's demands. In this step relaxation is shorter, imagery is set according to competition length, and self-talk is specific to the competitive situation. This step lasts about 15 sessions, each of them approximately 50 to 60 minutes.

4. *Transformation:* The athlete mentally prepares for the upcoming competition. All the skills that the athlete learned and rehearsed in the laboratory are transferred and integrated into the actual training setting by using a portable BFB device. This process allows the athlete to be prepared for future competitions by acquiring self-regulation abilities and mental readiness. This step lasts about

15 sessions and is provided during different parts of the training.

5. *Realization:* In this step, BFB is used in different settings, such as the field, pool, gym, bus, and boat at sea. In addition, the BFB is accompanied with relaxation, concentration, and imagery, which are used in different parts of the competition, such as before the start, between combats, after warm-up, and at the end of competition. The process of this step begins by applying the skills during less significant competitions, and gradually requesting the athlete to apply the skills in more significant events.

Self-regulation test (SRT) is given to the athlete before the beginning of the program and before each step. The goal is to examine the self-regulation level of the athlete. Recently, practitioners have been integrating the W5SA with the athlete's physical training, incorporating it within the periodization concept.

Neurofeedback

Neurofeedback (NFB) or EEG BFB relates to changes in electrocortical activity of the brain as the physiological measure of emotional and cognitive processes. The historical development of NFB began in clinical settings using alpha-type training. Later, research focusing on performance enhancement using neurofeedback of alpha activity in the left hemisphere, which is usually associated with expertise. Moreover, some research suggested that alpha range can be used as an indicator of attention processing. In sport, NFB is applied for the purpose of optimizing athletic performance by the athlete being able to master self-control and self-regulation strategies. For example, the first NFB study in sport examined the left–right hemispheric activity in rifle marksmanship. Neurofeedback training in sport is used in models for decreasing arousal or increased relaxation skills (alpha–theta type training) and for increasing attention–performance relationships (theta–beta type training).

BFB in Exercise Psychology

The major goal of using BFB in exercise psychology is to understand exercise behavior and the mechanisms that have an effect on participation rate and exercise adherence. In line with this goal, research has focused on the effect of self-monitoring and self-regulation of exercise intensity for fitness enjoyment, as well as adherence rate. Results have indicated that the positive effects of BFBT on achieving optimal exercise intensity for health and well-being can be accomplished during a relatively short time period.

Professional BFB Organizations, Journals, and Equipment

Professional Organizations

There are four major international BFB organizations that provide annual meetings, workshops, and publications: (1) The Association for Applied Psychophysiology and Biofeedback (AAPB) in North America (www.aapb.org); (2) The Biofeedback Foundation of Europe (BFE; www.bfe.org); (3) The International Society for Neurofeedback and Research (ISNR; www.isnr.org); and (4) The Biofeedback Certification International Alliance (BCIA; www.bcia.org), which provides biofeedback certification according to the Professional Standards and Ethical Principles.

Professional Journals

There are two major scholarly journals: (1) *Applied Psychophysiology and Biofeedback* (APB), formerly known as *Biofeedback and Self-Regulation*, and (2) *Biofeedback.* Both are supported by the AAPB.

BFB Equipment

There is a variety of biofeedback equipment that can be used in laboratory and field settings, depending on the intervention goal. Advanced technology and awareness of the possibilities of BFBT have led to the innovative and improvement of BFB electrodes, noncontact monitor tools, telemetric systems, and computer programs. For more detail, see the chapter "Psychophysiology: Equipment in Research and Practice," by Derek T. Y. Mann and Chris M. Janelle in A. Edmonds and G. Tenenbaum (Eds.), *Case Studies in Applied Psychophysiology: Neurofeedback and Biofeedback Treatments for Advances in Human Performance* (2012).

BFBT has many potential applications, such as in education, music, and the military.

Boris Blumenstein and Iris Orbach

See also Concentration Skills; Electroencephalograph (EEG); Electromyography (EMG); Imagery;

Psychological Skills Training; Psychophysiology; Relaxation; Self-Regulation; Stress Management

Further Readings

Association for Applied Psychophysiology and Biofeedback. (2011). Innovations in the application of biofeedback and neurofeedback for optimal performance [Special issue]. *Biofeedback, 39*(3).

Blumenstein, B., Bar-Eli, M., & Tenenbaum, G. (Eds.). (2002). *Brain and body in sport and exercise: Biofeedback applications in sport performance enhancement.* New York: Wiley.

Edmonds, A., & Tenenbaum, G. (Eds.). (2012). *Case studies in applied psychophysiology: Neurofeedback and biofeedback treatments for advances in human performance.* Chichester, UK: Wiley-Blackwell.

Leonards, J. (2003). Sport psychophysiology: The current status of biofeedback with athletes. *Biofeedback, 31*(4), 20–23.

Vernon, D. J. (2005). Can neurofeedback training enhance performance? An evaluation of the evidence with implications for future research. *Applied Psychophysiology and Biofeedback, 30*(4), 347–364.

Wilson, V., & Gunkelman, J. (2001). Neurofeedback in sport. *Biofeedback, 29*(1), 16–18.

Zaichkowsky, L. (2009). A case for new sport psychology: Applied psychophysiology and fMRI neuroscience. In R. Schinke (Ed.), *Contemporary sport psychology* (pp. 21–32). New York: Nova Science.

BIOPSYCHOSOCIAL MODEL OF INJURY

There are several prevailing models that connect psychological factors and sport injury, each with slightly different perspective on relevant biological, psychological, or social factors. Moreover, prevailing models have typically focused either on incorporating psychosocial factors in predicting and preventing sport injury incidence or upon identifying psychosocial factors associated with injury recovery and rehabilitation outcomes. Extensive reviews of these models have been written by Jean Williams and Mark Andersen, Britton Brewer, and Diane Wiese-Bjornstal. This entry provides an overview of the mediating biological pathways and physiological mechanisms linking psychosocial stress to athletic injury and, where appropriate, other adverse health consequences.

Both historical and recent conceptualizations of psychosocial stress posit wide-ranging biological effects on health. In this regard, Frank Perna and colleagues have argued that emotional, behavioral, and physiological aspects of stress response must be considered together with attention disruption to fully capture potential pathways mediating the relationship between psychosocial stress and adverse health including athletic injury. Additionally, since the physical demands of training volume and intense exercise required in competitive athletics are known to have adverse temporal effects on immune, neuroendocrine, and skeletal muscle repair response, a primary tenet of a biopsychosocial model of injury is that psychosocial distress may act synergistically with high-intensity, high-volume sports training to widen a window of susceptibility to illness or injury.

The biopsychosocial model of stress athletic injury and health (BMSAIH) is offered below to illustrate pathways between stress demands and athlete health (see Figure 1). The BMSAIH expands the Andersen and Williams model of psychosocial stress and athletic injury in three essential ways: (1) It clarifies mediating physiological pathways between athletes' stress response and adverse health outcomes (e.g., sport injury); (2) it considers other health outcomes and behavioral factors that impact sport participation as well as injury; and (3) it integrates the impact of exercise training upon athletes' health.

The BMSAIH should be considered an independent extension of Andersen and Williams's classic model of stress and athletic injury, which is reviewed elsewhere (see also the entry "Injury, Psychological Susceptibility to"). Similar to other generic models of stress and adverse health consequences, the Andersen and Williams model posited that a stress response mediated the effect of stressor(s) on the health outcome, athletic injury, with the stress response being composed of physiological and cognitive features (attentional perturbations such as peripheral narrowing) thought to predispose an athlete to injury. While the stress response was conceptualized as being both physiological and cognitive in nature, the original model and the preponderance of studies have principally only researched cognitive features (disturbances in attention and recognition of sport-related cues) thought to predispose an athlete to injury. Yet, the relationship between psychosocial stress and athletic injury appears stronger for overuse injuries

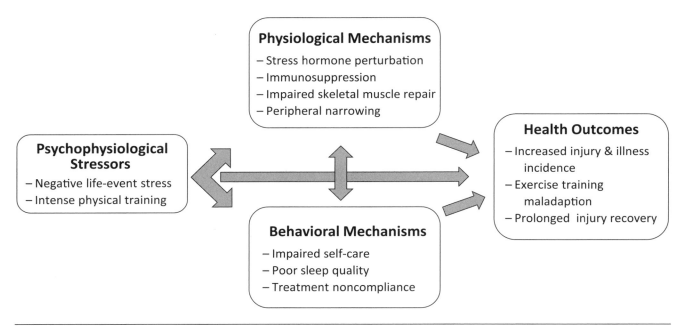

Figure I   A Biopsychosocial Model of Stress and Athletic Injury and Health (BMSAIH)
Source: R. N. Appaneal & F. M. Perna.

that are likely less dependent on cognitive processing and more likely related to physiological processes affecting exercise training adaptation and recovery. The stress-injury model also proposed a number of factors, such as personality, history of stress, and coping resources, that may moderate a stress response, but there was less clarity and exposition of mediating pathways, particularly those related to stress physiology, by which stress response may increase risk of injury.

Stress Response Mechanisms

Negative life stress and attendant emotional distress, through autonomic nervous system (ANS) response pathways, is thought to exacerbate the adverse effects of prolonged high-intensity and high-volume exercise. Specifically, psychological stress causes activation of the ANS yielding the release of catecholamines like epinephrine, norepinephrine, neuropeptides, and glucocorticoids (cortisol). Because target organs, such as heart, vasculature, muscle, and immune tissue, contain efferent nerves and have receptors for catecholamine and glucocorticoids, ANS activation affects target organs either by direct innervation of the parasympathetic and sympathetic nervous systems (PNS and SNS, respectively) or by hormonal action via activation of the hypothalamic-pituitary-adrenal-cortex

(HPAC) and cortisol release. Cognitive features related to a person's appraisal of the severity of a stressor and the capacity to cope with a stressor is known to exacerbate or prolong emotional reactivity and concomitant physiological response. Direct innervation, particularly by the SNS and catecholamine release, and hormonal action (e.g., cortisol release) thus provide the mechanistic links used to explain how the brain and associated cognitive–affective processes attendant to psychological stress may influence stress physiology and other physical systems, particularly those of relevance to athlete health like immune and skeletal muscle.

Because the ANS may operate either through direct innervation or hormonal action, there are a variety of possible neuroendocrine and hormonal patterns (differential responses to stress) that have evolved to characterize the stress response since Hans Selye first proposed the general adaptation syndrome, an undifferentiated response to stress. Moreover, specific ANS patterns are known to be influenced by features of cognitive appraisal particularly being dependent if an individual views a life event as a negative stressor or as a challenge. Thus, it is recognized that ANS activation in response to stress is not always deleterious, and indeed, is necessary. For example, it has long been known that ANS activation, particularly of the SNS, is associated with performance of physical and cognitive tasks. Similarly, HPAC activity and cortisol release are known to potentiate the actions of epinephrine in the completion of physical tasks and, when not prolonged, cortisol initiates a cascade leading to anabolic activity necessary for muscle repair following intense exercise.

A thorough discussion of possible hormonal response patterns in response to stress is beyond the scope of this entry but can be found in work by Trent Petrie and Frank Perna. In short, three hormonal patterns are thought to result in adverse health effects. These are thought to occur when individuals (a) experience frequent negative life stress and concomitant frequent activation of the SNS and HPAC pathways involving principally the release of epinephrine and cortisol to a lesser extent, (b) are hypersensitive to stressors and have an atypically high SNS and epinephrine response out of proportion to the magnitude of a stressor, and (c) experience chronic stressors and emotional distress with a prolonged activation of the HPAC and heightened cortisol release. The latter scenario involving measurement of enduring effects of negative life events, either in isolation or with their association with cortisol response, has received the most attention.

In addition to stress mechanisms described above, HPAC activation and possible concomitant behavioral disruptions (e.g., sleep disturbance) resulting from heightened negative affect may act in synergy with the demands of heavy exercise to increase risk of illness and injury. For example, poor sleep has been associated with prolonged elevation in evening cortisol, immune decrements, and lessened growth hormone release, all of which may inhibit muscle repair following acute exercise. Negative emotion-linked increases in stress hormones (cortisol) and behavioral perturbation may thus widen or prolong a window of susceptibility for illness and injury that is created by high-intensity and high-volume training. That is, psychological distress may impair muscle growth and repair processes by prolonging the presence of post-exercise catabolic hormones like cortisol that also impair immunity and inhibit the secretion and action of anabolic factors, such as growth hormone and insulin-like growth factors. Due to cortisol's immunosuppressive and muscle catabolic effects, prolonged training-induced cortisol elevation may create favorable conditions for viral infection, athletic injury, and exercise training maladaptation.

Similarly, elevated negative mood state, particularly fatigue and depression, has been used to identify overtrained athletes. Depressed mood has also been related to impaired immune function, and this effect may be mediated by cortisol elevation. Although the physiological strain of exercise training is largely responsible for cortisol and mood fluctuation, studies suggest that psychological life-event stress (LES) may also modulate cortisol and health parameters in athletes. For example, elite athletes with high LES, in comparison to low LES athletes, have been reported to experience prolonged post-exercise cortisol elevation, which was prospectively correlated with a greater frequency of physical symptom, such as muscle pain, back tightness, or flu-like symptoms. Elevated LES has also been prospectively related to increased risk of athletic injury and viral infection (e.g., common cold). In essence, the BMSAIH suggests that health effects of psychosocial stress would be most pronounced when an athlete was either in or just removed from a high-volume or high-intensity period of training, and that sport training cycle should be considered to optimally measure the association between psychosocial stress and athletic injury and adverse health.

Taken together, the literature indicates that independent from intensity and volume of sports training, psychological stress likely contributes to athletes' neuroendocrine and immune activity, which may be a mediating pathway linking stress to increased risk for adverse health effects including athletic injury. However, the effects of psychosocial stress on health may be more pronounced during periods of high-volume and intense exercise training. Because athletes must train at high volumes and intensities to make the physiological adaptations necessary for competitive success, commercially available exercise recovery monitoring systems have appeared on the competitive sports milieu and have been extensively reviewed by Michael Kellman. These systems include the assessment of physical, emotional, and social–contextual stress responses, as athletes must maintain a delicate balance between demands and recovery to stay healthy, avoid injury, and ultimately perform optimally. However, athletes' efforts to balance training and recovery occur within a sport culture that often undervalues the importance of psychosocial factors, and perhaps also recovery. As a result, the culture of competitive sport reinforces an imbalance between psychosocial and sport training factors, which ultimately may affect training adaptation, injury, and overall health. Sport psychology personnel trained to assist athletes with life-event, precompetitive, and post-injury stress are also widely available. However, the efficacy of psychosocial intervention to reduce injury risk, facilitate exercise-training adaptation, and enhance athlete health has been less extensively investigated.

Psychological Interventions

In the athletic domain, cognitive–behavioral stress management (CBSM) intervention in the form of psychological skills training is well known to reduce competitive anxiety and enhance athletic performance. CBSM has also been shown to reduce pain and speed recovery and return to play following arthroscopic surgery among injured recreational athletes. In a handful of randomized controlled trials, CBSM improved exercise training adaptation in the form of lessened fatigue, depressed mood, and cortisol curve during a high-volume training period among competitive rowers. Further, CBSM intervention has also been shown to reduce actual incidence of athletic injury and illness. One of these trials conducted by Perna and colleagues specifically tested if intervention effects on cortisol and affect mediated health outcomes. Findings demonstrated that rowers in a CBSM condition had significantly fewer days injured or ill and half the number of health and training center visits compared with controls. Mediation analyses indicated that modulation of affect and cortisol accounted for approximately one half and one fifth, respectively, of the intervention effect on days injured or ill. Though limited, the extant literature provides compelling support for the potential value of intervention to lessen risk of athletic injury and illness and to facilitate sports-training adaptation. Future research should seek to further elucidate the physiological pathways underpinning the psychosocial stress and health relationship, and explore biopsychosocial mechanisms that may be responsible for intervention effects on athlete health.

Renee N. Appaneal and Frank M. Perna

See also Autonomic Nervous System; Injury, Psychological Susceptibility to; Stress Management; Stress Reactivity

Further Readings

Brewer, B. W. (2010). The role of psychological factors in sport injury rehabilitation outcomes. *International Review of Sport and Exercise Psychology, 3*(1), 40–61.

Clow, A., & Hucklebridge, F. (2001). The impact of psychological stress on immune function in the athletic population. *Exercise Immunology Review, 7,* 5–17.

Kellmann, M. (2010). Preventing overtraining in athletes in high-intensity sports and stress/recovery monitoring. *Scandinavian Journal of Medicine & Science in Sports, 20*(Suppl. 2), 95–102.

Perna, F. M., Antoni, M. H., Baum, A., Gordon, P., & Schneiderman, N. (2003). Cognitive behavioral stress management effects on injury and illness among competitive athletes: A randomized clinical trial. *Annals of Behavioral Medicine, 25,* 66–73.

Perna, F. M., Antoni, M. H., Kumar, M., Cruess, D. H., & Schneiderman, N. (1998). Cognitive-behavioral intervention effects on mood and cortisol during exercise training. *Annals of Behavioral Medicine, 20,* 92–98.

Perna, F. M., & McDowell, S. L. (1995). Role of psychological stress in cortisol recovery from exhaustive exercise among elite athletes. *International Journal of Behavioral Medicine, 2*(1),13–26.

Perna, F. M., Schneiderman, N., & LaPerriere, A. (1997). Psychological stress, exercise, and immunity. *International Journal of Sports Medicine, 18*(Suppl. 1), S78–S83.

Petrie, T. A., & Perna, F. M. (2004). Psychology of injury: Theory, research, and practice. In T. Morris & J. J. Summers (Eds.), *Sport psychology: Theory, application, and issues* (2nd ed., pp. 547–551). Hoboken, NJ: Wiley.

Wiese-Bjornstal, D. M. (2010). Psychology and socioculture affect injury risk, response, and recovery in high-intensity athletes: A consensus statement. *Scandinavian Journal of Medicine & Science in Sports, 20,* 103–111.

Williams, J. M., & Andersen, M. B. (2007). Psychosocial antecedents of sport injury and interventions for risk reduction. In G. Tenenbaum & R. C. Eklund (Eds.), *Handbook of sport psychology* (3rd ed., pp. 379–403). Hoboken, NJ: Wiley.

BODY AWARENESS

Body awareness is described as awareness of, and attentiveness to, one's internal bodily processes and sensations. It is a sensitivity to normal bodily states that is separate from emotion yet originates from sensory proprioception and introspection and entails one's focus of attention toward the self.

Arguably, the most common perspectives used to understand body awareness are self-objectification, self-consciousness, and arousal. There is debate whether body awareness involves a somatic component of arousal or is distinct from somatic complaints. Some researchers have defined body awareness as separate from both emotion and somatic symptoms, whereas many sport and exercise researchers tend to define body awareness as somatic arousal.

From the perspective of self-objectification, it is argued that individuals, and in particular women, adopt an observer's perspective toward their bodies, and this objectification leads to an insensitivity to internal body cues. Also, individuals may be so vigilantly aware of the social cues and their outer body appearance that they deplete perceptual resources necessarily to attend to internal body sensations.

Similarly, researchers suggest that individuals who experience exaggerated self-consciousness or preoccupations with self will also deplete resources to attend to internal cues. *Private self-consciousness*, which is defined as the ability to introspect and pay attention to one's inner thoughts and feelings, has been used as a measure of body awareness in sport and exercise psychology research given the limited measurement tools available.

There is consistent evidence that women are less likely than men to attend to bodily cues and internal physiological cues, such as heartbeat, stomach contractions, and blood-glucose levels. Women are less likely to use these cues in determining how they feel, and these cues are less likely to be determinants of their subjective experiences compared to men.

Many mind-to-body approaches are used to help enhance body awareness, including yoga and tai chi, mindfulness-based meditation, and mental training for sport. In yoga, the nonjudgmental awareness of the body helps to emphasize responsiveness to body sensations, while also fostering physical challenge. Resistance-training exercise has also improved body awareness when examined in a pre- and post-study of college students. The proprioceptive and interoceptive training within sport psychology mental training programs are also important for enhanced body awareness. Breathing and progressive relaxation exercises within multimodal competitive stress and anxiety mental training programs are also used to enhance body awareness.

From a theoretical perspective, reducing body shame, anxiety, and self-objectification though intervention strategies, such as cognitive behavioral therapy and cognitive dissonance, may also help increase body awareness.

There is some debate on the adaptive or maladaptive features of body awareness. To some researchers, body awareness leads to maladaptive cognitions, such as somatosensory amplification, distress and anxiety, and somatization. These maladaptive perspectives suggest that heightened body awareness can be an impetus to eating disorders and maladaptive dieting or exercise behaviors. Alternatively, other researchers and practitioners argue that an ability to recognize subtle bodily cues leads to adaptive behavioral strategies to manage such body cues. Sport psychology researchers and practitioners often fall into this latter frame of thought and report the benefits of body awareness for competition and training.

Specifically, researchers have found that body awareness increases prior to sport competition and that this response is adaptive to successful performance. Strong associations between body awareness and state anxiety have been reported among athletes. Among individuals practicing yoga, body awareness was associated with lower perceptions of self-objectification and higher body satisfaction. High body awareness has also been consistently linked with lower incidence of disordered eating attitudes and behaviors in athletes.

Drawing from the injury and pain literature, it is also possible that increases in body awareness can help in the management of pain and facilitate sport injury rehabilitation. The most plausible argument explaining the mechanism stems from a distraction or attentional redistribution hypothesis such that focusing on body sensations and cues will distract from exercise-induced symptoms and pain.

Catherine M. Sabiston

See also Body Image; Self-Conscious Emotions; Self-Objectification

Further Readings

Kinsbourne, M. (2000). The brain and body awareness. In T. F. Cash & T. Pruzinsky (Eds.), *Body image: A handbook of theory, research, and clinical practice* (pp. 22–29). New York: Guilford Press.

Kotlyn, K. F., Raglin, J. S., O'Connor, P. J., & Morgan, W. P. (1995). Influence of weight training on state anxiety, body awareness and blood pressure. *International Journal of Sports Medicine, 16,* 266–269.

Mehling, W. E., Gopisetty, V., Daubenmier, J., Price, C. J., Hecht, F. M., & Stewart, A. (2009). Body awareness: Construct and self-report measures. *PLoS ONE, 4*(5), e5614. doi: 10.1371/journal.pone.0005614

Stegnar, A. J., Tobar, D. A., & Kane, M. T. (1999). Generalizability of change scores on the body awareness scale. *Measurement in Physical Education and Exercise Science, 3,* 125–140.

Body Dissatisfaction

Body dissatisfaction is the negative subjective evaluation of one's body as it relates to body size, shape, muscularity or muscle tone, weight, and fitness. Body dissatisfaction is considered to be an important negative affective factor related to body image. Typically, dissatisfaction involves a perceived discrepancy between one's current body and one's ideal body that fosters negative emotions and discontent. Body dissatisfaction has been viewed as normative and has received growing research attention during recent decades. The surge in popularity is due in part to the increasing prevalence worldwide, as well as implications for the development of a range of maladaptive behaviors and emotions, such as decreases in self-esteem, self-regulations, physical activity, happiness, optimism, pride, and increases in disordered eating, depressive symptoms, and body-related shame and guilt.

Sociocultural Effects

Pressures for women to be thin and fit, and for men to be lean and muscular, can originate from numerous sources, including the media, parents, siblings, partners, and peers. These sources may provide direct or indirect pressures to attain the desirable physique.

Sociocultural pressures to attain a socially desirable physique are considered important risk factors for body dissatisfaction. In particular, media awareness, knowledge of ideals as presented by the media, or actions taken or comments made by family, partners, and friends to encourage a socially desirable physique are important facets of the sociocultural pressure to conform to the ideal body. Researchers have concluded that even short-term exposure to idealized media images of men and women's bodies can lead to increased body dissatisfaction in both sexes. Theory and research also support modeling and negative communication as vehicles through which family and peers may influence body dissatisfaction. Nonetheless, the relationship between mass media and body dissatisfaction is complex, multiply determined, and bidirectional. It is important to recognize that a number of individual differences (internalization of the ideal physique, social comparison tendency, identification with models, appearance information, and critical body image processing) may moderate sociocultural pressures.

Gender Differences

One of the most consistent findings in the literature is that women are significantly more dissatisfied with their bodies than men. Higher prevalence rates are reported for women compared to men across the lifespan and geographic region. Upward of 90% of girls and women are dissatisfied with at least one aspect of their physiques, with elevated body weight and size typically ranking the highest. Nonetheless, body dissatisfaction among men is on the rise. Some researchers have reported that over 90% of men also experience some degree of body dissatisfaction. Contrary to the findings for women, men's body dissatisfaction focuses on muscularity and involves both ends of the weight continuum. That is, some men want to lose weight, while others want to gain weight.

Despite apparent gender differences, it is important to note that the majority of body dissatisfaction measures focus on evaluations of weight and shape at the expense of muscularity. Therefore, most measures of body dissatisfaction do not adequately assess typical concerns of men. It is difficult to draw concrete conclusions regarding gender differences in body dissatisfaction until the full spectrum of appearance and fitness evaluations represented by both men and women is considered.

Age

Body dissatisfaction can manifest at a very early age. Survey findings suggest a significant proportion of young children express dissatisfaction with their bodies, but levels in childhood are relatively low compared with adolescence and adulthood. Generally, girls experience heightened body dissatisfaction at puberty, which intensifies during adolescence. The normal physical changes of increased weight and body fat push girls further away from the cultural ideal of a thin and fit physique. Typically, dissatisfaction in women remains relatively stable throughout adulthood. In older adulthood, some women report heightened dissatisfaction with physical functioning aspects of their bodies in addition to age-related deficits in appearance. The impact of aging on men is less consistent. Boys go through a short phase of relative dissatisfaction with appearance in early adolescence, but the physical changes associated with puberty shortly bring them closer to the masculine ideal (increased height and muscularity, broader shoulders). Similar to women, dissatisfaction plateaus during adulthood; however, some men may experience a period of discontent around middle age ("male menopause"). Similar to their female counterparts, males place greater investments in fitness and health as they age.

One of the issues in comparing different age groups with each other using a cross-sectional design is that historical or cultural ideals and experiences vary across time. Research in this area needs to use longitudinal studies that track cohorts over time as they age.

Sexual Orientation

Given the emphasis on appearance within the gay subculture, considerable research has shown that gay boys and men constitute a group particularly vulnerable to body dissatisfaction. Homosexual men tend to report higher levels of body dissatisfaction compared with heterosexual men, whereas homosexual women have reported less body dissatisfaction than heterosexual women.

Ethnicity

There are reported ethnic differences in body dissatisfaction among individuals from Western countries. This paradigm of ethnic differences suggests one's meaning of the body is based on cultural and social group contexts. Most studies investigating ethnic differences concentrate on women. Body dissatisfaction is most frequent in Caucasian women and less frequent in Black women; however, this difference is small. Although research published in the 1990s reported that Hispanic and Asian women are typically more satisfied with their bodies than Caucasian women, new evidence suggests that there are minimal or no differences between Caucasian women and women of other ethnic origins. Researchers targeting variations in body dissatisfaction across ethnic groups indicate that Hispanic women are slightly more dissatisfied with their bodies compared to Black women. There is less work on ethnic differences in men's dissatisfaction, although there is general agreement that Black men report higher levels of satisfaction than Caucasian men and have heavier body ideals for women and men than do Caucasian men. Overall, there may be less ethnic difference in dissatisfaction than was once thought.

Relationship Status

Generally, people in stable, long-term relationships are more satisfied with their bodies than those who are single. This applies to all ages. With regard to less formal relationships, body dissatisfaction is more prevalent among adolescents who report lower quality of friendship and perceive less social support and less acceptance by peers. Also, women across the lifespan have reported quality peer relationships and social support protect them from body dissatisfaction.

Pregnancy

Several studies have indicated that pregnant women have more positive views about their body than nonpregnant women. Even though pregnant women may still value the thin and fit cultural body ideal, their concerns about failing to match this ideal are typically reduced during this life event. Nonetheless, postpregnancy introduces many body image concerns focused on excess weight and lack of muscle tone. The prevailing emphasis on achieving prepregnancy weight and body shape may exacerbate body dissatisfaction.

Body Dissatisfaction, Sport, and Physical Activity

Generally, body dissatisfaction can act as both a motivator and deterrent for sport and physical activity participation. Several researchers have noted that participating in sport and exercise may serve as a protective function against feelings of body dissatisfaction. Physical activity can also improve older adults' perceptions of the body by increasing perceptions of mastery of the body and refocusing attention onto health, fitness, and body function and away from concerns about physical appearance. Nonetheless, the relationship between body dissatisfaction and physical activity varies with the sport and cultural context. Some aesthetic sports, such as gymnastics, cheerleading, and ballet, place high importance on the culturally derived ideal body. In these cases, it is not uncommon for individuals to experience higher levels of discontent related to their body. Furthermore, some athletes report lower body dissatisfaction in the context of their sport, whereby their physiques have functional sport-specific value but greater body dissatisfaction outside of sport, where their athletic physiques are inconsistent with ideal societal standards of appearance and body shape. Less is known about the dose–response relationship between physical activity and body dissatisfaction.

Catherine M. Sabiston and Andree Castonguay

See also Body Image; Self-Discrepancy; Social Comparison

Further Readings

Campbell, A., & Hausenblas, H. A. (2009). Effects of exercise interventions on body image: A meta-analysis. *Journal of Health Psychology, 14,* 780–793.

Cash, T. F., & Smolak, L. (2011). *Body image: A handbook of science, practice, and prevention.* New York: Guilford Press.

Grabe, S., & Hyde, J. S. (2006). Ethnicity and body dissatisfaction among women in the United States: A meta-analysis. *Psychological Bulletin, 132,* 622–640.

Swami, V., Frederick, D. A., Aavik, T., Alcalay, L., Allik, J., Anderson, D., et al. (2010). The attractive female body weight and female body dissatisfaction in 26 countries across 10 world regions: Results of the International Body Project I. *Personality and Social Psychology Bulletin, 36,* 309–326.

BODY DYSMORPHIC DISORDER, MUSCLE DYSMORPHIA

Most people would like to change something about their physical appearance, and this *normative discontent* is not usually indicative of a serious body image issue. However, some individuals may feel extreme preoccupation with an aspect of their appearance: they perceive to be flawed. Typically, this perception is inaccurate or exaggerated and indicative of body dysmorphia.

Body Dysmorphic Disorder

Characterized as a somatoform disorder in the *Diagnostic and Statistical Manual of Mental Disorders, 4th Edition, Text Revision (DSM-IV-TR)*, *body dysmorphic disorder* is described as a preoccupation with an imagined defect in appearance, which causes severe distress and impairment in daily functioning. Body dysmorphic disorder tends to co-occur with other psychiatric conditions, such as obsessive-compulsive disorder, depression, substance abuse, and eating disorders. The disorder is prevalent in settings where a high importance is placed on physical appearance, such as sport and exercise contexts and in particular aesthetic sports.

Individuals with this disorder are overcome with constant preoccupations that aspects of their appearance are deformed, when in reality, the perceived flaw is minimal or non-existent. Individuals tend to focus on a few body areas and spend much of the day thinking about the perceived flaws. These individuals typically have low self-esteem and are prone to rejection, low self-worth, and shame. Individuals tend to exhibit delusions of reference, which involves thinking that other people focus on and mock one's perceived flaws and defects. These individuals are highly motivated to examine, improve, seek assurance, and hide the perceived flaw and respond by engaging in obsessive-compulsive behaviors. In competitive sport settings, symptoms may manifest as withdrawal from teammates and constant need for reassurance from teammates and coaches. These coping behaviors may extend to excessive dieting, compulsive exercising, and seeking plastic surgery.

The etiology of body dysmorphic disorder is complex and multifactorial and includes genetic, neurobiological, sociocultural, and psychological influences. Particularly in competitive sport and exercise settings, sociocultural influences play a large role, including strong pressures from coaches, trainers, parents, and even media influences. For example, a genetically predisposed adolescent elite gymnast who presents with high tendencies for perfectionism may be heavily influenced by social pressures, and be at high risk for developing body dysmorphic disorder. Despite the probable influence of social and cultural factors, clinical features of body dysmorphic disorder are similar across different cultures, even though typically body image concerns are more prevalent in Western societies.

Symptoms of body dysmorphic disorder initially present themselves during adolescence; however, most individuals are not diagnosed for an extended period of time after initial onset because of shame and embarrassment associated with discussing the preoccupations. Aside from difficulties in diagnosis, treatment for body dysmorphic disorder is also challenging. Treatment options include pharmacotherapy, particularly the use of serotonin reuptake inhibitors, and cognitive behavioral therapy, focusing on exposure and systematic desensitization.

Muscle Dysmorphia

Body dysmorphic disorder is equally prevalent in males and females; however, a subset of the disorder, *muscle dysmorphia,* is reported more frequently among males. Muscle dysmorphia is a chronic preoccupation with insufficient muscularity and inadequate muscle mass. Individuals presenting with muscle dysmorphia perceive themselves as much thinner than they actually are, and experience pressure to increase muscle mass and strength, despite possessing a much higher muscle mass than the average male. This condition involves excessive attention to muscularity, distress over presenting the body to others, extreme weight training, and focus on diet. Impaired function in daily life is also an outcome of these compulsive behaviors, along with a high risk of abusing physique-enhancing supplements and drugs, particularly anabolic steroids.

Individuals with muscle dysmorphia experience heightened shame with their preoccupations and engage in physique protection by hiding perceived defects and avoiding situations of physique exposure. For example, individuals may avoid busy times of training at the fitness center to avoid being seen by muscular weight trainers or wear loose clothing to hide the shape and size of their physiques. Researchers have indicated that athletes who are body builders and weight lifters are particularly susceptible to muscle dysmorphia and are at significant risk of anabolic steroid abuse. In competitions where physique-altering drugs are prohibited, individuals are at an increased risk for developing eating disorders and manipulating resistance training programs to achieve higher muscle mass while maintaining leanness.

Various theoretical frameworks have been employed to understand the complexity of muscle dysmorphia. Psychological theories posit that individuals strive for high muscularity to compensate for feelings of inadequacy, low self-esteem, and issues with masculinity identity. Sociocultural theories suggest that individuals with muscle dysmorphia strive for muscular physiques to attain societal and media-driven ideals that equate masculinity with muscularity. Sociocultural theories may be useful to explain muscle dysmorphia in elite athletes and the prevalence of similar body-related disorders in sport culture. Athletes are more susceptible to muscle dysmorphia if they are involved in sports that predominantly require strength and power, such as weight lifting, or aesthetics involving muscularity (e.g., body building).

Significant stigma surrounds psychiatric disorders like body and muscle dysmorphia, especially among athletes. In sport and exercise settings especially, psychoeducation is important to increase awareness and diminish shame surrounding having these disorders. Informed coaches and trainers can play an important role in preventing, identifying, and aiding in treatment of body and muscle dysmorphia. Treatment options in sport settings are best dealt with using a biopsychosocial model, which uses pharmacological and psychological treatment, while respecting the importance of the social and cultural sport environment in which these disorders thrive.

Catherine M. Sabiston and Eva Pila

See also Self-Discrepancy; Social Physique Anxiety

Further Readings

American Psychiatric Association. (1994). *Diagnostic and statistical manual of mental disorders* (4th ed., text revision). Washington, DC: Author.

Phillips, K. A. (2001). *Somatoform and factitious disorders.* Washington, DC: American Psychiatric Publishing.

Pope, H. G., Phillips, K. A., & Olivardia, R. (2000). *The Adonis complex: The secret crisis of male body obsession.* New York: Free Press.

Tod, D., & Lavallee, D. (2010). Toward a conceptual understanding of muscle dysmorphia development and sustainment. *International Review of Sport and Exercise Psychology, 3,* 111–113.

BODY IMAGE

In modern Western society, there is increasing pressure for females to be thin, fit, and well-toned, and for males to be muscular and lean, regardless of age. These ideal shapes tend to be difficult to achieve for most people because they have become progressively unrealistic, and with the ever-increasing obesity rates, predominantly unattainable. Consequently, many individuals have become aware that their bodies fall short of the idealized physique and experience what researchers have coined as *normative discontent*. Researchers have shown that this normative discontent is associated with impaired psychological and physical well-being, and that it can be a precursor for maladaptive behavioral patterns, such as disordered eating and dieting; self-induced vomiting; use of diet pills, laxatives, and diuretics; physical inactivity or compulsive exercising; and smoking.

Body Image Defined and Measured

Although there is no universally accepted definition of body image, it is generally explored as one's feelings and views about one's physical features and attractiveness. Expanding on this definition, current conceptualizations of the multidimensional nature of body image suggest there are perceptual, cognitive, affective, and behavioral dimensions.

The perceptual dimension reflects the mental representation or reflections that an individual has of one's body appearance and functions. It relates to the level of (in)accuracy between a person's perceived characteristics and the actual characteristics, either in relation to specific body parts or to the body as a whole. Perceptual body image is measured using body image accuracy techniques, which can include having a person manipulate the size of a body on a computer screen to fit one's body shape and size, using a compass-like device to indicate how wide the individual perceives the body to be, or illustrating the perceived body shape and size on a figure drawing. Using these techniques, it is clear that one's perception of oneself can be quite different from one's actual self. The cognitive dimension reflects an individual's thoughts, beliefs, and evaluations of personal body appearance and function. This dimension has often been studied using questionnaires or interviews targeting the assessment of an individual's description and satisfaction or dissatisfaction with one's body shape, size, and function. The affective dimension reflects the body-related feelings and emotions that an individual experiences. Commonly assessed emotions that stem from one's body size, shape, and function include anxiety (e.g., social physique anxiety), shame, guilt, pride, embarrassment, and worry. These emotions are measured using self-report questionnaires and in individual interviews. Last, the behavioral dimension relates to the behavioral manifestations that occur as a result of one's positive or negative perceptions, affect, and cognitions focused on one's body size, shape, and function. Specific behaviors may include avoidance; actions used to divert attention away from the body; lifestyle actions, such as dieting and physical activity; steroid use; cosmetic surgery; and body checking strategies, such as weight monitoring, measuring areas of one's body (e.g., dimension of wrist, ankle, thigh, waist), or pinching oneself as a measure of fatness.

In general, each of these body image dimensions can have positive or negative connotations. Positively valenced body image in any dimension may infer accurate perceptions, positive or satisfied thoughts and feelings about the body, and predominantly adaptive actions or behaviors. Negative body image refers to distorted perceptions, predominantly negative thoughts and feelings, and maladaptive actions or behaviors that are driven by physical self-evaluations. Furthermore, when people have distorted, negative views of themselves, negative thoughts, beliefs, evaluations, and emotions may arise, which in turn can lead to what are considered unhealthy behaviors (e.g., crash dieting, excessive exercising). Thus, each body image dimension is related and important to consider in research and practice.

The Development of Body Image

Body image begins as early as preschool through socialization processes; awareness of attractiveness; social comparison; and exposure to body-related prompts, such as dolls and figurines, images, and television advertising and programming. Drawing from sociocultural perspectives, the most common determinants of body image include individual characteristics like sex, age, and weight status; interpersonal experiences with peer groups, social environments, interactions, and social comparisons; social norms and pressures, such as societal beliefs, body-related stereotypes, media messages, and the fashion industry; and life events like puberty, early or late maturation, or illness. Some of these factors can significantly increase the risk of negative body image, while others can protect against negative body image. For example, younger people and obese people are especially likely to report negative body image. Going through puberty can influence body image because of the physical changes that occur. Based on the tripartite model of body image development, parents, siblings, peers, and other persons in one's support network can directly or indirectly play a key role in the development of negative body image through social disapproval or rejection, unsupportive behaviors, and negative social interactions. Receiving criticisms from peers, for example, can trigger negative body image. Conversely, the degree to which people sense that significant others support them can promote positive body image. Drawing on Leon Festinger's social comparison theory, comparisons can have a positive or negative effect on body image such that individuals who make upward body-related comparisons to others (the bodies they focus on are closer to their idealized bodies than their own or considered better in some way) are more likely to have negative self-evaluations, and in turn poorer body image. In contrast, individuals who make downward comparisons tend to feel better about the appearance and shape of their own bodies.

Body Image and Exercise

Two general approaches have been taken to study the relationship between body image and exercise. In the first approach, researchers have been concerned with determining if body image leads to engagement or avoidance of exercise. In the second approach, researchers have been concerned with determining whether exercise has a beneficial effect on body image. Researchers have shown support for both these approaches.

Body Image as an Antecedent of Exercise

Exercise is often viewed as a strategy to control weight, which may improve body image. Indeed, many people turn to exercise to try to achieve their body ideals and improve their body images. It is well documented that people's motives to engage in exercise often reflect appearance-related motives. Specifically, common reasons given for

exercising include weight control, physical attractiveness, muscle tone, and fitness. However, in spite of finding that body image may be a driving force that motivates people to initiate exercise, it is important to note that theories of motivation outline the importance of engaging in a behavior for intrinsic reasons (e.g., positive health benefits, enjoyment, and fun) since it has the greatest potential for resulting in long-term adherence. From this perspective, body image motives might be a key strategy to get people to initiate exercise but may be insufficient to motivate continued involvement, especially if people do not observe the desired changes in their physical appearance.

In addition to exercise motivation, the associations between body image and other exercise-related outcomes, such as setting preferences, effort, and behavior have been examined. Some researchers have documented that people who report high levels of negative body image engaged in exercise more often than those who report low levels of negative body image. In contrast, other researchers have shown that people who report high levels of negative body image are less likely to exercise. This has led to the notion that body image can be either a motivator or deterrent to exercise. However, it is important to note that the majority of the research using this approach has been cross-sectional, and thus, claims of causation are inappropriate. Furthermore, these equivocal findings demonstrate the complexity of understanding the association between body image and exercise behavior. In an effort to explain these inconsistent findings, researchers are increasingly highlighting the need to consider variables that can affect the direction or magnitude of the association between body image and exercise (i.e., moderators) in future research. Some emerging candidate moderator variables include sex and gender stereotypes, self-objectification, social support, motivation, and emotion.

Body Image as an Outcome of Exercise

The hope of improving body image to reduce the negative consequences lies in the development of effective and efficacious interventions. Psychologists have successfully adopted and used cognitive behavioral techniques to improve body image. In parallel, many exercise researchers have examined the effect of exercise on body image due to the numerous health benefits of exercise.

Typically, these researchers have instructed study participants to engage in aerobic training, strength training, or a combination of both, and examined whether body image improves following either an exercise bout or entire program spanning several weeks. The results have been positive, suggesting a beneficial role of exercise in improving body image in both males and females. That is, exercise improves body image immediately after a workout session, and there is also some improvement in body image as a result of long-term participation in an exercise program. Also, both intensity and type of exercise seem to be important features to consider when studying body image as an outcome. Specifically, aerobic training (e.g., jogging, running) and strength training (e.g., weight lifting) improve body image, and the more intense the exercise, the greater the effect on body image. One caveat to this finding is that some researchers have found strength training may exacerbate body image concerns among women.

In light of the evidence, researchers have provided some insight into how exercise might improve body image. They have suggested that at least some of the positive effects of exercise on body image may stem from improved physical fitness, increased awareness of physical capabilities, and increased self-efficacy. For example, body image may improve after exercise because people feel more efficacious by mastering a new skill or more autonomous by gaining some control over their bodies. Thus, the general inference is that exercise interventions are promising. Furthermore, both exercise and cognitive behavioral therapy have been associated with improvements in body image; however, it is unclear if the combination of exercise with cognitive behavioral therapy is more effective than the use of either intervention alone since relatively little research addressing this possibility has been conducted.

Conclusion

Although research on body image in the field of sport and exercise psychology has come a long way, the definition and measurement of body image is an ongoing source of discussion in the literature. An important challenge faced by researchers examining body image in mainstream and sport and exercise psychology is to establish a comprehensive, precise, and universally accepted definition of body image that can be adopted by all researchers. This would have important implications for the way in which researchers conduct their studies and the refinement of current body image measures, and would enable direct comparisons of findings across studies—an important endeavor if researchers are to increase their understanding of body image and its association with biological, psychological, social, and behavioral factors.

Jennifer Brunet

See also Body Dissatisfaction; Body Dysmorphic Disorder, Muscle Dysmorphia; **Body Self-Esteem; Social Physique Anxiety**

Further Readings

Campbell, A., & Hausenblas, H. A. (2009). Effects of exercise interventions on body image: A meta-analysis. *Journal of Health Psychology, 14,* 780–793.

Cash, T. F. (2008). *The body image workbook.* Oakland, CA: New Harbinger.

Cash, T. F., & Pruzinsky, T. (Eds.). (2011). *Body image: A handbook of science, practice, and prevention.* New York: Guilford Press.

Grogan, S. (2008). *Body image: Understanding body dissatisfaction in men, women and children.* London: Routledge.

Hausenblas, H. A., & Fallon, E. A. (2006). Exercise and body image: A meta-analysis. *Psychology & Health, 21,* 33–47.

Heinberg, L. J., Thompson, J. K., & Matzon, J. L. (2001). Body image dissatisfaction as a motivator for healthy lifestyle change: Is some distress beneficial? In R. H. Striegel-Moore & L. Smolak (Eds.), *Eating disorders: Innovative directions in research and practice* (pp. 215–232). Washington, DC: American Psychological Association.

Tiggemann, M. (2004). Body image across the adult life span: Stability and change. *Body Image, 1,* 29–41.

BODY SELF-ESTEEM

Self-esteem, considered synonymous with self-worth, is a global and relatively stable construct that reflects a person's evaluation about self-concept, that is, the set of beliefs and cognitions about one's qualities, character, roles, and attributes. Self-esteem is a complex and multifaceted concept of the self, and arguably one of the most important facets of self-esteem in Westernized countries is a sense of self that is focused on the body or physique. Specifically, body self-esteem is a strong predictor of global self-esteem when individuals value how they look and feel physically—meaning how one feels about one's physique, form, and function is a predominant guide to how one feels about oneself more globally. *Body self-esteem*, also identified as physical self-worth or physical self-esteem, is defined as an evaluation about the appearance and functioning of one's body. Theorists consider that body self-esteem develops as a result of the evaluative perceptions that arise from the different domains, such as perceived sport competence, physical condition, attractiveness, and weight concern. In turn, these arise from the different subdomains. For instance, positive self-evaluations of upper body strength contribute to the corresponding subdomain of physical strength, which in turn would enhance body self-esteem. On the other hand, negative evaluations of soccer competence will decrease the related subdomain of sport competence, and then in physical self-esteem. In addition, it has been argued that although body self-esteem may be relatively stable over time, specific self-evaluations may fluctuate depending on the situational cues—an individual may feel better about personal physical stamina after completing a 10-mile run or worse if unable to complete this run.

Researchers suggest that it is during adolescence that body self-esteem becomes particularly salient as a result of the physical and social changes associated with this developmental stage. Furthermore, researchers have also shown that there are gender differences in body self-esteem during this period and across adulthood, whereby men have reported higher levels of body self-esteem than women. While there are various potential reasons for this, many researchers have proposed that the greater sociocultural pressures on women to be thin, their inability to attain this standard, and the negative stereotyping of those whose current body is discrepant from the idealized standard, may partly explain this difference. Nonetheless, high body self-esteem is desirable in both sexes because it has a powerful influence on men and women's psychological, physical, and social well-being. Essentially, individuals who have higher levels of body self-esteem are more likely to report higher well-being in these domains. As a result, researchers have highlighted the importance of exploring factors that may increase or maintain body self-esteem

because it has public health importance. One such factor is exercise.

Body Self-Esteem and Exercise Research

Given that exercise has been consistently associated with psychological benefits, there has been an enduring interest in establishing the potential benefits of exercise as a strategy for the enhancement of self-esteem, and more specifically body self-esteem. With the use of different measures like specific cognitive and affective questions (Body Esteem Scale) and figure ratings (silhouettes that gradually increase in size and shape), researchers have found that exercise and body self-esteem are reciprocally related across the lifespan and in many diverse populations. This means that individuals suffering from low body self-esteem will be less likely to be physically active, and that individuals being more physically active show higher body self-esteem levels.

Often in research studies focused on body self-esteem improvements, the exercise parameters assessed have differed markedly. Specifically, the duration and intensity of training sessions, the number of training sessions per week, or the length of the training program tested varied from one study to another. It is possible that body self-esteem improvements found following exercise might be restricted to one particular type (aerobic training, strength training) or intensity (light, moderate, vigorous). However, at this point, it is not possible to provide an indication for the specific doses or types of exercise necessary to enhance body self-esteem. Thus, these parameters of exercise seem to be an important consideration for future research.

Another important problem is that some researchers are still using measures of global self-esteem such as the Rosenberg Self-Esteem Scale. This approach implicitly assumes that the overall concept of self-esteem would be related to exercise, which may not be the case, and lead to the erroneous conclusions that exercise is ineffective in improving self-esteem. Although it is unclear the extent to which the inclusion of global measures in previous studies reduced the associations found between exercise and body self-esteem, the current availability of body specific self-esteem measures provides an opportunity to examine the associations between body self-esteem and exercise to avoid the risk of making false conclusions regarding the magnitude of the association. Therefore, it is important to move beyond global measures and adopt a more systematic assessment of body self-esteem since exercise might have a more meaningful influence on this aspect of self-esteem without affecting others related to global self-esteem.

Nevertheless, one conclusion that has come out consistently from this research is that people who report lower levels of self-esteem and body image before beginning an exercise program report the greatest improvements in body self-esteem. This is likely because people with higher initial levels of self-esteem have less to gain than those with lower initial levels. Furthermore, although males and females across the lifespan have reported increases in body self-esteem following exercise, there is evidence that youth and middle-age adults benefit the most. Last, the magnitude of the effect produced by exercise on body self-esteem has been shown to be greater for people who are considered overweight or obese (body mass index ≥ 25.0 kilograms/meter squared); suffering from an illness or disease; or have low self-confidence, poor body image, or low self-concept. Accordingly, these personal characteristics, as well as other potential effect modifiers, should be considered when exercise is to be used as a strategy to enhance body self-esteem.

Possible Reasons for the Benefits of Exercise on Body Self-Esteem

To date, few efforts have been made to understand how exercise increases or maintains body self-esteem. Delineating the pathways, also known as mediating variables, through which exercise might exert its effect on body self-esteem has potential for developing interventions, especially since many researchers assume that exercise does not directly increase self-esteem. For instance, if improved physical fitness is identified as a factor that is affected by exercise, and in turn increases body self-esteem, then exercise interventions directed to increasing physical fitness might increase the likelihood of enhancing body self-esteem. As a result, some researchers have placed a particular emphasis on elucidating the psychophysiological pathways through which exercise might lead to enhanced body self-esteem.

Some of the explanations offered in the literature for how exercise might enhance body esteem have a cognitive or psychological foundation, such as those presented in the Exercise and Self-Esteem Model (EXSEM). The EXSEM,

a hierarchically organized model that links exercise to physical self-perceptions and global self-esteem, represents a practical framework that has helped researchers understand how exercise influences body self-esteem. Based on the most recent version of the EXSEM, exercise can influence perceptions of self-efficacy (i.e., people's judgments regarding their ability to become or remain active), which in turn influence physical self-perceptions, such as physical condition, physical competence, body attractiveness, and physical strength. Finally, physical self-perceptions, as well as physical acceptance or the extent to which individuals accept their bodies, are believed to then influence body self-esteem, which is related to global self-esteem. Cross-sectional and longitudinal research based on the EXSEM model has shown that global self-esteem can be influenced both directly and indirectly by exercise through its influence on physical competence and acceptance. Moreover, there is also some support that exercise can increase perceptions of personal control (people's belief regarding the extent to which they are able to control or influence their behaviors and outcomes) and self-schemata (set of beliefs and ideas people hold about themselves), and this may presumably increase self-esteem. For example, as people exercise more often and regularly, they may gain confidence if they are successful at trying new activities or if they master the skills required to perform their exercises. These feelings of physical confidence may increase their body self-esteem, resulting in improvements in global self-esteem.

Other explanations put forward in the literature have a physiological foundation. For instance, improvements in physical parameters (e.g., body composition, body weight, shape, fitness) may account for the positive changes in body self-esteem resulting from exercise. However, the literature examining these various pathways is scarce, preventing researchers to draw firm conclusions. Thus, insofar as the pathways through which exercise might affect body self-esteem are concerned, more studies are needed to identify mediating variables that explain the effect exercise has on body self-esteem. Based on current theorizing, it is clear that there are likely multiple mediators that should be considered in seeking to develop interventions with stronger and more sustainable effects on body self-esteem. For instance, if self-efficacy and body composition are identified as mediators, it would be logical to develop interventions that target these particular variables.

Conclusion

Body self-esteem is a multifaceted construct that is central to people's sense of self concept and worth, well-being, and development. Researchers have provided empirical evidence to support the notion that exercise can be a key strategy used to enhance body self-esteem, as well as global self-esteem. However, the research conducted to date has highlighted that the relationship between these two variables is complex and requires further investigation. Indeed, two important tasks facing researchers at the present time are to determine which exercise parameters (i.e., type, dosage) are the best to enhance body self-esteem, and identify the psychophysiological pathways by which exercise exerts its effect on body self-esteem.

Jennifer Brunet

See also Body Dissatisfaction; Body Image; Self-Acceptance; Self-Appraisal/Assessment/Perception; Social Physique Anxiety

Further Readings

Fox, K. R. (2000). Self-esteem, self-perceptions, and exercise. *International Journal of Sport Psychology, 31,* 228–240.

Haugen, T., Säfvenbom, R., & Ommundsen, Y. (2011). Physical activity and global self-worth: The role of physical self-esteem indices and gender. *Mental Health and Physical Activity, 4,* 49–56.

Rosenberg, M., Schooler, C., Schoenbach, C., & Rosenberg, F. (1995). Global self-esteem and specific self-esteem: Different concepts, different outcomes. *American Sociological Review, 60,* 141–156.

Sonstroem, R. J. (1997). The physical self-system: A mediator of exercise and self-esteem. In K. R. Fox (Ed.), *The physical self: From motivation to well-being* (pp. 3–26). Champaign, IL: Human Kinetics.

Sonstroem, R. J., Harlow, L. L., & Josephs, L. (1994). Exercise and self-esteem: Validity of model expansion and exercise associations. *Journal of Sport & Exercise Psychology, 16,* 29–42.

BRAIN

Neural plasticity is the mechanism by which the brain encodes experience and learns new skills, behaviors, and habits in daily life and on the athletic field. Brain cells called *neurons* form a communication network that serves as the foundation of information processing in the brain. The neural network of the brain holds the capacity to rearrange and strengthen communication efficiency. It is through this process of rearrangement (neural plasticity) that we can experience changes in the way our minds think, feel, and act. This includes everything from changing your backswing in golf or tennis, to developing a new mental routine for shot preparation, or restoring function following biomechanical or nervous system injury. Thus, optimal performance, skill learning, and recovery are achieved when the capacity for neural plasticity is maximized. Research has shown that physical exercise increases the brain's capacity for plasticity, reflected in part by changes in brain structure and function following exercise training in animal models and humans. Since aging results in gradual neurodegeneration, or loss and dysfunction of brain cells, and decreased neuronal plasticity, aged samples (e.g., 60–80 years) form a platform for studying methods to increase brain plasticity. This entry reviews research on exercise effects on mental performance and the brain and highlights results with aged samples.

Exercise's Influence on Cognitive Performance

Since the 1960s, studies have shown that physically more active people perform better on tests of cognitive performance compared with physically less active peers. The first studies examined performers' ability to successfully complete dual tasks by primarily measuring simple response time, the speed to respond quickly and accurately to a flash of light, and discrimination time, the speed to press one key if stimulus A appears and another key if stimulus B appears. Over time, more complex cognitive processes have been examined, such as the ability to switch between tasks, the ability to selectively pay attention and block out distractions, or the ability to inhibit automated responses or habits. Importantly, in these early studies the physically active groups were comprised primarily of competitive athletes. This may present interpretive problems due to the possibility of self-selection, such that athletes may seek and continue sports participation, in part, because of their natural superiority in cognitive processes that benefit sport performance, such as fast response time or the ability to focus amidst distraction. Thus, the best understanding of the effects of physical activity and exercise on mental performance and the brain comes from studying samples that have been well-matched on all characteristics other than physical activity level.

Several reviews have now quantified the effects of physical exercise on mental performance across studies in meta-analyses. Meta-analyses attempt to aggregate results from many studies and group results from similar variables together for the purpose of identifying and comparing replicable effects across studies at either the level of measurement (Does the effect replicate for a specific task?) or construct (Does the effect replicate across tasks that are all theoretically deemed to measure the same construct?). For example, the effect size of exercise training on simple response time could be calculated in different studies that included training and pre- and post-tests of simple response time, and then an average could be computed across studies to determine if exercise results in a consistent improvement independent of any one study or laboratory.

Meta-analyses that have examined the question of how exercise training affects different domains of mental performance have demonstrated that exercise has a small to moderate effect on a range of cognitive abilities across the lifespan. In older adults, consistent benefits have been shown in *speed of processing*, as in simple response time; *visuospatial and selective attention,* such as the ability to compare line drawings or to selectively attend to stimuli or objects in the environment without distraction; *executive function,* a set of abilities related to inhibiting unwanted actions, multitasking, or juggling information in one's mind such as mentally carrying out long-division; and *declarative memory,* which refers to the ability to remember previous events like the face and name of someone you met at a party last week. Across studies with older adults ages 55 to 80 years, several moderating variables have been identified that may result in greater effects of exercise on mental performance. In regard to exercise type, a combination of strength and aerobic training seems to result in greater effects than either alone. In regard to participant characteristics, women seem to benefit more than men and participants between ages 66 and 70 years may benefit more than younger or older adults. In regard to duration, 30- to 45-minute exercise sessions over 6 months

have produced a larger benefit than shorter training periods. Since many of these studies included previously sedentary participants, it does not take long for benefits to occur. Yet the question of how long benefits last and what type of exercise is optimal for maintenance of cognitive benefits is open for future research. It is also important to note that moderating variables such as these remain an active area of research in exercise neuroscience.

Exercise's Influence on Human Brain Structure

Exercise impacts performance in part through enhancement of structural properties of the brain. For example, aging typically results in shrinkage of brain volume in the frontal and temporal association cortices. This can be measured using *in vivo* brain imaging technology called magnetic resonance imaging (MRI). However, studies have shown that greater physical activity (e.g., distance walked) or moderate aerobic exercise training over 6 months (walking at 60%–70% HR max) among older adults is associated with greater gray matter volume in the frontal and temporal cortices and greater white matter volume in the frontal cortex. Gray matter refers to where neurons expend their energy for information processing and form their connections with communication points called *synapses*. White matter represents the part of neurons that transmit neuronal activity between different areas of the brain and is composed primarily of myelin, which insulates the transmission "wires" (known as *axons*) of neurons and increases the speed of neural communication.

Increases in gray matter from exercise could therefore be from increases in the number of connective branches a neuron forms to communicate with other neurons. In some brain regions like the hippocampus, exercise may actually accelerate normal generation of new neurons (*neurogenesis*). In contrast, changes in white matter could result from increased myelination production or repair or from increases in the number of axons that branch out from the neuron. Increases in the number and thickness of blood vessels could also contribute to increases in brain volume as measured in humans; blood vessels traverse through gray and white matter and are not well identified on typical brain scans that have been used in most studies to date. However, there is evidence that exercise training increases cerebral blood flow in the hippocampus in humans, which is consistent with animal studies. One reason enhanced blood flow is important is because energy for neuronal processing, and therefore information processing, is transmitted to brain cells through increases in blood flow. Therefore, greater resting cerebral blood flow is thought to predict greater responsiveness to the energy demands of information processing.

In sum, while aging results in gray and white matter volume decline in the frontal and temporal association areas, aerobic exercise has been shown to attenuate this atrophy through mechanisms of neuroplasticity that increase the connective branching of neurons, volume of insulating myelination, density of synaptic connections, and through increased birth and survival of brain cells in the hippocampus. Future research will continue to examine the cellular and molecular mechanisms of changes in human brain volume after exercise training.

Exercise's Influence on Human Brain Function

Contrasted to brain structure, brain function refers to how well neurons and their support system can coordinate activity to support ongoing thoughts, emotions, perceptions, and behaviors. Using MRI, the effects of exercise on brain function have been studied by either examining how well different parts of the brain respond to demand for information processing, which we call task-evoked functional MRI (fMRI), or by examining how well different regions in the brain activate in teams (functional networks) that we know support coordinated mental performance. Some studies have also used more direct neuronal stimulation methods like transcranial magnetic stimulation (TMS) to study the link between regular exercise and synaptic plasticity.

When examined with task-evoked fMRI, aging studies have examined activation during executive function tasks. Executive function tasks are of interest because they are known to engage the prefrontal cortices, which are areas of the brain that become dysfunctional with increasing age. In turn, studies have found that more aerobically fit older adults have more prefrontal brain activation during executive function performance. For example, one study found that greater aerobic fitness was associated with greater prefrontal activation during the Stroop task, which requires responding to the ink color of a word regardless of what the word says. Because of the automaticity of reading, the Stroop task is cognitively demanding and it requires coordinated brain activity in prefrontal and visual cortex. Importantly, greater fitness was only associated with greater prefrontal activity and not visual cortex activity.

Similarly, a training study found that 6 months of walking training in sedentary older adults resulted in increased prefrontal cortex activity during a task requiring attentional focus and inhibitory control, and that greater prefrontal activity was coupled with greater task performance. These studies support that aerobic exercise benefits mental performance in part through enhancement of prefrontal cortex function. Recent research also supports a beneficial effect of resistance training on brain activation associated with inhibition and memory processes that rely on areas outside the prefrontal cortex, suggesting resistance training may play a complementary role to aerobic training in supporting brain function across the lifespan.

Evidence also exists demonstrating that aerobic exercise is associated with greater coordination of brain activity—in regard to both broad brain networks and to synaptic plasticity in specific neuronal circuits. Brain networks are teams of physically distant regions that work in coordination and provide a system for the brain to carry out highly specific, local processes that feed up to coordinated, complex processes; neural plasticity is the foundation for these functional networks to maintain coordinated teamwork. In one study, older adults with greater aerobic fitness had greater functional coactivation in a brain network known as the *default network,* whose deterioration has significant implications for cognitive aging, risk for dementia, and a host of developmental psychiatric disorders. Exercise effects were strongest in the lateral and ventromedial prefrontal regions and the temporal cortex, including the hippocampus. Importantly, this research also suggests that greater functional coordination in the default network is associated with some of the cognitive benefits that are linked to aerobic fitness, suggesting this network may be an important component of how exercise improves cognition and decreases risk for dementia in late life. It may also suggest that exercise would be beneficial for developmental disorders related to impaired default network function.

Finally, there is evidence that greater aerobic fitness is associated with greater TMS-induced synaptic plasticity. The basis of learning is the brain's ability to form new neural connections or to strengthen existing pathways based on experience. One way to study this is to pair stimulation of a hand muscle with electromagnetic stimulation of a corresponding region of motor cortex. The capacity for synaptic plasticity in this circuit can be measured by the increase in reactivity of the hand muscle to activation of the motor cortex following paired training. One study showed that more active adults had greater synaptic plasticity in the specific motor circuit studied. Although this was a cross-sectional study, it presents complementary evidence for the link between aerobic fitness and enhanced synaptic plasticity that may be a generalizable mechanism for the effect of exercise on coordinated brain function and improved learning and performance.

Overall, there is exciting evidence for exercise's potential to attenuate age-related brain dysfunction, and these results have implications for improving the brain's capacity to learn and respond adaptively to injury at any age. However, the mechanisms for how this happens are not fully understood and future research should be guided by the need to understand the cellular and molecular basis of these benefits.

Michelle W. Voss

See also Brain Imaging; Cognitive Function; Information Processing; Interventions for Exercise and Physical Activity; Learning; Neuroscience, Exercise, and Cognitive Function; Sedentary Behavior; Skill Acquisition

Further Readings

Colcombe, S., & Kramer, A. F. (2003). Fitness effects on the cognitive function of older adults: A meta-analytic study. *Psychological Science, 14*(2), 125–130.

Cirillo, J., Lavender, A. P., Ridding, M. C., & Semmler, J. G. (2009). Motor cortex plasticity induced by paired associative stimulation is enhanced in physically active individuals. *The Journal of Physiology, 587*(24), 5831–5842.

Hillman, C. H., Erickson, K. I., & Kramer, A. F. (2008). Be smart, exercise your heart: Exercise effects on brain and cognition. *Nature Reviews Neuroscience, 9*(1), 58–65.

Thomas, A. G., Dennis, A., Bandettini, P. A., & Johansen-Berg, H. (2012). The effects of aerobic activity on brain structure. *Frontiers in Psychology, 3*, 86.

Voss, M. W., Nagamatsu, L. S., Liu-Ambrose, T., & Kramer, A. F. (2011). Exercise, brain, and cognition across the lifespan. *Journal of Applied Physiology, 111*, 1505–1513.

BRAIN IMAGING

Neuroimaging includes various techniques that either directly or indirectly image the structure and the function of the human brain. Thus, neuroimaging can be divided into two categories: structural imaging and functional imaging.

Structural imaging examines the structure of the brain (like gray and white matter) and the possible changes that occur in these structures with factors such as learning and aging. Popular methods to investigate changes in brain structure include voxel-based morphometry (VBM), which enables investigation of changes in the brain's anatomy, and diffusion tensor imaging (DTI), which enables examination of image neural tracts by measuring the restricted diffusion of water in the brain.

In contrast, functional imaging is used to observe the working brain. Functional brain imaging offers new insights into topics that lie at the heart of sport psychology. For example, research on motor imagery has reached a new level demonstrating that motor imagery is based on neural activation of core motor areas in the brain. This widely accepted finding has dramatically influenced approaches to motor rehabilitation.

Imaging of the living brain has to deal with the fundamental problem of the scale of observation. Research on the mirror neuron system (MNS), for example, is based on single-cell recordings in the monkey brain. However, cognitive neuroscience is typically interested in examining the relevance and interconnectivity of defined whole brain areas during specific tasks. In the case of the MNS, the role of the parietofrontal circuit for action recognition has been uncovered.

Functional imaging enables researchers to identify brain regions whose activation is associated with specific action-linked processes, such as action observation or action imitation processes. Possible methods for this are positron emission tomography (PET) and functional magnetic resonance imaging (fMRI). In PET studies, radioactive-marked molecules (e.g., radioactive-markered glucose) are administered into the participant's blood right before the study. The tomograph detects the radiation and therefore shows exactly where the molecules are being used in the brain. On the other hand, fMRI does not need an injection and is based on the different magnetic properties of the human blood. Both methods examine metabolic brain activity.

In sports and motor neuroscience, most published work uses fMRI because it has good temporal and spatial resolution properties. PET is used less often for research because radioactive-marked molecules have to be administered. Therefore, the fMRI will be described in more detail.

In humans, fMRI has proven to be an efficient method to study task-relevant brain activation. The resting brain is not silent and shows neural activity even during sleep. For this reason, fMRI studies attempt to understand brain activation by examining differences of brain activities between two or more tasks, such as action observation and motor imagery. Research on the functions of brain areas for specific tasks relies heavily on cytoarchitectonic results (structural information about anatomical regions of interest in the brain, based on the cellular composition) and on research with patients with defined cortical lesions.

To map neural activity, fMRI uses the change of blood oxygen flow within the brain. More precisely, the measurements rely on the different magnetic properties of oxygen-rich and oxygen-poor blood. Oxygen-rich blood is diamagnetic and therefore has less impact on the magnetic field, whereas oxygen-poor blood is paramagnetic, which leads to stronger interferences in the magnetic field. Thus, the strength of the measured signal depends on the degree of the oxygenation of the blood. The dependency between the image quality and the oxygen saturation of the blood is called *blood oxygenation level dependency* (BOLD). Changing blood flow and the related BOLD response is directly associated with neural activation in a certain brain region.

During fMRI scanning, it is necessary for participants to lie in a strong, permanent magnetic field with high homogeneity. Certain nuclei in the human body, the hydrogen nuclei, provide magnetic properties. Being in a strong magnetic field, hydrogen nuclei behave like a compass needle; they all align with the magnetic field. During fMRI scanning, radiofrequency impulses are applied to the aligned magnetic system. This results in a change of the orientation of the hydrogen nuclei. After the radio pulse ceases, the hydrogen nuclei return to their original orientation by emitting energy, which is detected by an antenna of the system. The source of this signal is specified by magnetic field gradients that vary the strength of the magnetic field and hence allow determination of the specific signal source and position. The position of the brain in the magnetic field is defined at the very beginning of the experiment. Therefore, it is crucial for the later analysis of the data that the participants do not move their head during the experiment. Otherwise a mislocalization of a detected increased activation may be possible.

Experimental Designs

Generally, science starts with a research question that in turn generates (neuroanatomical) hypotheses, which can then be tested by performing an experiment. For fMRI, the experimental strategy is to observe the brain's response (the BOLD response) to certain kinds of stimulation: for example, an observation task with different body movements. Over the last decade, three design types have dominated fMRI studies: the *blocked design*, the *event-related design*, and the *mixed design*. These designs vary in terms of stimulus presentation and timing. The blocked design is characterized by presenting a time interval with stimuli of only one condition, alternating this with intervals representing stimuli of other conditions. The main advantage of this type of paradigm is increased statistical power and robustness. In contrast, the event-related design presents random short-duration events drawn from the different conditions within the experiment, providing superior temporal resolution characteristics. This approach permits the temporal characterization of BOLD signal changes. A mixed design contains features of both these design types.

After completed data collection, the critical question is whether there are differences or commonalities between the different experimental conditions. To test for this, several types of comparison are possible. One central comparison strategy is the subtraction method, in which the BOLD response for the experimental condition has subtracted from it the BOLD response acquired from the control condition. The factorial strategy is an alternative to the subtraction strategy in which all experimental conditions are processed as experimental factors. This strategy also allows testing for interactions between the conditions. Some experimental tasks show different levels of difficulty. Given this, a parametric design can be used to test whether there is an increase of the BOLD effect that systematically varies with an increase of task difficulty. Each of the comparison strategies aims to detect differences between experimental conditions. In contrast, a conjunction analysis offers the possibility to detect the commonalities between the BOLD patterns of two conditions by calculating the intersection between the two conditions.

Implications

Functional magnetic resonance imaging (fMRI) has already had a strong impact on research in fields, such as action observation, motor imagery, and attention, and has great potential to impact other key topics in sport psychology and motor control as interactive actions, emotion, and empathy. Recently, imaging genetics has started to reveal new directions for brain imaging. Genes have an effect on neural activity on the molecular level. Different concentrations of neurotransmitters moderate neural activity in different cognitive tasks. Brain imaging may help to elucidate this complex interaction between genes and neural activity.

The striking development of functional brain imaging has been driven by the technical advances of the last 20 years; fMRI has become a standard tool in cognitive neuroscience. It is complemented by magnetoencephalograpy (MEG), which records magnetic fields produced by electrical currents in the working human brain; near infrared spectroscopy (NIRS), which measures changes in cerebral blood flow, similar to fMRI but vulnerable to movement, only useful on the cortex, and does not reach deeper regions; and electroencephalography (EEG), which measures electrical activity along the scalp. EEG also offers tools for functional brain imaging with low-resolution brain electromagnetic tomography (LORETA). These methods differ with respect to the fundamental limitations concerning the range of active movements feasible during data recording, with EEG and NIRS offering an advantage in this regard.

There has been no doubt that the advent of new methods of brain imaging, data recording, and data analysis has facilitated progress in understanding cognitive processes. Neuroimaging must build on, rather than replace, the importance of well-designed research with strong theory-driven hypotheses.

Jörn Munzert and Britta Lorey

See also Biofeedback, Neurofeedback; Brain; Cognitive Function; Imagery; Perception; Psychophysiology; Social Neuroscience

Further Readings

Amaro, E., Jr., & Barker, G. J. (2006). Study design in fMRI: Basic principles. *Brain and Cognition, 60,* 220–232.

Baars, B. J., & Romsøy, T. (2007). The tools: Imaging the living brain. In B. J. Baars & N. M. Gage (Eds.), *Cognition, brain, and consciousness: Introduction to cognitive neuroscience* (pp. 87–120). Amsterdam: Elsevier.

Eickhoff, S. B., Lotze, M., Wietek, B., Amunts, K., Enck, P., & Zilles, K. (2006). Segregation of visceral and somatosensory afferents: An fMRI and cytoarchitectonic mapping study. *NeuroImage, 31,* 1004–1014.

Huettel, S. A., Song, A. W., & McCarthy, G. (2008). *Functional magnetic resonance imaging* (2nd ed.). Sunderland, MA: Sinauer Associates.

Logothetis, N. K., Pauls, J., Augath, M., Trinath, T., & Oeltermann, A. (2001). Neurophysiological investigation of the basis of the fMRI signal. *Nature, 412,* 150–157.

BREATHING EXERCISES

Breathing strategies are often used as the basis for several advanced relaxation techniques, including progressive muscular relaxation, meditation, and calming imagery. However, breathing strategies act as an important technique in their own right to help physically and mentally relax the performer. Provided here is a synopsis of breathing exercises, based on the guidelines by Jean M. Williams, that includes diaphragmatic breathing, rhythmical breathing, and sighing when exhaling as strategies commonly advocated by applied sport psychologists to help relax athletes.

Diaphragmatic Breathing

Sometimes called complete breathing, diaphragmatic breathing is a physical relaxation strategy oriented around filling the lungs to capacity from bottom to top and emptying the lungs in a slow, controlled, and complete manner. Athletes should use a deep, long, and slow inhalation through the nose to completely fill the lungs. To help athletes achieve this, applied sport psychologists should ask the athlete to view their lungs as a three-section cavity. First, the athlete should inhale and simultaneously relax the stomach, pulling their diaphragm muscles down to fill the lower section of their lungs. Second, the rib cage should be lifted, the chest cavity expanded to fill the mid-section of the lungs, and then the shoulder blades widened to fill the lungs to the top. A slow, continuous, smooth, and controlled inhalation should be used throughout by the performer. The exhalation phase is just as important to invoking a relaxed state; here, the athlete should reverse the process described above by exhaling the top of the lungs first, then the chest cavity, and finally the lower section. Emphasis should be given to expelling air from the bottom of the lungs to complete a full exhalation, with a reduction in muscular tension and anxieties being associated with the air leaving the lungs. Throughout the exhalation phase, the muscles of the diaphragm and those surrounding the stomach should be used to help push the air from the lungs to facilitate a complete emptying of lung capacity. Athletes should be asked to associate a feeling of calmness and quietness with the final exhalation stage of the breath cycle to help invoke a completely relaxed state.

Rhythmical Breathing

Rhythmical breathing acts as an extension to diaphragmatic breathing where ratios of holding one's breath during inhalation and exhalation are suggested to control breath rate and help keep physical tension and mental anxieties under control. To create a symmetrical rhythm within their breathing cycle, athletes should inhale to a specific count of time (e.g., 3 seconds), hold their breath for the same time count, exhale to the same time count, and pause for the same count before repeating the cycle. Once proficient in this symmetrical rhythmical breathing technique, a different ratio of time count between inhalation to exhalation should be explored to help invoke a more relaxed state. For example, using a ratio of 1:2, athletes should take a symmetrical rhythmical first breath (i.e., a 1:1 ratio, inhale for 3 seconds and exhale for 3 seconds); then, on the next inhalation, they should inhale to the same count of 3 seconds and extend

the exhalation phase over a 6-second period (i.e., a 1:2 ratio). To achieve this, the performer should be encouraged to exhale more slowly and with greater control and awareness of this phase of the breath cycle. Alternative ratios should be explored by the performer to help create greater control and awareness of the inhalation–exhalation phases of the breath cycle to help create a powerful sense of control over the rhythm of breathing and thus the relaxed state of the athlete. The benefits of adopting a rhythmical breathing rate include lowered heart rate, better oxygen utilization, and lowered muscular tension and mental anxiety.

Sighing When Exhaling

This breathing strategy is a very simple, quick approach that can be used to help relax athletes. Specifically, if tension is perceived by athletes, they should exhale fully and powerfully through the mouth with an audible sigh, and then inhale slowly and quietly through the nose. The performer should repeat the process using the muscles around the rib cage to fully expel the air in the lungs so that tension within the body is reduced.

Conclusions

The strategies outlined in this entry illustrate how breathing control can help athletes achieve a relaxed state. In general, studies testing intervention effects have noted the positive effects of breathing strategies on enhancing performance. Further, these findings are relatively consistent across different sports and different competitive level athletes, from elite to non-elite. Additionally, studies that have assessed the psychological skill use of athletes have noted that elite performers tend to use relaxation strategies (including breathing exercises) more readily when preparing for performance than their non-elite counterparts. However, research has yet to establish whether one particular breathing strategy or a specific combination of various breathing strategies is more effective than another at helping to relax the athlete. Therefore, the broad recommendations that emerge from the applied research are that applied sport psychologists should teach the performers a range of breathing strategies and allow them to explore which is most useful for them given their needs. Performers should practice these breathing strategies in nonsporting stress-inducing situations (e.g., waiting in line in a shop, dealing with a difficult situation at work) before progressing to test the efficacy of the given strategy in a sporting context. Ideally, the strategies should be practiced in training environments before being utilized in the competitive arena.

Owen Thomas and Richard Neil

See also Centering; Mindfulness; Relaxation; Stress Management

Further Readings

Hanton, S., Thomas, O., & Mellalieu, S. (2009). Management of competitive stress in elite sport. In B. W. Brewer (Ed.), *Handbook of sport medicine and science: Sport psychology* (pp. 30–42). Chichester, UK: Wiley-Blackwell.

Vealey, R. S. (2007). Mental skills training in sport. In G. Tenenbaum & R. C. Eklund (Eds.), *Handbook of sport psychology* (pp. 287–309). Hoboken, NJ: Wiley.

Williams, J. M. (2010). Relaxation and energizing techniques for regulation of arousal. In J. M. Williams (Ed.), *Applied sport psychology: Personal growth to peak performance* (6th ed., pp. 247–266). New York: McGraw-Hill.

Burnout

Modern sport culture is replete with qualities thought to make burnout prevalent, including high training volumes and competitive demands, near year-round training, and in some sports, specialization at young ages. Given this sport landscape and the concerns raised by sport scientists and others involved in the sport community (coaches and administrators), the importance of athlete burnout is now widely recognized. This entry defines athlete burnout, describes its epidemiological significance, discusses potential causes, and concludes by addressing preventive strategies.

Defining Athlete Burnout

The term *burnout* is used in a variety of contexts in everyday discourse. Although some of these meanings converge with scientific uses of the term, others do not. Burnout is sometimes used synonymously with the term *sport drop-out*. However, not all athletes who drop out of sport do so because of burnout; athletes may leave sport for any of a myriad of reasons. Although some athletes who do experience burnout will discontinue sport, others may maintain their involvement. Others may compete at a lower, less demanding, level or they may choose to participate in a different sport. Thus, the term *burnout* should not be used interchangeably with the term *sport drop-out*.

Within the scientific community, burnout has a more precise meaning than that often used in everyday language. The most widely accepted definition casts athlete burnout as a psychological syndrome of emotional and physical exhaustion, a reduced sense of accomplishment, and sport devaluation. Athletes experiencing burnout may be emotionally exhausted from dealing with continual stresses of competition, training, and other demands for their time (work, school). They may also feel physically exhausted from high training loads. Another key factor involved in burnout is a reduced sense of accomplishment in which athletes question and doubt their sport skills and ability to be successful. They may feel they are training hard yet making minimal progress toward their goals. Finally, sport devaluation is represented by a psychological detachment from sport in which athletes may stop caring about sport and their performance to the point of developing a resentful attitude toward sport.

Epidemiological Significance

Although the modern culture of sport has characteristics that suggest burnout may be on the rise, the actual prevalence of burnout is unknown. Research surveying current athletes suggests that a low percentage of athletes (e.g., 2%–10%) have relatively high scores on a self-report burnout measure as assessed via the Athlete Burnout Questionnaire, or psychological characteristics suggesting they may be experiencing burnout. Research surveying current athletes suggests that a low percentage (e.g., 2%–10%) have characteristics suggesting they are experiencing burnout. However, surveying current athletes may underestimate its occurrence as some athletes who experience burnout may have left sport or have been absent from practice when the questionnaire was administered.

Even if burnout is not very prevalent, it has epidemiological significance because of the millions of sport participants across the globe and the negative toll it has on individuals suffering from it. Although minimal research has examined its consequences, burnout can potentially have negative impact on all spheres of an athlete's life, both within and outside of sport. Within sport, burnout is thought to lead to performance decrements, decreased motivation, and possibly sport discontinuation. Beyond sport, it can hurt physical and psychological well-being as well as negatively impact personal relationships.

If athletes do experience burnout, it is not something that will dissipate after a short break from sport—rather burnout is often chronic in nature. Consequently, it is important to structure sport in a way that prevents burnout rather than attempting to treat it once it occurs given its relatively enduring state. Developing effective prevention strategies is predicated on first understanding what causes burnout.

Potential Causes of Burnout

It is widely accepted that burnout is a reaction to chronic stress and occurs when demands associated with sport participation exceed or tax an individual's resources over an extended time period. Thus, burnout is linked to an imbalance between demands and resources.

Demands involve all the stressors involved in sport. These stressors, at least in many sports, stem from the physical demands associated with training. In some cases, burnout may be the result of overtraining characterized by overly high training volumes (duration x intensity) coupled with inadequate recovery. In addition, the time demands associated with sport can also be a contributing factor to burnout, in which athletes feel that sport takes too much time and results in their missing out on other life opportunities. Finally, the pressure associated with competition may be another source of stress associated with burnout.

A variety of external influences, such as pressure from coaches and parents, may also be sources of chronic stress associated with burnout. For example, overinvolved parents may create excessive pressure that predisposes athletes to burnout. On a more subtle level, parents who are supportive of their child's sport experience, but whose family life centers around sport, may also predispose athletes to burnout. Additional parental characteristics associated with burnout include setting high standards for their children coupled with being critical of their children and their performances.

Finally, coaches, through their leadership style and interactions with athletes, may also create a sport culture or team atmosphere that may make burnout more likely. Athletes who play for coaches who are perceived as being socially supportive, empathetic, and who provide praise, instructions, and training and a democratic coaching style have lower burnout compared with other athletes. In contrast, autocratic and aversive-style coaches who create a fear of failure in athletes may make burnout more likely.

Finally, the demands associated with sport can come from internal sources. Some athletes have personality qualities that make them vulnerable to burnout. For example, athletes who are perfectionistic, characterized by excessively high performance standards and self-doubt, are at risk of burnout. Related to perfectionism, athletes who base their self-esteem on performance accomplishments are more likely to experience chronic stress and burnout. Also, athletes who are pessimistic are more likely to experience burnout compared to those who are optimistic. Finally, athletes who are *trait anxious*, defined as predisposition to experience high levels of anxiety, are more likely to experience burnout than those with low trait anxiety.

Although burnout is a response to chronic stress, not all athletes who are in demanding sport environments experience burnout. Coping resources also play a role in the burnout process. Resources are the internal and external factors athletes have available that help them effectively manage stress. They include external factors such as social support and participation in activities that facilitate recovery. They also include internal resources such as self-awareness, strong self-regulatory skills, and effective lifestyle management skills that include healthy eating habits and good sleep habits. For example, having a good life balance wherein athletes are involved in more than just sport and potentially the strong use of mental skills training techniques may also serve as coping resources. In addition, athletes who experience low levels of life stress outside of sport are theoretically less vulnerable to burnout compared with those who experience a great deal of stress outside of sport.

At this point, it is widely recognized that burnout, especially exhaustion, is a reaction to chronic stress. Consequently, identifying stress related factors associated with burnout is important to understanding this phenomenon. However, there is more to the burnout process than a simple reaction to chronic stress. Burnout is only experienced when highly committed athletes become disillusioned and frustrated with their sport involvement. Given that burnout is intricately connected to commitment and motivational processes as well as stress, researchers have developed a commitment perspective on burnout, drawing from the organizational psychology and relationship literatures.

On a positive note, athletes can be committed to sport because they are passionate about it. These athletes want to be involved, find it enjoyable, and concomitantly experience high benefits and low costs. Because of their favorable outlook, they are likely to invest a great deal of time and energy into sport and perceive that it is more attractive than alternative options. These athletes are not theoretically likely to burn out as they experience enjoyment-based commitment.

There is another side to commitment. Although commitment can be influenced by positive pulls (e.g., passion, enjoyment, satisfaction), it can also be affected by nonpositive pushes (e.g., too much invested to quit, lack of attractive alternatives, social pressure to continue involvement). In other words, athletes can be committed for a combination of reasons related to *wanting to be* involved and feeling they *have to be* involved. Entrapment-based commitment occurs when athletes begin to have a more negative view toward sport (e.g., decreasing positive pulls) but maintain their involvement because they feel they have to continue (i.e., increasing nonpositive pushes). These athletes feel they are trapped and stifled by sport while missing out on other life opportunities. This is evident by decreasing enjoyment coupled with decreasing benefits and increasing costs. Despite this, they maintain involvement because of feeling locked into the role of being an athlete. They may feel there is too much invested to quit; perceive few attractive alternatives to being an athlete; or perceive that other people, such as coaches, teammates, or parents, expect them to maintain their involvement.

In addition to these sources of entrapment, two additional factors that may result in athletes, especially adolescent sport participants, feeling trapped by sport include a unidimensional identity and low perceived control. In normal development, adolescents sample a variety of activities and roles in the process of forming their personal identities. The teenage years are also characterized by the development of personal autonomy. However, sport participation, especially high-level involvement, can result in athletes prematurely developing a unidiemsional identity, which increases the risk of burnout. In addition, although they may have chosen initially to participate, in some situations, adults control their sport experience, resulting in feelings of low control over the sport involvement. Having a unidimensional identity whereby their sense of self is based exclusively on being an athlete, as well as low perceived autonomy, may result in athletes experiencing sport entrapment and their feeling trapped into the role of being an athlete. This theoretically increases the risk of burnout.

Converging with a commitment perspective, athletes who are passionate about sport view it as important and invest a great deal of time and energy into sport. Much like commitment, passion is not something athletes simply have or do not have, rather there are different types. One type is an obsessive passion for sport that is associated with higher burnout scores, at least in some research. The other type, harmonious passion, is characterized by a more intrinsically motivated type of passion associated with lower burnout scores.

Given that burnout is linked to an erosion of motivation, researchers are using common motivation theories, such as self-determination, and achievement motivation theories to better understand the burnout process and what potentially might predispose athletes to it. According to self-determination, the fulfillment of basic psychological needs, including perceived competence (positive perception of skills and abilities), autonomy (sense of say and control over their sport involvement), and relatedness (sense of belonging and acceptance), is associated with higher levels of well-being. The fulfillment of these basic needs is also connected with quality motivation such as high levels of intrinsic motivation, whereby athletes participate for the inherent pleasure and satisfaction derived from sport participation. In contrast, need thwarting is associated with indices of ill-being, including burnout. Burnout and the lack of need fulfillment are also associated with low-quality motivation. On the extreme level, this can include being amotivated (without motivation). On a less extreme level, lower quality motivation characterizes athletes who participate not because they want to but, rather, because they feel they have to be involved in sport. This can be due to either external pressure by a coach or parent or internal pressures of feelings of obligation to remain involved.

Another common motivation theory, achievement motivation, which has been used to understand burnout, focuses on whether athletes and the team atmosphere are mastery oriented or outcome oriented. With a mastery team climate, success is defined in terms of effort, learning, and improvement. In contrast, outcome-oriented team climates focus on social comparison and doing better than others. In a mastery-oriented climate, mistakes are viewed as part of the learning process, whereas in an outcome-oriented climate, they are viewed negatively and punished. Although studying burnout from an achievement goal perspective has not received extensive investigation, mastery-oriented team climates are generally thought to be associated with lower burnout scores compared to athletes who view the team climate as more outcome oriented.

Preventing Burnout

Nearly all of the scientific literature on burnout has been either correlational or qualitative in nature. The focus of the correlational research has been to examine the association of scores on a burnout measure with other variables that are theoretically related to or potential causes of burnout. The qualitative studies have focused on in-depth interviews of athletes who experienced burnout to better understand the burnout process. At this point, very few, if any, studies have evaluated the effectiveness of interventions designed to prevent or treat burnout. Thus, the knowledge based on intervention strategies is not well developed and comments on preventive strategies are provided tentatively.

As a starting point for understanding potential interventions designed to minimize burnout, public health frameworks provide a launching pad. Primary prevention strategies involve changing the sport culture or environment to eliminate or modify factors that potentially cause burnout. Interventions designed to help individuals manage or cope with the stress associated with sport are titled secondary prevention. Finally, interventions helping athletes already suffering from burnout are regarded as a tertiary prevention strategy with a focus on treatment or rehabilitation. As stated in the adage "an ounce of prevention is worth a pound of cure," interventions designed to prevent burnout are more effective than treating burnout once it occurs given its chronic nature.

At this point of knowledge development, one viable strategy to prevent burnout is to target theory-based variables associated with burnout in the intervention design. These can range from individual characteristics associated with stress-related processes (e.g., perfectionism) to the social–organizational structure of sport (e.g., coach and parent behaviors, how sport is structured, and training demands and recovery).

Given that burnout is a reaction to chronic stress, a common belief is that is that teaching athletes stress management skills will help prevent burnout. For example, helping athletes learn effective time management as well as lifestyle management skills will help them deal more effectively with the demands of being an athlete. In addition, an increased focus on recovery activities, as well as helping athletes to achieve a balanced lifestyle, will also help prevent burnout. Mental skills training techniques, such as effective goal setting, self-talk, and relaxation skills may also be effective. If athletes can learn to effectively cope with stress, then burnout will be less likely.

Although stress management strategies have a role in preventing burnout, it is premature to conclude that teaching athletes stress management skills geared at the individual will be the most effective intervention approach. In fact, researchers in organizational psychology argue that teaching individuals stress management strategies have not been very effective in reducing burnout. This is because social–environmental factors have a larger role in work burnout than individual factors. The same is likely true for athletes. Thus, interventions that target the sport environment will be more efficacious than those that target the individual and focus on helping athletes effectively manage stress. Taken one step further, some scholars suggest that teaching athletes how to cope with stress is analogous to treating burnout with a bandage. Rather than addressing the underlying cause of burnout, which is how sport is structured, teaching stress management only addresses the surface of the problem.

In addition to teaching stress management as part of life skill development, interventions need to address social–environmental modifications designed to create a more positive sport experience for athletes. Consequently, commitment and motivation theories should play a role in designing effective interventions targeting burnout. For example, strategies could be developed to help ensure that sport fulfills the basic psychological needs of perceived competence, autonomy, and relatedness. In addition, coaches who create a mastery-oriented team climate will help prevent burnout. Sport could be structured in a way that empowers athletes by developing multifaceted identities and that gives them control over their sport experiences. Finally, interventions designed to enhance enjoyment-based commitment and minimized feelings of entrapment should be central components of interventions. Given that burnout is a complex process, interventions that are multimodal in nature will be the most effective.

Conclusion

Although most athletes do not experience burnout, it is nonetheless a significant issue within contemporary sport culture. Although the term *burnout* conjures a variety of images, it is best defined as a psychological syndrome involving exhaustion, sport devaluation, and a reduced sense of accomplishment. Burnout is a complex issue that involves both stress- and motivation-related processes. Given its complexity, research addressing antecedents, underlying processes, and consequences associated with burnout will serve as the foundation for designing effective interventions. Interventions designed to prevent burnout should be multimodal and target both stress and motivation processes.

Thomas D. Raedeke

See also Affective Disorders; Emotional Reactivity; Injury, Psychological Susceptibility to; Overtraining Syndrome; Stress Reactivity; Underrecovery Syndrome

Further Readings

Coakley, J. (1992). Burnout among adolescent athletes: A personal failure or social problem? *Sociology of Sport Journal, 9,* 271–285.

Eklund, R. C., & Cresswell, S. L. (2007). Athlete burnout. In G. Tenenbaum & R. C. Eklund (Eds.), *Handbook of sport psychology* (3rd ed., pp. 621–641). Hoboken, NJ: Wiley.

Raedeke, T. D. (1997). Is athlete burnout more than just stress? A sport commitment perspective. *Journal of Sport & Exercise Psychology, 19,* 396–417.

Raedeke, T. D., & Smith, A. L. (2009). *The Athlete Burnout Questionnaire Test manual.*

Smith, R. E. (1986). Toward a cognitive-affective model of athletic burnout. *Journal of Sport Psychology, 8,* 36–50.

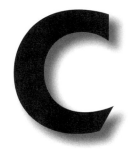

CALO-RE Taxonomy of Behavior Change Techniques

The Coventry, Aberdeen, and London—Refined (CALO-RE) taxonomy of behavior change techniques builds on initial work on classifying psychological techniques used in intervention to change behavior, with a particular emphasis on physical activity and healthy eating. The taxonomy aims to provide a common language for the organization, identification, and adoption of behavior change techniques in interventions. The taxonomy is a tool for researchers designing effective interventions that work and practitioners wishing to identify the techniques that will be most effective in changing physical activity behavior. The taxonomy is based on Charles Abraham and Susan Michie's initial taxonomy of behavior change techniques refined to eliminate inconsistencies. The taxonomy provides a reference guide for each technique and the psychological constructs it purports to change. Forty-three techniques are specified in CALO-RE. Each has a specific definition derived from systematic reviews of intervention research independently coded and verified by leading experts. The definitions also specify exclusions and exceptions ensuring that the techniques do not overlap. The CALO-RE taxonomy does not specify the theories from which the techniques are derived; this information was supplied by Abraham and Michie. The taxonomy provides a standardized set of common terms to facilitate understanding of interventions, enable better evaluation of the effectiveness of specific intervention techniques, and provide insight into the psychological mediators that explain the process by which the technique works in changing behavior.

Behavior Change Theory and the Taxonomy

A vast array of psychological factors, such as self-efficacy, attitudes, motivation, intentions, and risk perceptions, have been found to be linked to physical activity behavior. Such antecedents are important as it is assumed that such variables can be manipulated or changed through techniques communicated to individuals by various means like one-to-one consultations or via the media. While interventions targeting psychological factors have led to increased physical activity participation, their effectiveness has been shown to be relatively modest. A key reason is that interventions do not adequately identify the intervention techniques that will be successful in changing the psychological constructs known to be correlated with physical activity. This means that the techniques used may not be completely effective in changing behavior as they do not lead to a change in the psychological constructs, known as psychological mediators, associated with physical activity. Another problem in intervention research is that the reporting of the intervention components adopted to change physical activity behavior is inadequate. This limits the extent to which other researchers will be able to replicate the findings and limits the inferences that those aiming to synthesize research can make with regard to the effectiveness of specific techniques in changing the psychological constructs and changing behavior. A final problem is that many interventions adopt multiple behavior change techniques that seek to target multiple psychological mediators. While adoption of multiple techniques can be effective in bringing about behavior change, it limits researchers' ability to identify which of the techniques was responsible for bringing about the change. Researchers will, therefore, be unable to arrive at a definitive conclusion as to which of the intervention techniques are *doing the work* in changing behavior.

These issues have led to calls for (1) identifying and classifying the intervention techniques that target specific antecedents of physical activity through a mapping process, (2) improved reporting of behavior change techniques within reports of intervention trials, and (3) improvements in the design of interventions to provide tests of individual techniques identified in the mapping process on physical activity behavior change. Recent developments in the taxonomy of behavior change techniques have led to a direct mapping of specific techniques on to the psychological antecedents of behavior change. This has provided researchers and practitioners with a menu of strategies from which to choose when designing interventions as well as identifying any overlaps and gaps.

Methods and Development

The lists that Abraham and Michie used to develop their taxonomy mixed general theoretical approaches, modes of delivery, and intervention settings. Therefore, a refined taxonomy of 26 clearly defined behavior change techniques was developed so as to overcome these issues and allow reliable coding of interventions. Three systematic reviews were then completed to assess whether the behavior change techniques could be used to identify core components of behavior change interventions. The 26 behavior change technique definitions resulted in 93% agreement between raters, and acceptable interrater reliability levels for most of the definitions.

Since the publication of the original behavior change technique taxonomy, which has been widely adopted and used in reviews, researchers have identified further opportunities to improve the classification. Researchers at Coventry, Aberdeen, and London collaborated to identify limitations, such as lack of clarity or disagreement between raters, with Abraham and Michie's

original taxonomy, and to introduce further classifications. Research teams adopted an iterative process of coding one or two research articles, calculating interrater reliability coefficients, and revising the taxonomy accordingly through group discussion. This process resulted in the CALO-RE taxonomy, which has fewer conceptual problems and less overlap between items and is more comprehensive.

The Techniques

The 40 behavior change techniques identified in the CALO-RE taxonomy define and differentiate techniques, offering researchers and practitioners a clear guide as to which techniques may be adopted to change physical activity behavior in interventions. There is no guidance on which techniques to adopt or which will be more effective; the purpose is for identification and classification only. An outline of each technique is provided in the next section along with exercise-specific examples of what each technique might look like in an intervention to promote exercise and physical activity.

1. Information provision (general). In this technique, general (not specific) information is provided about physical activity and its possible outcomes. (A poster might provide a statement that "physical activity is enjoyable and fun for all.")

2. Information provision (to the individual). In this technique, specific information relevant to the individual about physical activity and its possible outcomes, consequences, benefits, and costs is given. (A physician might inform a patient that "if you participate in regular physical activity, it will help you to get your weight down and help you to feel less stressed at work.")

3. Information provision (others' approval). In this technique, information is provided about what others' might think of their physical activity. (An exercise specialist might tell a referred patient: "You will find that your family and friends will be very supportive of your new exercise program; they will see a fitter, healthier you!")

4. Information provision (others' behavior). In this technique, information concerning what others typically do with respect to exercise is provided. (A leaflet might inform a potential middle-age person thinking of taking up physical activity that "people over 50 years of age often take up exercise having not ever exercised in the past.")

5. Goal setting (behavior). In this technique, encouragement to begin or maintain behavior change is provided. It does not involve precise planning to do the behavior. (A goal may be to "exercise more next week.")

6. Goal setting (outcome). In this technique, the individual is encouraged to set general goals achievable through performance of the behavior, but distinct from the behavior itself. (A consultant might highlight blood pressure reduction and losing weight as achievable goals derived from regular exercise.)

7. Action planning. In this technique, detailed plans are made including when (e.g., frequency) and where (e.g., in what situation) to act. It is vital that there is a clear link between plans and behavioral responses to specific situational cues. Such plans are often expressed in *if–then* formats. (A business executive's plan might be, "If it is 5 p.m. and everyone is starting to leave the office, then I will collect my gym bag and head for the fitness center.")

8. Identifying barriers and problem resolution. In this technique, after the formation of a clear plan, individuals are tasked with identifying possible barriers to performance and solutions to the possible problems. Barriers may be cognitive, emotional, social, or physical ("I feel too tired to exercise on Fridays—therefore, I will go to sleep earlier on Thursday nights.")

9. Setting graded tasks. In this technique, the target behavior is broken into smaller, more manageable tasks, allowing successful progression in small increments—for instance, writing down a sequence of small steps to accomplish the overall behavior over time.

10. Review of behavioral goals. In this technique, individuals are prompted to review the successful accomplishment of previously set goals and contingencies and further plans made for instances in which goals were missed. (An individual may report not being able to exercise 5 times a week due to other commitments, so reschedules allotted

times to exercise at more convenient times or fits it into a work schedule by walking to work.)

11. Review of outcome goals. In this technique, an individual will review the attainment of previously set outcome goals and be given an opportunity to revise the goals. (At a routine check-up, a physician might encourage an exerciser to revise the blood pressure or weight goal and modify the physical activity regime accordingly to enhance chances for success.)

12. Effort or progress contingent rewards. In this technique, the person uses rewards or praise for *attempts* at achieving the goal. This is not reward for engaging in the behavior itself and is not contingent on actual success. (A trainer might say to an exerciser, "Well done, you have really tried hard to attain your goal of three visits to the gym this week.")

13. Successful behavior-contingent rewards. In this technique, rewards for successful performance of the target behavior are provided. The reward may be material or verbal but must be based explicitly engaging in the behavior itself—for instance, providing a reward or incentive for doing some physical activity, regardless of outcome.

14. Shaping. In this technique, graded contingent rewards are provided for movement toward completion of the target behavior. The individual may reward oneself for any increase in physical activity behavior in the first instance (e.g., jogging for 10 minutes as opposed to no activity). The reward schedule becomes progressively more restricted in later weeks (e.g., rewarding only for 20 minutes of jogging).

15. Generalization of target behavior. In this technique, the person is encouraged to find opportunities to try it in other situations, to ensure the behavior does not become situation specific. (After following a walking program for 2 weeks, a personal trainer will ask the client to try swimming for the same amount of time at the local swimming pool.)

16. Self-monitoring of behavior. In this technique, the person is asked to keep a detailed record of activity and use it as a means to change or modify behavior. This could take the form of a questionnaire or diary focusing on duration, time, and situation in which the physical activity was attempted or completed.

17. Self-monitoring of behavioral outcome. This technique is similar to point 16, but focus is on measurable outcomes of the behavior (e.g., blood pressure or weight reduction).

18. Focus on past success. In this technique, individuals reflect on successful past experience with physical activity as a means to increase motivation to be active in the future. (A person is encouraged to list or write down past successful experiences with physical activity.)

19. Provide feedback on performance. In this technique, individuals receive feedback regarding a recent physical activity success with the aim of increasing motivation to be more active in future. This may take the form of an exercise trainer commenting on, supporting, or critiquing a client's physical activity goals.

20. Informing when *and* where *to perform the behavior.* In this technique, individuals are offered advice and ideas on when and where physical activity could be performed (e.g., providing suggestions on local exercise classes or gyms, local recreation parks, or even to and from the workplace).

21. Instruction on how *to perform the behavior.* In this technique, a person is instructed on exactly how to effectively perform a behavior (e.g., advice on technique in the gym or instruction on correct frequency or duration of cycling to work).

22. Demonstrate behavior. In this technique, the person is shown how to perform an activity. (A gym instructor might give a customer a demonstration of a particular exercise or piece of equipment.)

23. Training to use prompts. In this technique, individuals are given instruction on use of cues as a reminder to perform a behavior. (Encouraging exercisers to use frequently occurring everyday events like a particular time of day or mobile phone alerts, reminds them of the need to initiate their physical activity routine.)

24. Environmental restructuring. In this technique, the individuals are prompted to make changes to their environment in order to facilitate changes in behavior (e.g., informing friends so that they may help prompt physical activity or removing tempting snacks or treats to help maintain weight loss).

25. Agreement of behavioral contract. In this technique, a written agreement between the individual and the practitioner with respect to behavior change is established. (A trainer and client may sign a contract explicitly stating the agreed activities or exercises so there is an explicit record and a sense of commitment on the part of the practitioner and client.)

26. Prompt practice. In this technique, the person is reminded to rehearse and repeat the behavior, or situations that lead to the behavior, helping make the behavior more automated or habitual (e.g., providing people with means to rehearse when they are going to do their exercise routine).

27. Use of follow-up prompts. In this technique, a set of reminders is delivered to a person that has started a behavior change routine in order to help remind them to continue. Over time, as the person becomes better at performing the behavior, reminders and prompts are reduced. These could include providing people with a personal alarm, e-mail, text message, or other reminder to help them recall their physical activity regimen or goal.

28. Facilitate social comparison. In this technique, individuals are encouraged to draw comparisons with others' behavior to increase motivation through modeling. (A person is encouraged to observe other regular exercisers to provide a positive example of technique or commitment.)

29. Plan social support. In this technique, the person is prompted to elicit social support from other people and close relations in order to facilitate successful completion of the behavior. This may take the form of joining clubs or groups involved in physical activity.

30. Prompt identification as role model. In this technique, the person is encouraged to view oneself as an example or role model to others for the behavior. This includes opportunities for the person to persuade others to adopt the behavior because of the benefits inherent in it (e.g., urging friends and family to engage in more physical activity).

31. Prompt anticipated regret. In this technique, expectations of shame, regret, or guilt for failure to accomplish the goal are induced. (The exercise specialist might encourage an exerciser to think about how guilty one would feel if one missed the next gym session.)

32. Fear arousal. In this technique, fear-inducing information aimed at motivating change is provided. (If weight loss is a goal, practitioners might highlight the health risks of being overweight or obese.)

33. Prompt self-talk. In this technique, the person is encouraged to use self-talk before and during activity to provide verbal encouragement and support. (An exercise practitioner might encourage individuals to use mantras or motivational words when they are finding their exercise routine difficult.)

34. Prompt use of imagery. In this technique, the person is provided with instruction on how to use visualization techniques and imagery to facilitate successful completion of the behavior (e.g., imagining completing a given walking distance or lifting heavier weights).

35. Relapse prevention. In this technique, the person is prompted to focus on situations or occasions in which one may relapse, and then develop methods to increase chances of success. (A person following a jogging routine may highlight bad weather as a possible barrier to maintaining the exercise; encouragement to use a treadmill in the gym on cold or rainy days would be a solution.)

36. Stress management. In this technique, the person is encouraged to focus on reducing related stress and improving emotional control in order to reduce these as a barrier and promote health. (A counselor or helper may provide therapy to an individual attempting to increase activity levels in order to reduce the effect of negative emotions on their behavior.)

37. Motivational interviewing. In this technique, specific interviewing techniques to prompt changes by minimizing resistance and resolving ambivalence to change are used. (A therapist may need to express empathy and provide opportunities for the client to express personal reasons to take up exercise.)

38. Time management. In this technique, the person is assisted in managing time efficiently to be able to engage in the desired activity (e.g., using a diary or organizer to plan time).

39. Communication skills training. In this technique, individuals are directed toward improving communication skills and improving interactions with others concerning the behavior. This often involves group work and focuses on listening skills and assertive oration. (An exercise specialist may encourage clients to engage in brief role play, encouraging an exercise partner to come to the gym or go to the local swimming pool with them.)

40. Stimulate anticipation of future rewards. In this technique, individuals are encouraged to consider future rewards associated with the outcome(s), without necessarily reinforcing behavior change (e.g., getting people to consider the possible gains of exercise, including extrinsic rewards like money and intrinsic rewards like satisfaction).

Implications of CALO-RE

The CALO-RE taxonomy provides a comprehensive and standardized protocol for the identification, reporting, and appraisal of behavior-change interventions for health behaviors, including physical activity. The taxonomy provides a common language for the scientific communication of theoretical-based interventions, which not only helps researchers effectively describe, interpret, and code behavioral-change strategies in interventions that directly link to theoretical constructs, but also establishes a basis for practitioners to accurately evaluate and apply behavior change techniques derived from previous research. The taxonomy assists in the systematic accumulation of knowledge of behavior change techniques from previous research trials and improves the precision for the implementation of multiple theoretical frameworks applied for the promotion of physical activity.

The development of the taxonomy offers a number of avenues for future research and applied practice in behavior-change interventions for physical activity. First, CALO-RE provides a rigorous and systematic procedure that helps correctly map theoretical constructs into behavioral change techniques, so it becomes more realistic to test the effectiveness of individual theoretical components within an intervention. Second, interventions can be optimized by identifying and eliminating overlapping or redundant elements of the behavioral change techniques driven by multiple theoretical components or frameworks. Third, the enhanced connection between theoretical knowledge and behavioral change techniques may enable researchers to reveal the underlying mechanisms of the intention and behaviors of physical activity.

Martin S. Hagger, David A. Keatley,
and Derwin K.-C. Chan

See also Enjoyment, as a Mediator of Exercise Behavior Change; Interventions for Exercise and Physical Activity; Multiple Behavior Change; Self-Efficacy; Self-Regulation; Social Cognitive Theory

Further Readings

Abraham, C., & Michie, S. (2008). A taxonomy of behavior change techniques used in interventions. *Health Psychology, 27*(3), 379–387.

Bartholomew, L. K., & Mullen, P. D. (2011). Five roles for using theory and evidence in the design and testing of behavior change interventions. *Journal of Public Health Dentistry, 71*(Suppl. 1), S20–S33.

Dombrowski, S. U., Sniehotta, F. F., Avenell, A., Johnston, M., MacLennan, G., & Araújo-Soares, A. (2011). Identifying active ingredients in complex behavioural interventions for obese adults with additional risk factors: A systematic review. *Health Psychology Review, 6*(1), 7–32.

Michie, S., Ashford, S., Sniehotta, F. F., Dombrowski, S. U., Bishop, A., & French, D. P. (2011). A refined taxonomy of behaviour change techniques to help people change their physical activity and healthy eating behaviours: The CALO-RE taxonomy. *Psychology & Health, 26*(11), 1479–1498.

Schaalma, H., & Kok, G. (2009). Decoding health education interventions: The times are a-changin'. *Psychology & Health, 24*(1), 5–9.

Webb, T. L., Sniehotta, F. F., & Michie, S. (2010). Using theories of behaviour change to inform interventions for addictive behaviours. *Addiction, 105*(11), 1879–1892.

Cardiac Function

Cardiac function refers to the contraction of cardiac muscle, which works as a pump to send blood throughout the circulatory system to provide adequate blood flow to organs and tissues. The heart achieves this by contracting its muscular walls around a closed chamber to generate sufficient pressure to propel blood from the left ventricle, through the aortic valve, into the aorta, and throughout the body. To accomplish this, the heart must maintain systolic and diastolic blood pressure and cardiac output (amount of blood ejected from the heart in one minute). Each time the heart beats, a volume of blood is ejected. This stroke volume (SV), times the number of beats per minute (heart rate [HR]), equals the cardiac output (CO). Normal, resting CO differs among individuals of different size. The resting CO of someone who weighs 240 pounds is greater than the cardiac output found in a person who weighs 120 pounds. Thus, measured values for CO are expressed as a flow (liters per minute [L/min]) per body surface area (m²). When cardiac output is expressed in this way, it is termed *cardiac index* and has the units of $L/min/m^2$. The surface area is estimated from calculations based on body weight and height (body surface area = $0.007184 \times W^{0.425} \times H^{0.725}$). Cardiac index normally ranges from 2.6 to 4.2 $L/min/m^2$.

There are numerous measures that can assess cardiac function. More extensive analyses include simple and noninvasive to more complicated and invasive tests of cardiac function. Noninvasive tests include chest x-ray analysis, electrocardiography (ECG), and echocardiography. Invasive tests include cardiac catheterization, Thallium scanning, and for patients with coronary artery disease, pharmacologic or exercise stress ECG, pharmacologic or exercise stress myocardial perfusion imaging (MPI), electron beam computed tomography (EBCT), and positron emission tomography (PET). These techniques allow for the determination of global cardiac muscle function analyses, volumetric analyses (calculation of left ventricular functional parameters like end-diastole volumes and ejection fraction), and regional wall motion abnormalities. In addition, the function of the heart as a pump can be determined by the force of ventricular muscles during systole and is directly affected by the preload and contractility of the heart. Preload is the *load* on the cardiac muscle during diastole (relaxation). This preload (end-diastolic volume) alters the ability of the heart to change its force of contraction and therefore increases stroke volume. This response to changes in venous return is called the Frank-Starling mechanism. Contractility can also be increased with an increase in calcium release into the cell. This can occur in response to catecholamines (epinephrine and norepinephrine), which are released by the sympathetic nervous system. Cardiac activation is often a result of sympathetic activation from the central nervous system.

Blood pressure indirectly provides a measure of cardiac function. As blood is pumped out of the left ventricle into the arteries, pressure is generated. The mean arterial pressure (MAP; the average pressure within an artery over a complete cycle of one heartbeat) is determined by the CO, systemic vascular resistance (SVR), and central venous pressure (CVP): MAP = (CO × SVR) + CVP. At normal resting heart rates, MAP can be approximated by the following equation: MAP = DBP + 1/3(SBP-DBP). MAP can indicate a level of cardiac function at rest.

In sport and exercise psychology, measures of cardiac function provide specific information regarding the effects of stress, both physical and psychological, on cardiac function. Elevations in cardiac function in physically healthy individuals indicate sympathetic nervous system activation. This can occur in response to perceived threat in a competitive challenge or in response to meeting the physical demands of movement. In addition, measures of cardiac function are often used to identify the physiological demand or intensity of an activity. This can be done to ensure that the activity is appropriate and safe and to examine changes in cardiac function following physical training, treatment, or an intervention.

Edmund O. Acevedo

See also Autonomic Nervous System; Biofeedback/ Neurofeedback; Neuroscience, Exercise, and Cognitive Function; Psychophysiology; Stress Reactivity

Further Readings

Berntson, G. G., Quigley, K. S., & Lozano, D. (2007). Cardiovascular psychophysiology. In J. T. Cacioppo, L. G.Tassinary, & G. G. Berntson (Eds.), *Handbook of psychophysiology* (3rd ed., pp. 60–92). New York: Cambridge University Press.

Boutcher, S. H., & Hamer, M. (2006). Psychobiological reactivity, physical activity, and cardiovascular health. In E. O. Acevedo & P. Ekkekakis (Eds.), *Psychobiology of physical activity* (pp. 161–176). Champaign, IL: Human Kinetics.

Klabunde, R. E. (2012). *Cardiovascular physiology concepts* (2nd ed., pp. 60–99). Baltimore, MD: Lippincott, Williams & Wilkins.

CAREER ASSISTANCE PROGRAMS

In order to prepare athletes for and support them during transitions, career assistance programs (CAPs) have been developed by elite sport organizations like a national sport governing body, universities, and private organizations. These CAPs generally consist of an integrated and comprehensive combination of workshops, seminars, educational modules, individual counseling, and referral networks providing individualized or group-oriented multidisciplinary support services to athletes with regard to their athletic participation, developmental and lifestyle issues, and educational and vocational development. Target groups for CAPs include prospective junior athletes, student–athletes, elite senior athletes, and retiring or retired athletes.

Some of the early established CAPs include the International Olympic Job Opportunities Program (OJOP), the Canadian Olympic Athlete Career Centre (OACC), and the Athlete Career and Educational Program (ACE). The OJOP was initiated in Australia, South Africa, and the United States to develop and create job opportunities for (potential) Olympians, by identifying job positions and providing a professional network, career analysis services, personal aptitude tests, and interview skills training. The OACC assisted athletes through the retirement transition by providing career and education planning, such as preretirement planning, clarification of career planning needs, life skills training, transition workshops, and a shadow program. The ACE provides career and education services for Australia's elite athletes, including career counseling and planning, personal development training courses, educational guidance, employment preparation, career referral networks, transitional support, online services, referrals, and lifestyle management. High Performance Sport New Zealand's Athlete Life Programme allows its elite athletes to work with an athlete life advisor to manage their sport lifestyle, career and education, personal leadership skills, and finances to minimize constraints and maximize opportunities that have the potential to impact sport performance.

During the past decade, several countries around Europe also established CAPs. In the United Kingdom, UKSport developed the Performance Lifestyle support service providing athletes the necessary skills to cope with the special demands of being an elite performer and to better prepare them for their life after sport. The British Athletes' Lifestyle Assessment Needs in Career and Education (BALANCE) was designed to identify adjustment difficulties on 12 specific factors related to career retirement, including identity as an athlete, degree of occupational planning, transferable skills, the availability of career transition support services, experience with transitions, and social support and mentoring. In France, the National Institute of Sport, Expertise, and Performance (INSEP) developed a project (*Projet de vie du sportif de haut niveau*), which includes career management support, support aimed at supporting elite athletes' social and cultural life, vocational support, and lifestyle management. In Belgium, the Vrije Universiteit Brussel developed the career support program (*Carrièrebegeleiding*) for Bloso, the Flemish governmental administration in charge of elite sport. This CAP is based on a developmental lifespan perspective on the athletic career delineating normative (predicted and anticipated) transitional challenges that athletes will face throughout, as well as after, their athletic career and that will influence their development. It provides career assistance services focusing on the major transitions and career stages of the athletic (high-ability, elite athletes), the academic (primary, secondary, higher), the vocational (elite student–athletes, professional athletes), and the postathletic career (retiring and retired athletes). In 1988, the Vrije Universiteit Brussel was also the first Belgian university to establish a top-level sport and study department focused exclusively on supporting elite student–athletes to achieve academic and athletic excellence by providing services related to education and career management and life skills training. In Sweden, a particular emphasis is put on the combination of elite sports and education through a close collaboration between elite sport and educational institutions (e.g., national and certified elite sport schools). In the Netherlands, the Dutch Olympic Committee and Dutch Sports Federation (NOC*NSF) focus on providing services related to the combination of school and elite sport with specialized secondary and vocational schools and centers for elite sport and education, as well as for coping with career transitions and the postathletic career. This includes the project *Goud op de werkvloer* (Gold on the work floor), which, in collaboration with a private employment firm, aims at

optimizing the vocational development of (retired) elite athletes and includes an active mediation between athletes and employers via, among others, specific job interview sessions for athletes, and the provision of flexible work conditions. In Spain, centers of high performance sport (Centro de Alto Rendimiento; CAR) provide specific services to talented and elite athletes. For example, the CAR Sant Cugat assists athletes in combining training and education (mentoring, tutoring), with access to employment (working experience) and personal development (retirement, finances). In Finland, the Finnish Olympic Committee collaborates with the Ministry of Education and Culture and a private employment firm in the Athlete Career Program (ACP). This CAP supports athletes in their combination of education and an athletic career and in (eventually) entering the labor market, as well as in finding a balance between sport and education and other areas of life and in coping with transitions during their athletic career.

Finally, it is noteworthy that the significance of CAPs has also been recognized at the European level. As part of a hearing on future European Union policy on sport, members of the European Parliament discussed the need to establish career assistance services for talented, elite, and retired athletes. Using the developmental lifespan perspective on the athletic career, recommendations and good practices were presented on the combination of a sporting career with education or work, on athletic retirement, and on the postathletic career. In parallel, the Sport Unit of the Directorate–General for Education and Culture of the European Commission developed, in consultation with European experts on elite sport, career development and career assistance services, specific guidelines to support the dual career of talented and elite athletes in the European Union member states. These include guidelines on, among others, sport academies and high-performance training centers, education (secondary, vocational, higher, and distance learning), health (medical support), employment (combination of work and sport; transition to a new job), finances (scholarships), and supporting services (career assistance; educational guidance).

Career Assistance Services

In light of the growing need for the provision of services to athletes, CAPs have been established worldwide. A survey among 27 CAP providers from Europe, North America, Oceania, Asia, and Africa showed that career assistance services generally served two aims: (1) providing assistance with transitions occurring during the athletic career and (2) providing assistance with the end of the athletic career and transition into the postathletic career. The services provided by these CAPs generally included education management, life skills training and lifestyle management, career management, financial management, and health management.

Sport psychologists were found to be part of the service provision at these CAPs, and were in general related to performance issues, life skills, and lifestyle management. In 82% of these CAPs, services were directed toward senior athletes, 70% toward retired athletes, and 59% toward junior athletes. The services provided by sport psychologists to senior athletes were related to goal setting (in 78% of CAPs), time management (in 74% of CAPs), media skills (in 70% of CAPs), coping and organizational skills (both in 67% of CAPs), and communication (in 63% of CAPs). With retired athletes, sport psychologists worked on the transition out of elite sport (in 74% of CAPs); goal setting (in 44% of CAPs); and communication, time management, problem solving, and organizational skills (all in 41% of CAPs). Sport psychologists provided junior athletes with services related to goal setting and time management (both in 63% of CAPs), communication (in 58% of CAPs), and media (in 56% of CAPs). Finally, sport psychologists were also found to provide clinical services to senior (in 41% of CAPs), retired (in 37% of CAPs), or junior athletes (in 33% of CAPs).

These findings reveal that sport psychology support provision aimed at enhancing junior, elite, and retired athletes' coping with transitional challenges has become an essential part of career assistance services.

Conclusion

The developmental lifespan perspective on the athletic career delineates the normative transitional challenges athletes will face throughout as well as after their athletic career. In order to enhance athletes' ability to cope successfully with these transitions, career assistance services should be provided in a structured way, based upon a developmental (from young to former elite athlete) and holistic (development in different domains) approach.

Elite sport governing bodies, such as national Olympic committees and international sports federations, are encouraged to take leadership in not only acknowledging the influence of career transitions on elite athletes and Olympians, but also in the provision of multilevel career assistance via well-structured multidisciplinary CAPs.

Sport psychologists have been shown to play a significant role in the provision of career assistance services to talented and elite, as well as retired, athletes. Building on the provision of psychoeducational services aimed at enhancing athletes' coping with normative transitions (e.g., junior-to-senior transition, first national team selection, transiting out of secondary education, athletic retirement), sport psychologists can already provide for the long-term career development needs of talented, elite, and retired athletes. Further efforts should be made to develop sport psychology services assisting athletes to successfully prepare for and cope with nonnormative transitions, such as a season-ending injury, unanticipated deselection from the team, or loss of a personal coach.

Finally, while CAPs have generally been developed for athletes, elite sport governing bodies as well as sport psychologists should envisage providing career assistance services to elite coaches.

Paul Wylleman and Anke Reints

See also Career Paths; Career Transitions; Developmental Considerations; Identity; Parenting; Roles; Talent Development; Transition

Further Readings

Stambulova, N. (2010). Professional culture of career assistance to athletes: A look through contrasting lenses of career metaphors. In T. V. Ryba, R. J. Schinke, & G. Tenenbaum (Eds.), *Cultural turn in sport psychology* (pp. 285–314). Morgantown, WV: Fitness Information Technology.

Wylleman, P., Alfermann, D., & Lavallee, D. (2004). Career transitions in perspective. *Psychology of Sport and Exercise, 5,* 7–20. doi: 10.1016/S1469-0292(02)00049-3

Wylleman, P., De Knop, P., & Reints, A. (2011). Transitions in competitive sports. In N. L. Holt & M. Talbot (Eds.), *Lifelong engagement in sport and physical activity* (pp. 63–76). New York: Routledge.

Wylleman, P., De Knop, P., Verdet, M.-C., & Cecic-Erpic, S. (2006). Parenting and career transitions of elite athletes. In S. Jowett & D. Lavallee (Eds.), *Social psychology of sport* (pp. 233–247). Champaign, IL: Human Kinetics.

Wylleman, P., & Lavallee, D. (2004). A developmental perspective on transitions faced by athletes. In M. Weiss (Ed.), *Developmental sport and exercise psychology: A lifespan perspective* (pp. 507–527). Morgantown, WV: Fitness Information Technology.

Wylleman, P., Lavallee, D., & Theeboom, M. (2004). Successful athletic careers. In C. Spielberger (Ed.), *Encyclopedia of applied psychology* (pp. 511–518). San Diego, CA: Elsevier.

Wylleman, P., & Reints, A. (2010). A lifespan perspective on the career development of talented and elite athletes: Perspectives on high-intensity sports. *Scandinavian Journal of Medicine & Science in Sports, 20*(Suppl. 2), 101–107. doi: 10.1111/j.1600-0838 .2010.01194.x

CAREER PATHS

For individuals seeking a career in sport psychology (SP), there are numerous options for those who have earned master's and doctoral degrees in SP. Most individuals with master's degrees work in athletic academic advising, as teachers or coaches, as licensed professional counselors (LPCs) within certain specialized areas, or go on to pursue a doctoral degree. The two primary career paths for those with doctoral degrees are in the clinical or counseling psychology profession or in research and teaching in academia.

A master's degree in SP may lead to one of five main options (excluding pursuing a doctoral degree).

1. *Athletic academic advising.* Most U.S. universities are members of the National Collegiate Athletic Association (NCAA). All universities in the NCAA's Division I are required to operate athletic academic advising entities, which provide academic counseling for their student–athletes. Athletic academic advisers work with student–athletes on course scheduling, study skills, and time management, but may also address a variety of life skills with their student–athletes. The National Association of Academic Advisers for Athletics (www .nfoura.org) is the main professional association for athletic academic advising. An SP's background is an excellent preparation for this career.

2. *Teaching and coaching.* Depending on one's academic interests (psychology or other areas), an SP degree allows one to work potentially more effectively as a school teacher, coach, or both and may allow for private practice work in performance enhancement consulting. The master's degree may also potentially increase one's salary by having obtained a postgraduate degree.

3. *Fitness and performance training for the military.* A relatively new and very exciting career route is with the military through the Comprehensive Soldier Fitness–Performance and Resilience Enhancement Program. These individuals work at U.S. Army bases with soldiers to better prepare them for their combat experience, as well as with the soldiers and families when the soldiers return from combat (Wounded Warriors; transitioning back into the community).

4. *Licensed professional counseling.* Working as an LPC (termed differently in different states) requires a clinical or counseling psychology master's level degree. The trained individual is licensed, certified, or accredited, depending on the state, to work within psychology, and get paid, including third-party reimbursement.

5. *Consulting.* Positions developed by individuals to suit their skills—niche creation—may include performance enhancement consulting in educational sport psychology work with athletes and recreational sport participants. This could also involve work in a health club or fitness center, in a research position, or as a wellness or life coach. The possibilities are only limited by an individual's imagination.

Career paths for holders of a doctoral degree center on work as a licensed psychologist or work in academia. Obtaining a doctorate, either a doctor of philosophy (PhD) or a doctor of psychology (PsyD) degree in clinical or counseling psychology provides the clearest route toward becoming a licensed psychologist and being able to work competently, ethically, and effectively as a sport psychologist. Such individuals may be found in private practice (individual or group practice) or in a more formal position. Individuals in private practice generally see clients across a number of areas within clinical or counseling psychology and develop the sport component of their practice as an added area of expertise. Although very few individuals have been able to become sport psychologists with 100% of their clientele being sport and exercise participants, it remains a possibility. Such professionals see clients, individually or in groups, for areas that can encompass performance-related skills such as goal setting, arousal control, imagery, attentional control, and self-talk but also clinical issues such as eating disorders, substance abuse, anger management, relationship issues, and so on. They may conduct workshops on a variety of sport psychology-related topics for teams. It is more common for psychologists to work with nonsport populations for part of their practice and sport participants for the other part. This may be by choice or because of client demand in the geographical area in which the psychologist practices.

Making a living as a psychologist in private practice is challenging, and many individuals opt for more formal positions such as in a university setting, perhaps within an athletics department (there are a limited number of these opportunities), or more often, as part of a university or college counseling center working part of the time with athletes. There are many different models for how this can work, such as half-time in the counseling center and half-time in athletics. The more elite positions are those as sport psychologists with the United States Olympic Committee (there are six such positions in the United States, although there are, of course, positions available with Olympic teams in other countries) or with professional teams. However, even though there are hundreds of professional teams across the various sports and levels (including minor leagues), there are very few sport psychologists who have full-time positions. More commonly, sport psychologists in private practice (or in academia) consult with such teams as needed.

What qualifies licensed clinical or counseling psychologists to call themselves sport psychologists? Although ethical standards require one to only work within one's area(s) of competence, some clinical or counseling psychologists believe that, because they are avid exercise and sport participants, this automatically provides them with the expertise to work as a sport psychologist. However, although they may be excellent clinical or counseling psychologists, there is a body of knowledge and research that the profession of SP believes is necessary to work effectively as a sport psychologist. Division 47 (Exercise and Sport Psychology) of the American Psychological Association is working on guidelines to facilitate developing one's competency in SP. For the moment, the process of becoming a Certified Consultant within the Association for Applied Sport Psychology (CC-AASP) provides the clearest path for developing a level of competency. The CC-AASP process does not have a clinical or counseling focus but rather a performance-enhancement focus. The CC-AASP certification process, as well as AASP ethical guidelines, specify the performance enhancement focus of this certification. Thus, clinical or counseling psychologists and academic sport psychologists are aware of the limitations and extent of this certification.

There are a few clinical or counseling psychologists who work in academia, generally within psychology departments. The majority of individuals within academia in SP are found through the kinesiology route, which is another primary career path for those more interested in an academic career. Primarily within kinesiology (or exercise and sport sciences or physical education or other such names), individuals with doctoral degrees in sport psychology from such departments remain within the discipline and teach and conduct research. Many of these individuals have consulting practices outside of their primary job within academia. A few of these positions are found in psychology departments, but these individuals have usually earned their degrees in psychology departments. These academic sport psychologists teach a variety of SP related courses at the undergraduate and graduate levels, and conduct research across a wide variety of topics within the field. They also engage in service to their university as well as to the profession (becoming an officer in a sport psychology organization such as AASP).

Some individuals work as performance psychologists, some with clinical or counseling psychology degrees and many as licensed psychologists, in occupations where performance is critical to success. These individuals may work with companies such as Cirque du Soleil, the New York City Ballet, Wall Street traders, or with medical school students, police, and firefighters. Although this encyclopedia focuses on sport psychology, it should be noted that many of the skills learned within this field are generalizable across other performance settings and, depending on one's background, one can find success in these other performance domains. A number of books are available by those who have worked in these specialized settings, particularly dance and the performing arts. This area has become known as performance psychology, to acknowledge the emphasis on performance in general (in a variety of performance domains, especially the performing arts) rather than sport per se.

While the focus of many individuals (and most books in the field) is on sport psychology, particularly with high-level and elite athletes, there will be many opportunities in the future for work within exercise psychology. Increased attention is being paid to the high prevalence of obesity and sedentariness in the general public, and exercise psychologists can work effectively within health care settings to facilitate motivation and adherence to exercise and physical activity and counteract this trend, now widely recognized as a public health issue. These opportunities may come through academia or in private enterprise within health clubs or fitness centers, corporations, insurance companies, and other entities.

Although there are a few undergraduate programs in sport psychology, the main route to a career in the field, as noted earlier, is through graduate study. To become a clinical or counseling psychologist, the recommended route is to obtain a PhD or PsyD in clinical or counseling psychology, either as the next step after one's undergraduate program or after obtaining a master's in sport psychology from a kinesiology department. The academic route generally finds individuals with master's degrees in kinesiology or clinical or counseling psychology followed by a PhD in kinesiology, specializing in sport and exercise psychology. These individuals often work as performance enhancement consultants.

Deciding on the best career path can be a challenge, although the availability of numerous paths to one's goal can be advantageous for individuals with a variety of backgrounds. Full descriptions of a variety of educational programs are available, as well as other resources to assist the prospective sport psychologist, including extensive coverage of career opportunities in exercise and sport psychology and personal accounts by professionals in the field (see Further Readings).

Michael L. Sachs

See also Credentials

Further Readings

Bach, P. L. (2011). Taking the next step: What to ask as you review the directory. In M. L. Sachs, K. L. Burke, & S. L. Schweighardt (Eds.), *Directory of graduate programs in applied sport psychology* (10th ed., pp. xxv–xxxviii). Indianapolis, IN: Association for Applied Sport Psychology.

Hanton, S., & Mellalieu, S. D. (Eds.). (2012). *Professional practice in sport psychology: A review.* New York: Routledge/Taylor & Francis.

Lesyk, J. L. (1998). *Developing sport psychology within your clinical practice.* San Francisco: Jossey-Bass.

Sachs, M. L., Burke, K. L., & Schweighardt, S. L. (Eds.). (2011). *Directory of graduate programs in applied sport psychology* (10th ed.). Indianapolis, IN: Association for Applied Sport Psychology.

Sachs, M. L., Lutkenhouse, J., Rhodius, A., Watson, J., Pfenninger, G., Lesyk, J. L., et al. (2011). Career opportunities in the field of exercise and sport psychology. In M. L. Sachs, K. L. Burke, & S. L. Schweighardt (Eds.), *Directory of graduate programs in applied sport psychology* (10th ed., pp. 251–277). Indianapolis, IN: Association for Applied Sport Psychology.

Silva, J. M., III, Metzler, J. N., & Lerner, B. (2011). *Training professionals in the practice of sport psychology* (2nd ed.). Morgantown, WV: Fitness Information Technology.

CAREER TRANSITIONS

Career transitions are turning phases in athletes' career development. Therefore, they should be first defined in terms of their place in the career context. The broadest career term in psychology is a *life career* that encompasses an individual's life-long development and achievements in various activities and spheres of life that unfold in a particular historical and sociocultural context. In sport psychology, an *athletic career* is defined as (1) part of and a contribution to an athlete's life career, (2) a multiyear competitive sport involvement voluntarily chosen by an athlete and aimed at achieving a personal individual peak in athletic performance in one or several sport events, and (3) a sequence of career stages and transitions.

These definitions highlight the various views and facets of athletic careers. The first definition is based on *a whole person approach* that recognizes the athlete as a person doing sports and having broader life issues, such as education, work, family, friends, and other. The second definition emphasizes a free career choice, a long-term commitment, striving for upward career movement, and a possibility of having a specialized or a generalized career. In specialized careers, athletes compete in one sport during the entire career, whereas in generalized careers, they practice and compete in several sports, either simultaneously or successively. Athletic careers can also be of different levels, such as local, national, international, and professional, depending on the highest level in competitions achieved by the athlete. International amateur and professional careers are also called *elite careers*. In the third definition, an athletic career is viewed as a developmental process that includes proceeding through career stages and coping with *career transitions as turning phases* in development.

As noted by Dorothee Alfermann and Natalia Stambulova, models that describe athletes' career development identify the following *athletic career stages:* initiation, development, mastery or perfection, maintenance, and discontinuation of competitive sport involvement. In these models, the stage-by-stage transitions are marked by changes in (a) athletes' perception of and attitude toward sport and the degree to which they identify themselves with the athletic role; (b) time and energy investment into sports; (c) athletes' social environment and the role of coaches, parents and family, and peers in career development; and (d) the degree to which they have to sacrifice in other spheres of life to accomplish their sport goals.

The aforementioned whole person approach contributes to *a holistic lifespan perspective* in understanding athletes' career development as a multidimensional process combining stages and transitions in their athletic, psychological, psychosocial, and academic–vocational development.

Transition Process and Outcomes

The transition process, the factors involved, and the transition outcomes are considered in the various career transition explanatory models. For example, in Stambulova's athletic career transition model, a transition is viewed as a process of coping with a set of *transition demands,* in which athletes use various *coping strategies* like planning, practicing more than their opponents, or seeking professional support. Effectiveness of coping is thought to be dependent on a dynamic balance between the coping resources and barriers. *Resources* consist of the various internal and external factors that facilitate the transition, such as previous athletic and personal experiences or social and professional support available), while *barriers* include the various internal and external factors that interfere with the coping process, such as low self-efficacy, poor coaching, low quality equipment, or insufficient financial support. The model entails two primary transition outcomes: successful transition and crisis transition. *Successful transition* is a result of effective coping when the transition demands and the athletes' coping resources and strategies are evenly matched. *Crisis transition* is a result of ineffective coping when low resources, high barriers, and inappropriate coping strategies make it difficult to meet the transition demands. Crisis is also conceptualized as a transition that the athlete is unable to cope with independently and perceives a need for transition intervention. Furthermore, according to the model, the crisis transition can have two possible secondary outcomes: *delayed successful transition* (in case of effective intervention) and *unsuccessful transition* (in case of ineffective or lacking intervention) associated with *negative consequences* of avoiding coping with the crisis (e.g., premature dropout, neuroses, overtraining, eating disorders, and substance abuse). Career transition interventions outlined by the model include crisis-prevention, crisis-coping, and negative-consequences-coping interventions.

Major Types of Athletes' Career Transitions

Athletes' transitions are classified into athletic and nonathletic, as well as into normative and nonnormative.

Normative athletic transitions are relatively predictable and based on the logic of athletic development. Thus, the transition into organized sport, the transition to the development stage or more intensive training in chosen sport, the transition to the mastery stage or from junior to senior sports, the transition to professional sport, the transition to maintenance career stage, and the transition to the post-sport career are all examples of the normative athletic transitions.

Normative nonathletic transitions refer to athletes' transitions in psychological, psychosocial, and academic–vocational development, such as the transition from childhood to adolescence, the transition from living at home to living independently, the transition to college or university, and the transition to the workplace.

Nonnormative transitions are less predictable, such as transitions caused by injury, divorce, moving abroad, or changing team or coach.

The predictability of normative transitions creates an opportunity for athletes to prepare for them in advance, while the low predictability of nonnormative transitions explains why athletes find these more difficult to deal with.

Normative Athletic Transitions

Among the normative athletic transitions, the most research has been done on the *transition from the development to the mastery stage* (also known as the transition from junior to senior and elite sports) and the *transition to the post-sports career* (athletic retirement).

The growing interest in the junior-to-senior transition can be explained by both the difficulty and the importance of this transition for athletes wanting to achieve an elite or professional level in sports. Vanden Auweele et al. showed that only 17% of elite junior athletes made a successful transition to senior or elite sports in 5 years of observation. International research showed that athletes perceive this transition as a big step associated with much higher standards in practice and performance than they experienced before. Issues outside sports are also very important, with studies and social aspects proving the most demanding. Athletes' ambitions to succeed in this transition and meet the expectations of significant others, together with uncertainty about success in coping, lead to high stress and increased sensitivity to social influences. Therefore, social support, especially from coaches, plays a pivotal role in the transition process. Coaches believe that coping strategies such as thoughtful problem solving, acceptance of responsibility, self-control, and positive reappraisal are beneficial to the transition success. Research also confirmed that successful coping with the junior-to-senior transition is associated with athletes' personal maturation and identity development.

The transition to the post-sport career or athletic retirement is the one inevitable transition that mixes athletic context reasons for termination in sports, athletic career satisfaction, and support from sport organizations with nonathletic context relevant to starting a new life after sports. Retired athletes must accept retirement and adjust to the status of a former athlete, start or continue studies or work, reconsider their personal identity, and renew their lifestyles and social networks. The status of former elite athletes is typically lower than that of active sports heroes. Therefore, former athletes need to adjust to a substantial decrease in social recognition and support. Many of them channel their energy into education or work. Starting a new professional career is not only important for making a living, but also for the development of a new professional identity. Many athletes confirm that their social lives change greatly during this transition. They often keep their sport friends but need to involve more nonsport people into their social networks. Family becomes a very important part of the renewed lifestyle, especially if the athletic retirement transition is associated with the transition to parenthood. Athletes who plan retirement in advance, receive their education while still in sport, have multiple personal interests and identities, keep good family relationships, and feel in control of their lives usually adjust successfully to their post-sport careers within months. About 15% to 20% of athletes experience this transition as a crisis accompanied by unemployment, separation or divorce, health problems, alcohol abuse, and feelings of being empty, alone, and forgotten.

Normative Nonathletic Transitions

In terms of normative nonathletic transitions, researchers focus mainly on the transition from adolescence to young adulthood (around 18–19 years old), emphasizing the athletes' identity formation, and on their transitions within the educational system.

Adolescence is known as a crucial period for young people to answer the question "Who am I?" integrating their social roles and related identities. For athletes, their athlete role and athletic identity or the degree of personal identification with the athlete role are involved in this process. Researchers showed that high athletic identity works as a resource during most of the athletic career transitions (e.g., the junior-to-senior transition), but it turns into a barrier in the transition to the post-sport career. Athletes who develop multiple personal identities—athlete, student, employee, family member, friend—are less at risk for the athletic identity foreclosure (single-minded focus on sport) and, consequently, for the identity crisis (self-misinterpretation) in the transition to the post-sport career.

The identity research in athletes has stimulated an interest in the so-called *dual career* studies that focus on athletes combining sport with education and their transitions within the educational system. Relevant research deals with student–athletes at sport classes, sport boarding schools, and colleges and universities. These studies emphasize the benefits of athletes' dual careers, such as balanced lifestyle, reduced stress, good conditions for developing life skills, and higher employability after sport, but also highlight the related demands and challenges, especially when athletes experience simultaneous transitions to a new level in both education and sport. For example, North American research on the student–athletes' transition to college showed that the incoming students have to meet new academic requirements and the challenges of living far from home, create relationships, manage their time and energy, as well as adjust to demanding sport participation at the intercollegiate level, new teammates, and coaches. They also should be ready to cope with athletic career termination upon graduation from the college. European dual career studies are marked by the holistic life span perspective in investigating student–athletes' sport, education, and private life issues.

Nonnormative Career Transitions

As mentioned above, the nonnormative transitions are less predictable and more idiosyncratic than the normative ones. This type of athletes' transitions has been acknowledged but not extensively studied. Examples of athletic nonnormative transitions include injury; overtraining; deselection; moving abroad to play sport; and changing a club, a coach, or a sport partner. Selection for and participation in the Olympic Games are also seen as nonnormative athletic transitions. Athletes' quasi-normative (expected in principle, but not in terms of their timing in life) or nonnormative transitions outside sport are marriage, divorce, parenthood, moving to a big city, immigration, and others. The lower the predictability of a nonnormative transition, the more often athletes need professional assistance.

Helping Athletes in Career Transitions

The holistic lifespan perspective is currently an influential guide in *career assistance,* which is a rapidly developing discourse in applied sport psychology aimed at helping athletes with various issues related to their careers inside and outside of sports.

Helping athletes to cope with athletic and nonathletic, normative and nonnormative transitions is a central aspect in career assistance provided by career assistance programs or by private sport psychology consultants. Career transition interventions are planned based on the career development and transition frameworks, as well as on the thorough investigation of the athlete–client's background, current situation and needs, and future plans (for further information see Stambulova, 2012).

Two major perspectives in career transition interventions, the preventive–supportive and the crisis–negative consequences coping perspectives, have been identified.

Preventive–Supportive Perspective

The *preventive–supportive perspective* covers interventions aimed at enhancing athletes' awareness about forthcoming or current transition demands and aiding in the timely development of all the necessary resources for effective coping. These interventions may improve the athlete's readiness for a normative career transition or support the athlete during the transition process. The following are the brief definitions of relevant intervention types.

- **Career planning interventions** are counseling interventions aimed at helping athletes increase their self-awareness; set realistic career goals bridging their past, present, and future; and prepare in advance for the forthcoming transitions.

- **Life development interventions and life skills training** consist of needs assessment, education, and training with regard to sets of transferable life skills, such as effective communication, dealing with success and failure, time, energy, and stress management, that are applicable in both sports and other spheres of life.

- **Lifestyle management interventions** consist of counseling, education, and training aimed at helping athletes combine sport and other activities in life, prioritize between them, and manage time and energy in a way that helps athletes maintain good health and well-being.

• **Identity development interventions** include counseling, education, and training aimed at helping athletes in self-exploration and development of multiple personal identities to minimize the risk for the athletic identity foreclosure and one-sided development.

• **Cultural adaptation interventions** consist of needs assessment, counseling, education, and training aimed at helping athletes adjust to the new sociocultural environment when moving to another country to play sport or to do both sport and studies. Practitioners help athletes increase their awareness of the new culture and find consensus between their previous values, perceptions, and habits and ones required and expected by the new culture.

Crisis–Negative Consequences Coping Perspective

The *crisis–negative consequences coping perspective* covers interventions assisting athletes in analysis of their crisis or traumatic situations and finding the best available ways to cope. This perspective is represented by the following interventions:

• **Crisis-coping educational interventions** are aimed at helping athletes analyze the crisis situation, generate alternatives in coping, make an action plan, and increase their self-efficacy to cope with the crisis. These interventions are useful at the beginning phase of the crisis when athletes feel distressed and disoriented but still do not experience any clinical symptoms.

• **Clinical interventions** are applied when athletes experience clinical symptoms related to overtraining, neuroses, psychosomatic illnesses, substance abuse, negative identities, eating disorders, anger and aggression, grief, clinical depression, and suicidal thoughts, which often are negative consequences of not coping with previous or current transitions. These are mostly counseling interventions based on various psychotherapeutic approaches, such as psychoanalysis, existential therapy, or cognitive-behavioral therapy.

Tracing various types of career transition interventions, it is easy to see some obvious overlapping among them. For example, exploring new social roles as a part of identity development interventions also contributes to the athlete's lifestyle management and life skills training. Such overlaps are not surprising because all the interventions deal with various aspects of the transition process and adopt the whole person approach. These overlaps also facilitate combining various types of interventions to best meet the particular needs of each athlete.

Conclusion

The career transition area of research and practice in sport psychology has been built and structured mainly over the last two decades. Major developments in this area include sport-specific definitions of key concepts; classifications of athletes' transitions, related frameworks, and interventions; the holistic lifespan perspective and the body of knowledge about athletes' transitions and factors involved; career assistance; and practical experiences with related principles, values, intervention strategies, and tools. Future challenges for the topic can be seen in more ecological and culturally sensitive research on athletic and nonathletic, normative and nonnormative transitions using various methodologies and designs, such as narratives, longitude, cross-cultural, intervention, and case studies, and also in further promotion of career assistance services among athletes and coaches.

Natalia Stambulova

See also Career Paths; Coping; Talent Development; Transition

Further Readings

Alfermann, D., & Stambulova, N. (2007). Career transitions and career termination. In G. Tenenbaum & R. C. Eklund (Eds.), *Handbook of sport psychology* (3rd ed., pp. 712–736). New York: Wiley.

Lavallee, D., & Wylleman, P. (Eds.). (2000). *Career transitions in sport: International perspectives.* Morgantown, WV: Fitness Information Technology.

Schlossberg, N. K. (1981). A model for analyzing human adaptation to transition. *The Counseling Psychologist, 9,* 2–18.

Stambulova, N. (2012). Working with athletes in career transitions. In S. Hanton & S. Mellalieu (Eds.), *Professional practice in sport psychology: A review* (pp.165–194). London: Routledge.

Stambulova, N., & Alfermann, D. (2009). Putting culture into context: Cultural and cross-cultural perspectives in career development and transition research and practice. *International Journal of Sport & Exercise Psychology, 7,* 292–308.

Stambulova, N., Alfermann, D., Statler, T., & Côté, J. (2009). ISSP position stand: Career development and transitions of athletes. *International Journal of Sport & Exercise Psychology, 7*, 395–412.

Taylor, J., & Ogilvie, B. C. (2001). Career termination among athletes. In R. N. Singer, H. A. Hausenblas, & C. M. Janelle (Eds.), *Handbook of sport psychology* (2nd ed., pp. 672–691). New York: Wiley.

Vanden Auweele, Y., De Martelaer, K., Rzewnicki, R., De Knop, P., & Wylleman, P. (2004). Parents and coaches: A help or harm? Affective outcomes for children in sport. In Y. Vanden Auweele (Ed.), *Ethics in youth sport*. Leuven, Belgium: Lannoocampus.

Wylleman, P., & Lavallee, D. (2004). A developmental perspective on transitions faced by athletes. In M. Weiss (Ed.), *Developmental sport and exercise psychology: A lifespan perspective* (pp. 507–527). Morgantown, WV: Fitness Information Technology.

Caring Climate

Understanding and ultimately optimizing the experience of individuals involved in physical activity is a focal point in sport and exercise psychology. From a social cognitive perspective, perceptions of the psychological climate represent an individual's perceptions of what is valued, emphasized, and promoted in a particular setting. Recently, Maria Newton and colleagues have identified a facet of the psychological climate termed *the caring climate*. This entry will define and discuss the conceptual underpinnings of the caring climate, review the existing empirical literature, and provide suggestions for future research.

Newton and colleagues define the caring climate as the extent to which individuals perceive a particular setting to be interpersonally inviting, safe, supportive, and able to provide the experience of being valued and respected. Conceptualization of the caring climate is firmly ensconced in the work of educational philosopher Nel Noddings, who describes caring as a state of awareness by the one-caring characterized by engrossment and motivational displacement for the cared-for. Engrossment refers to open and nonselective receptivity demonstrated by fully accepting and listening to the cared-for. Motivational displacement refers to emphasizing the goals and aspirations of the cared-for in lieu of one's own needs. Thus, caring is relational in nature and characterized by the one-caring taking time and energy to express authentic concern and connection with the cared-for.

In sport and exercise settings, coaches, group exercise leaders, personal trainers, and fitness specialists predominantly play the role of the one-caring while participants (teammates, clients) are the cared-for. Importantly, however, perceptions of a caring climate occur reciprocally and among all participants within a setting; members of a team can care for other teammates, opponents, and their coach (acting as the ones-caring).

Conceptually, perceptions of a caring climate are proposed to be positively associated with motivational striving, moral engagement, quality of relationships, and mental health. Perceptions of a caring climate are somewhat similar to participants' sense of belonging and social and relatedness goals emphasized in a particular setting but are philosophically different. The caring climate taps into a social–emotional sense of safety, closeness, and the feeling of being compelled to be of assistance to others, all of which make caring a distinct construct.

Emerging literature suggests that caring is an important element of the psychological climate of a setting and influential in understanding and maximizing the experience of individuals involved in physical activity. Newton et al. (2007) created the Caring Climate Scale (CCS), which measures the extent to which individuals perceive a specific context to be caring. Example items include "the leaders care about kids" and "everyone likes kids for who they are."

Perceptions of a caring climate are related to indicators of positive engagement and developmental outcomes in sport. Mary Fry and Lori Gano-Overway reported that athletes who perceived their team to be caring were more likely to have positive attitudes toward their teammates and coach, indicate greater enjoyment of and commitment to their sport, and were more likely to report acting in a caring manner toward others. In a sample of primarily African American underserved adolescent athletes, Daniel Gould, Ryan Flett, and Larry Lauer (2012) reported that perceptions of a caring climate were linked to positive developmental outcomes, most notably teamwork and social skills.

Studies have established links between perceptions of caring climate and mental well-being and social behaviors, while also providing evidence for possible mechanisms that explain how caring operates to influence outcomes. Fry and colleagues found that perceptions of a caring climate have been associated with greater hope and happiness and less depression and sadness as well as increased prosocial behaviors and decreased antisocial behaviors. Gano-Overway and colleagues reported that a perceived caring climate influenced mental well-being and social behaviors through aspects of personal efficacy. When individuals are cared for, they are better able to monitor and regulate their emotions and feel more capable of empathizing with others. These beliefs result in greater personal well-being as well as more adaptive social behaviors.

While a majority of the research has focused on participant outcomes associated with perceptions of a caring climate, an interesting study by T. Michelle Magyar et al. explored the predictors of leaders' self-reported ability to create a caring climate. Leaders' emotional intelligence, specifically their ability to control their emotions and efficacy for implementing instruction, were significant and positive determinants of their own personal caring.

The importance of a caring climate in exercise settings is yet unknown and a warranted focus of future research. Extending the leadership findings is another intriguing area of future research. Lastly, well controlled intervention studies would be most beneficial in identifying the impact of creating a caring climate.

Maria Newton

Further Readings

Fry, M. D., & Gano-Overway, L. A. (2010). Exploring the contribution of the caring climate to the youth sport experience. *Journal of Applied Sport Psychology, 22,* 294–304.

Fry, M. D., Guivernau, M., Kim, M., Newton, M., Gano-Overway, L. A., & Magyar, T. M. (2012). Youth perceptions of a caring climate, emotional regulation, and psychological well-being. *Sport, Exercise, and Performance Psychology, 1,* 44–57.

Gano-Overway, L. A., Newton, M., Magyar, T. M., Fry, M. D., Kim, M., & Guivernau, M. R. (2009). Influence of caring youth sport contexts on efficacy-related beliefs and social behaviors. *Developmental Psychology, 45,* 329–340.

Gould, D., Flett, R., & Lauer, L. (2012). The relationship between psychosocial development and the sports climate experienced by underserved youth. *Psychology of Sport and Exercise, 13,* 80–87.

Magyar, T. M., Guivernau, T. N., Gano-Overway, L. M., Newton, M., Kim, M., Watson, D. L., et al. (2007). The influence of leader efficacy and emotional intelligence on personal caring in physical activity. *Journal of Teaching in Physical Education, 26,* 310–319.

Newton, M., Fry, M. D., Watson, D. L., Gano-Overway, L., Kim, M., Magyar, M., et al. (2007). Psychometric properties of the caring climate scale in a physical activity setting. *Revista de Psicologia del Deporte, 16,* 67–84.

Noddings, N. (2002). *The challenge to care in schools: An alternative approach to education.* New York: Teachers College Press.

CENTERING

Athletes are often faced with a variety of factors that can throw off their focus on the athletic task, such as worry, unexpected events, and physical exhaustion. Therefore, it is important for athletes to be able to focus or refocus their attention on the athletic task, despite frequently changing circumstances. In this regard, *centering* is a process by which individuals direct their attention to a central portion of the body while engaging in deep rhythmic breathing, with the purpose of merging one's attention and one's center of gravity, and thus gaining or regaining focus.

As a technique, centering was historically incorporated into the martial arts as long ago as the first century BCE. At that time, centering emphasized focused thought, muscle relaxation, and rhythmic breathing. Centering has been used more recently in modern-day sports. By helping athletes focus attention on a particular central part of the body (such as the abdomen) as they engage in deep rhythmic breathing patterns, athletes can achieve a feeling of physical and mental groundedness and togetherness, which is thought to subsequently promote enhanced focus to the athletic challenges they face. When centered, a sense of *quiet mind* is created, as diverse thoughts and emotions are replaced by a narrow focus on one's own breathing and body. The narrowing of focus helps block out distractions both within the athlete (e.g., worry) and in the environment (e.g., crowd noise) and allows the athlete to concentrate more fully on the task.

As with any other skill, effectively developing the capacity to center oneself requires training and practice. Simply attempting to occasionally get focused is not sufficient for the development of centering skills. For most individuals, learning to center one's body and mind takes concerted effort. As such, athletes are encouraged to frequently practice centering (in a variety of contexts, and even when tasks do not require a centered state) until centering competencies are developed. Centering training usually begins with 20- to 30-minute exercises, but, as greater competencies evolve, the time required to attain a centered state can be systematically reduced to several seconds. The technique can be used with eyes open or closed, and in a lying, sitting, or standing position. Therefore, once mastered, centering can be employed by athletes at any moment and in any context just prior to movement. For example, a golfer can quickly center prior to putting and a hockey player can reach a centered state just prior to a face-off.

During sport performance, there are two primary values of centering. The first value is to help the athlete minimize internal and external distractions by transitioning attention away from past-, present-, or future-oriented thoughts, emotional states, performance concerns, or plans, and toward the present moment. The second value is to help the athlete remain focused on the athletic task at hand. It is important to state that centering is often misconstrued as a method of relaxation, as the goal is often incorrectly assumed to be a reduction or elimination of emotions such as anxiety or anger or tense bodily states. Yet while the individual may feel more relaxed after centering, any increase in relaxation would be merely a secondary consequence. In actuality, centering is more similar to mindfulness meditative exercises, and in fact, centering historically originated from the same Asian philosophical traditions as mindfulness.

Mindfulness is a state of nonjudgmental awareness and acceptance of internal experiences, and mindfulness exercises help individuals consistently engage in behaviors that matter to them rather than abandoning their goals and athletic or general life values when negative thoughts, feelings, or physical sensations get in their way. In the proper use of centering, the individual is actually not seeking a state of relaxation or a reduction of any particular thoughts, emotions, or physiological states, but rather is seeking a focused preparatory state for competitive performance. From this perspective, centering is a means of self-regulating attention by bringing the mind to a quiet place in which attention is directed away from distractions and onto the body. Once attention is placed on the body and distractions are minimized, the athlete is then better able to focus on the competitive moment and required athletic tasks. While centering can be used as a stand-alone technique, it is often incorporated into a more comprehensive mindfulness training practice. Yet regardless of whether it is used alone or as a component of mindfulness training, centering can have a marked positive impact on the attentional processes of the athlete and subsequent athletic performance. In fact, research has found that a centered focus of attention is highly correlated with flow states and athletic performance success.

Zella E. Moore

See also Attention Training; Breathing Exercises; Flow; Mindfulness; Relaxation

Further Readings

Gardner, F. L., & Moore, Z. E. (2007). *The psychology of enhancing human performance: The Mindfulness-Acceptance-Commitment (MAC) approach.* New York: Springer.

Nideffer, R. M. (1981). *The ethics and practice of applied sport psychology.* Ithaca, NY: Mouvement Publications.

Rogerson, L. J., & Hrycaiko, D. W. (2002). Enhancing competitive performance of ice hockey goaltenders using centering and self-talk. *Journal of Applied Sport Psychology, 14,* 14–26.

CERTIFICATIONS

Professional certification serves to identify individuals who have obtained or maintained qualifications to perform a specific work responsibility or task. Furthermore, certification indirectly serves to safeguard the public interest by assuring that the public can identify qualified professionals. In the United States, the Association for Applied Sport Psychology (AASP) certifies master's and doctoral trained professionals as Certified Consultants (CC-AASP). CC-AASP professionals are qualified to assist with performance issues that affect people in all areas of sport and exercise. Although other certifications in sport psychology exist, this entry is focused on the CC-AASP certification because of its connection to the largest nonprofit international organization (AASP) committed to promoting the *science* and *practice* of sport and exercise psychology, and because the CC-AASP certification requirements are consistent with the American Psychological Association (APA) Division 47 Proficiency in Sport Psychology.

Certification and Licensure

Certification is the process by which a nongovernmental organization, in this case AASP, grants recognition to an individual who has met predetermined qualifications specified by that organization. The process of certification is voluntary. Certified individuals have demonstrated the level of knowledge and skill required in the profession, and the certification serves to identify the occupation, role, and skills to the public and stakeholders. Professional practice can be governed by legal requirements. When this is the case, professionals in practice must be licensed. Licensure is given to one by the state. *Licensure* is the state's grant of legal authority, pursuant to the state's police powers, to practice a profession within a designated scope of practice. States define, by statute, the tasks and scope of practice of a profession and provide that these tasks may be legally performed only by those who are licensed. Licensure prohibits anyone from practicing the profession who is not licensed, regardless of whether or not the individual has been certified by a private organization. To date, the scope of practice defined by AASP certification is not governed by legal requirements.

The most common services provided by CC-AASP professionals include educating individuals, groups, and organizations about the role of psychological factors in sport, exercise, and physical activity, and teaching participants specific mental, behavioral, psychosocial, and emotional control skills in these physical contexts. To date, these activities are not governed by legal requirements, thus there is no requirement for practicing professionals to be licensed to provide these services. Moreover, APA Division 47 Exercise and Sport Psychology has also identified the specific knowledge and training necessary for ethical professional practice in the exercise and sport context. The requirements for CC-AASP and the Division 47 Proficiency in Sport Psychology are consistent and provide clear descriptions of a model for appropriate training for service providers in applied sport and exercise psychology.

Certification assists in defining the professional and ethical responsibility of individuals participating in consulting in applied sport and exercise environments. In addition, certification offers the public a definition and example of the training necessary for quality service. This in turn provides greater public understanding of the importance and possible impact of the application of psychology to sport and exercise. An example of this import role for CC-AASP certification is that the United States Olympic Committee Sport Psychology Registry requires CC-AASP certification for inclusion on the registry to work with U.S. Olympic athletes.

Requirements for Competent and Ethical Practice

CC-AASP and Division 47 Proficiency in Sport Psychology requirements specify that extensive disciplinary knowledge in sport and exercise psychology is required for professionals to competently practice applied sport psychology. Although consistent, the two sets of requirements differ in that CC-AASP requirements rely upon clearly defined necessities in coursework, whereas the Division 47 Proficiency requirements specify content area necessities for the ethical practice in sport psychology. For both the CC-AASP and the Division 47 Proficiency in Sport Psychology requirements, professionals must have knowledge in the following areas: professional ethics and standards; biomechanical or physiological bases of physical activity; historical, philosophical, social, or motor behavior bases of physical activity; psychopathology and its assessment; counseling skills; research design, statistics, or psychological assessment; biological bases of behavior; cognitive-affective bases of behavior; and individual behavior. For CC-AASP, the majority of the courses must be taken at the graduate level and the individual must have completed a master's or doctoral program. Furthermore, adequate training must include demonstrated competence in the field with mentored structured experiences. Finally, applied sport psychology professionals must show evidence of continued learning to maintain professional expertise. A process of certification renewal exists in the case of CC-AASP to support this end. One important side note is that the Division 47 Proficiency in Sport Psychology has included the knowledge of organizational and system aspects of sport consulting as a content area that is not inherently embedded within the specified coursework requirements for CC-AASP. Nonetheless, the overall uniformity across CC-AASP and Division

47 Proficiency in Sport Psychology requirements supports a clear and consistent depiction of the professional expertise required to practice applied exercise and sport psychology.

Commentary on Necessity for Clearly Defined Expertise and Practice

The AASP certification process initiated in 1989 and has certified over 250 professionals. One could argue that, for a licensed mental health care practitioner, there is little motivation to become CC-AASP certified. Yet there is growing interest in Applied Sport Psychology, and ethical practitioners committed to competent professional practice continue to seek opportunities to learn more about sport and exercise psychology and document professional credentials. A goal would be to increase the number of Certified Consultants so that the number reaches a critical mass that provides an awareness of this credential to the general public. One challenge that exists for professionals in the field is the difficulty in meeting specific coursework requirements. As the academic discipline continues to grow, there is the possibility for accessing online courses. In addition, AASP may consider approving continuing education credits to fulfill knowledge requirements. These as well as other options must be sensitive to maintaining the quality and rigor of the certification coursework requirements. Aoyagi, Portenga, Poczwardowski, Cohen, and Statler (2012) have argued that another possibility for increasing access and feasibility of CC-AASP certification for professionals in the field is to consider a certification exam. Again, the intent would not be to reduce the rigor of the certification process; in fact, those seeking the exam option could still be required to have a graduate degree and specific coursework. However, the exam option would allow for standardized assessment of the core content knowledge while offering a more accessible option for practitioners. An exam might offer a feasible alternative to the current process without diminishing the quality or meaningfulness of the certification.

International Developments in Professional Practice

There is growing international interest in defining the appropriate knowledge and experience for the professional practice of applied exercise and sport psychology. The terms used to identify and define professional practice and credentials (*accredited, chartered, registered, certified, licensed*) vary from country to country. However, the criteria identify the unique professional expertise required in sport and exercise. For example, the British Association of Sport and Exercise Sciences has an accreditation for sport psychology with the title *Accredited Sport and Exercise Scientist*. In addition, the British Psychological Society Division of Sport and Exercise Psychology has criteria for individual professionals to become Chartered Sport and Exercise Psychologists. Furthermore, the Australia Psychology Society College of Sport Psychologists has qualifications beyond those required for basic registration that requires a minimum of 6 years of university training, plus 2 years of supervised practical experience in sport psychology. It is evident that credentials for the expertise are in demand and that this trend is likely to continue and extend across the globe.

Certification provides a clear definition of the qualifications necessary to practice sport and exercise psychology. CC-AASP certification is open to licensed clinical professional counselors, licensed clinical social workers, individuals with master's level (MS, MA, MEd, or EdM) counselor licensure, individuals with doctoral degrees (EdD, PsyD, or PhD) generally from Council for Accreditation of Counseling and Related Educational Programs (CACREP) or APA accredited programs, or individuals from MS or PhD programs in Exercise and Sport Psychology. CC-AASP is a credential (not a licensure) from a professional organization that oversees standards in practice and training. CC-AASP without licensure can limit professional opportunities to those that focus on performance enhancement or mental skills coaching. However, CC-AASP certified professionals who also hold a license are well equipped to help a range of individuals with a range of mental health problems often linked to human performance decrements. The CC-AASP credential is becoming increasingly meaningful within the world of sport and exercise psychology, and is often preferred by employers seeking sport and exercise psychology expertise.

Edmund O. Acevedo and
Cassandra D. Pasquariello

See also Consultant Effectiveness, Assessment of; Consulting; Credentials; Ethics; Services; Supervision; Training, Professional

Further Readings

American Psychological Association. (2013). *Public description of sport psychology*. Retrieved from http://www.apa.org/ed/graduate/specialize/sports.aspx

Aoyagi, M. W., Portenga, S. T., Poczwardowski, A., Cohen, A. B., & Statler, T. (2012). Reflections and directions: The profession of sport psychology past, present, and future. *Journal of Professional Psychology: Research and Practice, 43,* 32–38. doi: 10.1037/a0025676

Association for Applied Sport Psychology. (n.d.). *About applied sport and exercise psychology*. Retrieved from http://www.appliedsportpsych.org/about/about-applied-sport-psych

Association for Applied Sport Psychology. (n.d.). *Become a certified consultant*. Retrieved from http://www.appliedsportpsych.org/Consultants/become-certified

Australian Psychological Society, College of Sport and Exercise Psychologists. (2012). *How to join*. Retrieved from http://www.groups.psychology.org.au/csep/join

The British Association of Sport and Exerise Sciences. (n.d.). *Accreditation*. Retrieved from http://www.bases.org.uk/Accreditation/Accreditation

The British Psychological Society, Division of Sport and Exerxise Psychology. (n.d.). *How to join*. Retrieved from http://spex.bps.org.uk/spex/join/join_home.cfm

CHARACTER DEVELOPMENT

The term *character* has a long, complex, and controversial history. An old adage holds that "sport builds character" and historically the inclusion of sport programs in educational settings often has been justified through appeal to their supposed character-building efficacy. The following entry elaborates on the meaning of character and discusses how sport researchers have dealt with this complex concept.

What Is Character?

Etymologically, the term *character* comes from the Greek *charaktēr,* meaning "indelible mark." Over the centuries, the term evolved and took on various and shifting connotations, yet it continued to carry the meaning of enduring qualities that mark a person. Today, there is no shared agreement on the definition of character. Some, for example, use it simply as a synonym for personality, while others promote a more narrow interpretation of character, limiting it to the moral dimensions of personhood.

Following the lead of the Character Education Partnership, the nation's leading umbrella organization of character educators, we elaborate a middle-road view of character that defines it more broadly than moral character yet not as broadly as including all dimensions of personality. For present purposes, let us define character as the set of psychological characteristics that motivate and enable the individual to seek truth and goodness. Character is rooted in desire for what is true, right, and good, and a honed ability to translate that desire into effective action. The term *virtue* is often used to describe a quality of character when it is well established. In turn, let us describe character development as the learning and development that individuals undergo as they acquire and solidify the requisite dispositions, competencies, and skills of character.

Character is evident in action, but a person's character does not fully determine behavior. Action arises from complex interactions among personal and situational influences, and sometimes temptations or pressures may overpower the tendencies that arise from one's dispositions. Nonetheless, research has demonstrated that character can be an important influence on behavior across contexts and situations.

Character can be elucidated in terms of four forms or dimensions of character: intellectual character, moral character, civic character, and performance character. All four are rooted in stable dispositional tendencies. They are elaborated below.

Intellectual Character

In his influential book, *Intellectual Character,* Ron Ritchhart describes intellectual character as a set of dispositions that both shape and motivate intellectual behavior. The dispositions that make up intellectual character include curiosity, open-mindedness, and truth seeking. Those with well-developed intellectual character are curious about the world around them, think critically, and are constantly seeking a deeper understanding. Athletes with exemplary intellectual character, for example, may ponder questions such as how sports influence broader society; what responsibilities elite athletes bear; how race, gender, and class limit opportunities; and so on. While it may be hypothesized that intellectual character contributes to a range of positive actions in sport settings, sport researchers have left this dimension of character largely unexamined.

Moral Character

When people talk of character, most often they mean moral character. Moral character refers to those psychological characteristics that motivate and enable the individual to function as a competent moral agent. These include moral reasoning competency and perspective-taking ability, empathy and moral identity, value hierarchies, and moral belief systems. At root, moral character is grounded in a basic and fundamental desire to do what is good and right. A person of high moral character is one who has a disposition to focus on moral dimensions of situations and act consistently with considered moral convictions.

Often, moral character is most evident in situations where values collide and choices need to be made. For example, an athlete may believe that cheating is wrong and simultaneously want to gain the benefits of victory. If moral character is strong, the moral concerns will take precedence over the more self-aggrandizing thoughts. It is important to recognize, however, that even a person with well-developed moral character may not be completely consistent in thought and action. All people, it is reasonable to assume, fail to resist the temptation to depart from their better selves on occasion (see "Performance Character" below).

Civic Character

Civic character refers to those psychological characteristics that motivate and enable the people's active, prosocial involvement in the groups to which they belong. A person with strong civic character tends to be engaged in communities and society, seeking to improve them. People with strong civic character tend to think in terms of shared interests and the common good. An athlete who seeks voluntary leadership roles on the team, not for selfish reasons but to serve, is likely to have well-developed civic character.

Performance Character

A dimension of character that has received growing attention in recent years is performance character. This dimension of character refers to all of those psychological characteristics that motivate and enable the individual to function effectively, efficiently, and competently as a value-pursuing agent. People with strong performance character have an increased likelihood of accomplishing their goals. Performance character includes such qualities as determination, perseverance, resilience, optimism, courage, loyalty, and attention to detail. Performance character reflects skills of self-management. It is important to recognize, however, that the qualities that make up performance character, while sometimes called *virtues*, are in themselves neither good nor bad. Is it good, for example, to be loyal to an ignoble leader or persistent in trying to rob a bank? The value of performance character depends on the goals served. When combined with a well-developed moral character, performance character enables a person to resist distractions and temptations and act effectively in the moral domain.

Character Development

How the multiple dimensions of character develop is a topic of considerable dispute among developmental and educational psychologists. The two most influential schools of thought have their origins in behaviorist and constructivist approaches to psychology.

The Behaviorist Approach to Character Development

According to behaviorists, and those influenced by them (such as social learning theorists), character development is primarily under the molding influence of the environment. From this perspective, the dispositions that constitute character are products of reinforcement contingencies and modeling opportunities. For example, if an athlete frequently gets in fights with opponents, it is because the athlete has learned that the negative consequences to fighting are outweighed by the rewards like an intimidated opponent. Similarly, if an athlete upholds the ideals of sportsmanship, it is because that athlete, through years of experience, has learned that there are significant benefits, such as an enhanced reputation and praise from others, from acting in a prosocial manner.

Character educators who rely predominantly on the perspectives of behaviorists and social learning theorists place a great deal of emphasis on the role of authority figures, such as parents and coaches. It is these people who have the greatest power to control how rewards are distributed. By modeling desired behaviors and managing the costs and benefits that follow actions, behavior can be shaped and eventually dispositions established and reinforced.

In addition, direct teaching of character virtues is often advocated by behaviorists and neobehaviorists. For example, coaches are encouraged to explain what *respect* means, model it themselves, and then shape the behavior of their athletes by rewarding respectful behavior and punishing deviations. Critics maintain that the strategies recommended by behaviorists may work to modify behavior, but only in the short term. What happens when the modeling and reinforcements change? What happens, for example, when a new coach arrives who rewards winning rather than respectful behavior? Since the behaviorist's strategies don't address the core beliefs and values of the learner, they may create situational conformity to expectations without genuinely influencing character.

The influential work of Albert Bandura provides something of a bridge between the behavioral and social learning traditions of psychology and the constructivist approaches to be discussed next. His theoretical roots extend deeply into social learning theory, but over the past couple of decades he has increasingly incorporated cognitive mediators of behavior. Like other behavioral and social learning theorists, character, for Bandura, is rooted in environmental experiences, and society is the ultimate arbiter of what counts as moral. Bandura extends the paradigm, however, by suggesting that the person can develop and employ self-management skills that can provide stability to character despite changing contextual influences. Cognitive processes, however, can also derail character. Bandura discusses at length the cognitive processes of *moral disengagement* that function to provide self-justifying excuses for antisocial behavior.

The Constructivist Approach to Character Development

The constructivist approach to character development maintains that the child is not a blank slate ready to be written on through modeling and reinforcement. Rather, the child is a *meaning maker* who actively interprets experience and selects what aspects of the environment to attend to. When, for example, an adult rewards a child, the effect is not automatic. Rather, the child interprets the informational value of the adult's action and may

choose to comply with or rebel against the effort to shape personal behavior. Children's character is influenced as much by the child's own choices and initiative as through such external sources as modeling and reinforcement.

Character educators who draw from constructivist theories engage with the child on the level of meaning and relationship, not just the level of reward and punishment. They emphasize such processes as dialogue, group dynamics, and building communities where trust and care are nurtured. The foundation of character is in positive relationships where personal dispositions are forged through enduring patterns of interaction. When a person feels known, valued, included, and empowered, the person is more open to positive social influence.

Character Development and Sport

It is clear that the physical activities of sport—throwing, kicking, or hitting balls, running, jumping, and so forth—do not have any significant impact on character development. To the extent that sport experiences contribute to the development of character, it is because of the opportunities they provide to set and pursue goals, build meaningful and purpose-driven relationships, cooperate to achieve shared aims, experience and manage a range of intense emotions, and test ethical commitments through the challenges of competition. Perhaps more than any other widely shared activity, sports can provide many young people with a chance to build nurturing relationships with both peers and adults.

As historians and sociologists have pointed out, the specific virtues that sport is claimed to nurture have varied considerably from one historical period to the next. In 19th-century England, for example, team sports were a regular part of life in many boarding schools because it was believed that they would build those qualities useful to the elites of the far-flung British Empire. It was claimed that sports would develop leadership, strategic thinking, loyalty, courage, and other aspects of *manliness*. By the early 20th century in the United States, the character-building ideology continued, but with a different cast of virtues. With a large influx of immigrants and a growing urban economy, sports were seen as vehicles to prepare a compliant workforce with such dispositions as obedience, discipline, patriotism, and self-sacrifice.

The changing definitions of character highlight the need for researchers to carefully and operationally define the term. To date, most research on character in sport has focused on the moral dimension.

Research on specific aspects of moral character, such as moral reasoning capacity, has shed some light. There has been no research to support a positive role for sports in advancing moral reasoning, apart from a small number of intervention studies. A few studies have suggested that participation in some sports, particularly at the college level, may have negative effects on moral reasoning, though inconsistent results and methodological concerns prevent this from being considered a verified conclusion. The research on what has been called the *professionalization of values*, though, has demonstrated that the longer one participates in sport and the higher the competitive level, the lower *playing fair* is as a value relative to winning.

Research related to dimensions of performance character is more encouraging, but the evidence is indirect. For example, based on longitudinal investigations, it appears that participation in high school sports is associated with later educational attainment and lower drop-out rates. One likely explanation for these positive outcomes is that sports develop qualities like goal setting, time management, delay of gratification, sequential thinking, initiative, concentration, and attention focusing. These skills and dispositions, which are core to performance character, can lead to greater success in both sports and school. Additional research is needed, however, to investigate directly the hypothesized links and to examine potential mediating effects of such variables as sport type, coaching styles, and team culture issues.

One encouraging finding is that when character development is an intentional and explicit aim of physical activity programs and when leaders are trained to implement it, positive results can be obtained. Don Hellison, for example, has developed an influential approach to character development through physical activity and sport. In his model for developing personal and social responsibility, he combines a focus on both moral character and the self-control dimensions of performance character.

No doubt, many practitioners will continue to list character development as one goal for sports participation, and researchers will continue to investigate the promises and pitfalls of such a goal.

To move forward, both theory-based practitioners and practice-based researchers will need to work diligently to clarify their terms and elucidate their theoretical framework. Character will continue to be a disputed concept, but an important one nonetheless.

Brenda Light Bredemeier and David Light Shields

See also Fair Play; Moral Development; Moral Judgment; Moral Reasoning; Self-Regulation

Further Readings

Bredemeier, B., & Shields, D. (2006). Sports and character development. *Research Digest, President's Council on Physical Fitness and Sports, 7*(1), 1–8.

Clifford, C., & Feezell, R. M. (2010). *Sport and character: Reclaiming the principles of sportsmanship.* Champaign, IL: Human Kinetics.

Hellison, D. (2010). *Teaching personal and social responsibility through physical activity* (3rd ed.). Champaign, IL: Human Kinetics.

Lapsley, D. K., & Power, F. C. (2005). *Character psychology and character education.* Notre Dame, IN: University of Notre Dame Press.

Shields, D. L. (2011). Character as the aim of education. *Phi Delta Kappan, 92*(8), 48–53.

Shields, D. L., & Bredemeier, B. L. (1995). *Character development and physical activity.* Champaign, IL: Human Kinetics.

Shields, D. L., & Bredemeier, B. L. (2008). Sport and the development of character. In L. Nucci & D. Narvaez (Eds.), *Handbook of moral and character education* (pp. 500–519). New York: Routledge.

Shields, D. L., & Bredemeier, B. L. (2011). Coaching for civic character. *Journal of Research in Character Education, 9*(1), 25–33.

CHEATING

Cheating in sport is a violation of an explicit or implicit promise to follow the rules of a sporting activity. This promise is an honorable action that an athlete takes to assure the opponent, the fans, and all interested parties that the rules will be followed. An example of an explicit promise is the International Olympic Committee oath for athletes. The oath is taken by one athlete representing all athletes from their home nation. The oath states,

In the name of all the competitors, I promise that we shall take part in these Olympic Games, respecting and abiding by the rules which govern them, committing ourselves to a sport without doping and without drugs, in the true spirit of sportsmanship, for the glory of the sport and the honour of our teams. (http://registration.olympic .org/en/faq/detail/id/28)

An implicit promise to follow the rules is the unspoken, accepted conditions that a player agrees to do when playing. In many amateur sport competitions, the competitors, captains, or coaches meet before the game begins and shake hands. The handshake is an implied agreement that each will play well, will play by the rules, and wishes the other good luck.

Categories of Rules in Sport

The rules that athletes and coaches promise to follow come in three different categories, and athletes and coaches have numerous creative ways to violate intentionally both the spirit and the letter of these rules. The rules are *constitutive, regulatory,* and *sportsmanship.*

The constitutive rules give order and direction as to how the game is to be formed and how it is played. The constitutive rules are norm referenced and give boundaries to the game. For example, consider the rule as to how long a game is played. In softball, three outs per team make an inning, seven innings for a game; in American football, four quarters make a game, and each quarter is a specific number of minutes of play; in amateur basketball, 60 minutes is the allotted period of play divided into two halves.

The regulatory rules maintain and temper the integrity of play within the constitutive rules. Regulatory rules are very useful but less fundamental. For example, in softball a player who is at bat cannot run to a base until a pitched ball is either hit or the ball reaches the catcher's glove and four balls are called by the umpire. In American football, a player cannot leave the line of play until the offensive center hikes the ball to the quarterback. In amateur basketball, a player cannot advance the ball down the court without dribbling or passing the ball.

Players accept the constitutive and regulatory rules as the guideline and give an implicit or explicit (verbal agreement) promise to follow these rules. Inadvertent violation of the playing rules, if caught by officials, results in a foul or rule break in the game. Both the constitutive and regulatory rules are usually governed by umpires, referees, or game officials. Violation of a rule is not cheating. However, intentional violation to break the rules without being caught is a violation of the promise to accept the consequences of breaking a rule. An example of cheating of constitutive rules in American football is the faked injury to stop the play clock. If a referee deems an athlete is injured, the referee must stop the play clock until the injured athlete is attended to and removed from play. Even though a rule exists against faked injuries, a team may conspire to have an athlete pretend to be injured, especially if the play clock is running out. The time clock stops, the player is treated and removed from play, and in the meantime the team uses the extra time to set up the next play and perhaps win. An example of cheating of the regulatory rules is the baseball pitcher altering the condition of the ball. The regulatory rules are specific as to the size, shape, and condition of the ball. Pitchers often change the condition of the ball by scuffing the surface with an abrasive located in their glove, hand, or pocket, or place goo on the ball.

Sportsmanship and Gamesmanship

A player, coach, and team also implicitly promise to follow the spirit of sportsmanship, which includes accepting the philosophy of fair play: the reason for rules' existence. Fundamentally, the philosophy of fair play is to offer each team and competitor an equal opportunity to be successful. However, coaches often break their implied promises through clever and artful techniques. For example, in 1928 a football coach tried to find a method for his team to be more competitive on the field of play. He looked through the rule book and found no rules that limited placing artifacts on the players' jerseys, except a number on the back of the jersey. He cut footballs into halves, and sewed one half of a football on the front of all the backfield players' jerseys. When his quarterback handed the ball off to a backfield member, everyone in the backfield had a football on his uniform. Because no rule existed to prevent the artful strategy, the coach violated the spirit of fair play in the ideal sense and he cheated.

The artful strategy of trying to get around the rules or push the rules beyond the letter is called gamesmanship. Gamesmanship often borders on cheating. Most players accept some gamesmanship that occurs; however, there is an arbitrary line when gamesmanship becomes cheating. In officiated games, players learn to push that arbitrary line and not only play a game against their opponent but also play another game against the official. The players use the rules to their advantage and challenge the official to catch them violating the letter and spirit of the rules. Players learn how much they can get away with when pushing the rules by learning how tight the game will be called by the official(s). Officials therefore must know the rules as well as know the ethos of how the game is played. The *ethos*, the essential nature of the game and how rules are interpreted, gives direction as to how much latitude the official uses in determining how closely the rules are followed. For example, basketball is a no contact game; however, there is a great deal of contact that is accepted as part of playing the game. The ethos directs the officials to decide how much contact is accepted and what is not accepted. Within this game climate, knowing the difference between violating a rule and cheating becomes fuzzy. The players and officials thus rely greatly on the written rules, the spirit of the rules, and their game-to-game experience in deciding the difference.

Intentionally violating an organizational or institutional rule that governs the preparation for the game, including player training, is governed by a different set of rules. These sportsmanship rules are established by the governing body that oversees how games are played. The goal is to establish a culture of fair play in which all players come to the game with a fair chance of being successful in playing and winning the contest, all of which is also very arbitrary, depending on each team's resources and genetics of the players themselves. A bobsled team from the Caribbean island of Trinidad would have little chance at success considering that no bobsled track exists in Trinidad. However, Trinidad has fielded a bobsled team to the Olympic Games. The team's chance of success is not necessarily fair. Players thus are members of teams and both the player and the team agree explicitly to follow the rules established by the organization in preparation and training as well as the actual playing of game. When players and their teams intentionally violate these rules, cheating occurs.

The same issue occurs in the constitutive rules and regulatory game rules—players and teams work the rules to gain an advantage; rules then become more explicit and officials become more aggressive in monitoring whether players and teams are following the rules. A case in point is the rule against players ingesting or injecting banned performance-enhancing drugs or supplements to gain a physiological advantage. A player is always limited by genetic predisposition, and no matter how much practice takes place, that limit cannot be overcome without some external chemical aid. Thus, some players try to gain that additional advantage beyond their own physiological makeup and choose to take chemical supplementation to overcome their own limitations. The practice is almost as old as competitive sport. Since the purpose of play is about fair play, meaning that everyone should have the same degree of chance to perform well, most if not all governing bodies have specific lists of acceptable and unacceptable supplement usage. In order to monitor players, the organizations demand testing—including urine samples and in some cases blood samples—to check if players are following the rules. Whole industries have been developed to test, track, record, and monitor players; the World Anti-Doping Agency is one of them. However, again the problem is gamesmanship. The players are constantly looking for an advantage, and since each human body has limitations, the players are looking for nutritional or chemical supplementation to overcome physiological and genetic limitations. The line again becomes fuzzy—which supplements are acceptable and which are not.

All players supposedly are acquainted with cheating, but in some cases they choose to manipulate and stretch the rule. The way sports are played and played out often makes it difficult to admit that cheating is the intentional violation of a promise to play by both the spirit and the rules of the game. However, cheating is always the intentional action of breaking a promise and violating the rules.

Sharon Kay Stoll

See also Character Development; Ethics; Moral Development; Moral Reasoning; Moral Values and Attitudes; Sportspersonship

Further Readings

Lumpkin, A., Stoll, S. K., & Beller, J. M. (2011). *Practical ethics in sport management*. Jefferson City, NC: McFarland Press.

Pearson, K. M. (2002). Deception, sportsmanship, and ethics. In J. Boxhill (Ed.), *Sport ethics: An anthology* (Chap. 8). Chapel Hill, NC: Wiley-Blackwell.

Reall, M. J., Bailey, J. J., & Stoll, S. K. (1998). Moral reasoning "on hold" during a competitive game. *Journal of Business Ethics, 17,* 1205–1210.

Shields, D. L. (2009). *What is "decompetition" and why does it matter?* Retrieved from http://searchwarp.com/swa471691.htm

Simon, R. L. (2003). *Fair play: The ethics of sport* (2nd ed.). Boulder, CO: Westview Press.

Stoll, S. K. (2011). Athletics: The good it should do. *Journal of College and Character, 13*(4), 1–5.

Stoll, S. K., & Beller, J. M. (2000). Do sports build character? In J. R. Gerdy, *Sports in school: The future of an institution* (pp. 18–30). New York: Teachers College Press.

Stoll, S. K., & Beller, J. M. (2006). Ethical dilemmas. In R. Lapchick, *New game plan for college sport.* Lanham, MD: Rowman & Littlefield.

CHOKING

Researchers, spectators and performers alike are often intrigued, and sometimes shocked, if motivated people perform dramatically worse than usual in important, high-pressure situations. This can happen not only in sports but in almost any domain in which people are specifically motivated to do well, be it music, surgery, academic examinations, or even a driving test.

Choking, or *choking under pressure,* is a metaphorical expression frequently used in sport settings to describe occasions when severe unexpected decrements occur in performance under anxiety-provoking situations. Such occasions potentially can be invoked by the presence of an evaluative audience, the possibility for high reward, competition, or factors unique to each individual choker. Examples of choking in sport tend to be memorable and sometimes sports evolve their own domestic expression for the phenomenon.

There is no agreed definition of what it means to choke. Early definitions suggested that *choking* is inferior or suboptimal performance in response to high motivation to perform well, but recent researchers have argued that such a definition does not capture the acute, dramatic declines in performance that go beyond merely suboptimal performance. Most examination of choking has derived from empirical studies, which are unable to re-create the factors that cause choking in each individual, so some researchers have highlighted the need for a more idiographic, qualitative approach that is ecologically valid.

Why Does Choking Occur?

It seems likely that choking arises as a stress response associated with very high motivation to perform well. It also has been suggested that a choking event can have a long-term negative psychological impact on performers, leaving them vulnerable to further choking events in the future.

Historically, arousal theories have been used to explain performance decrements in anxiety-provoking situations, but these are merely descriptive models, which link arousal or drive with performance. They offer little explanation of the underlying mechanisms that result in performance decrements (or indeed performance peaks). The best known of the theories is probably the Yerkes–Dodson law (better known as inverted-U theory), which suggests that improved performance accompanies increased arousal until intermediate levels of arousal are reached. Further increases in arousal result in performance decrements. Such a model has a number of shortcomings with respect to the phenomenon of choking. For example, the model implies that if arousal becomes too high and performance declines, a performer can regain the previous level of performance merely by reducing arousal. The model also implies that changes in performance level are smooth and gradual as arousal increases (or decreases), which does not explain the acute, dramatic drops in performance that typify choking. To resolve these issues, some researchers have turned to René Thom's theory of catastrophes, which tries to explain abrupt shifts or *bifurcations* in behavior (e.g., landslides, bridge collapses, and even capsized ships) that are associated with relatively small, continuous changes in contributing factors. In particular, the researchers have examined cusp catastrophes to elucidate how physiological arousal and cognitive anxiety (worry) interact to cause high or low levels of performance in sport. The model suggests that high cognitive anxiety couples with increasing physiological arousal to cause abrupt catastrophic drops in performance or *choke*s.

A shift in emphasis has seen attention theories exploited to better understand the cognitive mechanisms that underlie the effects of performance pressure on performance. These theories propose that under anxiety-provoking conditions there may be a disruptive reallocation of attention, which subsequently triggers performance decrements. To a certain extent this approach is underpinned by *cue utilization theory,* which suggests that changes in attentional focus caused by performance pressure influence the degree to which an individual is able to process task-relevant information but not task-irrelevant information. Two current models that exploit attention theories propose that performance can be disrupted because attention either becomes distracted away from important aspects of performance or because attention becomes overly attracted to skill-focused aspects of performance.

Distraction Models

Distraction models propose that performance pressure causes a shift in attention, which results in unnecessary processing of information irrelevant to performance of the task, such as worry and self-doubt. Working memory is thought to support the storage and active maintenance of information over short durations and, as a consequence, to be involved in processing information related to task performance. Processing additional irrelevant information is therefore likely to decrease the attention resources available to working memory and subsequently compromise its ability to process task-relevant information that is crucial for effective performance.

One particular theory, which offers insight to how distraction mediates the relationship between anxiety and cognition in sport (although it was not developed specifically for sport) is *attentional control theory* (ACT). ACT is an extension of *processing efficiency theory* (PET), proposed by Michael Eysenck and his colleagues. ACT proposes that anxiety reduces goal-directed focus but increases stimulus-driven focus, allowing attention to more easily be distracted to threat-related stimuli and the processing of threat-related stimuli to be less easily inhibited. Unnecessary processing of threat-related internal stimuli like worry about the consequences of performance failure or external stimuli like irrelevant environmental factors can harm performance, but the theory proposes that performance effectiveness can be preserved by increasing task-related effort in order to augment the processing resources dedicated to the task. Consequently,

anxiety may not always reduce the quality of performance.

To a certain extent, this theory seems feasible. For example, there is no doubt that most soccer players become highly anxious before a penalty shootout at the World Cup. Their attention is distracted to threatening internal stimuli, such as "What will the press say if I miss?" or to threatening external stimuli, such as sudden realization that the goal is smaller than they recall (or the goalkeeper taller). Fewer resources are thus available to allocate to the task at hand and the probability of failed performance increases dramatically. But not all players do fail in penalty shootouts. Some players seem to counteract the effects of pressure on their penalty-taking performance with intense effort. Others appear unable to compensate; they choke, as the newspapers will later claim.

A problem with distraction theories, however, is that evidence from research on nonmotor, cognitive tasks such as mathematics problems, suggests that those tasks that rely heavily on working memory are most affected by worry associated with pressure. Most examples of choking in sport involve performance of well-practiced skills that do not rely heavily on working memory because they are procedural and run automatically. Consequently, the performance of skills in sport should be relatively immune to depleted working memory resources. A second explanatory model has therefore emerged, which suggests that pressure heightens self-consciousness about performing successfully, causing attention to become skill focused. Theories that take this approach have a wide variety of nomenclature that includes self-focus theory, explicit monitoring theory, conscious processing hypothesis, the constrained action hypothesis, and the theory of reinvestment.

Skill-Focused Models

Skill-focused models intimate that well-practiced skills in sport (and in other movement-related domains) can be disrupted not by depletion of working memory resources but by the misappropriation of spare working memory resources to consciously control performance that is best left to run automatically. In order to ensure that performance is effective, the performer explicitly tries to control the process of skill execution, which disrupts or inhibits automatic control processes and usually results in poor performance. Roy

Baumeister probably described this best when he simply argued that consciousness does not have access to enough of the task-relevant knowledge needed to run automated skills effectively.

Some of the best evidence for the model comes from studies that have shown that expert performers tend to be able to preserve the high quality of their performance when carrying out a concurrent task (such as tone recognition) that takes attention away from execution of the skill. Well-practiced skills require minimal working memory resources for effective performance, leaving resources spare for the concurrent task. Skilled performers, however, tend to display disrupted performance when carrying out a concurrent task that requires attention to execution of the skills (e.g., a task that requires indication of the position of the bat when a tone sounds). Evidence from studies, using the same or similar paradigms, shows that under pressure skilled performers also become more accurate at the secondary task (e.g., indicating the position of the bat when the tone sounded), indicating that pressure causes increased skill focus.

It has been argued that distraction models and skill-focus models lead to opposing predictions, but it is unlikely that the models are independent. A shift in attention under pressure, which disrupts automaticity by unnecessary processing of declarative knowledge that is redundant for performance, appears to encompass both distraction and skill-focus models.

Personality and Performance Under Pressure!

Some performers may be more susceptible to choking than others. Specific dispositional traits (relatively stable personality characteristics) may predispose performers to choking. Attentional control theory, for example, suggests that high trait anxious individuals are more likely than low trait anxious individuals to display disrupted performance under pressure, although these findings are confined to test-anxiety situations, rather than performance in sport. It has been suggested that high levels of chronic anxiety might not even be relevant in sport as these relatively public settings may not attract individuals with such traits.

One personality trait associated with skill-focus theories is self-consciousness. It has been claimed that people who are generally high in self-consciousness are likely to perform better under pressure than people who are low in self-consciousness, because they are accustomed to

performing with the high levels of self-focus that pressure causes. It is unclear whether this proposal is correct, given that some evidence shows that people generally high in self-consciousness are more likely to choke than people low in self-consciousness. The *theory of reinvestment* argues that not only self-consciousness but also the inclination to consciously control performance is subject to individual differences. Psychometric measures of a general disposition for reinvestment, or for movement specific reinvestment, have been developed. Both make reference to personality traits that include self-consciousness, rumination, and even slips of action, and both show that the performance of people who score high on such metrics is generally more negatively influenced by pressure than the performance of people who score low on such metrics.

Protecting Performance Under Pressure

Techniques that divert attention away from conscious control, perhaps to an external rather than an internal focus, or that improve the ability of the performer to maintain the correct focus of attention, may help to prevent choking. Methods that train control of attention, such as emotion control training or hypoegoic self-regulation (in which an individual learns deliberately to relinquish conscious control of behavior), potentially can help performers maintain the fluid automaticity of their performance under pressure. Alternatively, training that acclimatizes performers to heightened self-consciousness may inoculate them against pressure. Ritualized behaviors or routines may swamp working memory and prevent skill focus, as may concurrent secondary tasks. There is even evidence that performing faster than usual when under pressure may help performers to avoid skill focus, although as anyone who has ever tried this approach will attest, it is not so simple in the heat of battle. A more enduring approach may be to use implicit motor learning techniques to curtail construction of a task-relevant declarative knowledge base. The integrity of automatic control processes should be more secure if task-relevant declarative knowledge cannot be extracted from long-term memory for conscious control purposes.

Research directly or indirectly related to choking has expanded considerably over the past three decades. Investigation has shifted from a passive to a more active approach, progressing from qualitative discussion about entertaining anecdotal reports of performance failure under pressure to concrete empirical research. As long as observers continue to be intrigued and shocked when motivated people perform their skills dramatically worse than usual when the stakes are high, the research interest is likely to continue.

Rich Masters and Neha Malhotra

See also Attentional Focus; Attention–Performance Relationships; Automaticity; Competition; Effort; Expertise; Motor Learning; Skill Acquisition

Further Readings

Baumeister, R. F. (1986). A review of paradoxical performance effects: Choking under pressure in sports and mental tests. *European Journal of Social Psychology, 16*, 361–383.

Beilock, S. L., & Gray, R. (2007). Why do athletes choke under pressure? In G. Tenenbaum & R. C. Eklund (Eds.), *Handbook of sport psychology* (3rd ed., pp. 425–444). Hoboken, NJ: Wiley.

Eysenck, M. W., Derakshan, N., Santos, R., & Calvo, M. G. (2007). Anxiety and cognitive performance: Attentional control theory. *Emotion, 7*, 336–353.

Hardy, L., Beattie, S., & Woodman, T. (2007). Anxiety-induced performance catastrophes: Investigating effort required as an asymmetry factor. *British Journal of Psychology, 98*, 15–31.

Hill, D., Hanton, S., Fleming, S., & Matthews, N. (2009). A re-examination of choking in sport. *European Journal of Sport Science, 9*, 203–212.

Lewis, B. P., & Linder, D. E. (1997). Thinking about choking? Attentional processes and paradoxical performance. *Personality and Social Psychology Bulletin, 23*, 937–944.

Masters, R. S. W., & Maxwell, J. P. (2008). The theory of reinvestment. *International Review of Sport and Exercise Psychology, 1*, 160–183.

Masters, R. S. W., & Poolton, J. (2012). Advances in implicit motor learning. In N. J. Hodges & A. M. Williams (Eds.), *Skill acquisition in sport: Research, theory and practice* (2nd ed., pp. 59–75). London: Routledge.

Wulf, G. (2007). *Attention and motor skill learning*. Champaign, IL: Human Kinetics.

CHUNKING/DECHUNKING

Cognitive psychologists argue that over time, task-related knowledge is organized into information-rich representations or chunks, a process termed *chunking*. *Dechunking* refers to when well-developed chunks are broken down into a number of smaller chunks or bits of information. Chunking is a fundamental building block of human memory and underlies the learning of perceptual and motor skills. Dechunking is a mechanism that potentially underlies suboptimal performance. In this entry, the process by which information is chunked during learning is explained in general terms and in relation to both perceptual and motor skills. The process and implication of dechunking are then briefly discussed.

To operate effectively, humans must utilize information in the performance environment, but the human information-processing system has limitations. Specifically, the capacity to store and retrieve verbally coded, declarative knowledge is finite and small, and serial processing of such information is time consuming. Despite these limitations, people can successfully execute perceptual–motor skills in environments that are often complex, dynamic, and time constrained. Indeed, experts are defined by their ability to overcome the limitations of the information processing system. Their decisions depend upon rapid processing of large quantities of perceptual information. Their motor skills are executed in a smooth and automated fashion. Chunking underlies these capabilities.

Stage models of skill acquisition propose that early in learning bits of information pertaining to a task are stored, retrieved, and processed as declarative knowledge by a short-term information processor (working memory), which interfaces with long-term memory. With repeated on-task experience, meaningful associations emerge between recurring bits of information that are grouped together and coded as chunks. Over the course of practice, between-chunk associations develop and higher and higher level chunks are compiled, until large amounts of the information pertaining to a task are hierarchically organized into a single representative chunk. The demand on information processing resources lessens as each level of the hierarchical structure is formed, until higher level chunks take a procedural form that no longer requires the retrieval and processing of declarative knowledge. In the domain of sport and exercise, chunking takes two distinct forms: the chunking of perceptual information for response selection, and the chunking of the motor information needed to organize and execute a successful response.

The strategies and rules inherent within dynamic activities like team sports generally result in the availability of structured perceptual information, such as the relative position of teammates and opponents or the mechanics of an opponent's movements. Visual elements that meaningfully correlate gradually become recognized as distinct patterns. With increased exposure, relations between these patterns emerge and so they are compiled together, and from then on recognized as a single pattern. Empirically, the chunking process has been demonstrated by findings that show experts have superior capacity to recall patterns of game play after only a brief presentation of a structured, rather than transitory, unstructured game scenario. Chunking allows experts to quickly and accurately recognize patterns from within the unfolding events and this, in turn, permits both the rapid and accurate selection of an appropriate motor response.

A motor response is the outcome of the ordered execution of a sequence of movement components. In the early stage of motor learning, the sequencing and control of independent movement components is typically controlled at a conscious level, placing high demands on the available information processing resources. Consistent repetition of a pattern of movement through practice causes adjacent movement components to coalesce into chunks. Chunks in motor learning are defined by pauses between successive movement components. For example, sequential key pressing experiments show that latencies between successive key presses decrease with practice in a clear and consistent fashion such that longer pauses demarcate chunk boundaries. Pauses between adjacent motor chunks result in a segmented or jerky motor action. Continued practice builds a hierarchical structure, in which fewer chunks comprising longer sequences of movement components exist. As a result, the movement is both less jerky and places fewer demands on information processing resources. Eventually, all movement components are incorporated into a single representative motor chunk, which, when selected, results in the smooth, automatic production of complex sequences of movement.

Compared to the concept of chunking, dechunking is a less well established phenomenon. As chunking is associated with the learning or progression of skills, dechunking may be used to explain occurrences of skill regression or skill failure. Declarative knowledge accrued during learning likely remains retrievable from long-term memory after it has been chunked at a higher level. The retrieval and processing of previously chunked declarative knowledge represents the dechunking of optimal and automated representations and regression to a less efficient and less fluid mode of control. In the competitive environment, contingencies such as performance anxiety may trigger dechunking and result in skill failure. Alternatively, in the training environment athletes may purposefully attempt to revise the composition of high-level representations by first dechunking and then rechunking information.

In summary, the chunking of information is a consequence of the practice that underlies skill learning. It allows well-practiced performers to operate proficiently despite the temporal and capacity constraints of the information processing system. Dechunking describes a return to the retrieval and processing of hitherto chunked declarative knowledge.

Jamie Poolton and Rich Masters

See also Choking; Information Processing; Motor Learning; Pattern Recognition and Recall; Skill Acquisition

Further Readings

Anderson, J. R. (1982). Acquisition of cognitive skill. *Psychological Review, 89,* 369–406.

Gobet, F., & Simon, H. A. (1998). Expert chess memory: Revisiting the chunking hypothesis. *Memory, 6,* 225–255.

Miller, G. A. (1956). The magical number seven, plus or minus two: Some limits on our capacity for processing information. *Psychological Review, 63,* 81–97.

Rosenbaum, D. A., Kenny, S. B., & Derr, M. A. (1983). Hierarchical control of rapid movement sequences. *Journal of Experimental Psychology: Human Perception and Performance, 9,* 86–102.

COACH–ATHLETE RELATIONS

The coach–athlete relationship is a unique interpersonal relationship characterized by mutually and interconnected thoughts, feelings, and emotions between an athlete and a coach. There are different types of coach–athlete relationships, including traditional coach–athlete dyads (the coach and athlete are not related in any way other than their coaching relationship), married coach–athlete dyads, and family coach–athlete dyads.

The coach–athlete relationship is of importance to both the athlete and the coach as an effective coach–athlete relationship is crucial to the achievement of successful performance and interpersonal satisfaction. For example, research has indicated the quality of the coach–athlete relationships can influence coaches' passion for coaching, coaches' motivation and the motivational climate they create, athletes' perceptions of self-concept and self-esteem, levels of intrinsic motivation, and perceptions of performance. Further, the quality of the coach–athlete relationship can influence athletes' perceptions of fear of failure, and the likelihood of burnout or drop-out.

Understanding Coach–Athlete Relationships

Initial research examining coach–athlete relationships almost exclusively focused upon utilizing models of leadership to illustrate how coaches' behaviors and actions influence athletes' actions and behaviors. Packinthan Chelladurai's Multidimensional Model of Leadership is one theory that has been widely used to examine coach leadership and the subsequent influence it has upon athletes. This model consists of three aspects of coaching behavior: actual leader behavior, preferred leader behavior, and required leader behavior. Actual leader behavior incorporates the behaviors a coach displays based upon his experience, personality, and ability. Preferred behaviors are the behaviors that athletes would prefer the leader to display. Preferred behaviors can be influenced by various factors such as athlete's age and gender. For example, younger or less experienced athletes may prefer higher levels of relationship-oriented behaviors from coaches than older or more experienced athletes. Similarly, although research is not conclusive, male athletes may prefer more autocratic coach behaviors than female athletes. Required behaviors are behaviors that coaches employ due to environmental or situational constraints and demands. This model suggests that athletes' performance and satisfaction are attributed to the degree of congruence among the three aspects of leader behavior.

Taking a relational perspective to examining coach–athlete relationships, Sophia Jowett developed the 3 + 1C model. This model proposes that effective coach–athlete relationships are characterized by four interrelated dimensions: *closeness, commitment, complementarity,* and *coordination.* Closeness accounts for the emotional aspect of the relationship. It refers to the interpersonal feelings between the coach and the athlete, and includes aspects such as trust, respect, and caring for each other. Commitment describes the cognitive component of the relationship and reflects the coach's and athlete's thoughts regarding their intentions to maintain a close athletic relationship over time. Complementarity refers to the behaviors part of the relationship. Complementarity reflects the coach's and athlete's cooperative interactions during training and competition. Finally, coorientation accounts for the coach's and athlete's shared perspectives, which are developed as a result of open channels of communication. The quality of the relationship is influenced not only by how the coach and athlete directly perceive their relationship but also by how they believe each other perceive the connection.

Conflict in the Coach–Athlete Relationship

Conflict has been defined as experiencing discord between oneself and significant others. Two of the main reasons conflict arises between coaches and athletes are an incompatibility in the relationship and either party breaking the rules of the relationship. Incompatibility can arise within the coach–athlete relationship when differences emerge regarding goals, beliefs, attitudes, values, or behaviors. For example, if a coach and an athlete are striving to achieve different goals there is potential for conflict to arise as each party is working toward a different outcome. Similarly, changes in circumstances may contribute to a coach or an athlete breaking the agreed upon rules of their relationship. Such rules are the expectations for behavior each party holds for the other party, themselves, and the overall relationship. Such conflict can arise or be enhanced if the relationship is lacking in terms of open, honest communication.

Coach–Athlete Relationships in Youth Sport

The coach–athlete relationship within youth sport is often complicated by the involvement of parents. When children begin to take part in sport, parents are often heavily involved and coaches play a more marginal role. However, as children progress in sport, they increasingly rely on their coach as more hours are spent training. At this time, the role of parents often changes as parents assume a more background role. The changing roles between parents and coaches can be associated with conflict or power struggles. If such conflict arises, it can cause tension within the coach–athlete and parent–athlete relationship. Children can also become unhappy or distressed if they become caught in the conflict.

Nicholas L. Holt and Camilla J. Knight

See also Autonomy-Supportive Coaching; Caring Climate; Interdependence Theory and the Coach–Athlete Relationship; Parenting; Talent Development

Further Readings

Jowett, S. (2007). Understanding the coach-athlete relationship. In S. Jowett & D. Lavallee (Eds.), *Social psychology in sport* (pp. 3–14). Champaign, IL: Human Kinetics.

Jowett, S., Paull, G., Pensgaard, A. M., Hoegmo, P. M., & Risse, H. (2005). Coach-athlete relationship. In J. Taylor & G. Wilson (Eds.), *Applying sport psychology: Four perspectives* (pp. 153–170). Champaign, IL: Human Kinetics.

LaVoi, N. M. (2007). Interpersonal communication and conflict in the coach-athlete relationship. In S. Jowett & D. Lavallee (Eds.), *Social psychology in sport* (pp. 29–40). Champaign, IL: Human Kinetics.

Rhind, D. J. A., & Jowett, S. (2012). Working with coach-athlete relationships: Their quality and maintenance. In S. Hanton & S. D. Mellalieu (Eds.), *Professional practice in sport psychology: A review* (pp. 219–248). Oxon, UK: Routledge.

COACHING EFFICACY

Self-efficacy judgments are domain-specific beliefs held by individuals about their ability to successfully execute differing levels of performance given certain situational demands (a situation-specific self-confidence). *Coaching efficacy* is the extent to which a coach believes in the personal capacity to affect the learning and performance of the athletes. Efficacy beliefs of a head coach play a central role in several broader theoretical models of effective sport coaching. This entry provides a broad overview of related research and first introduces a conceptual model of coaching efficacy. Measurement models for coaching efficacy are then described. Potential sources and proposed outcomes of coaching

efficacy are then reviewed, and the entry concludes with a discussion of future research directions.

A Conceptual Model of Coaching Efficacy

For as long as there has been organized sport, coaches have played a key role in the motivation and performance of athletes. Perhaps surprisingly, it was not until 1999 that a formal conceptual model of coaching efficacy was put forth by Deborah Feltz, Melissa Chase, Sandra Moritz, and Phillip Sullivan. The proposed conceptual model of coaching efficacy was intended to address a gap in the sport-oriented literature and was based, in part, on Albert Bandura's self-efficacy theory as well as the teacher efficacy literature. An important caveat of the original conceptual model was that it focused on high school and lower division collegiate coaches.

The conceptual model of coaching efficacy consisted of three key elements: (1) proposed sources of coaching efficacy information, (2) dimensions of coaching efficacy, and (3) proposed outcomes of a coach's efficacy beliefs. Since 1999, confirmatory evidence has been provided for many of the core facets of the conceptual model of coaching efficacy. Evidence has also been provided that has prompted modifications to the initial framework. Other populations such as youth sport coaches have also since been studied, which has further contributed to a continually evolving framework.

Measurement of Coaching Efficacy

The coach must competently and confidently perform multiple roles to be an effective leader. These roles often include but are not limited to that of teacher, motivator, strategist, organizer, physical conditioning trainer, and character builder. This complex and multifaceted task suggests that a coach's own belief in the personal ability to successfully execute core tasks may be best reflected within a multidimensional measurement model. A standard first step in multidimensional measurement is to operationally define the most general construct of which multiple dimensions are thought to exist. Coaching efficacy, broadly defined, is the extent to which a coach believes in the personal capacity to affect the learning and performance of the athletes. Because coaching efficacy is a belief, for which only imperfect observed indicators can be collected, measurement of the construct generally has taken a latent variable approach.

Deborah Feltz et al. put forth the first formal measurement model (theory) of coaching efficacy in 1999: the Coaching Efficacy Scale (CES). The multidimensional model for the CES posited that four specific efficacies were related to one another and defined coaching efficacy. *Motivation efficacy* was defined as the confidence coaches have in their ability to affect the psychological mood and psychological skills of their athletes. *Game strategy efficacy* was defined as the confidence coaches have in their abilities to lead during competition. *Technique efficacy* was defined as the confidence coaches have in their instructional and diagnostic skills. *Character building efficacy* was defined as the confidence coaches have in their abilities to influence the personal development and positive attitude toward sport in their athletes.

An investigation published in 2005 regarding the psychometric properties of measures derived from the CES concluded that several modifications could be made to increase the precision of coaching efficacy measures produced by the CES. Two of the major suggested modifications were to delimit subsequent versions of the CES by level coached, and to make a few structural changes to the CES itself. In 2008, the Coaching Efficacy Scale II–High School Teams (CES II–HST) was published, and in 2011, the Coaching Efficacy Scale II–Youth Sport Teams (CES II-YST) was published. Within both the CES II–HST and the CES II–YST and as compared with the CES, a new dimension of coaching efficacy, physical conditioning efficacy, was added, revised operational definitions for two of the previous dimensions were put forth, and a majority of new or revised items were developed. *Physical conditioning* was defined as the confidence a coach has in the ability to prepare athletes physically for participation in the sport. *Technique efficacy* was redefined as the confidence a coach has in the ability to use instructional and diagnostic skills during practices. *Character building* was redefined as the confidence a coach has in the ability to positively influence athletes' character development through sport. Evidence has been provided, for both the CES II–HST and the CES II–YST, that the proposed measurement model closely and reliably resembles real data for both male and female coaches.

Sources of Coaching Efficacy

Albert Bandura proposed that self-efficacy beliefs are based on the complex cognitive processing of approximately four general categories of potential sources of information: (1) past performance accomplishments, (2) vicarious experiences, (3) verbal persuasion, and (4) physiological or emotional arousal. Past performance accomplishments have typically been identified as the strongest source of efficacy information. Deborah Feltz et al. worked from Bandura's general framework and put forth potential sources of coaching efficacy information, which included coaching preparation, coaching experience, prior success in coaching, perceived ability of team, and social support from various stakeholders (e.g., athletic director, community, students, faculty, and parents). Subsequent research has since built upon this aspect of the conceptual model of coaching efficacy and has added a few potential sources of coaching efficacy information. These include assistant coaching experience, relevant athletic experience of the coach, perceived improvement of athletes, social support from athletes, and imagery use by the coach.

Each of the proposed sources of coaching efficacy information outlined in the previous paragraph has been found to be an important predictor of at least one of the proposed dimensions of coaching efficacy at one or more levels of competition. There is some evidence, however, that the degree of importance for some of these sources of coaching efficacy information may vary somewhat by level coached and or gender of the coach. For example, coaching preparation and coaching experience have been found to be reliable sources of efficacy information at both the high school and youth sport levels but less so for collegiate coaches at Division II and III. Prior success (e.g., won–loss record in the previous year or career winning percentage) has been shown to be an important source of efficacy information for female coaches but less so for male coaches at the high school level. Finally, the current proposed collection of proposed sources of efficacy information appear to be more salient, on average, for some dimensions of coaching efficacy, such as game strategy efficacy, technique efficacy, and motivation efficacy, than for other dimensions of coaching efficacy like character building efficacy. That said, it is important to note that even for the most understood dimensions of coaching efficacy, most of the variability in even these dimensions has yet to be explained. This suggests that there may be more work to be done to discover new sources of coaching efficacy information in order to get a fuller understanding of the complex cognitive processes that underlie these beliefs.

Outcomes of Coaching Efficacy

Albert Bandura proposed that self-efficacy beliefs often are the primary determinant of people's behavior and thought patterns. Self-efficacy beliefs affect the choices a person makes (Do I attempt to take on a particular task?), the effort a person dedicates to a particular task (Will I give my best effort to this task?), and the persistence a person displays while working toward completion of a particular task (Given a setback, will I redouble my efforts toward accomplishing this task?). Self-efficacy beliefs also affect the goals that a person sets (Will I select a goal that pushes me to perform my very best?), the attributions a person makes (Given a setback, will I identify internal or external explanations for the outcome?), and the emotional reactions a person has (Given that I almost, but not quite, accomplished my goal and that I no longer have the opportunity to pursue this goal, will I feel proud of what I did accomplish?).

Deborah Feltz et al. worked from Bandura's general framework and highlighted potential outcomes of coaching efficacy, which included coaching behavior, player and team satisfaction, player and team performance, and player and team efficacy. More efficacious coaches as compared to less efficacious coaches, on average, are theorized to provide more effective feedback (e.g., more of a focus on encouragement and inclusive leadership and less of a focus on organizational issues and autocratic leadership) to athletes or teams, be more appropriately committed to coaching and suffer less burnout from coaching, have more satisfied athletes or teams (e.g., want to play for the same coach again next year), have athletes or teams more frequently perform at or above their current ability level, and serve as positive source of efficacy information for their athletes or teams (e.g., the coach is perceived as confident in the athlete or team). Interestingly, to date, motivation efficacy and character building efficacy have generally been the most consistent predictors of positive outcomes for athletes or teams. Thus, the more relationship-based dimensions of coaching efficacy as compared with the more technical dimensions of coaching efficacy, such as technique efficacy and game strategy efficacy, may be especially important to athletes

or teams. The predictive ability of physical conditioning efficacy has yet to be systematically studied.

Future Directions

Self-efficacy theory provides a strong theoretical base for the construction of the coaching efficacy construct. The conceptual model of coaching efficacy serves as a very useful and flexible sport-specific theoretical framework. The measurement of coaching efficacy has improved yielding better model-data fit in recent years, in part, because of the recent development of different instruments based on level coached. Clearly there exists a solid basis from which future scholarship can proceed in some way. Future directions that may prove especially fruitful may include a sharper focus on relevant subpopulations, such as gender of both the coach and the team and level coached, with regard to potential sources and outcomes of coaching efficacy, and longitudinal research designs that describe the dynamic nature of coaching efficacy.

Nicholas D. Myers

See also Collective Efficacy; Implicit/Self-Theories of Ability; Interdependence Theory and the Coach–Athlete Relationship; Modeling; Relational Efficacy Beliefs in Coach–Athlete Relations; Self-Efficacy; Social Cognitive Theory

Further Readings

Bandura, A. (1977). Self-efficacy: Toward a unifying theory of behavior change. *Psychological Review, 84,* 191–215.

Bandura, A. (1997). *Self-efficacy: The exercise of control.* New York: Freeman.

Feltz, D. L., Chase, M. A., Moritz, S E., & Sullivan, P. J. (1999). A conceptual model of coaching efficacy: Preliminary investigation and instrument development. *Journal of Educational Psychology, 91,* 765–776.

Feltz, D. L., Hepler, T. J., Roman, N., & Paiement, C. A. (2009). Coaching efficacy and youth sport coaches. *The Sport Psychologist, 23,* 24–41.

Feltz, D. L., Short, S. E., & Sullivan, P. J. (2008). *Self-efficacy in sport.* Champaign, IL: Human Kinetics.

Horn, T. S. (2002). Coaching effectiveness in the sports domain. In T. S. Horn (Ed.), *Advances in sport psychology* (2nd ed., pp. 309–354). Champaign, IL: Human Kinetics.

Myers, N. D., Chase, M. A., Pierce, S. W., & Martin, E. (2011). Coaching efficacy and exploratory structural equation modeling: A substantive-methodological synergy. *Journal of Sport & Exercise Psychology, 33*, 779–806.

Myers, N. D., Feltz, D. L., Chase, M. A., Reckase, M. D., & Hancock, G. R. (2008). The coaching efficacy scale II–high school teams (CES II-HST). *Educational and Psychological Measurement, 68*, 1059–1076.

COGNITIVE CAPABILITIES

In the domain of sport, the term *cognitive capabilities* refers to the athlete's aptitude to process, evaluate, select, and compare information. Cognitive capabilities are encompassed in the cognitive system and serve as a linkage between the perceptual and motor systems. Thus, these assume the role of interpreters, translating environmental stimuli into meaningful patterns for further processing. The main function of these analytical mental skills is problems solving and decision making. The list of cognitive capacities is broad and includes, but not limited to memory, perception, attention, anticipation, and situational assessment.

An example from tennis is provided here to demonstrate and clarify the importance of cognitive capabilities in the sport domain: A player returning a tennis serve is required to process environmental information, which stems from the player serving the ball (the height and positioning of the ball, hip angle, arm and racquet motion, etc.) and other potentially salient sources of information (prevailing wind direction, the court characteristics, the match score, etc.). The capacity to efficiently analyze this information and anticipate the final location, speed, and spin of the ball, and generate plausible return options) for instance, is indicative of the returner's cognitive capabilities.

Measuring and Capturing Cognitive Capabilities

The exploration of cognitive components evolved from cognitive psychology and the information-processing approach, in which the computer processor was used as a metaphor for the black box (the human processor). Thus, similarly to computers, cognitive capabilities were traditionally measured by speed (e.g., reaction time), quantity (e.g., size of knowledge base), and quality (e.g., decision optimization) information. These three cognitive characteristics systematically distinguish among athletes of different skill levels, even more so than physical and technical skills. Although sport activity is primarily defined as a motor task, the cognitive components appear to be the decisive factor in the attainment of expertise.

As a result of the limitations in observing cognitive capabilities, a combination of creative research designs and state of the art technology are required to study these processes. Initially, researchers focused on measuring basic memory functions by utilizing pattern recognition and recall tasks (see also the entry "Pattern Recognition and Recall"). These set of studies attempted to capture athletes' ability to recognize and recall static and dynamic game patterns and structures. Although experienced, skilled athletes exhibited superior performance over novices on these tasks, ensuing studies provided evidence that these capabilities are relatively easy to train and do not afford information to the underlying mechanisms leading to the acquisition of advanced cognitive capabilities. Thus, research paradigms and designs shifted to the examination of more domain-relevant and representative tasks, which have been used in the past 30 years.

An innovative assessment tool, the temporal and spatial occlusion paradigm, explores athletes' anticipatory capability in representative situations (see also the entry "Anticipation"). The paradigm consists of a domain-specific, sport action video sequence, presented to athletes of different skill levels. In the spatial occlusion paradigm, different areas of the display are blocked for part or the duration of the entire action sequence. While using temporal occlusion, the action sequence is occluded at a certain point in time and usually remains occluded until the end of the sequence. Participants are then required to predict the following events of the sequence, based on the limited information they received. Thus, by observing differences in performances among spatial areas and temporal points, insight is given to the key environmental stimuli needed for successful anticipation. Additionally, under this paradigm, skilled athletes are able to predict opponents' intentions early and accurately by utilizing cues more efficiently (see also the entry "Cue Utilization").

To assess visual search behaviors that lead to anticipation and enhance decision making, eye-tracking technologies are used. The introduction of this equipment enables researchers to measure variables, such as fixation areas, fixation duration, frequency, and search order or sequence.

Comparison between successful and unsuccessful performances allows researchers to identify effective search strategies and gaze behaviors. Although this technology provides detailed and imperative information, there are several limitations that should be considered: the calibration of the instruments, inference from gaze behaviors, size and mobility of the equipment, and connection issues.

Finally, with the use of retrospective and concurrent verbal reports, researchers are able to explore the intact thought process from stimuli detection to action generation. In this process-tracing research method, athletes provide detailed reports of their thoughts during or after performance. This procedure enables gaining insight and access to cognitive processes.

All of the above-mentioned capturing and measuring paradigms make use of the expert–novice paradigm in which performance comparisons were used to infer on the cognitive capabilities necessary for achieving successful performance. Extant research using these paradigms resulted in abundant and valuable knowledge related to skill level differences in cognitive capabilities.

Expert–Novice Differences

Expert athletes are able quickly and accurately to anticipate future events. They are capable of assessing a situation efficiently by integrating in-vivo information from the environment with stored information like knowledge base and long-term memory, utilizing an advanced memory structure termed *long-term working memory*. Specifically, long-term working memory facilitates the acquisition of mental representations and planning. Thus, by relying on advanced cognitive capabilities, elite athletes display superior decision-making skills. These decisions are characterized by flexibility, creativity, and adjustment to dynamic situations.

Cognitive capabilities are often divided into different sequential processes. Visual search behavior is the initial process and refers to where athletes gaze and what they attend to. The two prevailing strategies are context (attending to a large visual field) and target (attending to a narrow visual field) control. Novice athletes cannot utilize context control strategies because of limitations in the amount of information they can process. On the other hand, experts have the flexibility to shift from context to target-control strategies depending on environmental demands.

Furthermore, experts exhibit advanced cue utilization skills. This allows them to incorporate complex and expansive cues in the anticipation process, and predict what will occur next with higher probability and confidence. Skill level differences are also evident in the option generation and prioritization process. Primarily, experts generate more relevant options and efficiently prioritize them. This cognitive advantage is subsequently reflected in the action selection process, where the expert athlete is able to determine the action that will result in the best possible outcome. More importantly, experts have the capability to alter a previously selected action pattern on the fly. Finally, elite performers evaluate their performance with better precision, compared to low-level performers, and hence can detect errors in their performance (process and outcome) and adjust their actions accordingly in the upcoming situations.

Gershon Tenenbaum, Itay Basevitch,
and Oscar Gutierrez

See also Anticipation; Cue Utilization; Expertise; Information Processing; Pattern Recognition and Recall

Further Readings

Mann, D., Williams, A. M., Ward, P., & Janelle, C. M. (2007). Perceptual-cognitive expertise in sport: A meta-analysis. *Journal of Sport & Exercise Psychology, 29,* 457–478.

Tenenbaum, G. (2003). An integrated approach to decision making. In J. L. Starkes & K. A. Ericsson (Eds.), *Expert performance in sport: Advances in research on sport expertise* (pp. 191–218). Champaign, IL: Human Kinetics.

COGNITIVE FUNCTION

Cognitive function refers to the mental process of knowing or thinking. It involves all aspects of mental processes that enable individuals to perceive, recognize, process, and understand thoughts. Specifically, cognitive function involves processes such as action, attention, memory, learning, reasoning, planning, problem solving, decision making, and communication. These cognitive functions are not only important to daily life but are also recognized as main components in health-related quality of life.

Cognition: A Lifespan Spectrum

Although the major brain areas that are the core resource of cognition are set at birth, along with emerging and forming networks of brain cells, cognition and intelligence continuously develop throughout childhood, adolescence, and into young adulthood, thereafter declining gradually after adulthood. For example, with the exception of vocabulary, multiple cognitive functions, including the speed of information processing, reasoning, and memory, peak at 20 years of age and then decline linearly until the age of 70 years. Generally, compared to the entire population, an individual's cognitive function at 20 years is above the 75th percentile, at 50 years it is near the 50th percentile, and at 70 years, it is in approximately the 20th percentile. This decline of cognitive function is linked to cognitive impairment in later life, such as dementia and Alzheimer's disease.

As one can easily notice, the rate of cognitive development during early life and cognitive decline later in life exhibit marked interindividual variability. Environmental factors and an individual's experiences, including physical activity, intellectual engagement, social interaction, nutrition, and self-confidence, can positively influence these cognitive changes. Participation in physical activity is particularly emphasized in both lifespan phases by numerous social and health institutions and organizations, because increased physical activity has been related to multiple benefits affecting physical and mental health in children and older adults.

Physical Activity and Cognition: Different Perspectives

Early and Large-Scale Observational Studies

Physical activity and cognition were first investigated by Waneen Spirduso, Karen Francis, and Priscilla MacRae in the 1970s. While the researchers found that older adults demonstrated a longer reaction time of information processing in response to several cognitive tasks compared with younger adults, they also found that both older and younger adults showed differences based on participation in sports. The older adults who participated in sports regularly not only had a greatly increased cognitive speed compared to older sedentary adults, but also had similar cognitive performances as young sedentary adults, suggesting that participation in sports positively moderated the age-related cognitive decline.

The positive associations between physical activity and cognitive performance have also been shown in large-scale epidemiological studies. Generally, studies of older adults based on retrospective reports of physical activity have suggested protective effects against cognitive decline and cognitive impairment. However, these subjective measurements of physical activity are somewhat imprecise, and information regarding the modality, intensity, frequency, duration, and length of participation in physical activity is often deficient.

A study focusing on physical fitness, rather than physical activity, which involved approximately 900,000 California schoolchildren, demonstrated that increased physical fitness was significantly positively associated with enhanced reading and mathematics scores, regardless of gender and grade. Although a cause–effect relationship cannot be established from observational studies, the positive correlation between physical activity and cognition is promising.

Interventional Studies

Using experimental designs, particularly with randomized assignment into an exercise group or non-exercise control group, some studies have provided stronger evidence for a cause–effect relationship. Interestingly, while an older adult group with long-term physical activity improved in general cognitive performance, such as speed-, spatial-, controlled-, and executive function-related cognition compared with a sedentary control group, physical activity training also provided the greatest benefit to executive function. Executive function is a high-order type of cognition that is used to regulate, control, and manage multilevel basic information processing for purposeful and goal-directed behaviors. Therefore, older adults who participated in long-term physical activity demonstrated improved cognitive function in general, and selectively, particularly in executive function.

Long-term exercise may also benefit cognitive performance in overweight children. Research has indicated that participating in an exercise program 5 days per week over 15 weeks for 40 minutes per day at moderate intensity improves the planning aspect of cognition. It should be noted that performing this exercise protocol for 20 minutes per day had only a limited effect, suggesting that the duration of 40 minutes is the minimum threshold for cognitive function to be enhanced among children. Physical activity in school-based physical education, play during recess, classroom physical activity, and extracurricular physical activity, has either been found to be positively related to academic attitude, behavior, and achievement or to have no relationship, suggesting that participation in physical activity at school does not negatively affect student achievement.

Chronic Exercise Versus Acute Exercise

Besides studies that target long-term physical activity, known as *chronic exercise,* the effect of single bouts of physical activity, known as *acute exercise,* on cognitive function has also been investigated. Generally, when performing acute exercise, individuals with higher fitness and those who do 20 minutes or more of exercise per session show greater improvements in cognitive performance than those with low fitness and those who perform exercise of shorter durations. Similar to chronic exercise, which has been shown to benefit many types of cognition including information processing and attention, acute exercise also has a positive effect on executive function. Although the effect of acute exercise on cognition is of a somewhat short duration, higher but not extreme exercise intensity appears to prolong the positive effect to 60 minutes. The beneficial effects of acute physical activity on cognition have recently been extended to overweight children and children with attention deficit–hyperactivity disorder.

Although both chronic and acute exercise benefits cognitive function, the mechanisms are likely to be different. According to the cardiovascular fitness hypothesis, the improvement in cognitive performance following chronic exercise is mediated by gains in cardiovascular fitness. In support of this hypothesis, studies using sophisticated neuroscientific and psychophysiological methods (e.g., magnetic resonance imaging or event-related potentials) have indicated that both older adults and children with high fitness levels show larger brain volumes in areas implicated in cognitive function (including gray matter, white matter, specific cortical structures like the prefrontal cortex, and subcortical structures like the hippocampus) than their counterparts with low fitness levels. In contrast, the mechanism linking acute exercise and

cognition is believed to be exercise-induced arousal or enhanced allocation of attentional resources and improved efficiency of stimulus evaluation in response to a given cognitive task.

Exercise Mode

Exercise-cognition research primarily emphasizes aerobic exercise, possibly because this exercise mode is linked to cardiovascular fitness. However, a recent line of investigation has evaluated the effect of exercise types on cognitive function. Particularly with respect to older adults, studies have demonstrated that resistance exercise training may also improve cognition. It is speculated that the ability to improve cognition through resistance exercise is based upon the increase of certain neurotrophic factors, such as insulin-like growth factor I (IGF-I), which are upregulated in response to muscle contraction. IGF-I is not only negatively related to aging but has also been linked to the promotion of neurogenesis, neuronal survival, and synaptic plasticity, which collectively can lead to improved cognitive performance. Furthermore, given that acute resistance exercise elevates physiological arousal similar to acute aerobic exercise, it is believed that acute resistance exercise can also benefit cognition. Indeed, positive effects of resistance exercise have been observed in studies evaluating executive function among young and middle-age adults.

Coordinative exercises, such as gymnastics, martial arts, soccer, or dance, have also been linked to executive function in kindergarten children. It is believed that the adaptation of coordinative exercise, which involves complex movement and cognitive demand for goal-directed behavior, may improve neuromotor abilities in both the peripheral and central levels, which in turn may enhance cognitive performance. In addition to cardiovascular fitness, coordinative exercise may also advance cognitive functions by increasing motor fitness, including movement speed, balance, motor coordination, and flexibility. In fact, individuals with better motor fitness have demonstrated to activate more cognition-related brain regions during the cognitive tasks.

Conclusion

Although cognitive functions develop and deteriorate during an individual's lifespan, participation in physical activity may alter the rate of these changes. Large-scale observational and interventional studies have revealed a positive relationship between physical activity and cognitive function in older adults, as well as a positive correlation between school-based physical activity and academic achievement in children. In addition, chronic exercise has been shown to impact cognitive functions in general and also, more selectively, executive functions. Similarly, beneficial effects of acute exercise have also been identified, although the magnitude of these effects can be moderated by fitness status, exercise duration, exercise intensity, and the type of cognitive task. Notably, the biological mechanisms associating chronic and acute exercise with cognition are likely to be different. Along with the beneficial effects of aerobic exercise on cognition, studies have also demonstrated the potential of resistance exercise and coordinative exercise for enhancing cognitive activity. Taken together, this body of evidence indicates that physical activity has beneficial effects on cognitive function throughout an individual's lifespan.

Yu-Kai Chang

See also Brain; Brain Imaging; Decision Making; Information Processing; Memory; Mental Health; Neuroscience, Exercise, and Cognitive Function; Psychophysiology

Further Readings

Chang, Y.-K., Labban, J. D., Gapin, J. I., & Etnier, J. L. (2012). The effects of acute exercise on cognitive performance: A meta-analysis. *Brain Research, 1453,* 87–101.

Chang, Y.-K., Pan, C. Y., Chen, F. T., Tsai, C. L., & Huang, C. C. (2012). Effect of resistance exercise training on cognitive function in healthy older adults: A review. *Journal of Aging and Physical Activity, 20,* 497–516.

Etnier, J. L., & Chang, Y.-K. (2009). The effect of physical activity on executive function: A brief commentary on definitions, measurement issues, and the current state of the literature. *Journal of Sport & Exercise Psychology, 31,* 469–483.

Hillman, C. H., Kamijo, K., & Scudder, M. (2011). A review of chronic and acute physical activity participation on neuroelectric measures of brain health and cognition during childhood. *Preventive Medicine, 52*(Suppl. 1), S21–S28.

Kramer, A. F., & Erickson, K. I. (2007). Capitalizing on cortical plasticity: Influence of physical activity on cognition and brain function. *Trends in Cognitive Sciences, 11,* 342–348.

Spirduso, W., Francis, K., & MacRae, P. (2004). *Physical dimensions of aging* (2nd ed.). Champaign, IL: Human Kinetics.

Tomporowski, P. D., Lambourne, K., & Okumura, M. S. (2011). Physical activity interventions and children's mental function: An introduction and overview. *Preventive Medicine, 52*(Suppl. 1), S3–S9.

COGNITIVE RESTRUCTURING

Cognitive restructuring is a technique that is commonly taught to athletes by sport psychologists in which self-defeating thoughts and negative self-statements are identified and substituted with positive, adaptive self-statements, and coping thoughts. Cognitive restructuring was originally developed in clinical settings and has since been used by practitioners in various contexts (including sport) to address a range of issues related to performance, social anxiety, maladaptive perfectionism, aggressive behavior, depression, and low self-esteem.

Generally speaking, cognitive restructuring has been examined as part of a package of mental interventions. These typically include the setting of effective goals, visualization, relaxation strategies, and self-talk. Invariably, psychological skills packages are associated with improved athletic and sporting performance. For instance, the positive effects associated with psychological skills packages have been reported in sports as diverse as baseball, basketball, boxing, figure skating, golf, gymnastics, karate, skiing, tennis, and volleyball. Pertinently, systematic reviews of the effects of psychological skills on performance indicate that cognitive restructuring interventions often have large positive effects on performance, suggesting these interventions are particularly effective. As yet, few studies have involved direct tests of the mechanisms that might account for the positive performance effects associated with cognitive restructuring. However, there is a large body of evidence indicating that cognitive restructuring is associated with improvements in a variety of psychological variables such as increased self-efficacy, reduced cognitive and somatic anxiety, an increased ability to cope, as well as increased effort and motivation to succeed. As a word of caution, research suggests that the skills required to deliver cognitive restructuring interventions require many hours of training to master. Practitioners considering using cognitive restructuring should bear this in mind prior to delivering such interventions.

Cognitive restructuring is often described as a technique in its own right. In this way, cognitive restructuring involves four sequential steps: (1) identifying the individual's negative thoughts or self-statements during problematic situations, (2) identifying coping self-statements and rehearsing them, (3) replacing negative self-defeating statements with coping self-statements, and (4) identifying and rehearsing positively reinforcing self-statements. However, it is worth noting that cognitive restructuring is more commonly used within a rational emotive behavior therapy (REBT) or a cognitive-behavior therapy (CBT) framework.

Albert Ellis developed REBT in the 1950s. At its core, REBT attempts to apply rationality and logic to a person's beliefs. Rational beliefs, which are thought to be at the core of psychological health, are flexible, consistent with reality, logical, and self-enhancing. Irrational beliefs, which are thought to be at the core of psychological disturbance, are rigid, inconsistent with reality, illogical, and self-defeating. In the context of sport, irrational beliefs often underlie much of the stress and resulting self-defeating thoughts and feelings experienced by athletes prior to or during athletic performance. REBT teaches that it is the irrational beliefs and thinking, and not the event or circumstance that contributed to the irrational beliefs, that lead to negative emotions. Sport psychology practitioners can help athletes reduce their self-caused negative emotions by enabling them to identify and dispute their irrational beliefs via a process known as ABCD cognitive restructuring:

A: Athletes are asked to keep a diary of daily events that generate negative emotions. The athlete is asked to describe the facts of the events as they occurred.

B: The athlete is to record in the diary the exact content of the dysfunctional self-talk (said out loud or silently in private) that followed the activating events.

C: The athlete then records the resulting emotional or behavioral responses.

D: After completing the ABC steps across a designated number of days, the final step requires the athlete to identify which aspects of the self-talk are irrational or distorted and substitute more rational and productive thoughts in their place.

This process is practiced repeatedly until the substituted rational statement is internalized.

Cognitive-behavioral therapies are often an amalgamation of cognitive and behavioral procedures. While some treatments may emphasize cognitive more than behavioral techniques, and vice versa, these interventions typically share an appreciation for basic learning principles *and* the role that cognitions play in human behavior and affective experience. When cognitive restructuring is used within a CBT framework it is often considered a discrete part of a wider intervention. This is because cognitive-behavioral therapies are more directive, educational, and future focused than traditional psychotherapies. Cognitive restructuring is one of the skills taught to the client as part of the therapy but it is often accompanied by other cognitive-behavioral techniques like relaxation training.

James Hardy and James Bell

See also Affirmations; Positive Thinking; Self-Talk; Thought Stopping

Further Readings

Blagys, M. D., & Hilsenroth, M. J. (2002). Distinctive activities of cognitive-behavioral therapy: A review of the comparative psychotherapy process literature. *Clinical Psychology Review, 22,* 671–706.

Greenspan, M. J., & Feltz, D. L. (1989). Psychological interventions with athletes in competitive situations: A review. *The Sport Psychologist, 3,* 219–236.

Haney, C. J. (2004). Stress-management interventions for female athletes: Relaxation and cognitive restructuring. *International Journal of Sport Psychology, 35,* 109–118.

Zinsser, N., Bunker, L., & Williams, J. M. (2010). Cognitive techniques for building confidence and enhancing performance. In J. M. Williams (Ed.), *Applied sport psychology: Personal growth to peak performance* (6th ed., pp. 305–335). Boston: McGraw-Hill.

COGNITIVE STYLES

Broadly defined, *cognition* refers to mental operations involving information processing and thus includes processes such as perception, problem solving, memory recall, and decision making. The term *cognitive styles* refers to the different approaches people characteristically use in undertaking cognitive tasks. Considered to be a personality trait and representing both nature and nurture effects, cognitive styles are thought to influence individuals' values, attitudes, and social interactions. Examples of cognitive styles include (a) reflectiveness versus impulsiveness, (b) cognitive complexity versus simplicity, and (c) tolerance versus intolerance for unrealistic experiences. Individuals are thought to differ in their quickness to respond to stimuli, their ability to process complex cognitive information, and their acceptance of unexpected experiences. To explain variability in cognitive styles, scholars from various domains have generated a number of theoretical and applied explanations addressing differences in (a) hemispheric lateralization, (b) perception and information processing, (c) problem-solving approaches, and (d) field dependence or independence. Aligned with the idea of cognitive styles, there is the notion of learning styles, specifically, (a) different types of learning and (b) idiosyncratic modes of intelligence. This entry presents research findings on both cognitive and learning styles and their application to the sport psychology domain.

Neuroscience research has revealed that the right hemisphere of the brain controls holistic and pictorial processing while the left hemisphere is more centrally involved in analytical and logical operations. Accordingly, peoples' cognitive styles are expected to vary on a continuum ranging from primarily logical–analytical (left-hemisphere dominant) to predominantly holistic–pictorial functioning (right-hemisphere dominant). Furthermore, individuals' cognitive styles may be further categorized into two orthogonal dimensions: (1) holistic–analytic and (2) verbal–imagery. The holistic–analytic dimension refers to how individuals gather and store structured information. Holists retain a gestalt, global conceptualization, of information, whereas analytics deconstruct information into its subcomponents. The verbal–imagery dimension refers to how individuals decode structured information. Verbalizers decode information by using words and verbal associations, whereas visualizers create mental pictures to represent structured information. These styles or individual differences typically exist on a continuum, and most people do not fall clearly into one or other discrete style classification.

Moreover, people perceive and process information using different methods. Activists learn through active experimentation and by proactively engaging in new experiences. Theorists generate hypotheses and then engage in analytical thinking and deductive reasoning. Pragmatists prefer methods based on measurable goals and practical outcomes. Reflectors, in contrast, engage in conscious and deliberate processing before comprehending and storing new information. Theoretically, therefore, activists are likely to learn best when exposed to new experiences; theorists optimize their learning experiences when presented with testable concepts; pragmatists prefer simulations of real scenarios; and reflectors excel when working on observational reports and analyses.

People also differ in their tendencies toward solving problems by engaging in (a) adaptive or innovative solutions, and (b) convergent or divergent thinking approaches. Adaptors utilize existing paradigms to generate solutions for a given problem, whereas innovators create new paradigms to problem solving. Similarly, convergent thinkers generate a singular and accurate response to a given problem, whereas divergent thinkers generate multiple responses. Additional variability in information processing among human beings may also be explained through a tridimensional approach based on (1) emotional or relational, (2) mental, and (3) physical dimensions. The relational or emotional dimension refers to knowledge primarily gained through social interactions and verbal and nonverbal communication. The mental dimension pertains to information acquired via deliberate thinking, abstract conceptualization, objectification, and reflection. The physical dimension represents knowledge apprehended via action-oriented skills, such as playing a sport or musical instrument.

Field dependence or independence is another extensive studied cognitive style. According to cognitive control theory, field dependent individuals rely on external cues and tend to generate a macroglobal view of a given context. Conversely, field independent individuals rely on internal cues and focus on identifying detailed information of a given context. Furthermore, field-dependent individuals have a greater social orientation than field-independent individuals, who are more likely to be introverted. Although not conclusive, research has shown that demographic, cultural, and situational factors may also influence people's reliance on field dependence or independence styles. For example, children and older adults are more likely to be field-dependent than younger adults. Also,

Western societies are thought to be primarily field-independent, whereas non-Western cultures have been described as predominantly field dependent. Finally, research suggests that people may also vary their preferred cognitive style from task to task.

Research in the sport and exercise psychology domain has revealed personal differences in athletes' cognitive styles. For example, Robert M. Nideffer's theory of attentional and personal styles suggests that people vary in their preferred attentional focus. More specifically, athletes have been shown to vary in both the width (broad to narrow) and direction (internal or external) of their preferred attentional style. Furthermore, research findings in the athletic domain confirmed the central tenets of attribution theory, as different sport actors (athletes, coaches, or referees) have been shown to vary in their causal attributions accounting for their success or failure. Finally, studies assessing learning and motor performance, as a function of field dependence or independence, have not been conclusive. This is congruent with current understanding of expert performance in sports, which suggests that reliable superior performance is dependent upon the task- and domain-specific cognitive skills.

Cognitive styles have also been linked to learning preferences. More specifically, people tend to prefer some learning modalities, such as visual, auditory, and tactile or kinesthetic, over others. Visual learners rely primarily on diagrammatic and pictorial information to gain knowledge of a particular subject. Auditory learners gain knowledge by primarily attending to spoken and written information. Kinesthetic or tactile learners acquire new knowledge by experiencing new activities and performances. Accordingly, kinesthetic or tactile learners should be given the opportunity to try out their new skills. Auditory learners may benefit from class discussions, as well as thinking and reading aloud exercises. Learning styles, however, may not be as discretely different as originally categorized.

Recommended instructional activities for visual learners include use of maps, videos, and presentations. Finally, a combination of multimethods like visual auditory and kinesthetic methods may facilitate learning across the board. However, it is important to note that learning styles may not be as discretely different as originally categorized.

Congruent with the idea of preferred learning styles, psychologist Howard Gardner has proposed seven distinct intelligence modes underlying cognitive variability among human beings. Specifically, Gardner's' model is grounded on the notion that people possess idiosyncratic mental capabilities represented by the following seven domains: (1) visual and spatial, (2) verbal and linguistic, (3) logical and mathematical, (4) bodily and kinesthetic, (5) musical and rhythmical, (6) interpersonal, and (7) intrapersonal intelligence. According to this view, creative architects primarily operate under visual and spatial intelligence mode; accomplished writers rely on verbal and linguistic intelligence mode, and so forth.

In summary, people vary in their preferred methods of processing information. For example, hemispherical dominance may explain why some individuals are more analytical than others. Personality tendencies may explain why some people are labeled activists and others theorists. Moreover, people vary in types of intelligence: field dependence, independence, and preferred attention and attribution styles. Research findings revealed that some individuals learn through visual channels while others primarily rely on their listening skills. There are also innovators, adapters, convergent, and divergent thinkers. This extensive variety of cognitive styles and abilities illustrates the complexity of designing optimal learning environments. Therefore, educators and applied professionals, such as coaches, should consider people's cognitive idiosyncrasies when preparing their instructional activities and selecting domains of expertise. Consideration of multimethods may facilitate learning across the board and retention of new and difficult information.

Gershon Tenenbaum and Edson Filho

See also Decision Making; Information Processing; Perception

Further Readings

Gardner, H. (1983/2011). *Frames of mind: The theory of multiple intelligences.* New York: Basic Books.

Sternberg R. J., & Zhang L. (Eds.). (2001). *Perspectives on thinking, learning, and cognitive styles.* Mahwah, NJ: Lawrence Erlbaum.

Suedfeld, P. (2000). Cognitive styles: Personality. In A. E. Kazdin (Ed.), *Encyclopedia of psychology* (Vol. 2, pp. 166–169). New York: American Psychological Association & Oxford University Press.

Cognitive Task Analysis

Cognitive task analysis (CTA) refers to a suite of scientific methods designed to identify the cognitive skills, strategies, and knowledge required to perform tasks proficiently. The goal of CTA is to use this information to improve instruction, training, and technological design (e.g., decision aids) for the purposes of making work more efficient, productive, satisfying, and of a higher quality, or to accelerate proficiency.

Background and Historical Development

CTA has a long history, spanning multiple communities of practice, ranging from those studying perception and thinking, to those studying the behavioral aspects of work and, subsequently, skilled performance in applied settings. Prior to the 1980s, these communities included (in approximate chronological order) those practicing introspection, applied and industrial psychology, task analysis, ergonomics, human factors, and instructional design.

In the early 1900s, physical labor dominated many aspects of work, and physical issues, such as fatigue and injury risk, were of concern. Accordingly, task analytic methods were often behaviorally oriented—designed to decrease inefficiencies and to increase productivity. Classic examples of task analysis include Frederick W. Taylor's time–motion studies of factory workers, and Frank and Lillian Gilbreth's study of bricklayers. Although worker behavior was emphasized during early task analyses, the decomposition of tasks using such methods rarely excluded cognitive aspects of work. However, over time, as work became more reliant on higher order cognition, the focus of task analysis shifted.

Despite historical antecedents, the term CTA did not emerge until the 1980s, when it was used to understand the cognitive activities involved in man–machine systems. A key turning point was a Nuclear Regulatory Commission workshop in 1982 on Cognitive Modeling of Nuclear Plant Operators, attended by cognitive and human factors psychologists David Woods, Donald Norman, Thomas Sheridan, William Rouse, and Thomas Moran. The changing nature of technology in the workplace and the increasing complexity of work systems resulted in a greater emphasis on cognitive work and, therefore, a greater need for cognitively oriented task analytic methods.

From the 1980s, a system-oriented perspective to CTA prevailed, focused on understanding adaptive cognitive work in complex contexts. This *joint-cognitive systems* or *sociotechnical systems* perspective viewed cognitive work as an embedded phenomenon—inextricably tied to the context in which it occurs. In naturalistic contexts, (a) systems may comprise multiple (human and technological) components; (b) task goals are frequently ill-defined; (c) planning may only be possible at general levels of abstraction; (d) information may be limited; and (e) complexity, uncertainty, time-constraint, and stress are the norm. Cognition in these contexts is often emergent or distributed across individuals—and technology. Moreover, cognition is also constrained by broader professional, organizational, and institutional contexts, which influence the strategies, plans, goals, processes, and policies employed. Consequently, CTA has evolved as a means to study adaptive, resilient, and collaborative cognition in simulated environments and, especially, in the field.

CTA has been championed by the cognitive systems engineering and naturalistic decision-making communities, and cognitive scientists studying expertise, including cognitive anthropologists and ethnographers. The range of CTA methods is vast. Rather than present an exhaustive list of methods, the reader is referred to Beth Crandall, Gary Klein, and Robert R. Hoffman's 2006 book *Working Minds*. A more detailed description of one particular method, the Critical Decision Method, is provided later in this entry.

In general, CTA is most synonymous with knowledge elicitation and cognitive process-tracing data collection methods, of which there are several classes: self-reports, automated capture-based techniques, observation, and interviews. As with all empirical methods, there are strengths and limitations to each method. Self-reports, such as questionnaires, rating scales, and diaries, permit efficient data collection and interpretation, which can be automated by computer. However, valid psychometric scale development takes time and effort. Moreover, self-reports do not afford the opportunity for additional exploration of the data, which may be problematic given the possibility of participant self-presentation or amotivation.

Automated capture includes computer-based tasks or those implemented in simulated task environments (e.g., situation awareness global assessment technique; temporal or spatial occlusion). These methods allow direct capture of important cognitive behavior in situ, such as making a specific prediction or decision. However, they may require supplementary methods (e.g., *a priori* goal-directed task analysis, verbal reports, eye movements) to generate design recommendations. Additionally, they are costly to establish, require extensive system and scenario development, and have limited flexibility.

Observation like ethnographic immersion and shadowing provide first-hand information about how events unfold (and permits post hoc verification of information elicited via other methods). However, as with many CTA techniques, it requires domain knowledge to identify useful targets for data coding and interpretation. Observation is not always feasible (e.g., low-frequency, life-threatening events), can be intrusive and, per the Hawthorne effect, can change the behavior of those being observed.

Structured and semistructured interview techniques (e.g., *critical decision method* and *crystal ball technique*) that employ directed probes can reveal information that other methods would not. In addition to conducting naturalistic studies, interviews and observations can be combined with experiment-like tasks (e.g., 20 questions, card sorting) to generate useful insights into the cognitive processes underlying superior performance. However, trained interviewers are required, interviewees' memory is fallible, and the validity of retrospective reports has been questioned.

The Critical Decision Method

The critical decision method (CDM) was developed by Gary Klein, Robert Hoffman, and colleagues and is adapted from the critical incident technique (CIT) developed by John Flanagan and colleagues (including Paul Fitts)—which was designed to generate a functional description of, and identify the critical requirements for, on-the-job performance in military settings. Like the CIT, rather than probe for general knowledge, the CDM is a case-based, retrospective, semistructured interview method. It uses multiple *sweeps* to elicit a participant's thinking in a specific, nonroutine incident, in which they were an active decision maker and played a central role. A particular goal of the CDM is to focus the interviewee on the parts of the incident that most

affected their decision making and to elicit information about the macrocognitive functions and processes—such as situation assessment, sensemaking, (re)planning, and decision making—that supported proficient performance. Although elicitation is not limited to events that could be directly observed, the use of skilled individuals and specific, challenging, and recent events in which they were emotionally invested was hypothesized to scaffold memory recall based on their elaborate encoding of such incidents.

In the first sweep of the CDM, a brief (e.g., 30- to 60-second) outline of a specific incident is elicited (see below for pointers on framing the interview). In a second sweep, a detailed timeline is constructed to elaborate on the incident. This should highlight critical points where the interviewee made good or bad decisions; the goals or understanding changed; the situation itself changed; the interviewee acted, failed to act, or could have acted differently; or relied on personal expertise. Once delineated, the timeline is restated back to the interviewee to develop a shared understanding of the facts and to resolve inconsistencies.

In the third, progressively deepening, sweep, the interviewer tries to build a contextualized and comprehensive description of the incident from the interviewee's point of view. The goal is to identify the interviewee's knowledge, perceptions, expectations, options, goals, judgments, confusions, concerns, and uncertainties at each point. Targeted probe questions are used to investigate each point in turn. The CDM provides a list of useful probes for many different types of situations. For instance, probes for investigating decision points and shifts in situation assessment may include: "What was it about the situation that let you know what was going to happen?" and "What were your overriding concerns at that point?" Probes for investigating cues, expert strategies, and goals may include: "What were you noticing at that point?" "What information did you use in making this decision?" "What were you hoping to accomplish at this point?"

A fourth sweep can be used to gain additional insight into the interviewee's experience, skills, and knowledge using *what if* queries, for instance, to determine how a novice may have handled the situation differently. Although some probes require reflection on strategizing and decision making, which increases subjectivity and may affect reliability, they provide a rich source for hypotheses formation and theory development. With subsequent analysis, these data can be leveraged into design-based hypotheses, for training or technology development to aid future performance and learning.

From Elicitation to Design

To meet the goal of communicating results (e.g., from a set of CDM interviews) for improving system performance, CTA embraces a range of data analysis and knowledge representation methods. Quantitative and qualitative methods are leveraged to understand the data, including hit rates, reaction times, thematic or categorical analyses, chronological or protocol analyses, and conceptual and statistical or computational models.

As with all qualitative analyses, the goal of the CTA practitioner is to unravel the story contained in the data. After conducting data and quality control checks, analysis is used to identify and organize the cognitive elements so that patterns in the data can emerge. Importantly, elements should be informed by asking cognitive questions of the data, such as: What didn't they see? What information did they use? Where did they search? What were their concerns? What were they thinking about? At this stage, knowing the data is key and organizational procedures—such as categorizing, sorting, making lists, counting, and descriptive statistics—can be used to assist in this effort.

Once individual elements have been identified, the next goal is to identify the higher order data structure that describes the relationships between elements. This is done by generalizing across participants to describe regularities in the data (e.g., by looking for co- and re-occurrences, or their absence, that might signify a pattern); organizing elements into inclusive, overarching formats (e.g., create tables of difficult decisions, cues used, and strategies employed); looking for similarities or differences across groups (e.g., cues used by experts but not novices); and using statistical analyses to examine differences and relationships.

Following the data analysis, knowledge must be represented in a useful form. Fortunately, many forms of representation exist as a natural part of the analysis process. However, representations developed early in the process will be data driven, whereas those developed later should be meaning driven. Narrative-based representations (story summaries) can extend participants' verbalizations to highlight what is implicit in the data. Graphical chronologies like timelines that retain the order of events can be used to represent the multiple viewpoints of team members and permit subjective and objective accounts to be linked. Data organizers, such as decision requirements tables, permit multiple sources of information to be synthesized to form an integrated representation. Conceptual mapping tools (e.g., http://cmap .ihmc.us) allow knowledge structures to be graphically and hierarchically represented. Process diagrams like a decision ladder represent cognition in action and provide insights into aspects of cognitive complexity that might otherwise appear to be simple.

The selection of CTA methods should be driven by framing questions, including: What is the primary issue or problem to be addressed by the CTA? What is the deliverable? Inexperienced CTA practitioners frequently underspecify the project and adopt a method-driven, rather than problem-focused, approach. To overcome these biases and to direct project resources efficiently, practitioners should become familiar with the target domain, the study of micro- and macrocognition, and the range of CTA methods available, and they should conduct preliminary investigations to identify the most cognitively challenging task components.

Translating CTA into actual design is often the least well-executed and most ambiguous step. However, it need not be. Making explicit what will be delivered (training plan, intervention, or decision aids) and agreeing on this with the target users permits the original goal—positively changing (system) behavior—to be attained. To do this effectively, however, the CTA practitioner needs to identify the stakeholders involved, understand their goals and needs, and determine the intended use of the deliverable. Frequently, data exist that can help frame a CTA project—for instance, behavioral task analyses or documented evidence about training or system inadequacies. Generating outcomes without reference to these issues will likely result in design recommendations or tools that do not generate an effective—or even adequate—solution to the problem. Ultimately, the goal of any CTA is to use mixed methods to generate products that leverage expert data in a way that can improve performance.

Paul Ward

See also Cue Utilization; Decision Making; Expertise; Human Factors; Knowledge Structure; Simulation Training; Situational Awareness; Verbal Protocols

Further Readings

Crandall, B. W., Klein, G. A., & Hoffman, R. R. (2006). *Working minds: A practitioner's guide to cognitive task analysis.* Cambridge: MIT Press.

Hoffman, R. R., Crandall, B. W., & Shadbolt, N. (1998). Use of the critical decision method to elicit expert knowledge: A case study in the methodology of cognitive task analysis. *Human Factors, 40,* 254–276.

Hoffman, R. R., & Militello, L. (2008). *Perspectives on cognitive task analysis: Historical origins and modern communities of practice.* New York: Psychology Press.

Hoffman, R. R., Ward, P., Feltovich, P. J., DiBello, L., Fiore, S. M., & Andrews, D. (2013). *Accelerated expertise: Training for high proficiency in a complex world.* New York: Psychology Press.

Klein, G. A., Calderwood, R., & Clinton-Cirocco, A. (1986). Rapid decision making on the fire ground. *Human Factors and Ergonomics Society Annual Meeting Proceedings, 30,* 576–580.

Salmon, P. M., Stanton, N. A., Gibbon, A. C., Jenkins, D. P., & Walker, G. H. (2010). *Human factors methods and sports science: A practical guide.* Boca Raton, FL: CRC Press.

Schraagen, J. M., Chipman, S. F., & Shalin, V. L. (2000). *Cognitive task analysis.* Mahwah, NJ: Erlbaum.

COHESION

Cohesion represents the degree to which task and social bonds exist among group members, as well as the strength of individuals' attractions to the task and social activities of the group. This entry briefly highlights the history, characteristics, conceptualization, measurement, and correlates of cohesion within sport and exercise environments.

History

Interest in and discussion surrounding the concept of cohesion has a long history across a wide variety of academic domains, including sport, exercise, business, education, and the military. This has resulted in the development of a number of definitions, conceptualizations, and assessment tools. As examples, previous research has proposed that cohesion is represented by the factors keeping members in the group, the degree to which the group can resist disruption, the commitment displayed by group members, and individuals' attractions to other members and the group's tasks.

Characteristics

Despite the varied historical approaches to understanding cohesion, the 1985 work by Albert Carron, Neil Widmeyer, and Larry Brawley served to provide a strong foundation for research within the fields of sport and exercise psychology, and highlighted four characteristics of group cohesion:

Multidimensional. There are a number of facets to consider with respect to cohesion, including the orientation of the social cognitions individuals hold about their group (*perceptions of group integration* and *personal attractions to the group*), as well as the focus of those perceptions (*task and social objectives of the group*). Importantly, groups within one context like sport or across contexts like sport versus business may differ in terms of which factors are most important to group unity.

Dynamic. Another assumption about the nature of cohesion is that it is dynamic. Essentially, cohesion can change over the course of group development. From a practical perspective, this is encouraging as it suggests that effective interventions could facilitate more positive perceptions of group unity.

Instrumental. Whether for task or social objectives, groups form with some purpose in mind. Furthermore, individuals hold perceptions about the unity with which the group pursues these objectives.

Affective. The interactions and communication that occur in groups result in social relationships among members and a larger sense of social cohesion.

Conceptualization

A well-accepted conceptual model of cohesion was advanced by Carron et al. in 1985 in conjunction with the development of their Group Environment Questionnaire. This model draws distinctions with respect to the two aspects of cohesion outlined previously (refer to the *multidimensional* characteristic of cohesion). The first considers the general objectives of the group, and broadly assumes that these objectives can be classified as being either task or social in nature. Task objectives refer to those that focus on the productivity and performance of the group. In contrast, social objectives refer to those that focus on maintaining group harmony and interrelationships among the members.

A second distinction that is made in the conceptual model considers cohesion from the perspective of the group as a whole (group integration), as well as individual members' attractions to the group. Group integration refers to the degree of bonding, closeness, and unity displayed by the members, while individuals' attractions refer to the personal motivations and feelings that draw and keep members within the group.

Consideration of the general objectives of the group (task vs. social), as well as the group versus individual perspective, results in a four dimension model of cohesion: (1) group integration–task, the degree to which the group is united around task objectives (GI-T); (2) group integration–social, the degree to which the group is united around social objectives (GI-S); (3) individual attractions to the group–task, group members' personal perceptions about their involvement with task aspects of the group (ATG-T); and (4) individual attractions to the group–social, group members' personal perceptions about their involvement with social aspects of the group (ATG-S).

It should be noted that recent research has highlighted that the above conceptual model is most relevant to an adult population. Studies conducted with younger sport participants provided evidence that these individuals do not distinguish between *group integration* and *individual attractions to the group* perspectives. As a result, it has been suggested that researchers differentiate cohesion perceptions of children and youth based only on the general objectives of the group, that is, task versus social cohesion. This is reflected in the measures that have been developed in recent years, which are summarized in the subsequent section.

Measurement

A number of assessment tools exist that capture perceptions of cohesion held by a variety of different groups. The most recent versions are presented:

- *Group Environment Questionnaire* (GEQ). Developed in 1985 by Carron and colleagues, the GEQ directly corresponds with the four dimension conceptual model outlined earlier.
- *The Youth Sport Environment Questionnaire* (YSEQ). Early cohesion studies periodically assessed cohesion perceptions held by youth sport participants via the GEQ. However, researchers noted that some of the psychometric properties of the GEQ were questionable when used with this population. Others postulated that the advanced level of readability, use of negative phrasing for some items, and decreased applicability of the conceptual model may partially explain the experienced difficulties. As a result, Mark Eys, Todd Loughead, Bert Carron, and Steven Bray developed the YSEQ in 2009 specifically to assess youth (approximately 13–17 years of age) perceptions of cohesion.
- *The Child Sport Cohesion Questionnaire* (CSCQ). Further extending the ability to assess sport participants' perceptions of cohesion, Luc Martin and colleagues developed an assessment tool relevant to children 9–12 years of age.
- *Questionnaire sur l'Ambiance du Groupe* (QAG). The Group Environment Questionnaire has been translated into several languages. The work conducted by Jean-Philippe Heuzé and Paul Fontayne in 2002 highlighted the difficulties in translating the meaning of specific questions across cultures and languages, but also reinforced the salience of the four dimension conceptual model of cohesion for adult populations.
- *The Physical Activity Group Environment Questionnaire* (PAGEQ). With the intention of gauging *exercisers'* perceptions of group cohesion within physical activity contexts, Paul Estabrooks and Bert Carron developed the PAGEQ. Its structure is similar to the GEQ in terms of dimensionality and response options.

Correlates

The availability of assessment tools and interest in group dynamics has yielded a number of insights pertaining to the antecedents and consequences of cohesion. The following sections briefly highlight two major correlates of interest, performance and adherence, and list a number of individual and group variables that have been linked with cohesion.

Performance. The cohesion–performance relationship has been a major research interest for the field. Substantial evidence exists that this relationship is positive and bidirectional, that is, greater cohesion leads to better performance and better performance leads to greater cohesion. Furthermore, this relationship exists at all competitive levels, from recreational to competitive levels, and across sport types (e.g., interdependent versus independent sports). Finally, of all the moderators examined, only gender appears to moderate this relationship. Specifically, the positive cohesion–performance link is stronger for female athletes.

Adherence. Another major variable of interest is the adherence of sport and exercise group members. The sport studies that have been conducted suggest that members of highly cohesive teams drop out less during the competitive season, show up to games and practices on time, expend more effort, and indicate stronger intentions to return to their team the following season. Furthermore, athletes' actual return to their sport team the following year has been predicted by their perceptions of group cohesion in the previous season. Similar findings have been demonstrated in exercise contexts, in that those individuals who participate in a cohesive group environment are more likely to adhere to their exercise regimens and accrue positive outcomes.

Individual variables. Perceptions of greater group cohesion tend to have positive associations with important variables at the individual level. As examples, cohesion is positively associated with athletes' sport satisfaction and negatively associated with perceptions of state anxiety and depression.

Group variables. In addition to team performance, stronger perceptions of cohesion relate to other group-oriented concepts, such as improved role involvement like greater role clarity, normative expectations, and collective efficacy, as well as lower levels of group conflict.

Potential Downsides of Cohesion

While the presentation of group cohesion highlights the many positive associations that cohesion has with important sport and exercise variables, it is also critical to consider whether high cohesion creates challenges for groups. It is possible for highly cohesive groups to be more likely to have issues with groupthink (tendency for a group to apply normative pressures on its members within decision-making processes), deindividuation (loss of personal identity and self-awareness), and social loafing. In 2005, James Hardy and colleagues explored whether athletes perceived downsides of highly cohesive sport teams; their findings indicated that over half of the athletes identified specific issues on this topic. For example, a number of participants noted that high social cohesion among team members may challenge their ability to focus and commit to task goals.

Mark Eys

See also Conflict; Friendships/Peer Relations; Group Characteristics; Group Formation; Interdependence Theory and the Coach–Athlete Relationship; Roles; Shared Mental Models; Team Building

Further Readings

Carron, A. V., Colman, M. M., Wheeler, J., & Stevens, D. (2002). Cohesion and performance in sport: A meta-analysis. *Journal of Sport & Exercise Psychology, 24,* 168–188.

Carron, A. V., Widmeyer, W. N., & Brawley, L. R. (1985). The development of an instrument to assess cohesion in sport teams: The Group Environment Questionnaire. *Journal of Sport Psychology, 7,* 244–266.

Eys, M. A., Loughead, T. M., Bray, S. R., & Carron, A. V. (2009). Development of a cohesion questionnaire for youth: The Youth Sport Environment Questionnaire. *Journal of Sport & Exercise Psychology, 31,* 390–408.

Hardy, J., Eys, M. A., & Carron, A. V. (2005). Exploring the potential disadvantages of high team cohesion. *Small Group Research, 36,* 166–187.

Martin, L. J., Carron, A. V., Eys, M. A., & Loughead, T. M. (2012). Development of a cohesion questionnaire for children's sport teams. *Group Dynamics: Theory, Research, and Practice, 16,* 68–79.

Senecal, J., Loughead, T. M., & Bloom, G. (2008). A season-long team-building intervention: Examining the effect of team goal setting on cohesion. *Journal of Sport & Exercise Psychology, 30,* 186–199.

Spink, K. S., Wilson, K. S., & Odnokon, P. (2010). Examining the relationship between cohesion and return to team in elite athletes. *Psychology of Sport and Exercise, 11,* 6–11.

COLLECTIVE EFFICACY

Albert Bandura defined *collective efficacy* (CE) as a group's shared belief in its conjoint capabilities to organize and execute the courses of action required to produce given levels of attainments, that is, situation-specific confidence in a group's ability. A commonly used definition of CE in sport and exercise is a group's (e.g., a sport team or an exercise group) belief in its ability to produce given levels of attainment. Whether in sport, exercise, or human behavior more broadly, CE is believed to be a primary determinant of group behavior and thought patterns that occur within groups. The content of this entry focuses mainly on CE in sport due to spatial limitations (but can easily be generalized to other settings such as exercise), provides a broad overview of related research, and is organized as follows. First, a distinction between self-efficacy (SE) and CE is provided. Measurement of CE then is described. Potential sources and proposed outcomes of CE then are reviewed. Future directions conclude this entry.

Self-Efficacy Versus Collective Efficacy

Like SE, CE beliefs focus on *can do* and not *will do* perceptions that reside within individuals. A key distinction between these two types of efficacy beliefs is the target of the efficacy appraisal or unit of agency where SE is focused at the individual level (my confidence in *my ability* to . . .) and CE is focused at the group level (my confidence in *my group's ability* to . . .). The relevance of CE depends, in part, on the presence of a sufficient level of interdependence within the group with regard to the performance task.

As an example, which will be used periodically throughout the remainder of this entry, suppose that female athletes are nested within female teams and that both SE and CE are of interest in relation to athlete-level and team-level performance, respectively. A team member can have beliefs about her own ability in relation to a particular individual performance task (SE for individual performance) that may differ from her beliefs in the team's ability in relation to a particular team performance task (CE for team performance). Similarly, individual athletes within the same team may differ markedly in their assessment of the team's ability in relation to a particular team performance task (within-group variability of CE for team performance). For the purpose of this entry, let us assume that CE and team performance are of primary interest. It should be noted, however, that both types of efficacy beliefs and both types of performance tasks could be studied simultaneously and that doing so would probably better reflect actual behavior and thought patterns that occur within interdependent groups in practice.

Measurement of Collective Efficacy

Kevin Spink and Deborah Feltz encouraged the study of CE in sport in the early 1990s, several years after the study of SE in sport was well established. These two seminal studies did not define, and therefore measure, CE in the same way. In one of the studies, the definition of CE focused on the fact that groups often have collective expectations for success (e.g., What placing do you expect to attain in this performance task?). In the other study, the definition of CE focused on a group's belief in its conjoint capabilities to produce given levels of attainment (e.g., Rate your confidence right now that your team can outskate your upcoming opponent team). Both of these studies used a task-specific measurement approach, where unique items were developed with respect to the specific performance task under study. From these seminal studies, CE in sport has since been assessed in a variety of ways.

There are at least four task-specific methods that have been used to assess CE in sport. The first method involves measuring each athlete's SE beliefs in relation to a particular performance (e.g., how confident are *you in your ability* to . . .) and then combining team members' SE measures in some way to form a single CE ($\rightarrow$CE) measure (SE$\rightarrow$CE) for each team. The second method involves measuring each athlete's CE beliefs (assumed to reside in the individual athlete; CEI) in relation to a particular performance (e.g., how confident are *you in your team's ability* to . . .) and then combining team members' CE measures in some way to form a single CE measure (CEI$\rightarrow$CE) for each team. The third method involves measuring each athlete's perception of the team's CE beliefs (assumed to reside in the team; CET) in relation to a particular performance (e.g., how confident is the *team in its ability* to . . .) and then combining team members' CE measures in some way to form a single CE measure (CET$\rightarrow$CE) for each team. The fourth method involves using a group discussion format to obtain a single, group-level (CEG) measure of CE. The CEI→CE method and the CET→CE method have become the most widely used and are largely accepted as valid. A task-invariant instrument, the CE Questionnaire for Sports, also exists but this instrument appears to be used relatively infrequently to date.

Sources of Collective Efficacy

Albert Bandura proposed that CE beliefs, just like SE beliefs, are based on the complex cognitive processing of approximately four general categories of potential sources of information: past performance accomplishments, vicarious experiences, verbal persuasion, and physiological or emotional arousal. Neither vicarious experience (e.g., team modeling) nor physiological or emotional arousal (e.g., team burnout) have been formally studied as potential sources of CE information in sport. Researchers in sport psychology have identified several sport-specific sources of CE information and a few of these are briefly summarized below.

Past performance accomplishments have typically been identified as the strongest source of CE information and have been the most studied to date. There is evidence that past performance, in addition to directly affecting CE, may also affect SE, which in turn can affect CE. Another efficacy belief that may serve as a source of CE information is role efficacy. Role efficacy has been defined as an athlete's confidence in his or her capabilities to successfully carry out formal interdependent role responsibilities within a group.

Verbal persuasion has been shown to be an effective way to increase CE. For example, a motivational pregame speech delivered by a coach has been shown to increase CE. More generally, teams that exist within a more task-oriented motivational climate as compared to teams that exist within a more ego-oriented climate are believed to have greater CE due, in part, to the positive reinforcements that exist in such environments for more malleable outcomes than won–loss (e.g., improvement, hard work, teamwork). Finally, a coach's behavior (e.g., communication style) in general is a key source of CE information.

There are a few proposed sources of CE information in sport that do not fit neatly into any of the four general categories of potential sources of information but may nonetheless be important.

Team size has been shown to be an important factor but the direction and magnitude of the relationship seems to depend strongly on the specific type(s) of performance task(s) being studied. Length of time that a team has been together is another potentially important factor given that CE beliefs take time to form (recall, for example, the role of past performances). Length of time a team has been together may also be related to more general team development issues, which in turn may be related CE beliefs.

Outcomes of Collective Efficacy

Albert Bandura proposed that CE beliefs often are a primary determinant of group behavior and thought patterns that occur within groups. CE beliefs affect the choices a group makes (Do we attempt to take on a particular task?), the effort a group dedicates to a particular task (Will we give our best effort to this task?), and the persistence a group displays while working toward completion of a particular task (Given a setback, will we redouble our efforts toward accomplishing this task?). CE beliefs also affect the goals that a group sets (Will we select a goal that pushes our team to perform our very best?), the attributions a group makes (Given a setback, will we identify internal or external explanations for the outcome?), and the emotional reactions a group has (Given that we almost, but not quite, accomplished our goal and that we no longer have the opportunity to pursue this goal, will we feel proud of what we did accomplish?).

The effect of CE on team performance or team functioning has been the most studied outcome in sport. Much of the earlier work was done in controlled laboratory settings, while much of the more recent work has been done in less controlled field settings. A key advantage of the laboratory setting stems from the ability to randomly assign participants to groups (e.g., high efficacy vs. low). A key advantage of the field setting stems from the ability to collect data from real teams that are engaging in a task that is likely to be important to the team members. Regardless of the setting, a positive effect of CE on team performance has typically been observed.

Potential team-level outcomes of CE other than team performance have also been studied and a few of these are briefly summarized below. Team cohesion and CE have frequently been studied simultaneously. Team cohesion has been defined as a dynamic process that is reflected in the tendency of a group to stick together and remain united in the pursuit of its instrumental objectives or for the satisfaction of member affective needs. In general, stronger CE beliefs have been found to be a positive predictor of team cohesion. CE as a predictor of team attributions has also been studied. In general, athletes who have strong CE beliefs also believe that their team's performance is something that could be controlled by the team, that is, the attribution for the outcome was internal to the team.

Future Directions

SE theory provides a strong theoretical base for the construction of the CE construct. Albert Bandura's model of CE serves as a very useful starting point for the nature, sources, and consequences of CE in sport. The definition and therefore the measurement of CE in sport have both become more consistent across time. Clearly there is an emerging basis from which future scholarship likely can proceed in some way. A future direction that may prove fruitful is to develop sport-specific and conceptual model(s) of CE that expand potential sources of CE information as well as potential outcomes of CE.

Nicholas D. Myers

See also Coaching Efficacy; Cohesion; Group Characteristics; Interdependence Theory and the Coach–Athlete Relationship; Relational Efficacy Beliefs in Coach–Athlete Relations; Self-Efficacy; Social Cognitive Theory; Team Building

Further Readings

Bandura, A. (1997). *Self-efficacy: The exercise of control.* New York: Freeman.

Feltz, D. L., & Lirgg, C. D. (1998). Perceived team and player efficacy in hockey. *Journal of Applied Psychology, 83,* 557–564.

Feltz, D. L., Short, S. E., & Sullivan, P. J. (2008). *Self-efficacy in sport.* Champaign, IL: Human Kinetics.

Maddux, J. E. (1999). The collective construction of collective efficacy: Comment on Paskevich, Brawley, Dorsch, and Widmeyer. *Group Dynamics: Theory, Research, and Practice, 3,* 223–226.

Myers, N. D., & Feltz, D. L. (2007). From self-efficacy to collective efficacy in sport: Transitional methodological issues. In G. Tenenbaum & R. C.

Eklund (Eds.), *The handbook of sport psychology* (3rd ed., pp. 799–819). New York: Wiley.

Myers, N. D., Payment, C. A., & Feltz, D. L. (2004). Reciprocal relationships between collective efficacy and team performance in women's ice hockey. *Group Dynamics: Theory, Research, and Practice, 8,* 182–195.

Spink, K. S. (1990b). Group cohesion and collective efficacy of volleyball teams. *Journal of Sport & Exercise Psychology, 12,* 301–311.

Watson, C. B., Chemers, M. M., & Preiser, N. (2001). Collective efficacy: A multilevel analysis. *Personality and Social Psychology Bulletin, 27,* 1056–1068.

COLLECTIVISM/INDIVIDUALISM

Clients in sport and exercise psychology contexts are from a diversity of cultural backgrounds. The terms *individualism* and *collectivism* have recently been integrated within sport psychology as elements of one criterion by which to understand the client's cultural standpoint. Individualism has often been associated with mainstream clients who are white and from the Western hemisphere. In contrast, people generally characterized as collective in their approach to self and world have often been depicted as South American or Asian in origin, or as having been born and raised in collective-minded communities such as an Israeli kibbutz or an aboriginal reserve. To assume, however, that every athlete born and raised in a collective community must be group minded, or that every client socialized in an individualist context must be driven by personal objectives would of course be too simplistic.

Socialization

A person's inclination to view the self or collective at the center of interpersonal exchanges is a matter of many personal factors and not necessarily the effect of such broad considerations as one's geographic origin, skin color, or religion. For example, there are white, mainstream, North American athletes who are collectively inclined, just as there are fitness enthusiasts from Latin American or Asian cultures with an individualistic mindset as they approach their physical exercise. Clients must be understood in their own right and not on the basis of stereotypes. However, it should also be observed that some clients are inclined toward the values of individualism, where others are somewhat or fully collective in their approach to performance.

Individualism

What differentiates someone with an orientation that begins with self from another with a collective inclination? A person who is situated more toward individualism in one or more areas of life would often use language that places one's self at the center of discussions, such as when the elite athlete is interviewed by the media and attributes personal accomplishments exclusively to personal efforts and personal abilities. Individualism is also typified through the use of theoretically informed objectives, including self-determination, self-efficacy, self-concept, and self-esteem, as well as the behaviors that manifest the intentions underpinning each term. Decisions are often informed more by personal objectives than those from within one's communities of affiliation, whether geographic, peer group, religious, or professional. Personal goals are derived from personal interests, ending in personalized accomplishments.

Collectivism

The collectively inclined person, in contrast, seeks position in relation to one or several groups, with the views and practices of the group(s) informing, and in some instances, determining personal decisions and behaviors. The decision to become an elite athlete might be informed by how that career path contributes to those living in one's community. Thereafter, the collectively inclined client might opt to return to that community and share experiences and skills with others for the collective's betterment, such as when a national team athlete or professional athlete returns to the cultural community to become a coach, or when one studies physical education and then returns to one's locale to work a physical educator. Hence, the person's decision to act in a certain manner or develop targeted skills will align with the development of the group as a whole and also informed by the community's stakeholders. The importance of social support, both in its reception and provision, becomes particularly salient for people socialized with a collective mindset.

Research Applications

There are research strategies that illustrate inclinations toward individual and collective values.

Consider qualitative strategies that reflect an emphasis on the individual, including personal interviews and single-subject case studies. Practices that are individualist are best used with participants holding like-minded cultural norms. When working with people who are more collectively inclined, one might consider group interviews to encourage group exchange and the convergence of ideas. Within research, the objective would be either to conceive of strategies that match where participants reside on the aforementioned continuum or at least to approach research studies with an awareness that orthodox research practices for individualist participants might cause discomfort among collectively inclined participants, and vice versa.

Conclusion

There are strategies that could be employed to better understand where the client resides in terms of self in relation to the collective. Perhaps the most basic suggestion is to listen with care to the client in terms of how the client describes, and therefore positions, him- or herself in relation to others. When motives seem to be informed by a community perspective, the sport or exercise psychologist can seek further clarification about where the client is from, what the values are within the community of origin, and whether these values are held dear by the client. Conversely, also through listening, when the client's description of self centralizes personal accomplishments, again, the practitioner might follow up with questions that clarify the client's origins and socialization.

Robert J. Schinke

See also Assimilation; Attribution Theory; Cultural Competence; Cultural Safety; Decision Making; Diversity; Race; Self-Presentation; Self-Talk; Team Communication

Further Readings

Blodgett, A. T., Schinke, R. J., Fisher, L. A., George, C., Peltier, D., Ritchie, S., et al. (2008). From practice to praxis: Community-based strategies for Aboriginal youth sport. *Journal of Sport & Social Issues, 32,* 393–414.

Hanrahan, S. J. (2004). Sport psychology and indigenous performing arts. *Sport Psychologist, 18,* 60–74.

Kim, B. J., Williams, L., & Gill, D. L. (2003). A cross-cultural study of achievement orientation and intrinsic motivation in young USA and Korean athletes.

International Journal of Sport Psychology, 34, 168–184.

Kontos, A. P., & Arguello, E. (2009). Sport psychology consulting with Latin American athletes. In R. J. Schinke (Ed.), *Contemporary sport psychology* (pp. 181–196). Hauppage, NY: Nova Science.

Peters, H. J., & Williams, J. M. (2006). Moving cultural background to the foreground: An investigation of self-talk, performance, and persistence following feedback. *Journal of Applied Sport Psychology, 18,* 240–253.

Schinke, R. J., Michel, G., Gauthier, A. P., Pickard, P., Danielson, R., Peltier, D., et al. (2006). The adaptation to the mainstream in elite sport: A Canadian Aboriginal perspective. *Sport Psychologist, 20,* 435–448.

Vélez, C. G. (1982). Mexicano/Hispano support systems and confianza: Theoretical issues of cultural adaptation. In R. Valle & W. Vega (Eds.), *Hispanic natural support systems: Mental health promotion perspectives* (pp. 45–54). Sacramento: State of California, Department of Mental Health.

COMMITMENT

Sport commitment is a central motivational construct because it goes right to the heart of athletes' persistent pursuit of their sport. Simply put, it is a psychological state explaining why athletes do what they do. There are two types of sport commitment: enthusiastic and constrained. *Enthusiastic commitment* (EC) is the psychological construct representing the desire and resolve to persist in a sport over time. Conceptualized recently to provide a more complete picture of commitment, *constrained commitment* (CC) is the psychological construct representing perceptions of obligation to persist in a sport over time. Knowledge of the sources of both types of commitment is critical to understanding the commitment process. These sources are presented as part of the sport commitment model (SCM) detailed next.

The SCM explains the complex process of commitment by encompassing the sources of both types of commitment, and their predicted behavioral consequence: actual persistence in one's sport. The SCM has been tested, modified, clarified, and expanded from the time it was first introduced in the literature in 1993. Many researchers have contributed to this progress, and using the combination of quantitative survey and qualitative interview methods has increased significantly the depth with which we understand what it is that creates commitment.

The sources of commitment are presented in this entry in the following manner. First, every source in the SCM is defined. Next, the hypothesized or explored relationships between the sources and EC and then CC are summarized.

Sources of Commitment: Construct Definitions

Sport Enjoyment—the positive emotional response to a sport experience that reflects generalized feelings of joy.

Valuable Opportunities—important opportunities that are only present through continued involvement in a sport, such as traveling to competitions or playing in a future World Cup.

Personal Investments-Loss—personal resources put into a sport that cannot be recovered if participation is discontinued. Example investments include time and effort expended.

Personal Investments-Quantity—the amount of personal resources put into a sport.

Emotional Social Support—the encouragement, caring, and empathy received from significant people to the athlete such as parents, coaches, and teammates.

Informational Social Support—the provision of useful information, guidance, or advice received from significant people.

Desire to Excel–Mastery Achievement—striving to improve and achieve mastery in a sport.

Desire to Excel–Social Achievement—striving to win and establish superiority over opponents in a sport.

Other Priorities—attractive or pressing alternatives that conflict with continued sport participation such as work, educational pursuits, and family.

Social Constraints—social expectations or norms that create perceptions of obligation for the athlete to remain in a sport; for example, anticipating the disappointment of parents or coaches if the athlete dropped out of the sport.

Sources of Commitment: SCM Predictions

Sources of Enthusiastic Commitment

The SCM hypothesizes that many sources are positive predictors of EC and, thereby, strengthen it, while one source is negatively related to EC and, hence, lessens it. The following sources are contended to strengthen EC: sport enjoyment, valuable opportunities; both types of personal investments (loss and quantity), social support (emotional and informational), and desire to excel (mastery and social achievement); and social constraints.

SCM conceptualizes other priorities to be negatively related to EC and, therefore, the source lessens or chips away at this type of commitment. In fact, to keep this negative effect from happening, rich interview data show that many elite athletes, and their families, actively employ strategies to eliminate any conflict with other priorities in their lives. This allows playing to remain the top priority.

Sources of Constrained Commitment

The research is limited when CC is studied within the general framework of the SCM. Hence, with three exceptions, the current sources of EC will need to be explored to see how they relate to CC. In a few studies, personal investments, other priorities, and social constraints were found to be positive predictors of CC. Future research will help us understand why some athletes feel trapped in their sport.

Progress with the SCM continues. Based on what has been learned from research to date, a significantly updated English version of the Sport Commitment Questionnaire has been developed, and adapted into Spanish and Portuguese to stimulate cross-cultural research. There also is considerable interest in adapting the questionnaire into other languages.

Tara K. Scanlan and Graig M. Chow

See also Adherence; Effort; Enjoyment; Talent Development

Further Readings

Scanlan, T. K., Chow, G. M., Sousa, C., Scanlan, L. A., & Knifsend, C. A. (2013). The development of the Sport Commitment Questionnaire 2 (English version). Manuscript submitted for publication.

Scanlan, T. K., Russell, D. G., Magyar, T. M., & Scanlan, L. A. (2009). Project on Elite Athlete Commitment (PEAK): III. An examination of the external validity across gender, and the expansion and clarification of the Sport Commitment Model. *Journal of Sport & Exercise Psychology, 31*, 685–705.

Scanlan, T. K., Russell, D. G., Scanlan, L. A., Klunchoo, T., & Chow, G. M. (in press). Project on Elite Athlete Commitment (PEAK): IV: Identification of new candidate commitment sources for the Sport Commitment Model. *Journal of Sport & Exercise Psychology*.

Scanlan, T. K., Simons, J. P., Carpenter, P. J., Schmidt, G. W., & Keeler, B. (1993). The Sport Commitment Model: Measurement development for the youth sport domain. *Journal of Sport & Exercise Psychology, 15*, 16–38.

Wilson, P. M., Rodgers, W. M., Carpenter, P. J., Hall, C., Hardy, J., & Fraser, S. N. (2004). The relationship between commitment and exercise behavior. *Psychology of Sport and Exercise, 5*, 405–421.

Young, B. W., & Medic, N. (2011). Examining social influences on the sport commitment of Masters swimmers. *Psychology of Sport and Exercise, 12*, 168–175.

COMPETENCE MOTIVATION THEORY

Competence motivation theory is a conceptual framework designed to explain individuals' motivation to participate, persist, and work hard in any particular achievement context. The central thesis of the theory is that individuals are attracted to participation in activities at which they feel competent or capable. The theory can be used by researchers and practitioners in sport and exercise psychology fields to identify why and how children, adolescents, and adults can be encouraged to participate and to exert effort in these achievement contexts.

In the following entry, the research and theory on competence motivation within the physical domain are reviewed. This begins with a brief historical overview of the theory and its constructs. Following that, the results of the research on the following segments are summarized: (a) correlates of competence motivation, (b) developmental trends in perceived competence, and (c) the impact of significant others on competence motivation.

Historical Overview

Most scholars identify Robert White's classic paper on motivation reconsidered as the forerunner of competence motivation theory. In this 1959 publication, White coined the term *effectance* and defined it as a tendency to explore and influence one's environment. White argued that organisms are intrinsically motivated to engage in interactions with their physical and social environments. If such attempts result in success (production of an observable effect on the environment), then that individual receives intrinsic rewards like feelings of efficacy and pleasure and is motivated to continue effectance efforts. White's theory of competence motivation was considered a novel approach in that it differed significantly from the traditional drive theories of human behavior and from the psychoanalytic instinct theory proposed and popularized by Sigmund Freud.

In the late 1970s, Susan Harter extended White's theory to develop a more complete framework that she initially identified as effectance motivation theory but was later more commonly referred to as competence motivation theory. Consistent with White, Harter also centered enjoyment as the reason why individuals are motivated to interact with their environment, but she added a number of other components. First, she introduced the idea that individuals' effectance or competence motivation can vary across achievement domains (e.g., cognitive, physical, social). Within each domain, individuals are motivated to engage in mastery attempts for the purpose of developing or demonstrating competence. If their mastery attempts result in success at an optimally challenging task and if they receive socioemotional support from significant individuals for such task success, then they will experience perceptions of competence (belief in their abilities in that domain) along with perceptions of performance control (belief in their ability to control their performance). High perceptions of competence and control, in turn, result in feelings of pleasure that lead to maintenance of or increases in effectance (competence) motivation. In contrast to White, Harter also proposed a negatively oriented path that specified that individuals who engage in mastery attempts but meet with failure at optimally challenging tasks or lack of reinforcement or disapproval from significant social agents will experience decreased perceptions of competence and control in that achievement domain, along with anxiety and shame. This combination of events will lead to decreased effectance motivation in that particular domain.

Harter also added a developmental dimension to her theoretical framework by suggesting that children who are successful in their initial mastery attempts and who get positive and effective reinforcement from significant adults will (with sufficient cognitive maturation) internalize both a self-reward system and a set of mastery goals. Due to this internalization of standards for optimal challenge in that domain, such adolescents will no longer be dependent on social agents to evaluate their performance or to motivate them to continue their mastery attempts. Correspondingly, children who are either continually unsuccessful in their early mastery attempts or who get disapproving or no feedback from significant adults will not only develop low perceptions of competence and control in that achievement domain but will continue, as adolescents and adults, to be dependent on external sources both to evaluate their performance and to motivate them to continue their participation in that domain.

The publication of Harter's early work stimulated much research during the next 2 decades in the academic, social, and physical domains. More recently, interest in competence motivation theory has waned somewhat, likely because the construct of competence has been subsumed within other theories of motivation, such as achievement goal and self-determination. However, in 2005, Andrew J. Elliot and Carol Dweck proposed a more central role for competence and recommended that the term *achievement motivation* be changed to *competence motivation*. Their arguments were based on the idea that competence motivation (a) is broadly present in daily life activities, (b) has a large and influential effect on individuals' emotional and psychosocial well-being, (c) is operative across the lifespan (from infancy through older age), and (d) has relevance across cultures.

Research on Competence Motivation Theory in the Physical Achievement Domain

Correlates of Competence Motivation

The initial studies by researchers in sport psychology provided support for the model itself but also for the importance of competence as a motivational construct. Specifically, individuals who perceive themselves as having high competence in any particular sport or physical activity context exhibit higher intrinsic motivation to participate in that activity and experience more positive affective reactions (e.g., pleasure, satisfaction, enjoyment) when participating than do their peers who hold lower perceptions of competence.

Correspondingly, perceived competence levels can also affect or predict individuals' behavior. Children and adolescents in a variety of physical contexts (e.g., physical education classes, sport teams) who perceive themselves as having high competence are more apt to continue their participation and to exhibit higher levels of effort, persistence, and preference for more challenging tasks, whereas their peers who perceive low levels of competence exhibit lower levels of such task-oriented behaviors and are, subsequently, at greater risk of discontinuation. More recent studies have indicated that perceptions of competence are also tied to physical activity behaviors; children with high perceived physical competence exhibit higher frequency and intensity of daily physical activity levels. Such connections have also been demonstrated in intervention studies; children who successfully engage in physical activity programs show increases in perceived physical competence, which, in turn, increases both their motivation to be physically active and their actual physical activity levels. Interestingly, perceptions of physical competence have also been shown to be relevant for older adults, as those who have high perceptions of physical competence are more physically active and also exhibit higher perceived quality-of-life attitudes than do their peers who have lower perceptions of physical competence. Finally, high perceptions of competence in individuals across the lifespan have been consistently linked to higher levels of global self-worth or self-esteem. These results, again, point to the importance of individuals possessing high perceptions of ability or competence in at least one valued achievement domain in order to have an overall high regard for the self.

Developmental Trends in Relation to Perceived Competence

Two lifespan changes are particularly relevant to the physical domain. First, the number of domains in which individuals evaluate their competence appears to increase with age. That is, young children (4–7 years) tend to perceive competence in only two domains (general competence and social competence). However, older children (8–13 years) exhibit a somewhat more diversified perception of competence that spans five different achievement domains (academic, athletic, social, physical appearance, and behavioral). During the adolescent years, the number increases to include three additional ones (close friendship, romantic relationships, and job competence). Other, smaller, developmental changes continue to occur across the adult years.

Second, research in both the cognitive and physical domains has indicated that the sources of information that individuals use to evaluate their competence change with increased maturation. For younger children (4–7 years), the primary sources of information are few in number and very concrete, for example, feedback from significant adults and simple task accomplishment. Thus, such a child might say, "I am really good at throwing because I can throw this ball all the way to that wall," or "I know that I am a really good thrower because my teacher says so." During the middle to late childhood years (7–12 years), the number of sources children use to evaluate their competence increases somewhat, but the sources remain quite concrete. It is during this period that peer comparison and performance outcomes (winning or losing) become more relevant. During the adolescent years (13–18 years), the number of sources again increases, and most adolescents have the cognitive capacity to use a broader range of sources that include both internal (e.g., achievement of self-set goals) and external (e.g., feedback from others, performance outcomes, peer comparison) sources. Going back again to the early Harter model, it may be important for adolescents to reach a stage where they do use multiple sources and where they are able to use more internalized sources like personal satisfaction rather than remaining dependent on single sources like peer comparison or on externally available sources such as coaches' evaluation of their performance.

The Impact of Significant Others on Competence Motivation

As indicated in the original Harter model, significant others, such as parents, teachers, coaches, and peers play a major role in the development of individuals' perceptions of physical competence and effectance motivation. In particular, parents may serve as the first important social agents. They can, for example, affect their children's perceptions of competence through modeling (children observing their parents' own engagement in, and enjoyment of, mastery attempts). However, an equally important role that parents may play is in the feedback they provide in response to their child's early engagement in mastery attempts. Obviously, positive feedback like "Good work, Maria!" is better than negative or no feedback. But, it is also the content of parents' feedback that appears important. Specifically, a child who participates for the first time in a tee-ball league will learn from the parents' feedback not only whether mastery attempts in such a domain are valued but also *how* the performance should be evaluated. That is, does the parent provide feedback that evaluates the child's performance based on (a) the performance outcome ("Good job, Susan. You got to first base again."), (b) peer comparison ("You have to work harder in practice. You let Chase beat you again today."), or (c) personal mastery of a skill ("Good work in practice today, Joshua. I see that you learned how to catch the ball.")?

A second group of adults who can have a significant impact on individuals' perceptions of competence and effectance motivation in the physical domain are coaches, physical education teachers, and physical activity directors. Although positive feedback from such individuals is certainly more facilitative of high perceived competence in students and athletes, teachers and coaches also need to ensure that such positive feedback is appropriate. That is, for very young children (4–7 years), positive and general feedback ("Good job, Enrico!") may be good. But for older children and adolescents (12 years and up), coaches and teachers should be sure that their praise is appropriate. That is, if a coach provides a 12-year-old player who just got to first base on a pitcher's error with exaggerated praise ("Wow, Robert, that was truly just an excellent performance."), the athlete's competence may not be enhanced as he may realize that the praise is not consistent with the performance. In such a situation, the receiver of that inappropriate praise may actually perceive low competence as he assumes that the coach thinks he is really bad at batting if that is the level of performance that is rewarded. Thus, the coach could better respond by providing more contingent praise ("Robert, you really did a good job in not swinging at those bad pitches.")

In addition, coaches and teachers who provide skill-relevant, informational, and corrective feedback to athletes in response to their performance attempts ("That was a good hit, Samantha. But next time, you should extend your elbow a little bit more. That will give you even more power.") will do more to enhance young athletes' perceptions of competence and control than will feedback statements that are evaluative only and which provide no corrective information ("That was a good play, Samantha," or "You struck out again, Domingo!")

Another social group that may be particularly important in regard to children's and adolescents' perceptions of competence in particular achievement domains is peers (friends, classmates and teammates). Research studies have demonstrated that peer acceptance (the degree to which children and adolescents feel accepted and valued by their peers) and the number and quality of friendships can enhance perceptions of competence and can result in continued motivation to participate in that achievement activity. Correspondingly, the type of feedback that peers provide has also been shown to affect individuals' levels of competitive anxiety, sport motivation, and enjoyment.

Conclusion

The central thesis of competence motivation theory is that individuals are attracted to participate in activities at which they feel competent or capable. In physical activity domains, then, if the goal is for people to be motivated to be physically active or to strive for performance excellence, it will be necessary to design environments that will enhance their perceptions of competence. Based on the research and theory to date, enhanced perceptions of competence can be achieved when individuals experience success at optimally challenging tasks and when they receive positive, encouraging, consistent, and information-based feedback from significant others within that environment.

Thelma S. Horn

See also Achievement Goal Theory; Achievement Motive Theory; Hierarchical Self; Self-Determination Theory

Further Readings

Elliot, A. J., & Dweck, C. S. (Eds.). (2005). *Handbook of competence and motivation*. New York: Guilford Press.

Harter, S. (1978). Effectance motivation reconsidered: Toward a developmental model. *Human Development, 1*, 34–64.

Horn, T. S. (2004). Developmental perspectives on self-perceptions in children and adolescents. In M. R. Weiss (Ed.), *Developmental sport and exercise psychology: A lifespan perspective* (pp. 101–143). Morgantown, WV: Fitness Information Technology.

Horn, T. S., & Harris, A. (2002). Perceived competence in young athletes: Research findings and recommendations for coaches and parents. In F. L. Smoll & R. E. Smith (Eds.), *Children and youth in sport: A biopsychosocial perspective* (2nd ed., pp. 435–464). Dubuque, IA: Kendall/Hunt.

Weiss, M. R., & Amorose, A. J. (2008). Motivational orientations and sport behavior. In T. S. Horn (Ed.), *Advances in sport psychology* (3rd ed., pp. 115–155). Champaign, IL: Human Kinetics.

White, R. W. (1959). Motivation reconsidered: The concept of competence. *Psychological Review, 66,* 297–333.

COMPETITION

Competition is often described as a contest, or a process of contesting, between two or more parties (organisms, individuals, or groups) for a scarce resource or good. The scarcity can result from nature or history, such as competition for limited food, or it can be created artificially, such as the good of winning a game. As the term is most often used, competition is the opposite of cooperation. Since competition is a central dynamic in most if not all sports, competition is of keen interest to sport scientists. In this entry, various forms of competition are described, the social science research on competition is reviewed, and theory and research on competitiveness is summarized.

What Is Competition?

Competition comes in many forms and is relevant to many fields of study. Economic, political, biological, evolutionary, and sport competition, for example, each have unique characteristics, along with some commonalities. Competition occurs between and among nonhuman organisms, individuals, teams, organizations, cultures, and nations, to name only some of the most obvious. Competition can be direct or indirect, subtle or intense, formal or informal. It can be zero sum, resulting in winners and losers, or allow for many variations of outcome distributions.

To define competition, most social psychologists have focused on the goal structure of situations. Morton Deutsch, for example, defined *competition* in terms of "negative social interdependence." A situation is competitive if the progress or success of one party interferes with the progress or likelihood of success of other parties.

Rainer Martens proposed a definition of competition from a sport psychology perspective. For Martens, competition is a form of social evaluation; it entails comparison of individual or team performances against one another or against an objective standard of excellence. In Martens's view, people compete because humans have an innate motive to evaluate their ability. A competitive situation is one that allows for the evaluation process through providing a rule structure that (a) defines the goal toward which action is directed and (b) defines the allowable means to try to achieve the goal.

Competition: The Social Science Research

Psychologists have studied the effects of competition for more than a hundred years. In the late 1890s, in what is often called the first sport psychology study, Norman Triplett found that cyclists performed faster when they were racing against other cyclists than when they were racing against the clock. Despite this promising initial start, subsequent research has demonstrated that for most types of tasks in most situations, competition leads to poorer performance. The exceptions are simple tasks or rudimentary skills, the performance of which can be facilitated through competition.

In his extensive if somewhat polemical review of the literature in *No Contest: The Case Against Competition,* Alfie Kohn concluded that competition is associated with a range of negative outcomes. As noted above, in most situations it hinders optimal performance. Competition, both interpersonal and intergroup, has also been associated with increased hostility, aggression, and prejudice. It tends to interfere with developing positive and stable self-esteem; it creates stress and anxiety, along with their negative health consequences; and it promotes conformity and reliance on external evaluation.

Many researchers, such as David and Roger Johnson, acknowledge the extensive literature demonstrating these negative consequences, but still maintain that competition can be useful. Writers in this tradition seek to distinguish healthy from unhealthy, beneficial from destructive, and productive from harmful forms of competition. Unfortunately, the distinctions are often unclear and are based more on differences of degree than of kind.

A different approach has been advanced by David Shields and Brenda Bredemeier, who offer a qualitative distinction between competition and the forms of contesting that lead to negative outcomes. They define *competition* as striving for excellence in a contest situation. According to this view, competition entails a combination of a contest structure with a personal orientation toward seeking excellence through the mutual challenge that opponents provide to each other. They introduce a new term, *decompetition,* to describe a situation in which a contest is metaphorically understood as a battle for superiority or extrinsic reward. They suggest that it is the different motivations and goals associated with decompetition that account for the negative findings prevalent in the literature.

What Is Competitiveness?

When people compete, they strive to obtain a limited goal and to compare favorably to others similarly striving. In sports, the contest-specific goal, of course, is to win. The amount of preparation, focus, determination, and energy that a person puts into striving to win is often referred to as their competitiveness. Competitive people have a strong desire to achieve and succeed, thereby demonstrating their competency to themselves and others. There are two main instruments that have been developed to measure competitiveness in sport.

Robin Vealey used achievement-goal theory to help her define and operationalize competitiveness. Correspondingly, competitiveness can take two different forms, depending on what goal the athlete is trying to achieve. Athletes can be outcome oriented (winning) or performance oriented (performing masterfully) or both. When Vealey developed the Competitive Orientation Inventory (COI), she placed the two orientations in opposition. The format of the instrument consists of a 16-cell matrix in which four levels of performance (very good, above average, below average, and very poor) are intersected with four outcomes (an easy win, a close win, a close loss, and a big loss). For each of the resultant 16 cells, the athlete indicates their level of satisfaction. Those athletes who indicate high satisfaction when they win, irrespective of how well they played, score high on outcome-oriented competitiveness; in contrast, those who are most satisfied with playing well score high on performance-oriented competitiveness.

Another widely used assessment of competitiveness, called the Sport Orientation Questionnaire (SOQ), was developed by Diane Gill and Thomas Deeter. The measure assesses three orientations: competitiveness, goal orientation (a focus on personal standards), and a win orientation. The concept of *competitiveness* is defined as a desire to enter and strive for success in sport competition. For example, respondents are asked to indicate their extent of agreement with "I thrive on competition," and "The best test of my ability is competing against others."

Researchers have investigated competitiveness both as a dependent and as an independent variable. For example, researchers have generally found male athletes to be more competitive than female athletes, elite athletes to be more competitive than recreational athletes, and U.S. athletes to be more competitive than those from more collectivist cultures. In turn, competitiveness seems to predict sport involvement, poor sportsmanship, higher alcohol consumption, and sexually aggressive attitudes.

Brenda Light Bredemeier and
David Light Shields

See also Achievement Goal Theory; Aggression; Conflict; Interdependence Theory and the Coach–Athlete Relationship

Further Readings

Gill, D. L., & Deeter, T. E. (1988). Development of the Sport Orientation Questionnaire. *Research Quarterly for Exercise and Sport, 59,* 191–202.

Kohn, A. (1992). *No contest: The case against competition* (Rev. ed.). Boston: Houghton Mifflin.

Martens, R. (1976). Competition: In need of a theory. In D. M. Landers (Ed.), *Social problems in athletics* (pp. 9–17). Urbana: University of Illinois Press.

Shields, D., & Bredemeier, B. (2011). Contest, competition, and metaphor. *Journal of the Philosophy of Sport, 38,* 27–38.

Vealey, R. S. (1986). Conceptualization of sport-confidence and competitive orientation: Preliminary investigation and instrument development. *Journal of Sport Psychology, 8,* 221–246.

CONCENTRATION

In sport psychology, concentration refers to focusing on sensory or mental events coupled with mental effort. It therefore relates primarily to the selective attention dimension in which individuals are able to selectively process some sources of information while ignoring others. It has its roots in the oft-cited quote from William James's 1890 book *The Principles of Psychology* (Vol. 1):

> Everyone knows what attention is. It is the taking possession by the mind, in clear and vivid form, of one out of what seem several simultaneously possible objects or trains of thought. Focalization, concentration, of consciousness are of its essence. It implies withdrawal from some things in order to deal effectively with others. (pp. 403–404)

Within sport psychology, research interest in concentration is predominantly focused in two areas. First is the study of skill failure under pressure, or choking; there is strong evidence that skill failure can result from *reinvestment* of conscious control processes. Second, researchers have investigated the efficacy of external and internal foci of attention during learning and in skilled performance.

Measurement

Researchers have used a range of psychophysiological tools, as well as self-report measures, to infer attentional states. These include heart rate measurement, electroencephalography (EEG), functional magnetic resonance imaging (fMRI), and ratings of the extent of focus on a particular information source in experimental paradigms. In addition, dual-task paradigms have been used to measure performers' awareness of task-relevant and extraneous information, most notably in the study of choking. Self-report measures include the Test of Attentional and Interpersonal Style (TAIS), which was devised by Robert Nideffer to assess a range of personality measures, a subset of which were linked to his proposed two-dimensional model of attention. This model distinguishes between direction of attention (external, internal) and breadth of attention (broad, narrow) creating four combinations. The scale contains groups of items to measure positive attributes of attention (effective integration and effective narrowing) and items to measure negative attributes (overloading and underinclusion). Other scales that are more specifically focused include the Self-Consciousness Scale, which measures individual propensity for attending to the self, and the Reinvestment Scale (and its movement-specific and decision-specific versions), which measures the tendency to exert conscious control over movements or the decision making process.

Concentration and Choking

There is good evidence that skill failure in self-paced skills such as golf putting, basketball free throws, rugby goal kicks, and static target shooting is caused by the performers concentrating on deliberately and consciously controlling their movements. Much of the research work examining this issue has assessed the performer's attentional state in the few seconds prior to skill execution using a variety of experimental paradigms. These experimental paradigms have included cross-sectional designs comparing individuals of different levels of ability or experience, and within-participant designs in which the performer's concentration is directly manipulated via explicit instruction or task-related instructions. Evidence from performance measures and indirect measures of attention indicates clear differences between high-skilled and less-skilled performers, and that skilled performance breaks down when individuals reinvest conscious control over largely automatic actions. For example, explicit monitoring of motor skills has been shown to have a detrimental effect on skilled performers but does not impair, and sometimes facilitates, novice performance. By contrast, experts are able to perform a concurrent secondary task with minimal impairment to primary task performance, whereas novice performance tends to get worse. Relatedly, there is within-group evidence that skilled performers' ability to report task-relevant and extraneous information relates to how well they have been performed on preceding trials. For example, baseball batters are better able to report bat position during a performance slump than when on a streak of good performance, implying their concentration is more directed to the swing motion during slumps.

A second line of research into concentration in sport concerns the efficacy of adopting either an external focus (on an implement or movement effects) or internal focus (on body movements) during learning and skilled performance. There is now a considerable body of evidence across a variety of tasks and using different age groups that an external focus is preferable for learning and evidence that this also extends to skilled performance. Further, the effect is moderated by distance so that a more distal external focus is more beneficial than a proximal focus. By studying task outcome alongside the movement kinematics and EMG activity, improvements in movement efficiency as well as accuracy have been reported resulting in more rapid skill acquisition and better retention. The *constrained action hypothesis* has been proposed to explain these findings, referring to the self-organizing nature of the motor system and the potential for an external focus of attention to facilitate high frequency unconscious adjustments. Conversely, an internal focus of attention is hypothesized to constrain the self-organizing nature of the motor system as the performer attempts to actively monitor and control the system.

Conclusion

The term *concentration* embodies one element of the multidimensional construct of attention. In the sport psychology literature, the term has been particularly important in the study of skill failure under pressure and in the realm of skill acquisition. Concentration strategies are a key component of the mental routines performers employ before executing self-paced skills. Proposed interventions for aiding performance, particularly under pressure, support the view that the information on which a performer concentrates in the few seconds before skill execution is a key determinant of performance.

Robin C. Jackson

See also Attention Theory; Attentional Focus; Choking

Further Readings

Gray, R. (2004). Attending to the execution of a complex sensorimotor skill: Expertise differences, choking, and slumps. *Journal of Experimental Psychology: Applied, 10,* 42–54.

Masters, R. S. W., Polman, R. C. J., & Hammond, N. V. (1993). Reinvestment: A dimension of personality implicated in skill breakdown under pressure. *Personality and Individual Differences, 14,* 655–666.

Milton, J., Solodkin, A., Hluštík, P., & Small, S. L. (2007). The mind of expert motor performance is cool and focused. *NeuroImage, 35,* 804–813.

Nideffer, R. M. (1976). Test of Attentional and Interpersonal Style. *Journal of Personality and Social Psychology, 34,* 394–404.

Singer, R. N. (2002). Preperformance state, routines, and automaticity: What does it take to realize expertise in self-paced events? *Journal of Sport & Exercise Psychology, 24,* 359–375.

Wulf, G., & Prinz, W. (2001). Directing attention to movement effects enhances learning: A review. *Psychonomic Bulletin & Review, 8,* 648–660.

Wulf, G., & Su, J. (2007). An external focus of attention enhances golf shot accuracy in beginners and experts. *Research Quarterly for Exercise and Sport, 78,* 384–389.

CONCENTRATION SKILLS

Several sources of evidence reveal that concentration, or the ability to focus on what is most important in any situation while ignoring distractions, is vital for success in sport. First, anecdotally, lapses in concentration can mean the difference between winning and losing at the Olympics. For example, at the 2008 Games in Beijing, rifle shooter Matthew Emmons missed an opportunity to win a gold medal in the 50m three-position target event due to a lapse in concentration. Leading his nearest rival Qiu Jian as he took his last shot, Emmons lost his focus and inexplicably misfired, finishing without a medal (in 4th place). A second source of evidence on the importance of concentration comes from research showing that the capacity to become absorbed in the present moment is a key component of peak performance experiences in sport (see also the entry "Flow"). Finally, experimental evidence suggests that athletes who have been trained to focus on task-relevant cues tend to perform better than those who have not received such training. Despite the preceding evidence, however, psychology researchers have struggled to answer two significant questions in this field. First, if concentration is so important, why do athletes appear to lose it so easily in competitive situations? Second, what are the building blocks of effective concentration skills in sport?

Why Do Athletes Lose Their Concentration?

According to a conceptual approach called *spotlight theory* (see also the entry "Attention Theory"), paying attention is like shining a mental beam at targets located either in the external (real) world or in the internal world of our thoughts and feelings. It is like the head-mounted torch that divers and miners wear in dark environments. Wherever they look, their target is illuminated. A practical implication of this theory is that concentration cannot be lost, although one's mental spotlight can be diverted easily to a target that is not relevant to the task at hand.

In competitive sport, an abundance of distractions can threaten to divert an athlete's mental spotlight from its intended target. Normally, these distractions fall into two main categories: external and internal. Whereas external distractions are objective stimuli that exist in the world around us, internal distractions include a vast array of thoughts, feelings, or bodily sensations like fatigue that can disrupt our focus. Typical external distractions include factors such as spectator movements, sudden changes in ambient noise levels (e.g., the click of a camera), gamesmanship (e.g., trying to block a goalkeeper in soccer from seeing the ball at a corner kick) and unpredicted weather conditions (e.g., tennis players may get distracted when windy conditions affect their ball toss before serving). Typically, these distractions impair athletic performance. For example, the marathon runner Vanderlei De Lima was leading the race in the 2004 Olympics in Athens when an unstable spectator suddenly jumped out from the crowd and wrestled him to the ground. Stunned and distracted, De Lima eventually finished third in the event. Internal distractions stem mainly from thoughts such as wondering what might happen in the future, regretting what has happened in the past, or worrying about what other people might think, say, or do. A classic example of a costly internal distraction occurred in the case of the golfer Doug Sanders, who missed a putt of less than 3 feet, which prevented him from winning the 1970 British Open championship in St. Andrews, his first major tournament. Remarkably, Sanders's attentional lapse was precipitated by thinking too far ahead: He had made a victory speech in his mind before his final putt had been sunk. Unfortunately, little research has been conducted on the mechanisms by which internal distractions disrupt performance. Nevertheless, Daniel Wegner developed a model that attempted to explain why attentional lapses occur *ironically,* or precisely at the most inopportune moment for the person involved. Briefly, this model postulates that when our working memory system (which regulates our conscious awareness) becomes overloaded because we are anxious or tired, a particular form of ironic distractibility may occur. Specifically, trying *not* to think about something may paradoxically *increase* the prominence of this very thought in our consciousness. According to Wegner, this increased awareness of the very thing we try to suppress is called a *rebound effect* and applies to *actions* as well as thoughts. For example, in sport, ironies of action are evident when anxious penalty takers in

football try *not* to kick the ball at the goalkeeper but end up doing so or alternatively, when tired golfers try *not* to overshoot the ball when putting, but again, end up doing so.

Building Blocks of Effective Concentration Skills

Research suggests that there at least four building blocks of effective concentration skills in sport.

Deciding to Concentrate

To begin with, athletes must make a conscious decision to invest mental effort in their performance. Just as researchers have distinguished between deliberate practice (a purposeful activity in which the learner tried to improve a specific skill under the guidance of an expert coach) and mindless practice (whereby the learner flits from one skill to another without any plan), we can distinguish between *deciding* to concentrate and merely hoping that it will happen. To implement this principle, many athletes establish imaginary *switch on* and *switch off* zones in their competitive environment. For example, entering the locker room before a game may serve as a trigger for footballers to turn on their concentration before a match. Likewise, in an intense game, tennis players may use a between-points routine of wiping their face with a towel at the back of the tennis court to safely switch off from thinking about the previous point.

Having Only One Thought at a Time

Next, the *one thought* principle is the idea that one can focus consciously on only one thing at a time. This principle comes from research on the bandwidth of attention or the number of items in working memory on which one can focus effectively. Studies on this topic suggest that people's focus of attention may be limited to just one item. Extrapolating from this finding, it seems plausible that the ideal thought for a sports performer should be a single word that triggers the appropriate feeling or tempo of the action to be executed (e.g., *smooth* for a golf swing) rather than a complicated set of instructions (e.g., bend your knees and go from low to high) (see also the entry "Attention Training").

Focusing Only on Factors Under One's Control

Third, research shows that people's concentration wanders when they think too far ahead or otherwise focus on factors that are irrelevant to the job at hand. To counteract this tendency, athletes should focus only on actions that are under their control; for example, a penalty taker in soccer should focus only on where the player wants the ball to go, not on the position of the goalkeeper.

Focusing Outward When Nervous

The final building block of effective concentration is the idea that anxious athletes should focus *outward* on actions, not inward on doubts. This outward focus is necessary because anxiety tends to make people self-critical and hypervigilant, primed to detect any sign of what they may fear.

Aidan Moran

See also Attention Theory; Attention Training; Concentration; Flow

Further Readings

Kremer, J. M. D., Moran, A. P, Walker, G., & Craig, C. (2012). *Key concepts in sport psychology*. London: Sage.

Moran, A. P. (1996). *The psychology of concentration in sport performers: A cognitive analysis*. Hove, East Sussex, UK: Psychology Press.

Moran, A. P. (2012). Concentration: Attention and performance. In S. M. Murphy (Ed.), *The Oxford handbook of sport and performance psychology* (pp. 117–130). New York: Oxford University Press.

Moran, A. P. (2012). *Sport and exercise psychology: A critical introduction* (2nd ed.). London: Routledge.

Wegner, D. M. (2009). How to think, say, or do precisely the worst thing for any occasion. *Science, 325*, 48–51.

CONFLICT

In 1954, Muzafer Sherif, O. J. Harvey, B. Jack White, William R. Hood, and Carolyn W. Sherif undertook a project that allowed them to examine inter- and intragroup relationships in a naturalistic setting. This classic field-based experimental study, known as the Robbers Cave Experiment because of its location (Robbers Cave State Park in Oklahoma), involved 22 boys (mean age 11 years, 1 month) with similar appearances and backgrounds. The children were assigned to one of two groups (they named themselves the "Rattlers" and "Eagles"), with each group unaware of the

other's existence, and were transported separately to opposite sides of the camp. This segregation enabled the initiation of the first of three experimental stages: *in-group formation, friction,* and *integration*. In the first stage (in-group formation), through camping situations, the researchers witnessed spontaneous friendship choices and the development of status hierarchies (e.g., leadership roles, group norms) within the two groups. After a week, the groups were made aware of each other's presence in the camp and quickly developed an us-versus-them mentality (in-group favoritism and out-group rejection). This marked the beginning of the second stage (friction) in which direct competition activities involving camp chores and sports were implemented. Initially, these activities led to minimal tension between groups; however, in a short time, this tension escalated to the point where the researchers were required to intervene. Interestingly, this intergroup hostility also resulted in greater intragroup solidarity. In order to decrease intergroup conflict, the third stage (integration) involved a variety of noncompetitive scenarios in which the groups played games and ate meals together. When these scenarios failed to decrease hostilities, the members of both teams were required to engage in a series of collaborative tasks that required the pursuit of a series of *superordinate goals,* and only when members of both teams worked together in this way did the tension and intergroup conflict dissipate.

The Robbers Cave example is a useful representation of what is known as intergroup conflict. Conflict can be generally described as a situation in which one party believes its goals or objectives to be adversely influenced by another. Conflict involves a minimum of two individuals and refers to disagreements or friction involving verbal or nonverbal actions and emotions. This can occur between members of opposing groups (intergroup) or between members within a group (intragroup). In light of the pervasiveness of groups across diverse life contexts, it is perhaps unsurprising that individuals are constantly placed in situations where collaboration and competition, either within or between groups, is necessary; and where interactions are inevitable, so too, is conflict. Sport represents one prominent social context in which conflict is particularly evident.

In sport, a common criterion for success is to defeat one's opponent. Naturally, this leads to competition and occasionally highly overt intergroup conflict between the competing parties. Intragroup conflict on the other hand, is often much less obvious. Although team members share common goals and must interact in order to achieve these goals, individuals frequently compete with one another for personal accolades or recognition within the team. Such intragroup conflict can develop from interactions between teammates as well as those that occur between a coach and athletes. The former (intragroup conflict between teammates) represents the primary focus of this entry. The relationships (and potential incongruence) between coaches and their athletes are covered in greater detail within other entries in the encyclopedia. (See, for example, "Attachment Theory and Coaching"; "Autonomy-Supportive Coaching"; "Coach–Athlete Relations"; and "Relational Efficacy Beliefs in Coach–Athlete Relations.")

Conceptual Framework for Intragroup Conflict

A prominent conceptual framework that differentiates between types of intragroup conflict that may exist was advanced by the organizational psychologist Karen Jehn. Based on her model, intragroup conflict is considered to be multidimensional in nature, consisting of relationship, task, and process dimensions. *Relationship conflict* refers to incompatibilities or disagreements relating to social attachments. *Task conflict*, on the other hand, results from differences in beliefs or opinions in relation to the instrumental (performance-related) objectives of the group. Finally, *process conflict* involves controversies or arguments relating to *how* established objectives will be carried out. This occurs when parties have differing beliefs and expectations with regard to the roles and responsibilities for different members of the group and the processes by which they carry out their specific assignments. In the organizational psychology literature, the process conflict dimension has been the focus of debate, with some suggesting that it is not a distinct dimension in itself but, rather, represents a specific form of task conflict. The other two dimensions, task and relationship conflicts, however, are widely accepted.

In the sport literature, even though research on intragroup conflict is in its infancy, the presence of these two dimensions has also been supported. Jehn contended that relationship conflict

is detrimental to group processes and outcomes, whereas task conflict is not necessarily debilitative, and if resolved may in fact result in improvements in team performance. This is also the case in sport settings. To elaborate, task conflict can provide an outlet for athletes to voice their opinions and provide insight into different viewpoints and beliefs. Take, for example, a pitcher and a back catcher in baseball who disagree on the type of pitches that should be thrown. If task conflict arises, and both parties are able to voice their opinions, a superior strategy may be derived and consensus can subsequently improve the commitment from both athletes with regard to the pitches chosen.

Research with youth sport participants has found that friendship conflict (similar to relationship conflict) is positively correlated with athlete anxiety, and negatively correlated with perceptions of friendship quality. Furthermore, research with youth girls has found the presence of friendship conflict to inhibit the development of friendships and social support. At the university level, athletes have been found, in general, to be adversely affected by intragroup conflict. They indicate that task and relationship conflicts are inevitable in the sport domain, and the tendency for these conflicts to arise increases when athletes exhibit self-centered behavior in relation to both the task (e.g., not involving certain teammates in practices or game systems) and relationships (e.g., not reciprocating support offered by teammates). Although both types of conflict have been found to hinder team performance, in certain instances, if task conflict is moderate in nature and managed at an early stage, it can have positive consequences.

In recognition of this potential facilitative role for task-related conflict, a preliminary study by Phillip Sullivan and Deborah Feltz distinguished between *constructive* and *destructive* conflict *styles* in sport teams. An example of a constructive conflict style might involve an individual tackling disagreements by actively involving all affected parties and working to derive a mutually beneficial result, whereas a destructive conflict style might involve teasing a teammate or making the teammate feel guilty. The results of this work indicated that although destructive conflict was negatively related to task and social cohesion, constructive conflict (in particular by using integrative tactics) was positively related to social cohesion. This is significant because cohesion is positively related to many important psychological variables, such as participant satisfaction, motivation, and adherence.

Strategies for Preventing and Resolving Intragroup Conflict

In acknowledgement of the potential deleterious effects of destructive intragroup conflict (especially relationship conflict), the *prevention* (proactive approach) and *resolution* (reactive approach) of these debilitative intragroup dynamics becomes increasingly important for optimal group functioning. However, because conflict can arise for many different reasons and in many different situations, there is no one best established method to alleviate such conflict. Nevertheless, there is evidence from the group dynamics literature of the existence of effective conflict prevention and resolution strategies. The most ideal situation is to *prevent* elevated levels of intragroup conflict from developing in the first place. Because conflict arises when differing parties perceive their objectives as being negatively influenced or impeded by another party, one method to successfully prevent intragroup conflict involves targeting athletes' understanding of their own and their teammates' preferences for interdependent interaction. By having open lines of communication and conducting *role playing* activities, team members are able to see (a) how their personal preferences directly affect their teammates, and (b) why their teammates might act in different ways to themselves. By helping athletes to better understand themselves and their teammates (empathy is developed), they are better able to adapt and connect with one another.

Another successful way to prevent intragroup conflict is through the implementation of peer-mentoring systems. During a sport season, athletes are often in close proximity to one another and although this can foster positive social interactions and team cohesion, there is also the potential for increased task and relationship conflict. By assigning partners, athletes are encouraged to provide feedback to one another, discuss situations that may cause conflict, and consider strategies to prevent such interpersonal conflict. Through this process, athletes are better equipped to handle and address the idiosyncrasies of their teammates.

Nevertheless, when conflict does arise and is allowed to go unresolved, it has the potential to intensify and cause problems for the team at important times during the season. Identification and intervention at an early stage are important for two reasons. First, emotions are not as intense at an early stage and resolution is easier than if the conflict is allowed to fester. Second, and based on the literature that suggests there are positive benefits relating to conflict resolution, if conflict is resolved early, there is potential for the added advantage of different viewpoints and strategies to be voiced that could eventually result in improved group functioning.

From an interventionist perspective, conflict resolution can be approached in a negative or positive manner, and by taking a passive or active approach, resulting in four types of conflict management: (1) *avoiding* (negative and passive), (2) *fighting* (negative and active), (3) *yielding* (positive and passive), and (4) *cooperating* (positive and active). The latter (cooperating) of these has generally been found to be the most effective in guiding conflict resolution. One strategy for resolving conflict that utilizes a positive and active approach is through the use of a third party mediator. Ideally, this mediator should be a formal (captain or assistant captain) or informal (senior athlete) leader who is not directly involved with either of the conflicting parties. It is also possible, however, that using teammates as mediators can lead to further conflict because the mediator can be forced to take sides. In certain instances, a coach can act as a mediator, although on occasions athletes may be reluctant to involve the coach in this process. An alternative is the use of a sport psychology consultant. These options should be implemented based on the needs of the athletes or team as well as the context of the conflict.

Another somewhat related conflict resolution strategy involves clear-the-air team meetings. The difference between team meetings and the third party mediator approach is that the whole team participates in the discussion rather than only the parties involved. These meetings can be executed with (a) only the athletes (without an authority figure), (b) a coach as the mediator, or (c) a sport psychology consultant as the mediator. In these sessions, athletes are encouraged to voice their opinions and discuss issues pertinent to the group. Through this process, athletes take ownership of the conflict resolution and develop perceptions of autonomy and empowerment.

Conclusion

To summarize, intragroup conflict is inevitable in sport. Based on the extant literature, conflict can be resolved and the negative outcomes can be minimized if handled properly. In addition, the resolution of task conflict in certain instances can lead to positive outcomes such as increased teammate understanding and cooperation and, subsequently, group functioning. In order for this to occur, conflict should be handled at an early stage and ideally in a collaborative manner.

Luc J. Martin and Mark R. Beauchamp

See also Cohesion; Collectivism/Individualism; Competition; Friendships/Peer Relations; Self-Categorization Theory; Social Identity Theory; Team Building; Team Communication

Further Readings

Beauchamp, M. R., Lothian, J. M., & Timson, S. E. (2008). Understanding self and others: A personality preference-based intervention with an elite co-acting sport team. *Sport & Exercise Psychology Review, 4,* 4–20.

Copeland, B. W., & Wida, K. (1996). Resolving team conflict: Coaching strategies to prevent negative behavior. *Journal of Physical Education, Recreation & Dance, 67,* 52–54.

Holt, N. L., Knight, C. J., & Zukiwski, P. (2012). Female athletes' perceptions of teammate conflict in sport: Implications for sport psychology consultants. *The Sport Psychologist, 26,* 135–154.

Jehn, K. A. (1995). A multimethod examination of the benefits and detriments of intragroup conflict. *Administrative Science Quarterly, 40,* 256–282.

Jehn, K. A. (1997). A qualitative analysis of conflict types and dimensions in organizational groups. *Administrative Science Quarterly, 42,* 530–557.

Sherif, M., Harvey, O. J., White, B. J., Hood, W. R., & Sherif, C. W. (1961). *Intergroup cooperation and conflict: The Robbers Cave Experiment.* Norman, OK: Institute of Group Relations.

Sullivan, P. J., & Feltz, D. L. (2001). The relationship between intrateam conflict and cohesion within hockey teams. *Small Group Research, 32,* 342–355.

CONFORMITY

Conformity refers to the process of matching one's actions or beliefs with the behavior and norms of those around us. Research into the nature of this phenomenon was popularized by prominent social psychologists in the early to mid-20th century such as Muzafer Sherif and Solomon Asch. Today, there exists a well-established literature base regarding the different types of conformity that individuals display, the conditions under which conformity is (and is not) likely to occur, and the various desirable and undesirable consequences of conforming behavior.

Types of Conformity

Two interrelated types of conformity are described in the literature, which differ according to their underlying cause. On the one hand, *informational* conformity occurs when we are uncertain about the most appropriate behavior in a given situation, and we conform to those around us in order to bring about correct courses of action. Imagine, for instance, the uninitiated exerciser who observes more experienced individuals using the weights machine in the gym, before trying to mirror their technique when the time comes to use the equipment oneself. In the case of informational conformity, individuals most often look to put their trust in those who are viewed as highly credible, and tend to genuinely believe that they are adopting the most effective strategy. In sport, informational conformity has been documented in relation to performance appraisals, whereby gymnastics judges have been shown to display more consistent scoring patterns when they have been made aware of one another's previous ratings (even despite knowing their subsequent scores will not be revealed). On the other hand, *normative* (or instrumental) conformity is underpinned by a desire to integrate with others and occurs when we acquiesce in order to be liked or accepted. In this case, individuals may not have genuine faith that their chosen behavior or belief is correct, but they conform nonetheless as a display of public compliance. For example, new players on a sports team may feel it is in their best interest to join in when their new teammates are complaining about their coach, despite having no personal grievances against the coach.

Although informational and normative conformity typically occur when one conforms to the will of the many, this is not always the case. In some instances, it is possible that the direction of influence may be reversed, and that the majority (the group) may conform to the opinions and behaviors of a single individual. This notion of *minority influence* dictates that when a high-status person makes a particularly compelling case for a course of action, that person may successfully shape the behavior of teammates. In sport for instance, it is easy to imagine how a group of rookies might willingly conform to the behavior of someone who occupies a position of authority on the team, such as a captain or senior player.

Individual and Situational Influences

From an individual standpoint, there is less pressure on high-status individuals to conform within the group. For example, members of a sports team might implicitly accept that although their flamboyant star player consistently performs well in competition, that player is not expected to practice as hard as the rest of the group through the week. There is also evidence that conformity to group norms increases when individuals hold strong perceptions of team cohesion or unity, and that gender may interact with task characteristics to shape conformity behavior. Specifically, females have been shown to conform more than males when performing "masculine" tasks, whereas males tend to display greater conformity on "feminine" tasks. In terms of situational and societal influences, people from collectivist (relative to individualist) cultures appear to be more likely to conform to others' behavior, and it has been recognized that conformity is more likely as task difficulty increases. It has also been shown that individuals display a greater tendency to conform when the size of the unanimous majority (to which they are conforming) is large. Finally, priming research has demonstrated that the subconscious activation of affiliation goals and conformity-related concepts may also be responsible for promoting conformity. For example, simply viewing conforming (e.g., a picture of an accountant) versus nonconforming (e.g., a picture of a skinhead punk) images has been shown to impact conformity-related behavior.

Potential Benefits and Pitfalls

Conformity behavior is driven by a need for certainty and inclusion in one's social interactions. By adopting both the *correct* (informational conformity) and *desired* (normative conformity) behavior, individuals not only bring their actions in line with the other members of their group, they also satisfy their need for belongingness and collective identity, as well as experience improved self-esteem. In addition, they may also foster more positive social relationships by eliciting favorable responses toward themselves from the other group members.

That said, researchers have also documented what may be viewed as adaptive outcomes associated with nonconformity (a heightened perception of uniqueness and personal identity), and conformity behavior is not without its potential drawbacks. The concept of *groupthink*, which has been studied extensively in organizational and political contexts (though less so in sport), provides an interesting illustration of the dangers associated with conformity behavior. Groupthink occurs when a team's desire for conformity interferes with the necessary processing of alternative ideas, viewpoints, and decision-making options, and several famous historical and contemporary events have been described as prototypical examples of this phenomenon: decisions associated with the 1941 attack on Pearl Harbor, the 2003 invasion of Iraq, and the escalation of the current global financial crisis. Groupthink is most prevalent within highly cohesive networks that do not possess norms encouraging free speech, dissent, expressiveness, and sharing of opinions. This concept is typically characterized by, among other things, overestimations of the group's capabilities ("We're a much better team than these guys."), closed-mindedness ("They'll never play as well against us as they did last week."), illusions of unanimity and invulnerability ("We're all agreed, there's nothing to fear from this opponent."), and indeed a pressure to conform ("Everyone else is fine, what are you worrying about?")

Ben Jackson

See also Cohesion; Group Characteristics; Norms; Self-Categorization Theory; Status

Further Readings

Boen, F., van Hoye, K., Vanden Auweele, Y., Feys, J., & Smits, T. (2008). Open feedback in gymnastic judging causes conformity bias based on informational influencing. *Journal of Sports Sciences, 26,* 621–628.

Carron, A. V., Hausenblas, H. A., & Eys, M. A. (2005). *Group dynamics in sport* (3rd ed.). Morgantown, WV: Fitness Information Technology.

Cialdini, R. B., & Goldstein, N. J. (2004). Social influence: Compliance and conformity. *Annual Review of Psychology, 55,* 591–621.

Prapavessis, H., & Carron, A. V. (1997). Sacrifice, cohesion, and conformity to norms in sport teams. *Group Dynamics: Theory, Research, and Practice, 1,* 231–240.

CONSULTANT EFFECTIVENESS, ASSESSMENT OF

Sport psychology professionals maintain an ethical obligation to ensure services are helping clients (and conversely, not harming them), and thus allowing clients the opportunity to provide feedback is a key element of effective service provision.

Components of Evaluation

There are a variety of subjective (or self-report) and objective measures available that consultants can select to evaluate the effectiveness of any consultation. Self-report forms typically include items focused on characteristics of the consultant, positive and negative experiences with the consultation, impact on team and individual performance, ratings of individual intervention components, time spent on aspects of the consultation, and specific information learned. Items can ask clients to rate their agreement or disagreement with particular statements, or they may ask clients to rate satisfaction (from "not at all satisfied" to "very satisfied") with specific intervention components. Often, these forms allow open space for athletes to express confidential feedback regarding any aspect of the consultation. It may also be useful to solicit similar feedback from the coaching and other support staff, assuming they were involved as clients in a team consultation. These self-report data solicited from athletes and coaches can be critical to helping consultants understand if the clients' needs are being met, and if there is a desire to continue services in the future. It is best practice to have someone else besides the consultant administer these subjective forms so clients can feel free to express their true opinions.

These subjective measures of effectiveness can be complemented with objective measures to provide a more comprehensive evaluation model. Depending on the nature of the consultation, the professional may choose a specific behavior (e.g., improved first-serve percentage or reduced penalty minutes) or performance indicator (e.g., defensive points against, running or swimming time in a specific event) that is a relevant dependent variable in the consultation. If the consultant intends to share this behavioral or performance data at a scientific meeting or in the form of a scholarly publication, an informed consent for research prior to data collection must be obtained. If the data remain internal to the consultation, then a brief discussion of the measurement approach and intervals for data collection is sufficient. The key dependent variables in any consultation emerge from a joint discussion between client and consultant based around the question, "How would we know if the time spent on sport psychology services was worth the effort?"

Timing of Evaluation

Most professionals suggest that postseason (or termination) evaluations are necessary to meet the minimum requirement for evaluation. However, best practice guidance from the literature suggests that an ongoing evaluation with regular tracking of performance and behavioral data is a more useful and effective approach. Thus, subsequent to a needs assessment and the identification of individual client or team needs, the parties can put into place a transparent system that allows everyone to track progress toward objective goals. Additionally, consultants may want to gather self-reported feedback from all involved parties at regular intervals throughout the consultation, at least once in the middle and once at the end of the experience.

In sum, a comprehensive approach to evaluation has the potential to generate empirical support for the efficacy of sport psychology interventions and strengthen the field as a whole. Without the checks and balances provided through a comprehensive evaluation system, sport psychology practice can seem like a trial-and-error process, and will likely prove less efficient and potentially less effective for the consumer.

Sam J. Zizzi

See also Consulting; Ethics; Interventions; Psychological Skills Training

Further Readings

Anderson, A. G., Miles, A., Mahoney, C., & Robinson, P. (2002). Evaluating the effectiveness of applied sport psychology practice: Making the case for a case study approach. *The Sport Psychologist, 16,* 432–453.

Association for the Advancement of Applied Sport Psychology. (n.d.). *Ethics code: AASP ethical principles and standards.* Retrieved June 12, 2012, from http://appliedsportpsych.org/about/ethics/code

Gould, D., Murphy, S., Tammen, V., & May, J. (1991). An evaluation of US Olympic sport psychology consultant effectiveness. *The Sport Psychologist, 5*(2), 111–127.

Grove, J. R., Norton, P. J., Van Raalte, J. L., & Brewer, B. W. (1999). Stages of change as an outcome measure in the evaluation of mental skills training programs. *The Sport Psychologist, 13,* 22–41.

Partington, J., & Orlick, T. (1987). The sport psychology consultant evaluation form. *The Sport Psychologist, 1,* 309–317.

Consulting

Consulting may be described as a temporary relationship that is developed when an individual or entity seeks information or advice. Consultation may occur at the individual, group, or organizational level. It is intended to help the designated client function more effectively and efficiently within a specific setting.

Although consultation is a helping relationship, it differs from psychotherapy, counseling, or coaching along a number of dimensions. Psychotherapy (or counseling—used interchangeably for the purpose of this article) is often described as directed toward remediation, restoration, or recovery of former functioning. In contrast, consultation is designed to improve or enhance functioning and performance. It is intended to resolve a problem or assist in the development of performance excellence, as compared to changing an individual's overall functioning. Although the relationship between consultant and client may be an important means to the end (e.g., positive results), the relationship per se is not the focus of consultation. Psychotherapy is bounded by strict rules regarding confidentiality, and services almost always occur within a therapist's office. Issues of confidentiality within consulting are more complex, in part because multiple players may be involved; services often take place within the client's work setting.

In a strictly *medical model* of psychotherapy, the practitioner performs an assessment from which a diagnosis is derived. This in turn determines the practitioner's plan for treatment. Treatment is hierarchical in nature: The therapist, by virtue of knowledge and regulation, is in a position of power in relation to the client or patient.

Consultation may share many of these elements, such the sequential aspects of data gathering, evaluation, and decision making in regard to the most useful intervention. As with psychotherapy, this process may take place via interview alone, or may be augmented by the use of relevant assessment instruments. At the same time, the method of interaction and presentation may be much more collaborative. Assumptions are made that the client has the requisite skills to perform the job; it is the consultant's role to assist in the specific enhancement of that job.

At times and in some settings, the term *coaching* is used interchangeably with consulting. Often, however, a coach is in the position of a teacher, imparting knowledge about specific skill development. Consulting, in contrast, usually implies that the consultant will assist in providing information or assist with application rather than specific work skill development.

Psychotherapy and coaching are often dyadic in nature, involving an interaction of two people. Consultation can be considered triadic, involving consultant, consultee, and client. The consultee may be the contracting organization, interested in having the consultant work directly with the client. Alternatively, consultants at times work directly only with the consultee concerning the client; knowledge of the client in this situation may be indirect.

As a consultant, one is typically hired or retained as an outsider rather than a staff member who is part of the organizational structure. The advantage to this role relationship is that the consultant is less bound by some of the constraints that an employee may experience; the consultant may feel freer to offer advice, recommendations, or suggestions even if these might prove unpopular. On the other hand, the system, or organization, has no obligation to accept the advice proffered.

Use of Title

In contrast to counseling, psychotherapy, or psychology, which may be regulated by law for the protection of clients, the term *consultant* is not regulated. The term is widely used; it does not imply any specific training or ethical duty. For that reason, it can be viewed as positive, neutral, or because it is so widely used in some settings, might be considered pejorative.

Applications to Sport Psychology

A *sport psychology consultant* is a professional with expertise in understanding systemic structures, interpersonal interactions, or mental skills for optimal performance, brought in for specific assistance over a limited period of time. For example, such a consultant might work with a university athletic director to develop services that would assist athletes in stress management, might assist a coach in developing learning strategies regarding optimal methods for team teaching, might be brought in to work with a team on leadership skills or team cohesion, or might work with an athlete on mental skills development.

Within sport settings, the term *therapist* may imply psychopathology; the term *consultant* may not hold the same negative connotation. Although consulting and coaching may be similar, within sport settings the term *coach*, without modification, may be confusing. On the other hand, when modified in a specific way, such as *mental skills coach*, it may have greater acceptability.

Sport psychology consultants receive graduate training in both psychology and the sport sciences in order to offer requisite consultation with regard to cognitive and behavioral skills for performance enhancement or optimal performance. As with more generic consultation, the actual work may occur at the individual, team, community, or organizational level. Because there are various routes to competent practice, potential practitioners and potential clients in North America should be guided by the criteria for becoming a certified consultant through the Association for Applied Sport Psychology and the proficiency in sport psychology of the American Psychological Association.

Kate F. Hays

See also Decision-Making Styles in Coaching; Ethics; Expertise; Leadership in Sport: Mutidimensional Model; Leadership in Sport: Transactional and Transformational; Psychological Skills Training

Further Readings

American Psychological Association. (2013). *Public description of sport psychology*. Retrieved from http://www.apa.org/ed/graduate/specialize/sports.aspx

Aoyagi, M. W., Portenga, S. T., Poczwardowski, A., Cohen, A., & Statler, T. (2012). Reflections and directions: The profession of sport psychology: past, present, and future. *Professional Psychology: Research & Practice, 53,* 32–38.

Association for Applied Sport Psychology. (n.d.). *About certified consultants.* Retrieved from http://www.appliedsportpsych.org/Consultants/About-Certified-Consultants

Lowman, R. L. (Ed.). (2002). *The California School of Organizational Studies handbook of organizational consulting psychology: A comprehensive guide to theory, skills, and techniques.* San Francisco: Jossey-Bass.

O'Roark, A. M., Lloyd, P. J., & Cooper, S. E. (2005). *Guidelines for education and training at the doctoral and postdoctoral level in consulting psychology/ organizational consulting.* Washington, DC: American Psychological Association. Retrieved from http://www.apa.org/about/policy/education-training.pdf

Sachs, M. L., Lutkenhouse, J., Rhodius, A., Watson, J., Pfenninger, G., Lesyk, J. L., et al. (2011). Career opportunities in the field of exercise and sport psychology. In M. L. Sachs, K. L. Burke, & S. L. Schweighardt (Eds.), *Directory of graduate programs in applied sport psychology* (10th ed., pp. 251–277). Indianapolis, IN: Association for Applied Sport Psychology.

Control Theory

Concepts from *control theory* date back to the early 1900s; however, the origination of control theory is usually ascribed to the publication of Norbert Wiener's 1948 acclaimed work, *Cybernetics: Control and Communication in the Animal and the Machine.* To describe control theory simply, one could generalize that it is premised in understanding and describing self-regulating systems. In the decades following its conception, control theory and various elements of control theory were used to guide work in an array of diverse disciplines, including engineering, economics, mathematics, and medicine. It wasn't until the early 1980s that Charles Carver and Michael Scheier presented control theory within the context of human behavior and psychology, and more specifically the regulation of health behavior through health psychology. Although introduced to human behavior in the 1980s, control theory has not been readily adopted in fields of health and exercise behavior. As described by Carver and Scheier, this could be in part because of the acceptance and prolific use of learning theories to understand human behavior, or potentially a hesitancy to consider a theory developed outside the realm of human or animal behavior. Regardless, the work of Carver and Sheier to apply control theory to human behavior and health psychology is the impetus that opens the door for application of control theory concepts in understanding exercise and physical activity behaviors. The purpose of this entry is twofold: first, to describe concepts of control theory as applied to health and specifically exercise and physical activity behaviors; and second, to discuss how these concepts have been and could be used in understanding and changing exercise and physical activity behaviors.

Although most terms used in this entry will be defined at the time of introduction, there are a few that should be more specifically discussed at this point. First, given the original work in control theory and subsequent application, it should be noted that control theory is also referred to as *cybernetic theory* or *cybernetics* in the literature. Clarification of the terms *exercise* and *physical activity* is also needed. While these terms are often used interchangeably, each is distinct. *Physical activity* refers to any movement of the body produced by skeletal muscle contraction that is associated with energy expenditure beyond a person's basal level. *Exercise,* on the other hand, is considered a subcategory of physical activity and refers to any planned, structured, and repetitive physical activity carried out for the purpose of improving or maintaining at least one physical fitness component (cardiorespiratory endurance; muscular strength, endurance, and power; flexibility; balance; body composition; movement speed; or reaction time). For this entry the term *exercise* will be used, although principles of control theory are also pertinent to explaining and changing broader physical activity behavior as well.

The Negative Feedback Loop

The foundational concept of control theory lies in what is referred to as the *negative feedback loop.* The feedback loop contains several important features, beginning with an *input function* (a point where present conditions are evaluated by an individual), also called *perception.* Information gathered during perception is then compared against a

reference value (also called the *standard of comparison*) by a *comparator.* This reference value represents a predetermined value of a condition, such as a predetermined behavioral or health goal. In this loop, the role of the comparator is similar to the concept of self-monitoring, where there is an assessment of current behaviors, any potential external influences, and progress toward an established standard (a goal). If a discrepancy is detected during this comparison between the assessment of present conditions and the reference value, a *behavior* is then performed (also called *output function*) to reduce the discrepancy by creating change in the present condition so as to have an *impact on the environment* (anything external to the person or system). This change in the environment then leads to a new perception by the individual and subsequent comparison against the established reference value. The feedback loop also includes what is referred to as *disturbance,* which is any change external to the individual or system (environment) that influences the feedback loop independently of the person's own action, specifically entering the loop through environmental impact. This feedback loop is a closed circuit whereby the environment, person (system), and behavior all influence and are influenced by one another, similar to Albert Bandura's construct of reciprocal determinism within the social cognitive theory. One important note to make here is that the purpose of the feedback loop is not to create a behavior, but rather to ensure that a predetermined, desired condition (as set by the reference value) is maintained through the comparison of the perception and reference value. Therefore, if a discrepancy is not detected, no change in behavior is needed.

An example of this feedback loop can be demonstrated by considering a person who is jogging in one's neighborhood. Once on a jog throughout the neighborhood, most people primarily aim to remain in a safe portion of the road, clear of cars and other hazards. This maintenance is usually determined and addressed through visual monitoring of the road for traffic and by establishing ample room to jog safely between regular traffic and the curb or edge of the pavement. What would happen if a large moving truck approaches the jogger or if a shoulder that was once part of the road disappears? In using control theory with either of these scenarios, the jogger would detect a discrepancy between the perception of currently jogging in the road given these disturbances and the established safe jogging space reference value. For an avid jogger, this discrepancy would be quickly addressed by the jogger swiftly jumping off the street to continue jogging in a neighbor's front lawn until the moving truck passed or the shoulder reappeared. As is apparent in this example, during any given jog numerous disturbances that require behavioral actions to eliminate associated discrepancies could occur.

Reference Point/Standard of Comparison

Given that the feedback loop heavily relies on a standard of comparison, it is important to understand the derivation and nature of the *reference point*. As conceptualized by Carver and Scheier, the reference point is dynamic and determined within the context of William T. Powers's hierarchical system of goals. In this hierarchy, there are both higher order and lower order goals. Achievement of the lower order goals is intimately related with and essential for the achievement of the higher order goals. In this hierarchy, a higher order goal provides the reference values for feedback loops at the next lower order level. The highest order level within this hierarchical system is referred to as a *system concept,* as it represents both personal characteristics that one wants to embody as an idealized self-image and an attempt for one to minimize sensed discrepancies between how they currently are versus the ideal they desire to be. The second highest order level, *principle control,* specifies principles to use as reference in relation to the system concept; however, these are still qualities and are not specific to any one behavior. In the next lower order level in the hierarchy, referred to as *program control,* actions are identified although specific steps to accomplish these actions are not completely defined since specificity of some steps depends on situational circumstances. Subsequent lower order levels continue to monitor discrepancies between actuality and goals based on the next higher order feedback loop. Therefore, each level within the hierarchy has independent feedback loops that establish and adjust reference points for the feedback loop of the next lower order level, thereby demonstrating the dynamic nature of the goal system.

Again, the jogging example helps illustrate this hierarchical goal system. In this example, the individual is a 26-year-old female, Elizabeth,

who views herself as a good friend and daughter, which represent the *system concept.* Given this view, Elizabeth usually attempts to behave in such a manner that her perception of her present-self matches this reference point, demonstrating self-regulation within this level. One example of how Elizabeth could accomplish this is to make certain that her mother feels special. This becomes the next lower order level reference point or goal, referred to as *principle control* since it is applicable to many behaviors, and thus could happen in many different ways. To self-regulate with such a broad reference point, *program control* feedback loops are then established at the next lower order level where the principle level goal is operationalized to specific behaviors.

In this example, Elizabeth can make her mother feel special by wearing her original wedding dress for her own wedding. However, she needs to be at a lower weight so that she can wear her mother's dress, which can be accomplished by exercising daily (30–60 minutes/day). Although her behavior is generally defined at this point (exercising), it also includes a series of implicit *if–then* decisions based on the circumstances she encounters. Elizabeth's normal 45-minute jog would keep her within the perimeter of her neighborhood; however, if a close friend called and needed to talk she might leave the neighborhood and jog over to her friend's house. On a different day, it could be raining, and she might choose to go up to the school gym and ride a stationary bike instead of jogging. Each of these decisions is made to ensure that the goal of exercising 30 to 60 minutes daily is met, and each variation from the normal occurs to promote conformity to any of her other goals (e.g., not getting sick or ensuring she is a good friend). In each level of the goal hierarchy, the higher order feedback loop specifies the reference point for the next lower order level, whereby behavioral output is required for successful self-regulation in maintaining each reference point, and reference points are dynamic in that they reflect the feedback loop of the higher order goal.

Control Theory and Exercise Behavior

As previously mentioned, the application of control theory to exercise behavior is limited, although concepts found within control theory, especially those consistent with other behavioral and learning theories, such as social cognitive theory, self-regulation and the transtheroetical model, and processes of change, are consistently applied to and related with exercise. Some of the most prominent concepts congruent with control theory that have been applied to exercise are self-monitoring, specific goal setting, goal review, the idea of tiered goals (goal staircase), and performance feedback provision. In fact, research supports self-regulatory strategies as both direct and indirect predictors of exercise behavior across the lifespan. Additionally, interventions that use self-monitoring alone or with at least one other control theory concept (defined by some researchers as immediate goal setting, performance feedback, and review of behavioral goals) have demonstrated a significantly greater effect on physical activity behavior change than those that didn't include any of these self-regulatory strategies.

Conclusion

In reading about how control theory concepts have been applied to exercise behavior, it is evident that these concepts fall into the broader theoretical context of self-regulation. Where self-regulation is defined as goal-directed behavior, exercising control over self in terms of maintaining or achieving a preferred standard, or feedback loops, it is only successful when it succeeds at both monitoring current conditions and behavior in relation to a goal (reference point) and making changes and adjustments as desired (based on a hierarchy of goals). In this context, control theory concepts are consistently supported as invaluable to understanding and initiating exercise behavior. However, given that research has heavily focused on predictors of initiating behavior, the roles of self-regulation and control theory concepts might differ when trying to understand and improve the maintenance of exercise behavior and habit formation.

In comparing control theory with many other prominent behavioral theories, two additional points need to be made. First, where many value-expectancy and learning theories postulate that behavior change is influenced by self-reinforcement via reward for goal achievement and punishment when goals are not achieved, the control theory does not. Rather, as described earlier, control theory operates on the notion that humans inherently self-regulate through the goal-striving (reference point striving), discrepancy-reduction cycle. In this, reinforcement is only useful if it provides information (knowledge of results) that can help in the perception–goal comparison. Second, the concept of outcome expectations is also not directly addressed here. However, this idea is widely included throughout prominent theories and works in tandem with control theory.

While control theory has much overlap with other current and prominent health behavioral theories, control theories have been met with some criticism and misunderstanding. Some of this can be explained through the historical perspectives described earlier through the prominent application of learning theories and the hesitancy to consider a theory based on a machine model. However, a more macrolevel distinction between control theory and other current health behavior theories lies in the concept of reinforcement. Where many value-expectancy and learning theories postulate that behavior change is influenced by self-reinforcement via reward for goal achievement and punishment when goals are not achieved, the control theory does not. Rather, as described earlier, control theory operates on the notion that humans inherently self-regulate through the goal-striving (reference point striving), discrepancy-reduction feedback loops. In this, reinforcement is only useful if it provides information (knowledge of results) that can be integrated and used within a feedback loop.

Although prominent control theory concepts pertaining to exercise have been addressed within this entry, it should be noted that control theories include additional concepts and interested readers should see the Further Readings list below.

M. Renée Umstattd Meyer

See also Goal Setting; Self-Monitoring; Self-Regulation; Social Cognitive Theory

Further Readings

Carver, C. S., & Scheier, M. F. (1981). *Attention and self-regulation: A control-theory approach to human behavior.* New York: Springer-Verlag.

Carver, C. S., & Scheier, M. F. (1982). Control theory: A useful conceptual framework for personality-social, clinical, and health psychology. *Psychological Bulletin, 92*(1), 111–135.

Michie, S., Abraham, C., Whittington, C., McAteer, J., & Gupta, S. (2009). Effective techniques in healthy eating and physical activity interventions: A meta-regression. *Health Psychology, 28*(6), 690–701.

COORDINATION

Coordination is something we all take for granted—at least until it breaks down under extreme stress (as it does sometimes in competition) or following an insult or disease to the brain, or even when body parts are injured or replaced. So to understand coordination scientifically, we must somehow *make the familiar strange*—akin perhaps to the proverbial falling apple that led to Newton's great insights about gravity. Coordination is not just physics, even though we may apply physical methods to try to understand it. Nor is it just psychology, even though methods of cognitive science such as reaction time are used to assess how coordination is planned before movements are even initiated. To understand coordination is a very deep problem, maybe as deep as understanding life itself. The reason is that coordination is not just any kind of order in space and time. It concerns how very many component parts and processes on many different levels of organization relate in an orderly fashion to produce a recognizable function or accomplish some particular task. *Coordination* may thus be defined as a *functional* ordering among interacting components in space and time. Coming in many guises, coordination represents one of the most striking features of living organisms. It's everywhere we look—whether in the regulatory interactions among genes that affect how cells become organs; the tumbling of a bacterium; the coordinated responses of organisms to constantly varying environmental stimuli; the coordination among nerve cells and muscles that produce basic forms of locomotion; the coordination among cell assemblies of the brain that underlies our ability to think, decide, remember, and act; the miraculous coordination between the lungs, larynx, lips, and tongue that belies a child's first word; the learned coordination among fingers and brain that allows the skilled pianist to play a concerto; the coordination of motion and emotion when making a key play in sport settings when the game is on the line; or the coordination between people like rowers in a racing eight and players in a rugby team, working together to achieve a common goal. From the micro to the macro, from genes and cells to brains, people, and society, everything involves coordination.

Basic Principles of Coordination

Although the details of coordination are bound to be different at different levels of biological organization, for different organisms and for different functions, might there also be some basic principles of coordination that transcend these differences? The behavioral physiologist Erich von Holst certainly thought this was so. In his essay "On the Nature of Order in the Central Nervous System" (1937), von Holst surveyed the wide occurrence of three basic kinds of coordination in the neural and rhythmic activities of animals, from respiration to voluntary movements, from worms to human beings. One he called *absolute coordination*, a long-recognized form in which component parts operate with the same frequency and with specific reciprocal phase relationships, just like a marching band or people clapping after a performance. Another, extremely rare, form that von Holst didn't give a name to concerned the complete *lack of interaction* between component parts as in the locomotion of centipedes and millipedes in whom a certain number of (middle) legs had been amputated (no reference to the game of cricket intended!). Persistent practice, von Holst thought, as in playing the piano or the violin, could also lead to complete independence among the fingers of the two hands. The third, possibly most important basic form, von Holst termed *relative coordination*. Here the activities of the individual component parts are neither completely independent of each other nor linked in a fixed mutual relationship. For example, the fins of a fish may not always oscillate at the same frequency and can flexibly slip in and out of preferred phase relationships as internal and surrounding conditions change. Relative coordination provides a glimpse of the tensions between two opposing tendencies that are present in all forms of complex coordination, the tendency of the components to keep separate (segregation) and the tendency to cooperate together (integration). Back in the days when chain reflexes were thought to govern coordinated behavior, the phenomenon of relative coordination hinted at the importance of intrinsic pattern-generating processes in the central nervous system. Since these early days, great strides have been made in identifying the cellular mechanisms involved in neuronal circuits underlying the generation of rhythmic patterns of coordination. Moreover, in the last 30 years or so, a theoretical framework called *coordination dynamics* has emerged to explain all of von Holst's basic coordination types, mixtures among them, and more generally how coordination emerges, adapts, persists and changes in complex biological systems. Principles of coordination dynamics have been shown to govern patterns of coordination (a) within a moving limb and between moving limbs; (b) between the articulators during speech production; (c) between limb movements and tactile, visual, and auditory stimuli; (d) between people interacting with each other spontaneously or intentionally; (e) between humans and avatars; (f) between humans and other species, as in riding a horse; and (g) within and between the neural substrates that underlie the coordinated behavior of human beings as observed using modern brain imaging methods.

Key Concepts

Some of the key concepts that are allowing a deeper understanding of coordination are self-organization, collective variables, degeneracy, synergy, informational coupling, and intrinsic dynamics. *Self-organization* refers to the fact that patterns of coordinated behavior can arise solely as a result of the dynamics of the system, with no homunculus-like agent inside telling the parts what to do and when to do it. The *self* in the word comes from the fact that the system organizes itself. What is important is setting up the conditions for such self-organized pattern formation to occur. The latter is defined, not in terms of the many individual parts or degrees of freedom, but rather in terms of *collective variables* that arise as a result of the many interactions that are going on. Collective variables are low dimensional, hence simpler descriptions of a complex system. They are meaningful quantities for the system's proper functioning. Collective variables are important to identify because they span different domains, such as sensory and motor, brain and body, perception and action, which are usually defined as separate. Collective variables thus refer to the coupling between different things and processes. *Degeneracy* is an important concept in biology

and means that at every conceivable level of description, the same outcome or function can be achieved in many ways using different components and different combinations among them. Thus, for example, in coordinated movements such as reaching for a cup, many different neural pathways and muscular configurations can combine to achieve the same goal. The mechanism that nature seems to use to handle degeneracy is that it synergizes. *Synergies* are context-sensitive *functional* groupings of elements that are temporarily assembled to act as a single coherent unit. Depending on context, synergies may accomplish different coordinative functions using some of the same components (e.g., the jaw, tongue and teeth to speak and chew) and the same function using different components (e.g. "hand" writing with a pen attached to the big toe). The hallmark of a synergy is that during the course of ordinary function a perturbation to any part of the synergy is immediately compensated for by remotely linked parts in such a way as to accomplish a task or preserve functional integrity. Synergies are important because they are the functional units of coordination at all levels of biological organization. A nice example is the so-called coxless pair in rowing where each oarsman has a single opposing oar. The boat can only go straight across the river if each rower pulls his own weight. If one slacks off, the boat will go in circles and the joint goal of the pair will not be accomplished. This kind of cooperative, mutually beneficial interdependency among the interacting parts of a coupled system to achieve a common objective is ubiquitous in nature. It is a signature of *functional synergy*. Relatedly, the coordination between different things (e.g., parts of the body, regions of the brain) and between different kinds of things (e.g., the organism and the environment, two people, and so forth) depends on information exchange, usually bidirectional in nature ("I talk to you; you talk to me."). Interacting components and features can thus be coupled by material forces, by light, by sound, by touch, by smell, and by intention to accomplish an objective. Such meaningful information transcends the medium through which the parts communicate; it is context specific to the particular form that coordination takes in different task settings. In the coordinated systems of life and movement, the component parts and processes are seldom coupled purely mechanically; they are *informationally coupled*. Information is not lying out there as mere data, coded in some symbolic form; information is meaningful to the extent that it modifies, and is modified by the intrinsic, self-organizing dynamics.

Intrinsic Dynamics and Learning

This brings us to the important question of how new patterns of coordination are learned. Much evidence now indicates that this depends on the predispositions and capabilities of the individual learner *before* learning begins. This is sometimes quite difficult for scientists to quantify. Nevertheless, such predispositions constitute the learner's behavioral repertoire at a given point in time: the learner's *intrinsic dynamics*. As any inspiring coach or teacher knows, the great benefit of identifying the learner's intrinsic dynamics is that one knows *what* to modify. Any new information (say a task to be learned, an intention to change behavior) has to be expressed in terms of the learner's intrinsic dynamics, otherwise change is not possible. Indeed, the mechanisms through which coordination changes and the nature of the change with learning itself depend crucially on the initial individual repertoire before new learning begins. In this view of coordination, information is not really information unless it modifies the dynamics.

J. A. Scott Kelso

See also Anticipation; Cognitive Function; Competition; Dynamical Systems; Generalized Motor Program; Laws of Movement Learning and Control; Motor Development; Movement; Neuroscience, Exercise, and Cognitive Function

Further Readings

Fuchs, A., & Jirsa, V. K. (Eds.). (2008). *Coordination: Neural, behavioral and social dynamics.* Heidelberg, Germany: Springer.

Kelso, J. A. S. (1995/1997). *Dynamic patterns: The self-organization of brain and behavior.* Cambridge: MIT Press.

Kelso, J. A. S. (2009). Coordination dynamics. In R. A. Meyers (Ed.), *Encyclopedia of complexity and system science* (pp. 1537–1564). Heidelberg, Germany: Springer.

Kelso, J. A. S. (2009). Synergies: Atoms of brain and behavior. *Advances in Experimental Medicine and Biology, 629,* 83–91.

Kostrubiec, V., Zanone, P.-G., Fuchs, A., & Kelso, J. A. S. (2012). Beyond the blank slate: Routes to learning new coordination patterns depend on the intrinsic dynamics of the learner—experimental evidence and theoretical model. *Frontiers in Human Neuroscience, 6,* 212. doi: 10.3389/fnhum.2012.00222

Schöner, G., & Kelso, J. A. S. (1988). Dynamic pattern generation in behavioral and neural systems. *Science, 239,* 1513–1520.

Sheets-Johnstone, M. (2011). *The primacy of movement* (2nd ed.). Amsterdam/Philadelphia: John Benjamins.

COPING

Coping refers to conscious and effortful cognitions and behaviors used by the athlete to manage the perceived demands of a situation. Coping is of interest to sport and exercise psychologists because athletes are constantly under pressure to perform. Athletes' and coaches' expectations, injury, performance plateaus, poor performances, equipment failure, superior opponents, skill difficulty, and audiences can all trigger a process of stress and emotion. Athletes need to manage or cope with these demands and their own physiological, emotional, and psychological reactions. The most widely used approach to studying coping in sport is Richard Lazarus's process-oriented perspective called the cognitive–motivational–relational theory of emotion (CMRT). Lazarus's CMRT is a process-oriented perspective about the relationship between a person and one's environment that combines stressors, emotions, and coping as interrelated parts. In the following section of this entry, how athletes appraise stressors in their sporting environments is discussed. Next, how athletes cope with stressors is identified and trait versus state coping, coping effectiveness, and gender differences in coping are discussed. Finally, the development of coping skills and the way in which athletes learn to use coping skills in sport is examined.

Stressor Appraisals

Stressors are subjective appraisals of internal demands, such as personal expectations or internalized performance standards, or external demands like opponent's skill or external time standards that are taxing or exceeding the athlete's personal and social resources, such as their coping skills or social support available to deal with the stressor. These appraisals can be very rapid and automatic or more conscious and reflective and involve higher cognitive functioning. Thus, social learning, values, and beliefs, along with hardwired emotional responses linked to basic survival can all impact the appraisal process.

There are many types of appraisals that influence the stress and emotion process. Lazarus argued that individuals make primary and secondary appraisals about events or demands. Primary appraisals involve what is at stake to an athlete, especially if the demand is relevant to the athlete's personally meaningful goals, values, beliefs, personal resources, social environments, or intentions. An assessment of these factors can produce appraisals of harm or loss (social or personal damage has already occurred), threat (there is a possibility of damage in the future), challenge (difficulties to be overcome), or benefit (there is a possibility for gain). Take an example of a female basketball player who is injured in a game. The athlete appraises that the injury will prevent her from continuing to play, perform, and receive social recognition, resulting in an assessment of harm or loss. Threat appraisal also becomes activated when she realizes that the injury might prevent her from playing in future games, endangering her sport scholarship, other sport-related goals, and her athlete identity.

Secondary appraisals involve evaluating coping options or coping potential (Do I think I can cope with this event?), the controllability of the stressor, and perceived outcomes of the event (What will happen?). In the example above of the basketball player, the athlete's secondary appraisal may involve her evaluation that she can manage some of the initial distress and pain, she has access to excellent medical and rehabilitation services, she can work hard to recover during rehabilitation, and she has some control over rehabilitation process. She is, however, uncertain about the long-term outcome. Primary and secondary appraisals made by an athlete will have a major impact on how the athlete will cope.

Appraisals result in decisions that produce a relational meaning, which is the athlete's subjective evaluation of the relationship between oneself and the environment. Emotions arise or change based on these relational meanings (subjective evaluations) that an athlete constructs about one's person–environment relationship. For example, during tryouts, an athlete may appraise the relationship between self and the competitive environment as threatening since one may be cut from the team, resulting in the emotion of fear. If the athlete makes the team, the relationship between self and the environment has changed and the threatening situation has been resolved, resulting in the emotion of relief. Thus, athletes may need to manage a variety of negative and positive emotions, involving anger, anxiety, sadness, shame, guilt, envy, jealousy, hope, relief, fear, happiness, joy, and pride.

Stressor appraisals can vary from person to person because appraisals are influenced by the athlete's personal goals, values, and past experiences. Therefore, athletes may interpret stressors differently, and not all athletes will appraise the same situation or event as a stressor. However, some situational variables seem to consistently influence stressor appraisals such as the magnitude of the stressor or whether the stressor was anticipated or unanticipated. The magnitude of the stressor (e.g., major or minor) is related to the extent to which the event interferes with or is related to the athlete's goals and values. Minor stressors such as spilling water on one's uniform before a competition are likely to be less stressful than major stressors such as trying out for a team and being cut. Stressors that are anticipated or expected are considered less threatening than stressors that are unanticipated or unexpected. For example, consider a situation in which an athlete is facing an opponent who is stronger in ability. The athlete may expect to lose the match and, therefore, the stressor appraisal may be less threatening to goals and values. However, if the opponent is weaker in ability and our athlete does not expect to lose the competition, then a loss would be appraised as more harmful to goals and values since the loss was unexpected.

Coping Strategies

Coping refers to conscious and effortful cognitive and behavioral efforts to deal with the perceived demands of a situation. Some responses to stressful situations like defense mechanisms, crying, or yelling are considered unconscious, noneffortful, or involuntary responses, which fall outside the commonly accepted definition of coping. Researchers in sport have identified over 100 coping strategies, although many of these can be classified into more general categories. Common coping strategies in sport include arousal control, relaxation, concentrating on goals, time management, isolation, deflection, seeking social support, increasing effort, wishful thinking, venting, refocusing, information seeking, learning about opponents, practicing, increasing training, visualizing and imagery use, humor, prayer, substance use, denial, self-talk, maintaining positive focus, positive self-talk, and positive reappraisal. Coping strategies can affect various aspects of the stress and emotion process in athletes. These strategies can help athletes change the perceptions of demands (appraisal), recognize and communicate emotions, regulate arousal and impulses associated with emotional feelings, regulate competing demands, develop effective plans and actions, seek available resources, and develop better technical and physical skills.

There are different definitions and ways of conceptualizing coping. A popular macro-level approach, based on the work of psychologists Richard Lazarus and Susan Folkman, is to categorize various coping strategies under two general coping functions: problem-focused coping and emotion-focused coping. *Problem-focused coping* refers to cognitive or behavioral actions to deal with the demands of the situation like planning, increasing effort, or seeking informational support, whereas *emotion-focused coping* refers to cognitive or behavioral actions to deal with the emotions arising from the situation, such as acceptance, positive reappraisal or reinterpretation of the event, and seeking emotional support. Recent conceptualizations of coping in sport by psychologist Patrick Gaudreau and Jean-Pierre Blondin (2002) propose a distinction between engagement coping (e.g., increased effort, relaxation, thought control), disengagement coping (e.g., venting, physical or mental disengagement) and distraction coping (e.g., mental distraction, focusing attention on other tasks). Other approaches involve a microanalytic approach where researchers examine specific coping strategies used to deal with particular stressors.

Trait Coping Versus State Coping

There is some debate about whether athletes may have a preferred coping *style* or if coping fluctuates and changes across situations and contexts. It appears some athletes do cope in a consistent manner with similar stressors. For example, an athlete may cope with training stressors in a consistent manner, particularly if the features of the training session are similar: same coach, same teammates, or same drills. However, there is strong evidence that athletes do not cope consistently across all situations and contexts; as an example, athletes do not cope with competition stressors in the same way they cope with training stressors. There are several reasons for a lack of stability in coping. First, the stressors might be quite different across situations. Second, even for the same type of stressor, the individual might appraise the stressor differently at different times. Stressors are appraised in terms of their relevance to the athlete's goals, values, and the relational meaning the individual constructs about the relationship between oneself and the environment. If the features of a competition are deemed to be different from training sessions (e.g., a competition is considered "more important" than a training session), then the appraisal of competition demands will result in a different relational meaning for the athlete. This appraisal is likely to trigger a different emotion requiring a different combination of coping strategies. Therefore, athletes' inconsistency in coping across situations and contexts may be due to differences in the actual stressor faced as well as appraisal of the stressor.

Researchers of competitive anxiety have also suggested that the degree to which athletes perceive they have control over a stressor is a key factor influencing stressor appraisals, emotions, and the use of coping strategies. That is, athletes who perceive a stressor is controllable will likely interpret their emotions as facilitative for performance and are more likely to be able to cope with the stressor. Conversely, athletes who do not perceive they can control the stressor will interpret their emotions as debilitative for performance and are less likely to be able to cope with the stressor. Perceptions of control are also important for predicting athletes' use of coping strategies; athletes who perceive they are in control of the appraised stressor are more likely to use problem-focused or engagement-type coping strategies. Athletes who perceive they are not in control of the appraised stressors are more likely to use emotion-focused, disengagement-, or distraction-type coping strategies. Athletes' perceptions of control may change over time as they become more accustomed to coping with particular stressors. As athletes face similar stressors, they may develop enhanced perceptions of control and enhanced beliefs about their ability to cope with the stressor effectively.

Stressor appraisals and coping do not occur in isolation and are related to athletes' social environments. Athletes may appraise stressors related to a coach, teammate, opponent, referee, or parent—pressure to perform; criticism from coaches, teammates, or parents; receiving a bad call from a referee or official; or interpersonal conflicts. Athletes also frequently report social dimensions related to coping with stressors. In terms of coping, common strategies include seeking emotional support (e.g., turning to others for comfort) and informational support (e.g., seeking advice or guidance about a problem). Social support is helpful for athletes in that it can sometimes protect or buffer athletes from appraising stressors in sport, it can decrease the severity of athletes' appraisals, or it can enhance athletes' perceptions of their ability to deal with potential stressors.

Coping Effectiveness

A number of coping strategies can be used to deal with stressors; however, not all coping actions are effective in all situations. Some measures of effective coping are achieving performance outcomes, reducing anxiety or negative emotions, alleviating the stressor (e.g., resolving the problem), and improving overall well-being. There is, however, no clear answer as to what constitutes effective coping. A specific strategy may have a short-term effectiveness but produce problems in the long term. For example, ignoring the coach may help reduce the athlete's initial distress but cause long-term problems in the athlete–coach relationship. Some researchers have suggested that problem-focused or engagement coping is associated with achievement of performance goals and is an effective approach to coping with stressors, particularly controllable stressors. Some strategies like seeking support can serve as both a problem-focused and an emotion-focused coping strategy. For instance, an athlete may seek support from a teammate in order to learn a new drill or skill (seeking informational support as a problem-focused coping strategy), while at the same time using the opportunity to talk to the teammate about frustrations (venting and seeking emotional support as an emotion-focused coping strategy).

Researchers such as Susan Folkman, Judith Moskowitz, and Hugh Richards have advocated that coping effectiveness must account for the individual's personal goals, the situational context, and the individual's appraisal of the situation. For example, avoidance may be considered an ineffective coping strategy in some cases, yet in other circumstances it may be necessary and desirable to remove oneself from a stressful situation. Avoidance may be an effective coping strategy in the short term while the athlete determines an appropriate way to deal with the situation. By taking into account the athlete's goals, the situational context, and the athlete's appraisal of the situation, different coping strategies will be effective at different times and across different contexts. Effective coping should entail flexible coping, wherein athletes are able to use different coping strategies as situations change and unfold.

Gender Differences in Coping

Gender differences in sport coping are unclear. Some studies report no gender differences in athletes' coping, whereas others do report differences. Studies that find gender differences report different findings such as suggesting that female athletes use more support-seeking or help-seeking to deal with stressors and focus their efforts on managing their emotions, whereas male athletes are more likely to use problem-focused coping strategies, confrontational strategies, avoidance, and venting.

The issue of gender differences in coping is complex and there are several possible reasons for the equivocal findings to date. One suggestion is that males and females are socialized to cope with stressors in different ways that are considered acceptable: Females are encouraged or socialized to express emotions, whereas males are socialized to conceal emotions or engage in assertive coping behaviors. However, sport also may be considered a context that supports traditional masculine values such as competitiveness, assertiveness, and achievement. Consequently, female athletes may be less likely to cope in a traditionally feminine manner and may adopt more masculine-gendered coping behaviors.

Recent advancements in the examination of gender roles suggest two hypotheses to explain differences in male and female athletes' coping: the *dispositional hypothesis* and the *situational hypothesis*. According to the dispositional hypothesis, if male and female athletes appraise the same stressor in the same manner (e.g., equally relevant to their goals, values), gender differences in coping will emerge. For example, if a male and female athlete both appraised coach criticism as a stressor in a similar manner (e.g., equally threatening to each athlete's personal goals and values), the male athlete might cope by venting emotions, while the female athlete might cope by seeking emotional support from teammates. The situational hypothesis, on the other hand, suggests that the reason for gender differences in coping is because of differences in the way male and female athletes appraise stressors. According to the situational hypothesis, coach criticism might be appraised in a distinctly different manner by the male and female athletes. The male athlete might appraise the coach's criticism as unwarranted and he might feel that the coach was unfair, resulting in the athlete venting his emotions. Conversely, the female athlete might appraise the coach's criticism as accurate and feel embarrassed about her performance, and she may seek support from a teammate to avoid drawing any further attention to herself. Additionally, the athlete's appraisal of the intensity of the stressor is important in determining gender differences in coping: The male athlete may appraise the coach's criticism as less severe or intense than the female athlete does, which could also explain gender differences in coping. Therefore, it is important to understand the way in which male and female athletes appraise stressors before being able to determine gender differences in coping.

Development of Coping

Coping changes as athletes age and mature, and also as they gain more competitive experience in sport. Coping is also influenced by developmental changes in cognition and through socialization practices (e.g., the way athletes are encouraged to cope with stressors in sport by parents, coaches, or peers and teammates). Early adolescent athletes appear to appraise fewer stressors and appraise qualitatively different stressors than middle adolescent athletes. For example, early adolescent athletes report stressors related to making errors, opponents, team performance, and family concerns, while middle adolescents reported stressors related to making errors, team performance, coaches, social evaluation, contractual stressors, and playing at higher competitive levels. These differences in stressor appraisals likely reflect contextual differences in the athletes' competitive environments, where older athletes may be more concerned about their future careers as competitive

athletes. Therefore, athletes' stressor appraisals change in response to changes in their competitive context.

With regard to coping, older adolescent and young adult athletes appear to use a more diverse range of coping strategies than do younger adolescent athletes. Younger adolescent athletes appear to use more behavioral coping strategies like increasing effort, seeking support, or behavioral disengagement, while older adolescent athletes appear to use more cognitive forms of coping like reflection, cognitive reappraisal, positive self-talk, or mental disengagement. There are several explanations for the emergence of a greater variety of coping strategies among older adolescent athletes. As athletes age, they develop a greater capacity for abstract thinking and the ability to use cognitive coping strategies, in addition to primarily behavioral coping strategies. Second, younger athletes may have difficulty reflecting on their coping or discussing and reporting their coping attempts on measures such as surveys, questionnaires, or in interview settings. Increased self-awareness as athletes age and develop may contribute to older adolescents' reporting of greater coping repertoires. As athletes mature and develop, their coping repertoire becomes more diverse and the use of coping strategies is more differentiated; they use coping strategies specific to the perceived demands of the situation. Coping becomes more organized and flexible compared to younger athletes, and older athletes appear to be able to reflect upon their coping and evaluate the effectiveness of their coping, potentially learning from past coping experiences to deal with future stressors.

Learning Coping Skills

Athletes can learn the necessary cognitive and behavioral skills to effectively manage stress and emotion. Learning can occur through experience and training. Research has shown that adolescent athlete coping changes across different stages of development and at different levels of competition, and older athletes seem to have a wider repertoire of coping strategies than younger athletes. Increased exposure to stressors (e.g., playing more difficult opponents, higher training loads, learning more complex strategies) may enable some athletes to learn coping skills, although the support of coaches and parents seems necessary to allow athletes to develop their coping skills in a safe and supportive environment. Learning to cope may be associated with athletes' ability to anticipate stressors and plan ahead, for example by thinking about upcoming competitions and anticipating increased training demands. Learning to cope also may be associated with self-awareness and the ability to reflect upon past coping episodes in order to learn from prior experience. As athletes gain experience coping with stressors in sport, they may learn to apply particular coping strategies in response to the particular demands of the situation. Although some coping strategies may be more adaptive than others (e.g., substance abuse would be considered a maladaptive coping strategy), it is important to note that no single coping strategy will be universally effective in coping with all stressors. Instead, athletes should learn to apply strategies selectively based on the demands of the situation.

There are also a number of psychological skills or coping skills training programs that can facilitate the learning of coping skills. Coping training programs developed or modified for sport include stress inoculation training (athletes are given opportunities to practice a range of coping skills), COPE training (control, organize, plan, and execute coping skills), cognitive-affective stress management training (athletes develop a coping response involving relaxation and self-statements to manage stressful sport situations), self-compassion training (athletes learn to more accurately perceive and rectify maladaptive patterns of thought) and coping effectiveness training (athletes learn appraisal skills and a range of coping skills [see also the entry "Stress Management"]). Most of these programs involve an educational phase, a coping skill development phase, and a coping skill application phase. Enhancement of coping skills is also possible through many other psychological skills training and emotional regulation programs.

Conclusion

Coping represents a complex topic that is related to athletes' stressor appraisals, goals and values, emotions, beliefs, identity, and their resources and abilities to deal with the demands associated with sport. Because of the intricacy of the coping process, it is important to consider multiple antecedents and outcomes. There are situational, as well as individual (e.g., gender, developmental) differences in coping that require attention by researchers in order to evaluate what constitutes effective and adaptive coping in sport. Athletes' coping changes with development and can be improved through interventions and training, which represents an important area for improving athletes' performance and overall experience in sport.

Katherine Tamminen and Peter R. E. Crocker

See also Basic Emotions in Sport; Stress Management

Further Readings

Folkman, S., & Moskowitz, J. T. (2000). Positive affect and the other side of coping. *American Psychologist, 55,* 647–654.

Gaudreau, P., & Blondin, J.-P. (2002). Development of a questionnaire for the assessment of coping strategies employed by athletes in competitive sport settings. *Psychology of Sport and Exercise, 3,* 1–34.

Hoar, S. D., Kowalski, K. C., Gaudreau, P., & Crocker, P. R. E. (2006). A review of coping in sport. In S. Hanton & S. D. Mellalieu (Eds.), *Literature reviews in sport psychology* (pp. 47–90). New York: Nova Science.

Kaisler, M. H., & Polman, R. C. J. (2010). Gender and coping in sport: Do male and female athletes cope differently? In A. R. Nicholls (Ed.), *Coping in sport: Theory, methods, and related constructs* (pp. 79–93). New York: Nova Science.

Lazarus, R. S. (2000). Cognitive-motivational-relational theory of emotion. In Y. L. Hanin (Ed.), *Emotions in sport* (pp. 39–63). Champaign, IL: Human Kinetics.

Nicholls, A. R. (2010). Effective versus ineffective coping in sport. In A. R. Nicholls (Ed.), *Coping in sport: Theory, methods, and related constructs* (pp. 263–276). New York: Nova Science.

Richards, H. (2012). Coping processes in sport. In J. Thatcher, M. Jones, & D. Lavallee (Eds.), *Coping and emotion in sport* (pp. 1–32). New York: Routledge.

Skinner, E. A., & Zimmer-Gembeck, M. J. (2007). The development of coping. *Annual Review of Psychology, 57,* 119–144.

CREDENTIALS

To call oneself a psychologist (at least in the United States and Canada), or use the terms *psychologist, psychological, or psychology,* one must be licensed in the state or province in which one practices. However, if one works in academia, calling oneself a sport psychologist is an appropriate term to use as it is descriptive of one's role at one's academic institution. Credentials are aimed at demonstrating one's competency within the field. This competency is critical for the sport and exercise psychology profession. The term *competency* indicates that one has the educational background that provides the knowledge base to be an effective practitioner and has the experience, gained through one's educational program, to practice effectively. Consumers have the right to require competent practitioners; similarly, practitioners must demand that we and our colleagues have demonstrated levels of competence to earn the credentials discussed in this entry.

Competency underlies obtaining a credential as a sport and exercise psychologist. This competency is generally obtained through experiences in three areas. First, one obtains an academic degree, usually a doctoral (PhD, PsyD) degree, but in some cases a master's degree (MS, MA, MEd) is sufficient. Second, one would successfully complete specific coursework at an academic institution, usually as part of one's master's or doctoral degree, including psychology, kinesiology, and sport and exercise psychology–specific courses. Third, one would obtain experience within clinical or counseling settings. This would generally be mentored through applied experiences with individuals as well as teams in a variety of sports and settings. This experience provides an indication that one has obtained a base of knowledge in clinical or counseling psychology as well as the skills set and temperament to work effectively in a role as a sport and exercise psychologist. This knowledge base and skill set may encompass counseling and psychotherapy work with a variety of mental health issues, program development and evaluation, and psychological assessment.

Individuals who work as licensed professional counselors (LPC; the term used depends on the state, province, or country) have earned master's degrees in counseling or clinical psychology or related fields and are eligible for licensure, certification, or accreditation (the term used depends on the state, province, or country).They are qualified, if they meet the relevant criteria, to work as counselors and receive payment for such work, including third-party reimbursement.

Individuals with doctoral degrees may become licensed as psychologists in the United States and Canada (other countries may allow master's level practitioners to be called psychologists). This process generally requires a doctoral degree (e.g., PhD, PsyD) in psychology (or a related field), specific coursework, internship hours, and successfully passing state and national exams. States, provinces, and countries have generally similar standards, but they may differ. One must verify the specific standards for the jurisdiction in which one wishes to practice.

The primary credential in the sport and exercise psychology field is being a Certified Consultant within the Association for Applied Sport Psychology (CC-AASP). CC-AASP provides the clearest path for developing the level of competency required to work within a performance enhancement focus in sport and exercise psychology. The CC-AASP process does not have a clinical or counseling focus. CC-AASP requires attainment of numerous criteria, including a doctoral degree, 400 hours of mentored applied work (of which 100 must be directly with individuals, teams, or both), and a variety of coursework across areas within kinesiology and psychology. This coursework includes not only sport and exercise psychology specific courses but also coursework in other areas within kinesiology like motor learning and exercise physiology, as well as numerous areas within psychology, such as social, developmental, and learning. There is also the option of provisional certification with a master's degree, and full certification if one completes an additional 300 hours (above the 400) of mentored experience. There is a standard application process and review by the Certified Consultants Committee to determine whether one has met the criteria needed for CC-AASP status. There were approximately 300 Certified Consultants as of fall 2012. AASP is working toward publicizing the CC-AASP credential more widely so that potential clients (e.g., athletes, parents, coaches) will be aware of what to expect from a practitioner with CC-AASP credentials in terms of competency and experience.

The British Association of Sport and Exercise Sciences (BASES) has several accreditation programs for identifying competency within sport and exercise science, including a High Performance Sport accreditation. The basic one for sport and exercise psychologists is termed *Accreditation* and focuses on the ethical and professional standards of BASES members practicing in the exercise and sport sciences. An individual fulfilling the accreditation criteria is called a *BASES Accredited Sport and Exercise Scientist*. This involves a similar process to that of the CC-AASP in terms of mentored-applied work and coursework. Accreditation can be obtained with undergraduate and master's degrees—a doctoral degree is not required.

Division 47 (Exercise and Sport Psychology) of the American Psychological Association has established sport psychology as a proficiency within APA. Proficiency is seen as a specialization after one attains one's doctoral degree. The proficiency focuses on competence in working with athletes on their psychological skills, well-being, developmental and social components of participation in sport, and issues related to working within sports organizations. Division 47 within APA is taking steps to develop guidelines for meeting the proficiency.

The Australian Psychological Society (APS) offers a specialty area within sport and exercise psychology (one of nine specialty areas within the APS), and established the Australian College of Sport and Exercise Psychology (a "college" within APS) among its other branches. Sport and exercise psychologists are regarded as specializing in numerous areas, including performance enhancement, stress management, overtraining, team building and leadership, and psychological assessment. Attaining full membership as a sport psychologist requires at least 6 years of university education, plus 2 years of supervised practical experience within sport and exercise psychology. It should be noted that this is different from the United States and Canada, where the doctoral degree is generally seen as required to become a psychologist. Other countries may have specialty certifications as well.

Credentials for someone working in academia would generally encompass an advanced degree like a PhD or EdD in kinesiology or psychology, with an emphasis on sport and exercise psychology. This includes the standard teaching, research, and service roles of an academician. Someone providing performance enhancement consulting services needs to be mindful of the credentials previously identified with respect to certification. It is not uncommon for academicians to work with athletes or teams at their host college or university. While academicians generally do not acquire additional credentials per se (although one can become a fellow in one's professional organizations, such

as AASP and APA), one is expected to remain current in the field. Many professions (e.g., psychology, medicine) require continuing education hours each year. While academia generally does not require these as such, one is expected to be acquainted with the literature, attend conferences, and perhaps conduct research and present and publish the work. The goal is to be knowledgeable of the current literature within sport and exercise psychology.

Offering consulting services outside the college or university setting encompasses a different level of practice. In the United States, anyone can hang up a shingle and provide services as a consultant, a therapist, or another "unprotected" term (protected terms include, e.g., the term *psychologist*). The standard caveat, *Buyer beware*, is critical. While some of these practitioners may have acceptable levels of experience, it is preferable to identify someone with the credentials identified earlier (e.g., certification, licensure) if one is looking for a professional to provide services for oneself, one's athletes, one's team, or one's organization.

Michael L. Sachs

See also Career Paths; Certifications; Consultant Effectiveness, Assessment of; Consulting; Training, Professional

Further Readings

American Psychological Association, Division 47: http://www.apa47.org

Association for Applied Sport Psychology: http://www.appliedsportpsych.org

Australian Psychological Society, College of Sport and Exercise Psychologists. (2013). *About us*. Retrieved from http://www.groups.psychology.org.au/csep/about_us

The British Association of Sport and Exercise Sciences: http://www.bases.org.uk

Hanton, S., & Mellalieu, S. D. (Eds.). (2012). *Professional practice in sport psychology: A review*. New York: Routledge/Taylor and Francis.

Lesyk, J. L. (1998). *Developing sport psychology within your clinical practice*. San Francisco: Jossey-Bass.

Sachs, M. L., Lutkenhouse, J., Rhodius, A., Watson, J., Pfenninger, G., Lesyk, J. L., et al. (2011). Career opportunities in the field of exercise and sport psychology. In M. L. Sachs., K. L. Burke, & S. L. Schweighardt (Eds.), *Directory of graduate programs in applied sport psychology* (10th ed., pp. 251–277).

Indianapolis, IN: Association for Applied Sport Psychology.

Silva, J. M., III, Metzler, J. N., & Lerner, B. (2011). *Training professionals in the practice of sport psychology* (2nd ed.). Morgantown, WV: Fitness Information Technology.

CUE UTILIZATION

Whether out of envy or admiration, people have long been fascinated by the extraordinary skills of champion athletes such as Roger Federer (tennis), Michael Phelps (swimming), and Lionel Messi (soccer). Building on this interest, recent years have witnessed increasing collaboration among researchers from cognitive psychology, sport psychology, and cognitive neuroscience in studying the mental and neural processes that underlie *expertise*—or the growth of specialist knowledge and skills as a result of effortful experience—in sport. Such research has helped scientists understand how expert athletes manage to achieve certain remarkable feats in the face of severe time constraints and rapidly changing environmental conditions. For example, how can top tennis players hit winning returns of balls that travel toward them so fast (up to 250 kilometers, or more than 150 miles per hour) and cannot be seen clearly? This paradox is intriguing because in dynamic sports like tennis, the time taken for a ball to travel from one player to another is often shorter than the combined duration of an athlete's reaction time and movement time. Thus, how do top athletes respond effectively to fast-moving balls *before* they consciously perceive them?

The answer lies in *anticipation*. Specifically, recent studies of rapid reactive sports like tennis, baseball, and cricket show that expert performers can circumvent fundamental information-processing constraints by using clues (advance cues) from their opponents' movement patterns to anticipate the direction, trajectory, and likely landing point of balls speeding toward them. Such *cue utilization* (or the ability to extract and extrapolate from task-relevant information provided by opponents' behavior) gives athletes additional time to devise and execute appropriate responses to fast-moving balls. Clearly, expert athletes in fast-ball sports appear to have a *cognitive* (anticipation-based) rather than a

physical advantage over less skilled athletes. This conclusion raises two key questions. First, what methods do psychology researchers use to investigate cue-utilization processes in athletes? Second, what are the main research findings in this field?

Investigating Visual Cue Utilization Processes in Sport

Various research methods have been used to investigate expert–novice differences in the perceptual–cognitive skills of athletes. These methods include qualitative procedures (e.g., protocol analysis, involving recording what people say as they think aloud while solving problems in their specialist sport), as well as quantitative strategies such as *occlusion* tasks, where viewers have to make sport-specific predictions based on limited information, and *eye-tracking technology*, which measures the location and duration of perceivers' visual fixations elicited while viewing slides or movie clips of sporting scenes. The latter methods, which have proved fruitful in studying visual cue-utilization processes in athletes, are explained briefly as follows.

Occlusion Tasks

Occlusion tasks require people to make predictions, such as judging the likely direction of a shot in tennis, from sport scenes in which vital information is either obscured or incomplete. By analyzing how expert athletes differ from novices in their performance on these predictive tasks, researchers can establish the relative importance of different perceptual cues to likely outcomes. Normally, occlusion tasks can be either temporal or spatial. In temporal occlusion studies, participants have to guess what happens next when viewing film sequences in which certain important temporal information (e.g., disguising the flight-path of a ball) has been deliberately occluded. In spatial occlusion studies, specific portions of the visual scene are progressively removed or occluded from view, and their effects on viewers' accuracy scores are analyzed. The assumption of this latter approach is that if there is a performance decrement when a particular spatial area of a stimulus display like the hips or shoulders of a tennis player model during a simulated serve is occluded from participants, then that *area of interest* seems likely to be especially informative to viewers.

Eye-Tracking Methods

Eye-trackers (whether fixed or mobile) are designed to record the location, duration, number, and sequence of a perceivers' visual fixations as they look at slides or video film simulations of sport-relevant information in laboratory settings. Using such variables, eye-tracking researchers draw inferences about athletes' visual search behavior. For example, the location of a visual fixation is usually regarded as an index of the relative importance of a given cue within the display being viewed. Similarly, the number and duration of athletes' fixations in a particular region are believed to reflect the information-processing demands of the information displayed in that area.

Research Findings on Cue Utilization

A considerable volume of research on cue utilization processes in athletes has been conducted by sport psychology investigators using occlusion and eye-tracking methods. Three important findings of these studies may be summarized as follows. First, expert athletes are generally superior to novices in their ability to anticipate what their opponents will do next on the basis of advance visual cues extracted from their adversaries' postural movements and from the relative motion between opponents' bodily features. One advantage of this superiority in anticipation skills is that it gives expert athletes additional time to counteract the perceived intentions of their adversaries. Second, expert athletes appear to employ more efficient visual search strategies than those of novices when inspecting visual displays in their specialist sports. For example, elite performers tend to display fewer visual fixations than novices while viewing sport scenes, but these fixations are often of longer duration than those of their less skilled counterparts. In other words, experts tend to be drawn more than novices to information rich areas of interest in sport-related displays. Finally, expert athletes tend to be superior to novices in sporting pattern-recognition—using their greater knowledge of game-specific event probabilities to anticipate how a given scenario is likely to develop over time (see also the entry "Situational Awareness").

Despite these advances in our understanding of cue utilization processes in athletes, at least two unresolved issues remain. First, the theoretical mechanisms underlying expert–novice differences in anticipation skills remain largely unknown.

Therefore, the attempt to explain how expert athletes acquire, develop, and update their anticipatory advantages over less proficient counterparts is an urgent priority for future researchers in this field. Second, there is little consensus at present among researchers as to whether or not it is possible to effectively train perceptual–cognitive skills in athletes. As before, additional research is required to arbitrate empirically on this issue.

Aidan Moran

See also Anticipation, Expertise

Further Readings

Abernethy, B., Zawi, K., & Jackson, R. C. (2008). Expertise and attunement to kinematic constraints. *Perception, 37,* 931–948.

Müller, S., Abernethy, B., Eid, M., McBean, R., & Rose, M. (2010). Expertise and the spatio-temporal characteristics of anticipatory information pick-up from complex movement patterns. *Perception, 39,* 745–760.

Williams, A. M., & Ford, P. R. (2008). Expertise and expert performance in sport. *International Review of Sport & Exercise Psychology, 1,* 4–18.

Williams, A. M., Ford, P. R., Eccles, D. W., & Ward, P. (2011). Perceptual-cognitive expertise in sport and its acquisition: Implications for applied cognitive psychology. *Applied Cognitive Psychology, 25,* 432–442.

Wright, M. J., Bishop, D. T., Jackson, R. C., & Abernethy, B. (2010). Functional MRI reveals expert-novice differences during sport-related anticipation. *NeuroReport, 21,* 94–98.

CULTURAL COMPETENCE

Sport and exercise psychology has traditionally been understood to consist of a set of skills and theoretical underpinnings distanced from culture. These skills have been taught in postsecondary educational settings and presented in authoritative textbooks. Although readers might not at first recognize what rests beneath the surface of these writings, a closer look suggests that they are in fact culturally informed and in relation to one culture, suggestive of a very specific cultural competence, loosely referred to as European in origin. Thus, the practitioner or researcher who works within a group that conforms to mainstream cultural practices is engaged in culturally competent work, intended only for that population.

Culturally Competent Practice

Sport and exercise psychologists are becoming increasingly open to cultural sport psychologies whose approaches account for cultural uniqueness, in place of a single monolithic cross-cultural approach. There is now a greater understanding among a growing number of scholars in sport science that what motivates athletes and exercisers, in part, pertains to their cultural socialization. Underpinning much of the discussion of cultural sport psychology is the search for culturally relevant strategies for practitioners and researchers, targeting discrete groups and better understanding each group's uniqueness.

Cultural competence involves a narrower approach than multicultural competence, with one's focus placed upon what defines a given culture in terms of conventional practices. One might seek to become culturally competent in terms of the general practices of American Indians, Latin Americans, Indo-Canadians, Muslims in Kuwait, or another general grouping of people, residing in a geographic region at a specific moment in time (current practices). One might also seek to learn the current religious practices of Islam, Hinduism, Judaism, or Buddhism, generally, in advance of working with athletes who actively practice any of the above sets of beliefs.

Within sport and exercise psychology, the onus is on the practitioner and researcher to seek an understanding of the cultural other, partly in advance of consultation, and partly through an open exchange with the client and astute observation for confirmation of what ought to be appropriate cultural practices. There are several general dimensions that are found within cultural competency training. Included among these criteria are (a) what constitutes appropriate use of physical space between people during formal and informal conversations; (b) whether time is regarded in terms of a clock (clock-based time) or an event (event-based time); (c) whether university education, life education, or both types of learning are regarded as creditable; (d) eating practices; (e) appropriate dress; (f) views of gender definition, and on a continuum; (g) the practice of sustained or averted eye contact; (h) where a group resides in terms of individualism to collectivism; and (i) how often one should speak or listen within a conversation—contingent upon the nature of the discussion and one's place within.

Courses are often provided for professionals to inform them what constitutes culturally competent behavior. A common belief is that after one has completed a formal cultural competence education module, one has gained the necessary cultural skills to conduct appropriate cultural practices with competence. However, taking a course to learn the tenets of cultural competence is only the start of a larger educational process in which one seeks to hone the necessary skills and then correctly support the cultural identity of one's client base. Hence, application of the educational module and the successful integration of the teachings determine whether one is effectively skilled and thus culturally competent.

Research Applications

Within sport and exercise psychology research, there are also important cultural practices that must inform a culturally competent exchange, building on the aforementioned dimensions. Specific methodologies might lend themselves more closely to the general tenets of a given culture. For example, within a collectively minded culture, the use of participatory action research might feature appropriate consultation processes and engaged group discussion. Research protocols might also require a feast in advance of data collection. One's methods might also vary depending on the cultural group in question. For example, the researcher might use talking circles in place of conventional focus groups when engaging with select indigenous populations. Writing practices might also vary from a conventional presentation of data to storied writings and teachings, reflecting the cultural practices of the participants and their cultural community. Cultural competence within research contexts, then, must permit opportunities to feature participant-relevant practices, leading to the featuring of diverse perspectives and voices as opposed to cultural silencing.

Conclusion

Cultural competence denotes a general approach intended to provide researchers and practitioners with a set of useful rules in advance of work with a population unfamiliar to them. The understanding and honing of these skills is meant to undergird approaches to communication, the selection of appropriate motivational skills, and also investigative techniques. These general strategies are intended as a platform upon which specific culturally safe practices are negotiated with the intended audience. The dialectic between cultural competence and cultural safety fosters what becomes the meaningful approach, developed to centralize the identity of the client or the participant.

Robert J. Schinke

See also Certifications; Consultant Effectiveness, Assessment of; Ethics; Ethnicity; Feminism; Gender; Heterosexism, Homonegativism, and Transprejudice; Multiculturalism

Further Readings

American Psychological Association. (2002). *Guidelines on multicultural education, training, research, practice, and organizational change for psychologists.* Washington, DC: Author.

Kontos, A. P., & Breland-Noble, A. M. (2002). Racial/ethnic diversity in applied sport psychology: A multicultural introduction to working with athletes of color. *The Sport Psychologist, 16,* 296–315.

Martens, M. P., Mobley, M., & Zizzi, S. J. (2000). Multicultural training in applied sport psychology. *The Sport Psychologist, 14,* 81–97.

Riggs, D. W. (2004). Challenging the monoculturalism of psychology: Towards a more socially accountable pedagogy and practice. *Australian Psychologist, 39,* 118–126.

CULTURAL SAFETY

Over the course of the past 10 years, there has been considerable discussion devoted to multicultural competence within the counseling professions. These discussions are only now beginning to surface within sport and exercise psychology certification. The intent through multicultural training is to provide the intended clients with health services that more closely align with their specific cultural background. However, there is a distinction between garnering multicultural competencies and skills that pertain directly to a client in relation to the cultural experience. The divide between cultural competencies and the uniqueness of each client determines whether the services are culturally safe.

Culturally Unsafe Practices

There are a variety of culturally unsafe practices sometimes committed by the practitioner. Within the writing, one finds reference to the term *race blindness*: an act committed by people in authority who attempt to view and treat the diversity of their clients the same—using a one-size-fits-all cultural approach. There is an obvious distinction between *sameness* and *equality*, with the latter term conforming more closely to cultural safety. A second unsafe practice is for the practitioner to engage in acts of stereotyping, where clients are classified as part of larger groups, such as a nationality, race, gender, or religion. From overarching categories of classifications, the practitioner might move forward, employing general cultural guidelines, proposed as pertinent across the group. A third example of unsafe practice is for the sport and exercise psychology consultant to approach all consultation opportunities employing a mainstream sport psychology approach, mostly built from Western academics. From this third misstep, the consultant might entirely overlook the practices of a client from a marginalized background, perpetuating the marginalization.

Possible Considerations

Cultural safety requires a close match of the specific counseling skills and proposed motivational tools of the sport and exercise psychologist with the customs and practices of the client. For example, when working with a Canadian Aboriginal athlete in northern Canada, socialized with traditional indigenous customs, the sport psychology consultant might work in consultation with Aboriginal elders or enter into meetings that begin with the use of local Aboriginal sacred medicines, such as the burning of sweet grass. For each client that holds cultural values that differ from that of the sport psychology consultant, there are specific practices that need to be accounted for, outlined within another section pertaining to cultural competence. Beyond more general cultural guidelines, there must also be a closer consideration of the client's socialization and identity. The possibility of offending or disempowering a client exists within the diversity of exchanges encountered by sport psychology professionals. To offset culturally unsuitable applications, the practitioner must engage in a process of discovery that allows for specific practices and general guidelines pertinent to the client.

Garnering a Culturally Safe Approach

There are various ways to develop a closer understanding of clients in terms of their cultural identity. The most likely strategy is to meet with the client, and during an intake interview, learn more about the socialization through direct questions and observation. Questions might bring to light the client's religion and level of adherence, view of self in relation to family and community, value in terms of formal and informal education, dietary practices, and use of wording, among a wider range of considerations brought forth with open-ended questions. Via observation, the astute practitioner can learn from the client's eye contact the extent that sustaining or averting is suitable. In addition, the client will seat or re-seat at a specific distance from the practitioner, suggesting an appropriate physical distance that in turn suggests formality or informality. Clothing would also provide some visible indication of whether the client is traditional in relation to general cultural guidelines or assimilative of specific subcultural practices. One might learn about the client's cultural standpoint, also by engaging in collateral meetings with coaches or people the practitioner is referred to as offering collateral information, by the client. From collateral interviews, the practitioner learns more about the client's affiliations and motivational views.

Research Applications

Cultural safety is also relevant within research contexts. There are instances when the applied sport researcher interviews or observes participants from minority or oppressed cultures and subcultures. When entering into these exchanges, the researcher can seek to learn the specific research practices that align with the participant's standpoint. One example might be to interview participants with a collective inclination in groups, or have people threatened by personal interviews or cross-gender exchanges via research accompanied by a family member or friend. There is uniqueness within small local groups of participants that refine more general cultural considerations, such as among a community's early adolescents as contrasted with its elders. These details become parts of a culturally safe methodological approach, building trust and rapport with the intended participants.

Conclusion

Cultural competence is often gained through courses where people, including sport and exercise psychologists, might learn about, for example, Hispanic, Indo-American, or American Indian (indigenous) practices. Cultural competencies include general cultural practices within a larger cultural group. Cultural safety narrows cultural understanding to the local level, where the client is considered more closely in relation to his immediate context, peer affiliations, and familial socialization.

Robert J. Schinke

See also Identity; Participation Motives; Psychological Well-Being; Race; Racism/Whiteness; Self-Presentation; Sex Differences; Stereotyping, Cultural/Ethnic/Racial

Further Readings

McGannon, K. R., & Johnson, C. R. (2009). Strategies for reflective cultural sport psychology research. In R. J. Schinke & S. J. Hanrahan (Eds.), *Cultural sport psychology* (pp. 57–75). Champaign, IL: Human Kinetics.

Parham, W. D. (2005) Raising the bar: Developing an understanding of culturally, ethnically, and racially diverse athletes. In M. Andersen (Ed.), *Practicing sport psychology* (pp. 211–219). Champaign, IL: Human Kinetics.

Schinke, R. J., Hanrahan, S. J., Eys, M. A., Blodgett, A., Peltier, D., Ritchie, S., et al. (2008). The development of cross-cultural relations with a Canadian Aboriginal community through sport research. *Quest, 60,* 357–369.

Whaley, D. E. (2001). Feminist methods and methodologies in sport and exercise psychology: Issues of identity and difference. *The Sport Psychologist, 15,* 419–430.

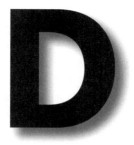

Decision Making

Decision making (DM) is the cognitive operation of selecting a response from a range of available responses in circumstances where an action is needed. DM usually takes place while interacting with either the external environment or internal desires and requirements. Decisions may be made by an individual or a group, which mediates between the environment and the behavior or performance. DM can operate slowly under conditions that lack environmental constraints and demands but must be fast under circumstances of pressure, stress, or temporal constraints. When circumstances permit, the brain processes the information needed for DM intentionally through a perceptual–cognitive linkage.

The environmental information needed for a decision to be made is perceived by the senses, mainly the visual system in sport-related environment. The visual system enables capture of environmental stimuli and perceives patterns in the visual field, and feedforward of this information to long-term memory (LTM) allows anticipatory decisions to be made or a response decision to be primed. Such a process is slow, deliberate, and intentional. It operates under conscious control and can be modified and altered if time allows. In contrast, an emergent-type of DM is spontaneous, automatic, self-organized, and relies on established perception–action couplings. Such a DM triggers responses that are either retrievable automatically from LTM (in experts who

have accumulated many hours of practice and experience) or used randomly with the possibility of a high rate of error (in novices who have acquired limited hours of practice and situational exposure). Repeated exposure to similar situations, stimuli, tasks, and environments may turn DM operations from a deliberate–slow process into an automatic–fast process. Experience and expertise allow DM to shift from an intentional and deliberate mode into an automatic mode of operation when the environmental conditions and constraints necessitate this shift. The ability to shift between different attention and DM modes enables the cognitive system to operate efficiently by increasing the probability of making the right decision at the right time and avoiding errors, detrimental to performance.

Approaches to Decision Making

DM has been given much attention in the military, business, economic, gambling, and statistics domains. While the approaches related to the types of DM in each of these domains differ, each of these approaches has some relevance to sport. We describe each of these approaches briefly before examining the DM concept in the sport domain. The *prescriptive approach* to DM (the prescriptive theoretical normative model) views the person as a goal- or outcome-oriented creature attempting to maximize effort toward goal attainment. In gambling, where uncertainty is an inherent condition, probabilistic estimates are used to arrive at an optimal solution (e.g., the winning DM).

The *cognitive-oriented approach* to DM relies on the supposition that the person's cognitive capabilities are limited. However, repeated exposure and domain-specific experience circumvents these limitations by allowing the decision maker to efficiently capture visual and logical patterns, deliver them to LTM via the operation of long-term working memory (LTWM), and accordingly retrieve responses that are stored in a rich network of mental representations.

The *naturalistic-descriptive approach* to DM (NDA) consists of both rational and irrational processes, and incorporates personal values, morals, motivation, personal state, and emotions; all affect the personal DM process. NDM models, such as the *image theory, explanation-based theory, recognition-primed DM* (RPD), and *cue-retrieval of action* attempted to account for the DM behaviors. Heuristics (e.g., a method of solving a problem for which no formula exists, based on informal methods or experience, and employing a form of trial and error iteration) have been offered within the NDA to account for the underlying mechanisms of DM in the real world. The RPD postulates that DM consists of cue identification, situational goals, alternative action generations, and expectations for possible alterations; and all are affected by experience. The more complex the situation is, the more practice is needed for adjustment to take place. This concept is based on mental representations (knowledge structure) for guiding, monitoring, and executing the decision process. The NDA is therefore a knowledge-driven discourse, which consists of accumulating both the *declarative* and *procedural* neural circuits necessary for DM in situations that vary in complexity and certainty. The RPD within the NDA is an approach that influenced the current concepts of DM in the sport and exercise domain.

Decision Making in Sport

The approach to DM employed in almost all sport research has been heavily influenced by the RPD naturalistic concept, but modified for the unique environment of each sport. For example, DM in rifle shooting pertains to attending to internal bodily cues and pulling the trigger at the right time. DM in dynamic and fast sports, such as soccer, football, hockey, basketball, handball, volleyball, water polo, and racquetball, is dependent on

visual–spatial attention strategy (mainly visual), cue-priming, attention flexibility, selectivity, pattern recognition, anticipatory mechanisms, and the ability to assign probabilities to sequential events (to prime responses), all of which are governed by mental representations, the neural schemas containing declarative and procedural knowledge. Extensive exposure to the sport environment may result in the intentional conscious control of information processing and DM being replaced, at least in part, by more automatic control processes that allow the attention system to be more flexible and seek information from more than one source in parallel. Thus, the efficiency of the information processing system in making decisions is dependent on the richness and structure of the knowledge system (the mental representations network). The ability to encode information via the perceptual system, deliver it to the higher level processing system via LTWM, and process and retrieve responses are all a function of the extent to which the knowledge system is well developed and structured.

When an athlete chokes under pressure, a breakdown in the mental representation network occurs, and the perceptual–cognitive–motor linkage becomes dysfunctional. Specifically, under conditions of emotional or temporal pressure, the perceptual–cognitive system ceases to function appropriately and the probability of an erroneous decision being made increases substantially. Thus, coping with stress must be taken into account within the DM conceptualization.

Competitive sport events are laden with social and emotional stressors. Information processing under pressure may be affected in that attention is narrowed, which inhibits recognition and selection of essential environment cues. In turn, the cognitive system has limited resources to establish visual and meaningful patterns and prime a response. Instead, the cognitive system becomes overloaded with interfering thoughts, and attempts to control emotions are accompanied by declined self-efficacy. Under such stressful conditions, DM is expected to suffer because of the inability to prime and trigger the appropriate response, and this, in turn, is likely to result in performance decline. Existing evidence supports the notion that the quality of DM depends on how pressure is appraised and interpreted and what coping strategies and self-regulation are applied by the athlete in an effort to maintain the operating efficiency of the perceptual–cognitive system.

Gershon Tenenbaum and Lael Gershgoren

See also Anticipation; Attention Theory; Attention Training; Attentional Focus; Attention–Performance Relationships; Expertise; Information Processing

Further Readings

Tenenbaum, G. (2003). Expert athletes: An integrated approach to decision making. In J. L. Starkes & K. A. Ericsson (Eds.), *Expert performance in sports: Advances in research on sport expertise* (pp. 192–218). Champaign, IL: Human Kinetics.

Tenenbaum, G. (2004). Decision making in sport. In C. Spielberger (Ed.), *Encyclopedia of applied psychology* (Vol. 1, pp. 575–584). San Diego, CA: Elsevier.

Tenenbaum, G., & Bar-Eli, M. (1993). Decision making in sport. In R. N. Singer, M. Murphey, & L. K. Tennant (Eds.), *Handbook on research in sport psychology* (pp. 171–192). New York: Macmillan.

Zsambok, C. E., & Klein, G. (Eds.). (1997). *Naturalistic decision making*. Mahwah, NJ: Erlbaum.

DECISION-MAKING STYLES IN COACHING

A critical component of coaching is decision making, which is the process of selecting an alternative from among many choices to achieve a desired end. Decisions may involve the training programs; selection of team members; deployment of various strategies, practice, and tournament schedules; choice of uniforms; and such other serious and simple matters. In fact, every act of the coach dealing with the team or athletes is an instance of decision making with a profound impact on the team and the members. From this perspective, it can be confidently stated that successful coaching is in essence the art and science of decision making.

While this perspective is generally understood and agreed upon, there is considerable debate over the extent to which the coach should allow members to participate in decision making. This entry focuses on the specific issue of participation in decision making.

Decision-Making Processes

There are two processes in decision making. The cognitive process is focused on the rationality of the decision, which means selecting the best means to achieve a given end. Rationality is best assured when the decision maker defines the goal (or the problem) clearly, generates all possible alternatives to achieve the stated end, evaluates the alternatives, and chooses the best alternative. The social process refers to the extent to which members are allowed to participate in decision making. It must be stressed that the focus in the social process is not on the substance of the final decision but on who should be involved in making that decision.

Advantages and Disadvantages of Participative Decision Making

Coaches need to be aware of benefits inherent in member participation in decision making. First, there is more information and insight in a group than in an individual, which would result in the generation of more and meaningful alternatives and subsequent evaluation of them. Second, when the problem is explained and the solutions are discussed in a group setting, the members understand the problem and the rationale behind the choice of a solution. Third, members feel that it is *their* decision, and that sense of ownership would spur them to execute the decision more effectively. Finally, such participation contributes to the personal growth of the members, their feelings of self-worth and self-confidence and the development of their problem-solving skills.

Coaches must also be aware of the disadvantages of participative decision making before permitting the athletes to participate in decision making. Participative decision making takes a long time not only because of the complexity of the problem and the factors associated with it but also because members tend to engage in tangential discussions and to argue over trivial issues. A second issue is that the group may not be as effective as the best individual in the group in solving complex problems where a number of factors have to be kept in perspective and series of steps have to be taken to link all the factors involved and gain a gestalt, or overall, view of the issue. As Harold Kelley and John Thibaut have noted, a group may be more proficient than an individual in solving a crossword puzzle because the members can suggest several words to fill up the blanks and each word can be checked against the criteria. Also, it is only necessary to be concerned with one word at a time. But construction of the puzzle involves looking at the whole set of words and associated criteria and ensuring they are all linked in a coherent and logical manner. In this case, the best individual in the group can do a better job than the group as a whole. An example of a complex problem from sport would be that of drawing up a set of plays in football. This would require that the relative abilities of team members and opponents, the sequence of events, and the various options and their consequences all be held in perspective. The coach with all relevant information is more likely to be better at this task than a group of players.

Further, the group needs to be integrated before they can effectively participate in making decisions. It must be recognized that every athlete is self-oriented and therefore would be competing with teammates for opportunities and rewards within the team context (e.g., playing time). In this scenario, it is conceivable that there could be internal rivalries and conflicts, which may not bode well for participative decision making.

It is not uncommon to hear the complaint that coaches in general are autocratic in decision making. In fact some coaches acknowledge that they are autocratic and that they need to be. In the movie *Remember the Titans*, Coach Herman Boone, referring to his football team, says, "This is not a democracy. It is a dictatorship. I am the law." In his view, coaching football is a situation that does not allow for much participative decision making. This perspective can be extended to specific problems faced by a coach in any sport. That is, some of the problems would call for participative decision making while some other problems may call for autocratic decisions. For example, there is no time for participative decision making during a timeout in basketball. Hence, the coach has to make autocratic decisions. In essence then, it is the nature of the problem to be solved that defines the extent to which the coach will allow members to influence the decision. Following the model proposed by Victor Vroom and associates, we carried out some research in the context of sport. Our research framework begins with describing the problem in terms of five attributes as follows:

1. Quality Requirement

The solutions to some problems have to be optimal while some other problems may not call for high-quality decisions. For example, selecting team members is more critical than the decision on the style of the uniforms.

2. Coach Information

Rationality of a decision is based on the quality and reliability of the information available. Thus, the extent of athlete participation in decision making is contingent on the coach not having the information and the athletes having it. If the players do not possess the information, engaging them in decision making would tantamount to "pooling of ignorance."

3. Problem Complexity

As noted earlier, when a problem is complex, the coach with the necessary information is more likely to make the optimal decision than the team as a whole. For example, the selection of plays for a football team should be based on the knowledge of the relative abilities of team members and opponents, the sequence of plays, and the various options and their consequences. Thus, the coach is likely to make more optimal decisions than the team.

4. Group Acceptance

Most of the decisions have to be implemented by the members of the team. Thus, it is necessary that the athletes accept a decision as optimal and executable. For instance, the strategy of a full court press in basketball should be perceived by the players as useful and well within their capacity. Such acceptance is easily generated when members participate in the decision to employ full court press as and when necessary.

5. Team Integration

This attribute refers to the quality of interpersonal relations and cohesion among the team members. Participative decision making would be fruitful only when the team is integrated. If it is not integrated, decision participation may weaken the already fragile team consensus and team spirit.

The configuration of these five attributes in a given problem situation would indicate the extent to which the coach would allow the athletes to participate in decision making regarding that problem. The various levels of member participation (or decision styles, as we had labeled them) are described as follows.

Decision Styles

Autocratic I. The coach makes the decision using the information available at the time.

Autocratic II. The coach obtains the necessary information from relevant players and then decides. The coach may or may not tell the players what the problem is. The role played by the players is simply providing the information they have.

Consultative I. The coach consults with relevant players individually and then decides. Coach's decision may or may not reflect players' influence.

Consultative II. Coach consults with all players as a group and makes the decision, which may or may not reflect players' influence.

Group. Coach shares the problem with the players and the coach and the players jointly make the decision without the coach exercising his or her authority.

The results of two studies conducted by Pakianathan Chelladurai, Terry Haggerty, and Peter Baxter in 1989 and Chelladurai and Cheng Quek in 1995 are reported here. Our approach was to present to the respondents a set of cases representing all possible configurations of the presence or absence (or high or low) of the five problem attributes, which resulted in 32 cases (2 × 2 × 2 × 2 × 2). Following each case, the set of five decision styles described above was presented for the respondents to indicate the one style they would choose or prefer in that particular case.

The participants in the 1989 study were 22 coaches (males = 15; females = 7) and 99 players (males = 53; females = 46) from university basketball teams in Ontario, Canada. The coaches indicated their choice of a decision style in specific situations, and the athletes expressed their preferences of a particular decision style in the same situations. Although there were differences among the three groups (coaches, male, and female players), the AI style (coach making decision alone) was chosen more often than any other style by each group. The CII style (consultation with all players

on a group basis) was the second most popular choice in all three groups. While the participative style (G) was chosen less than 20% of the time in all three groups, the combination of AI, AII, and CI (because they involve minimal influence from the members) resulted in 64.8% for coaches, 59.4% for male players, and 57.3% for female players. The study in 1995 was concerned with the decision-style choices of 51 coaches of high school boys' basketball teams in and around Toronto, Canada. With these coaches, A1 was the most preferred choice (32.5%) and CI style was the least preferred choice (9.7%).

The results of these two studies and earlier ones show that the respondents chose or preferred different decision styles according to situational characteristics. It is also noteworthy that players of both genders and coaches were influenced more or less to the same degree by the variations in the problem situation. These results support Vroom's assertion that we should view the situation as either democratic or autocratic rather than dubbing the leaders or coaches as democratic or autocratic.

Commentary

Based on the preferences of players for more autocratic decision making than participative decision making, the coaches should not be faulted for being autocratic. That is, the coaching context is relatively more autocratic than participative. However, coaches should be able to analyze a problem situation correctly and decide on the extent to allow participative decision making. Further, they should also realize that participative decisions require different skills than coaching per se. The coach should make the problem clear to the group, control the discussion to be focused on the problem than on tangential issues, and help the group reach a good decision, and in the whole process, should avoid influencing the decision in any way. Thus, the coach needs to consciously develop the skills to conduct participative decision making.

Packianathan Chelladurai

See also Athlete Leadership; Autonomy-Supportive Coaching; Coach–Athlete Relations; Decision Making; Group Characteristics; Leadership in Sport: Trait Perspectives; Team Building; Team Communication

Further Readings

Chelladurai, P., Haggerty, T. R., & Baxter, P. R. (1989). Decision style choices of university basketball coaches and players. *Journal of Sport & Exercise Psychology, 11*, 201–215.

Chelladurai, P., & Quek, C. B. (1995). Decision style choices of high school basketball coaches: The effects of situational and coach characteristics. *Journal of Sport Behavior, 18*(2), 91–108.

Kelley, H. K., & Thibaut, J. W. (1969). Group problem solving. In G. Lindzey & E. Aronson (Eds.), *The handbook of social psychology* (2nd ed.). Reading, MA: Addison-Wesley.

Vroom, V. H. (2000). Leadership and the decision-making process. *Organizational Dynamics, 28*(4), 82–94.

Vroom, V. H. (2003). Educating managers for decision making and leadership. *Management Decision, 41*(10), 968–978.

DEVELOPMENTAL CONSIDERATIONS

Development refers to physical, cognitive, emotional, and psychological changes across the life span. Considering development within sport and exercise contexts allows for more realistic expectations regarding participants' attitudes, perceptions, affect, and behavior and helps us account for important differences in physical activity settings. Theories commonly emphasize that development is a result of the interaction between personal and contextual factors. While the nature–nurture debate in the past was considered winnable, presently there is strong consensus that both individual factors (e.g., biological, cognitive, psychological) and environmental factors (e.g., interpersonal interactions, social relationships, roles, cultural norms) together influence the growth and development of individuals. In this entry, discussion of developmental changes acknowledges that changes are organized in character, are based on the earlier self, and engender a sense of continuity alongside transformation.

Each theory of development provides a different lens or perspective for explaining the important aspects of development, providing additional insights into why we grow and change the way that we do. Theories differ regarding *when* development occurs. Some earlier theorists like Sigmund Freud and Jean Piaget regarded childhood and adolescence as the primary time periods for growth, while others like Erik Erikson focus on change and development over the entire lifespan. Theories also differ regarding explanations of *how* we change and develop, with different perspectives emphasizing the driving force behind developmental change as either coming from outside or from within the individual. For example, learning theory (e.g., Albert Bandura) and behaviorism (e.g., B. F. Skinner, John B. Watson) assert that much of development is a result of the environments we are placed in, whether focusing on the behaviors that other people show or the reinforcement patterns they use. Other theorists suggested that characteristics contained within individuals are most important in influencing development, based on such biological factors as brain systems, neurotransmitters, or genes or personality traits. While research examining developmental differences in adulthood lags behind research examining development of youth, some of the most successful and well-accepted theories today embrace individual factors and contextual factors, as well as the interaction between the two, as important considerations to be made across the lifespan.

Development occurs within a context, but individuals are active in their own development and simultaneously act upon the context. For example, Uri Bronfenbrenner's bioecological model has provided a framework that has fostered a more ecologically valid (real world) consideration of development as the interrelated forces or systems (including the immediate social context and the cultural context) that influence and are influenced by the individual. A systems perspective integrates aspects of the individual as well as the context in explaining development, thus serving as a bridge in the nature versus nurture debate by acknowledging the mutually influential role of both. Other common theories in sport psychology (e.g., self-determination theory, achievement goal theory) similarly emphasize the importance of both individual factors like basic need satisfaction or goal orientations and contextual factors like autonomy-supportive behaviors or motivational climate as mutual predictors of behavior.

Development is both systematic by following general patterns within populations and idiographic by highlighting specific individual differences in pathways. Thus, variations in developmental trends will occur across individuals and across contexts. Below are several common trends in development identified in the sport and exercise literature, including physical activity levels, reasons for participation, social development, motivational orientations, and self-perceptions. Developmental considerations regarding contextual factors are also addressed in the following sections.

Developmental Trends

Physical Activity Level

Participation in sports and any physical activity peaks in early adolescence and then steadily declines. This is problematic as physical activity represents an opportunity to curb the increasing disease rate and biological declines that accompany aging. Physical activity habits developed in youth tend to be predictive of future behaviors. Adults over 65 represent a growing population and are the most sedentary segment of the population, yet they have received relatively little attention in the sport and exercise literature. Physical activity behaviors associated with age are highly reflective of the life context and the associated norms, values, and beliefs for different age groups (e.g., socialization, education, culture, employment).

Reasons for Participation in Sport or Physical Activity

Children and adolescents most often cite enjoyment, affiliation, and competence development as primary reasons for engaging in sport. Although children typically move in and out of particular sports to sample different activities, they also cite reasons for discontinuing sport that include overemphasis on winning, issues with the coach, lack of playing time, and lack of enjoyment. As children enter adolescence, they may also discontinue sport because of increasing competition and team selection or cuts. In contrast to engaging in youth sports, youth who exercise provide reasons more closely aligned with adults. Thus, adolescents initiate exercise largely for external factors, including to lose weight, for health benefits, to satisfy other's expectations (e.g., doctor's orders), or to decrease stress.

As there are fewer opportunities for adults to reap the many benefits of physical activity through sport involvement, there is a greater emphasis on exercise participation in adulthood. Adults cite health and fitness as important reasons for participation in physical activity. The majority of those who initiate exercise will discontinue in a relatively short amount of time. Those that do continue to exercise do so for more intrinsic reasons, such as enjoyment and developing value and identity for exercise. Competition and comparisons to others generally becomes less important with increasing age across adulthood, while self-referenced criteria are generally more consistent. Group involvement constitutes a motivating factor to both initiate and continue involvement. Adults who exercise in a group setting report more positive outcomes compared to those exercising alone. However, the majority of adults do not participate in regular exercise, demonstrating the difficulty of sustaining exercise involvement. Adults identify reasons for not exercising that reflect the demands and responsibility inherent in adulthood, including a lack of time, energy, knowledge, and value.

Although the level and intensity of physical activities generally decrease across adulthood, older adults can enjoy many physiological, psychological, and social benefits of being physically active. As physically active persons are less likely to experience cognitive decline and dementia later in life compared with sedentary persons, physical activity serves an added benefit for maintaining or reducing the risk of cognitive decline. Relevant concerns for this population tend to focus on functional movement and quality of life. Older adults' perceived ability to be active is as important as actual ability when predicting physical activity levels. Key physical activity motivators for older adults include enjoyment, social opportunities, maintaining or enhancing control over activities of daily living, and increasing self-confidence and perceptions of competence. Unfortunately, there are many barriers to participation that largely reflect lack of information and negative perceptions or attitudes toward physical activity for older adults.

Social and Emotional Development

A pervasive and persistent motivator across the lifespan is the social opportunities afforded by participation in sport, exercise, and physical activities. Initiating and maintaining social relationships and social connections constitute a core aspect of motivation and behavior in physical activity pursuits, yet affiliation alters in structure and function across the lifespan.

Childhood

The role of adults in the sport experience of children has garnered substantial attention. Parents largely direct their children's activities, exerting the primary social influence in early participation. Factors such as parent involvement, beliefs, and activity patterns are all influential on children's perceptions and behaviors regarding physical activity. However, other adult leaders like coaches and teachers also constitute important social influences. Important adults help shape the meaning of and understanding of emotions, such as pride, shame, and guilt.

Awareness of and reliance on peers increases through middle childhood and into adolescence. Young children view peers as others to share activities with, while peer group acceptance and belonging become important in middle childhood. Although the role of parents does not necessarily decline, there is a clear emergence of peers as an important source of social influence in middle childhood to early adolescence. Developing in early adolescence, interpersonal intimacy and close friendships are also important and serve an emotional function. This is increasingly important as the ability of emotions to be verbally acknowledged emerges.

Adolescence

Peer relationships, peer pressures, and general attention to one's social surroundings make adolescence a time of particular sensitivity toward peers. Peers therefore constitute a salient source of information about one's self (e.g., self-esteem, competence) and in developing attitudes, beliefs, and affective responses to sport and physical activities. Other markers of adolescent development are the formation of identity and of independence. In mid- to later adolescence, there is an increased awareness of and development of one's personal standards and expectations. Though social influences like parents and peers remain important, they are integrated with and accompanied by greater self-reflective ability and more internal judgments that reflect more abstract thoughts.

Adulthood

In the later adolescent years and into adulthood, romantic relationships are developed and constitute a primary social relationship. Unfortunately, there is sparse information about romantic relationships in the sport and exercise literature. As salient social relationships during adulthood, romantic relationships and spouses are an important potential source of influence on sport and exercise experiences, for example serving as sources of social support for exercise. Additionally, their own children become another source of influence for adults. By middle adulthood, social networks become stronger and more stable, aiding in the increased ability to manage emotions and enhanced coping skills to deal with a variety of life changes.

Older Adulthood

Social relationships change in structure and function in older adulthood. Career, family responsibilities, and social circles decrease, while close relationships and social ties take on increased relevance. Having friends and social opportunities predicts mental health in older adulthood. Sport and exercise provide a venue for social interactions and an opportunity to make and maintain social relationships. As such, the sport and exercise context can provide an important source of social support for this population.

Motivational Orientations

Young children do not differentiate the concepts of ability and effort. Thus, children tend to view self-referenced ways of defining success such as trying hard and task completion as markers for high perceived ability. By adopting this mastery-oriented approach to their activities, children embrace effort and personal improvement as signs of success. However, as children age, they become more able to differentiate the concepts of ability and effort. Whereas previously, trying hard signaled being good at an activity, comparisons against others become more meaningful and trying hard can actually signal less perceived ability than others. By early adolescence, individuals are more fully able to adopt a performance-oriented approach that emphasizes comparisons against others as ways of defining success.

In addition, across youth, participating in sport for intrinsic reasons declines. Children's enjoyment of sport and physical activity declines, as does the focus on self-regulation. Participation for external reasons (e.g., feeling controlled by others, feeling guilty) increases across childhood and early adolescence. These changes in motivation are linked to both contextual features as well as cognitive development.

Self-Perceptions

Research findings are inconsistent about changes in level of perceived physical competence across childhood and adolescence; however, accuracy of perceived physical competence increases across childhood and early adolescence. Young children tend to rely on important adults for competence information. In early adolescence, social comparisons are also used to form competence perceptions. Adolescents become increasingly able to use internal criteria to judge competence. The incorporation of more sources of information enables a more accurate determination of competence; as a result, perceived competence drops for some with age.

Perceptions of physical appearance are relevant from early adolescence across the lifespan. Early adolescents are keenly attuned to how others perceive them, and self-presentation concerns arise, such as social self-consciousness, sensitivity to early or late physical maturation rates, needs for social acceptance, and in particular body-image concerns. For example, girls cite reasons for not engaging in physical activities that often reflect being self-conscious of how the activity may negatively impact their appearance or social relationships. Self-presentation concerns, including body image, are associated with negative consequences, such as negative attitudes, low self-esteem, and avoidance of physical activity. Body-centered issues tend to persist across the lifespan, taking on different emphases at different life stages. There are changes in physical appearance across the lifespan, and although the importance of appearance tends to decline through adulthood, perceived physical appearance is a consistent predictor of self-esteem across the lifespan.

Contextual Factors

Youth Sports

Youth sport often aims to use a developmental model, treating the child as a whole person to be developed. However, the context of sport changes with age and level and generally shifts toward a more professional model emphasizing competition and outcome. When the motives of children do not match the experiences provided to them, such

as when a professional model is applied too early, there can be deleterious effects. As sport becomes more competitive and selective, there are not only changes to the social context but fewer opportunities for participation in organized sport. Because organized sport is a large source of physical activity for kids, as participation in organized sports declines, so do physical activity levels.

Motivational Climate or Coaching Style

Coaches are important influences in the youth sport context, as their philosophies and ways of responding to athletes influence youth athletes' psychological growth and development in sport. For example, coaches who create a mastery motivational climate provide goals and reinforcement to participants who improve over past performances, try hard, and work together. Coaches using a mastery motivational climate generally have athletes who show greater self-perceptions, more self-determined motivation, and general well-being. In contrast, coaches who use a performance motivational climate emphasize comparisons against others; youth in these contexts generally show less self-determined motivation, more anxiety, and lower physical activity.

Coaches who adopt a positive approach to providing feedback emphasize instruction, reinforcement, and encouragement toward their athletes. Utilizing the positive approach in a manner contingent with athletes' behavior predicts increased enjoyment, self-esteem, liking of coach and teammates, more prosocial attitudes and behaviors, increased likelihood of continued participation, and lower anxiety. The coach clearly provides an important influence on the development of attitudes, perceptions, and behavior during the childhood and adolescent years.

Physical Education

For youth, physical education (PE) is a physical activity context that is distinct from organized sport. Often compulsory in nature, PE includes a wider range of skill levels across youth participants. PE curricula traditionally focus on competitive, sport-based skills rather than on experiences that foster lifetime activities like fitness or recreation. This is problematic for youth who may have lower fitness, physical ability, or slower physical maturity. However, PE can serve as a context from which to develop adaptive beliefs and values that can foster lifelong physical activity habits with the right focus. PE teachers create a leadership structure and set the tone of the environment. Teachers who provide a more supportive, cooperative environment foster more positive experiences within PE that also translate into positive outcomes beyond the PE environment.

Positive Youth Development

Organized sport is a popular activity for children and youth, in part because sport participation is expected to impart character. Sportspersonship, teamwork, leadership, and fair play represent common idealized outcomes of competitive sport participation. However, research has not confirmed these common beliefs. In fact, it appears that increased involvement in competitive sport may come at a price for some. Older athletes are more accepting of cheating than younger athletes, rule violations are more accepted as competitive level increases, and collegiate athletes use more aggression than youth. In addition, beginning around age 12, athletes use lower levels of moral reasoning in sport than in daily life. However, these outcomes only represent average experiences. There are many examples of positive outcomes in sport, but most are predicated on intentional efforts to foster youth development.

Positive youth development (PYD) programs promote personal and social assets of youth to enhance physical and mental health, foster social and psychological well-being, increase academic achievement, and develop character. PYD programs generally emphasize the need to create an engaging, positive context encouraging long-term commitment, positive relationships with caring adult mentors, and opportunities to develop life skills such as social skills and problem-solving skills and to transfer skills to new contexts. Sport and physical activity contexts provide an optimal vehicle for PYD, as they can address physical and mental health and foster social and psychological well-being. Sport-based PYD programs therefore tend to promote more growth and development than do many traditional competitive sport programs that focus on sport-specific skills and competition.

Adult Exercise Settings

Adult exercise settings vary widely. Factors that enhance the exercise experience tend to stem from social and contextual factors. Social support and group cohesion foster positive norms, values, and overall motivation and behavioral adherence. Some exercise facilities cater to the needs of adults in order to minimize barriers to exercise. For example, it is common to provide child care; have extended hours of operation; provide multiple services in one location, such as a spa or restaurant; and offer a wide range of classes. Exercise facilities sometimes target certain groups, such as women-only gyms, in an effort to tailor the facility to the unique needs of certain segments of the adult population. Despite these efforts, exercise adherence remains a problem for most adults.

Person–Context Interactions

The trends noted earlier suggest that a sport or exercise context that emphasizes mastery, support, and developing assets will produce the most positive outcomes. However, there are certain individuals who will thrive in an environment that does not reflect these ideal conditions. For example, an adolescent who is competent, self-determined, and focused will likely thrive in a highly competitive environment (e.g., elite level competitive sports). Likewise, an adult may prefer to exercise alone despite the expectation that exercising in groups is preferable on average. Though the contextual features described earlier are generally advantageous, there is also a need to adapt contexts to specific individual or developmental needs of participants. While in general there are many changes in psychology-related variables across the lifespan, it is also clear that development needs to be viewed as an interaction between individuals in specific contexts.

Sarah Ullrich-French and Cheryl Stuntz

See also Character Development; Coach–Athlete Relations; Cognitive Capabilities; Ecological Theory; Friendships/Peer Relations; Motor Development; Quality of Life; Youth Sport, Participation Trends in

Further Readings

Bornstein, M. H., & Lamb, M. E. (Eds.). (2011). *Developmental science: An advanced textbook* (6th ed.). New York: Psychology Press.

Lerner, R. M. (2002). *Concepts and theories of human development* (3rd ed.). Mahwah, NJ: Lawrence Erlbaum.

Weiss, M. R. (2004). *Developmental sport and exercise psychology: A lifespan perspective*. Morgantown, WV: Fitness Information Technology.

Whaley, D. E. (2007). A life span developmental approach to studying sport and exercise behavior. In G. Tenenbaum & R. C. Eklund (Eds.), *Handbook of sport psychology* (3rd ed., pp. 645–661). Hoboken, NJ: Wiley.

DEVELOPMENTAL HISTORIES

In the context of sport, developmental histories provide information on an athlete's career with respect to practice activities related to their primary sport. In studies of elite athlete development, researchers have used carefully designed questionnaires or interview methods to ascertain information about the routes to success in sport. Methods for obtaining developmental histories vary with respect to the research question guiding their use and the breadth and depth of information required. Typically developmental histories provide insights into current and previous practice habits at various levels of detail.

Over the past 2 decades, developmental histories have become a commonly used method of ascertaining data on athletes' career histories. The interest in collecting developmental histories has stemmed largely from the seminal paper by K. Anders Ericsson, Ralf Krampe, and Clemens Tesch-Römer on the concept of *deliberate practice* and its centrality to expert performance. According to Ericsson et al., expert performance can be predicted based on the number of quality hours spent engaged in practice designed specifically to improve performance. There has therefore been a need to find methods for collecting reliable and valid data on the amount and quality of practice accrued over an athlete's career to test the validity of this proposition. Across a diverse range of sports, considerable support has been forthcoming. As a result of data collected from developmental histories, it has been shown that practice hours consistently differentiate across skill class (e.g., international versus national versus club level performers) and performance metrics (e.g., swimming or running times).

Recently there have been attempts to use developmental histories to understand how age of involvement in a primary sport impacts later success in the sport (either positively or negatively).

This has been studied with respect to ideas concerning early specialization versus early diverse involvement in many sports with an early focus on fun and enjoyment. The Developmental Model of Sport Participation, developed by Jean Côté, Jennifer Murphy-Mills, and Bruce Abernethy, has been used as a theoretical framework to study developmental pathways to success in sport. There has been mixed evidence in support of the suggestion that an early focus on play type of activities, potentially coupled with early sampling of various sports, positively impacts attainment of later success.

Data collected via developmental histories usually pertain to three general areas: *personal demographics* (including such variables as gender, age, education, family involvement in sport and living environment), *current practice profiles and levels of performance*, and *previous practice profiles and past successes*. Data are collected to inform as to the amount of hours per week spent practicing in the person's primary sport and sometimes in other sports or activities. This is usually evaluated with respect to the number of practice sessions per week, the number of weeks or months away from the sport (due to off-season or injury) as well as with respect to the current reasons for engagement in the activity (e.g., primarily for fun or for improvement). In addition, researchers have also tried to ascertain how much practice was supervised or coach-led like team practice versus self-directed or individual practice, as well as the extent of competition involvement. Once the researcher has a measure of the number of hours per week spent in practice, it is possible to estimate the number of hours accumulated in various types of practice activities across a 12-month period, that is, the number of hours per week multiplied by the number of weeks of participation (not including injury and off-season). Current levels of performance and areas of strength and weakness are then related to current amounts and types of practice.

Past levels of practice over an athlete's career are usually obtained through similar methods as for current practice but typically not in as much detail. Researchers usually solicit information about age of first involvement in the sport and age of serious commitment to the sport, and this information is either gathered for every year of involvement or in 2- to 3-year blocks (to make the recall process less arduous for the participant). In cases where data are not collected for every year of involvement, estimates of practice in the intervening years are calculated based on the previous and subsequent year entries and on the assumption that practice gradually increased in a linear fashion.

Retrospective, recall-based methods of data collection, as is the case with developmental histories, require some demonstration of accuracy on the part of the researcher (validity and reliability checks). There have been a number of different methods used to ensure that the data are accurate. With respect to reliability, the same questions have been asked a number of times within a questionnaire or interview session, usually under slightly different guises: one question asking how many hours a week are spent in team practice versus a table requiring the person to specify the number of sessions per week they attend team practice and the average length of each session. Reliability is also gained through test–retest methods. Typically, 1 to 3 months after initial data collection, a select number of participants are asked to fill in all or parts of the questionnaire again. With respect to validity (or truthfulness) of the reports, attempts have been made to measure practice composition during actual practice sessions (e.g., via video), semistructured interviews have been coupled with questionnaire-based methods, and parents or coaches have been asked to report on current and past practice habits of the athletes.

Nicola Jane Hodges

See also Expertise; Practice; Skill Acquisition; Talent Development; Youth Sport, Participation Trends in

Further Readings

Côté, J., Murphy-Mills, J., & Abernethy, B. (2012). The development of skill in sport. In A. M. Williams & N. J. Hodges (Eds.), *Skill acquisition in sport: Research, theory and practice* (2nd ed., pp. 269–286). London: Routledge.

Ericsson, K. A., Krampe, R. T., & Tesch-Römer, C. (1993). The role of deliberate practice in the acquisition of expert performance. *Psychological Review, 100,* 363–406.

Hodges, N. J., Kerr, T., Starkes, J. L., Weir, P., & Nanandiou, A. (2004). Predicting performance from deliberate practice hours for triathletes and swimmers: What, when and where is practice important? *Journal of Experimental Psychology: Applied, 10,* 219–237.

Ward, P., Hodges, N. J., Williams, A. M., & Starkes, J. L. (2007). The road to excellence in soccer: A developmental look at deliberate practice. *High Ability Studies, 18,* 119–153

Diet Drugs

The World Health Organization defines *obesity* and *overweight* as the excessive accumulation of body fat and warns that both conditions pose serious threats to health by increasing the risk for chronic diseases like diabetes, cancer, and cardiovascular diseases. Effective methods to counter obesity include changes in lifestyle, such as engagement in physical activity and exercise, as well as controlling one's weight through balanced dieting. Nevertheless, lifestyle modifications are not always easy to achieve. Therefore, scientists have called for effective antiobesity pharmacological treatments, or diet drugs. These drugs include both pharmacological and nonpharmacological agents that aid weight regulation by interfering with the processes of metabolism, reducing appetite, or influencing the absorption of calories or fat in the body. Pharmacological agents typically comprise substances that are purchased with medical prescription, whereas nonpharmacological agents refer to nonprescribed substances, such as dietary supplements and herbal products. While primarily intended to counter obesity, diet drugs are widely used by athletes and leisure-time exercisers to increase endurance, physical stamina, and leaner muscle mass. This entry presents an overview of commonly used diet drugs and addresses the potential role diet drugs play in weight control and athletic performance by focusing on their alleged health benefits and reported side effects.

Pharmacological Agents for Weight Loss

A wide range of diet drugs can be purchased in nutritional supplement stores, pharmacies, and through online retailers. However, regulatory authorities, such as the U.S. Food and Drug Agency (FDA), have only approved a handful of these substances. In professional sports, the World Anti-Doping Agency (WADA) and affiliated official sporting associations consider the use of diet drugs a doping practice.

Orlistat, sibutramine, and *rimonabant* are pharmacological agents used in dieting and weight-loss interventions. Orlistat is a gastric and pancreatic lipase inhibitor that aids weight control by reducing the absorption of dietary fat. Sibutramine is a monoamine reuptake inhibitor initially developed to treat depression. Unlike orlistat, sibutramine stimulates thermogenesis (the production of *heat* energy in the body) and acts in the human brain to increase satiety, which is the feeling that one is full. Rimonabant is a selective cannabinoid receptor antagonist that was approved in 2006 in Europe as an aid to exercise and weight-loss interventions. Clinical trials have shown that both orlistat and sibutramine are effective in weight loss, and their effects are increased if followed by lifestyle modification, such as exercising and dietary changes. There is limited evidence about the effectiveness of rimonabant in weight-loss interventions. However, following several reports about their side effects (e.g., increased cardiovascular risk, suicide ideation), sibutramine and rimonabant were suspended and withdrawn from the markets. Orlistat is the only currently licensed drug for dieting and weight-loss interventions.

Nonpharmacological Diet Drugs

Nonpharmacological diet drugs include herbal supplements with weight-loss properties and typically serve two purposes. They provide the body with nutrients that are scarce in low-caloric diets and stimulate weight loss. These supplements can be purchased over the counter and usually come in formulas or so-called proprietary blends containing vitamins, botanical derivatives (e.g., green tea, açai berry, guarana), caffeine, or even aspirin. *Ephedrine* is a well-known herbal diet drug and stimulant derived from the Chinese plant *Ephedra sinica* and was initially used for the development of amphetamine drugs. Several nutritional supplements contain ephedrine alkaloids. These supplements are assumed to counter obesity and increase athletic performance by stimulating thermogenesis. A meta-analytic study found that ephedrine use is associated with modest short-term weight loss, but there is no sufficient data to support the long-term effects of ephedrine on long-term weight loss and athletic performance. Most importantly, the concurrent use of ephedrine with others stimulants, such as caffeine, is associated with increased heart palpitations and psychiatric, autonomic, and gastrointestinal symptoms. Ephedrine was banned by the U.S. FDA in 2004 in response to consumer reports of adverse health effects, and is included in the 2012 list of prohibited substances issued by WADA.

Ephedra-Free Diet Drugs

Following the ban on ephedra-based products, the nutritional supplements industry introduced alternative ephedra-free diet drugs. These supplements come in formulas or so-called proprietary blends. Bitter orange or *Citrus aurantium* is assumed to be an effective and safe alternative to ephedrine, and is a rich source of adrenergic amines *synephrine* and *octopamine*. Synephrine and octopamine are similar to norepinephrine, and their thermogenic effects are heavily advertised. Although related research is still growing, the safety of octopamine and synephrine was challenged by evidence showing that their effects on cardiac function are similar to that of ephedra-based supplements. While synephrine is not considered a doping substance, octopamine is included in WADA's 2012 list of prohibited substances.

Conclusion

Dieting and weight management can effectively counter obesity. However, only a few pharmacological agents have been licensed for this purpose. Over-the-counter pharmacological and herbal-based dietary supplements with alleged health benefits and weight-control properties are easily accessible for individuals suffering from obesity, athletes, or leisure-time exercisers. Nevertheless, the safety of such products has either been challenged or still remains to be determined by empirical evidence. The development of regulation policies for diet drugs in professional sports is an ongoing and dynamic process.

Lambros Lazuras and Vassilis Barkoukis

See also Body Dissatisfaction; Obesity; Performance-Enhancing Drugs

Further Readings

Ara, R., Blake, L., Gray L., Hernández, M., Crowther, M., Dunkley, A., et al. (2012). What is the clinical effectiveness and cost-effectiveness of using drugs in treating obese patients in primary care? A systematic review. *Health Technology Assessment, 16*(5). doi: 10.3310/hta16050

Boesten, J. E., Kaper, J., Stoffers, H. E., Kroon, A. A., & van Schayck, O. C. (2012). Rimonabant improves obesity but not the overall cardiovascular risk and quality of life; results from CARDIO-REDUSE (CArdiometabolic Risk reDuctIOn by Rimonabant: The effectiveness in daily practice and its use). *Family Practice, 29,* 521–527.

Dwyer, J. T., Allison, D. B., & Coates, P. M. (2005). Dietary supplements in weight reduction. *Journal of the American Dietetic Association, 105,* 80–86.

Greenway, F. L. (2001). The safety and efficacy of pharmaceutical and herbal caffeine and ephedrine use as a weight loss agent. *Obesity Reviews, 2,* 199–211.

Padwal, R. S., & Majumdar, S. R. (2007). Drug treatments for obesity: Orlistat, sibutramine, and rimonabant. *Lancet, 369,* 71–77.

Rossato, L. G., Costa, V. M., Limberger, R. P., Bastos, M. L., & Remião, F. (2011). Synephrine: From trace concentrations to massive consumption in weight loss. *Food and Chemical Toxicology, 49,* 8–16.

Shekelle, P. G., Hardy, M. L., Morton, S. C., Maglione, M., Mojica, W. A., Suttorp, M. J., et al. (2003). Efficacy and safety of ephedra and ephedrine for weight loss and athletic performance: A meta-analysis. *Journal of the American Medical Association, 289,* 1537–1545.

Simpson, S. A., Shaw, C., & McNamara, R. (2011). What is the most effective way to maintain weight loss in adults? *British Medical Journal, 343,* d8042. doi: 10.1136/bmj.d8042

DISABILITY

What is disability? There are many ways to answer this question. But how sport and exercise psychologists define disability has profound implications. Either intentionally or unintentionally, their perspective of disability will shape how research is carried out, what is deemed valuable in applied practice, who is considered the expert, and what is to be done to enhance the lives of people with disabilities. Thus, sport and exercise psychologists cannot ignore this question. Within sport and exercise psychology there are several ways to understand what constitutes disability; this entry discusses four of them.

The Medical Model and the Social Model

Two popular models for understanding disability are the medical model and social model. The *medical model*, or what is sometimes referred to as the individual model of disability, is based on decades of Western thinking that defines disability

as largely an individual deficit. Documented in 1980 by the World Health Organization, *disability* was defined as impairment, the loss or abnormality of psychological, anatomical, or physiological function. In this sense, disability was defined as any restriction or lack of ability (resulting from an impairment) to perform an activity in the way or within the range considered normal for a person. Therefore, disability is *caused* by parts of the body that do not work *properly*. The medical model shaped much early social and welfare policy and furthermore has, deliberately and by default, informed a great deal of sport and exercise psychology work on disability. Consider the example of spinal cord injury (SCI) and athletic identity. In such a study, participants with SCI would be labeled as having a physical disability and the dominant focus of identity and sport participation questions would be on the individual; such a project would be particularly amenable to survey research. Disability, as defined by the SCI, is the same for all participants. It is a medical problem or matter.

In recent years, the medical model has been widely criticized. Critics argue that it relies exclusively on individualistic medical definitions and biophysical assumptions of *normality*. However, normality is a highly contentious concept; normality is influenced by various cultural and historical forces that, in turn, mean what is normal in one cultural or context might be defined as not normal in another. Moreover, the medical model paints an overly negative and tragic image of people with disabilities. Individuals are depicted as defective and therefore disability is seen as a personal tragedy that should be overcome. As a result, individuals with disabilities may be pitied, stigmatized, and subject to a number of negative consequences. In relation to the previous two criticisms, the medical model has been further criticized for locating *solutions* to the *problem* of disability within the individual. By consequence, the individual's impairment needs to be cured or dealt with by health and medical professionals. Disabled bodies, rather than society, are seen as the site where interventions should take place. The focus on the normalization of the body and compliance with medical standards creates a hierarchy of power in which individuals with disabilities lose autonomy over their bodies to medical experts; failure to follow medical advice identifies an individual as deviant, potentially leading to stigma and other negative outcomes. As a result, power and control is placed in the "expert hands" of the medical profession as opposed to people with disabilities themselves.

In the 1960s, the disability movement began to challenge the assumptions of disability put forth by the medical model; this challenge was fuelled by a new understanding of disability. The *social model* posits that disability is the result of sociostructural barriers that serve to exclude and restrict people with impairments. For example, in this model, inaccessible sporting facilities or negative attitudes from coaches produce disability as opposed to individual impairments. The social model contains several key elements. It claims that social structures and attitudes exclude people with disabilities from participation in certain activities, such as sport. Furthermore, the social model asserts that people with disabilities are an oppressed social group. It also distinguishes between the impairments that people have and the oppression that they experience within society. Therefore, the social model severs any causal link between impairment and disability. Disability is reconceptualized as having nothing to do with impairment and the body; rather, it is a social construction and a restriction of activity. Consider again the example of SCI and athletic identity. When framed from the social perspective, researchers might examine how individuals with SCI are either denied access to sporting opportunities based on physical impairments and thus cannot develop an athletic identity based on these oppressive, sociostructural barriers to sport.

The social model has had an important impact on the lives of people with disabilities, including elite athletes and people interested in engaging in leisure time physical activity. First, it enabled the identification of a political strategy to remove barriers and oppression. If people with impairments are *disabled* by society, as the social model proposed, then the priority is not to pursue a strategy of medical cure or psychological rehabilitation. Rather, it requires the removal of disabling barriers in order to promote the inclusion of people with impairments. This model has been instrumental in shaping antidiscrimination law. Indeed, the social model was a catalyst for the numerous legislative measures and policy initiatives to address the oppressive environments encountered by many persons with disabilities. For example, by law, it has meant that people with disabilities

should be able to access gyms, sport clubs, sporting stadiums, and so on.

The second impact of the social model was on people with disabilities themselves. Offering an alternative to the medical model of disability, the social model was and remains very liberating for many individuals with disabilities—it offers them a very different narrative of disability that enabled them to understand that they themselves were not at fault—society was. They did not need to change; society needed to change. They did not have to identify their impairments as tragic; rather, they could accept their body and lives as they chose. In such ways, the social model is a source of empowerment and a way to restore the autonomy of body and choice for people with impairments. The social model as a counternarrative has enabled people with hearing impairments to positively think of themselves as communicating in a different language compared to individuals without hearing impairments. As a result, they view themselves in affirmative ways and do not consider themselves as having a disability.

Critique of the Social Model

Despite the important impact the social model has had, recently this way of understanding disability has also been critiqued. First, it has been criticized as ignoring the cultural and experiential dimensions of disability. For example, with the emphasis on the removal of social barriers, matters like athletic identity, emotional regulation, stories of mental coping strategies, or psychological well-being are passed over.

Second, it is argued that the idea of a barrier-free world is constrained by the natural environment, is at times economically impractical and is not possible for all people with disability. Moreover, by accommodating some impairments, barriers may then be put in place for other bodies. For example, wheelchair users can find curb cuts useful to enable their movement through the built environment. However, blind people might find that the same curb cuts make it difficult for them to differentiate pavement from road, and leave them walking into the path of a vehicle. Wheeling their way to play in a local tennis tournament, wheelchair users might have difficulties with tactile paving, which gives locational cues to people with visual impairments.

Third, in separating impairment from disability, critics have been keen to stress that the social model overlooks the importance of the body and impairments in people's lives. Indeed, impairment is not simply biological but profoundly psychological and social too. Consider again the example of SCI. By providing ramps, accessible washrooms, adapted sport and so forth, social barriers are removed and thus, in theory, so should the experience of *disability*. Yet after injury, bodily changes can lead to a host of new issues previously unknown to the individual, including the experience of pain, chronic health conditions, a *new* body and a new method of mobility. Thus to reduce disability to solely sociostructural barriers is overly simplistic. In light of these critiques, other models of disability have very recently emerged but have not yet garnered much attention within the sport and exercise psychology literature.

The Social Relational Model

One such model is an extension of the social model: the *social relational model*. It defines *disability* as a form of social oppression that involves the social imposition of restrictions of activity on people with impairments *as well as* the socially engendered undermining of their psychoemotional well-being. Like the original social model, the social relational model takes account of the sociostructural barriers and restrictions that exclude and oppress persons with disabilities. However, the social relational model also accounts for the social processes and practices that place limits on the psychoemotional well-being of people with impairments. In addition, the social relational model underscores the importance of impairment. It sees impairment and disability as linked and interactive. For example, an able-bodied person may tell a spinal-injured wheelchair athlete that they cannot be a coach at their tennis club *because* they are impaired: The athlete cannot run around the court or stand to serve, so they should not be a tennis coach. In this case, damage may occur to the psychoemotional well-being, and concomitantly the identity as an athlete or coach, of the person with disabilities. The damage is not solely the result of structural barriers. Rather, any damage caused, and the oppression and restrictions of activity that go with this, is an effect of impairment that operates in and through social interaction. Accordingly, the social relational model brings the body and impairment into focus, recognizing the impaired body as a biological, experienced, and psychosocial entity while

maintaining that people with impairments can still be oppressed. It is an approach to understanding disability that keeps social oppression at the heart of matters and yet considers disability in a far more layered, complex, embodied way than was detailed in the social model. Consider once again the example of SCI and athletic identity. Research from the social relational model of disability could explore how participation in adapted sport at the elite level reduces felt stigma and embodied concerns in certain contexts and therefore increases the individual's perceived quality of life. Or, in relation to impression management, it might examine able-bodied people's attitudes toward both people with disabilities who are physically active and people with disabilities who are not.

The Interactional Model

In the *interactional model*, disability and how it is experienced is understood as a consequence of the complex relationship between factors intrinsic to individuals, and extrinsic factors arising from the wider context in which these individuals find themselves. Intrinsic factors include the nature and severity of individuals' impairments, their own attitudes to these impairments, their personal qualities and abilities, and personality. By contrast, extrinsic or contextual factors include the attitudes and reactions of other people; social support systems; the extent to which the environment is enabling or disabling; and wider social, cultural, and economic issues pertinent to disability in society. The interactional model is similar to the social relational model such that impaired bodies are brought back into the understanding of disability. Both models also consider the relational aspect of disability. Therefore, as with the social relational model, a researcher interested in SCI and athletic identity would explore how interactions and impairment intersect to create an identity. In particular, a project framed from this perspective could examine how interactions in specific contexts (like dialogue or conversations in the locker room) either produce or detract from certain identities, such as that of the athlete and that of the person with disabilities.

Relational and Interactional Models Compared

Although similar, there are differences between these two models. First, *relational* in the context of the interactional model refers to the relationship between intrinsic factors and extrinsic factors that produces *disability*. By contrast, *relational* in the context of the social relational model refers to the relationship of those socially constructed as problematically different, or disabled, as the result of bodily or cognitive variations from the normal and cultural criteria for normal. Furthermore in the interactional model, rather than reserving the word *disability* for impairment effects, oppression, or barriers, the term is used more broadly to describe the whole interplay of different factors that make up the experience of people with impairments. By contrast, impairment is a necessary though not sufficient element in a disability relationship within the interactional model. It is always the combination of a certain set of mental or physical attributes, in a particular environment, within a specified relationship, played out in broader cultural, historical, and political context that, when combined with impairment, create the experience for any individual. Whereas the social relational model places emphasis on oppression and doing things to challenge or eradicate it, the interactional model would suggest there are many things that could be addressed to improve quality of life. This might include physical activity to improve self-esteem, exercise to enhance body–self compassion, or sport to create meaningful friendships and opportunities for travel.

Narrative Inquiry and Narrative Analysis

Understandings of disability are shaped by the model a sport and exercise psychologist adopts. But in addition, the type of theoretical approach adopted also underpins and informs work within sport and exercise psychology on disability. One approach that is garnering interest within sport and exercise psychology disability research is *narrative inquiry*. The core premise of this approach is that a person is essentially a storytelling animal; stories structure our experiences. We make meaning or sense of things through storytelling, and stories act on and in us, often working to shape and inform human behavior. Such a narrative approach is, therefore, of some relevance to sport and exercise psychologists who as professionals are in the business of dealing with *experience*, *meaning*, and *human behavior*. In both applied practice and for research purposes, we often ask athletes with disabilities to share with us their personal accounts of key moments or phases in their career.

In so doing, we are inviting stories. These stories are not passive or uninformative. They are needed in order for people to represent experiences that remain inchoate until they can be given a narrative form. Stories not only offer and impose form to experience, they express experiences. They are one of the most powerful means we have for communicating to others events that have happened, along with our emotions, attitudes, beliefs, and identities. When people tell stories, these stories have the capacity to affect what we do or do not do, shaping who we are and might be. As such, there is much to be gained from inviting stories and then analyzing them.

Narrative analysis is an umbrella term for an eclectic mix of methods for making sense of, interpreting, and representing data that take the form of a story. It takes stories or storytelling as its primary source of data and examines the content, structure, performance, or context of the story or storytelling as a whole. The analytical interest is not simply on what is said in a story in terms of content. The language and telling itself is also examined along with the environments that give shape to narrative content, structure, and performance. That is, in a narrative analysis the interest moves between *what* is being said, *how*, and *why* a person or group tells and performs the story as they do, in certain places and under specific conditions. For example, the narrative analyst is interested in how a story is put together to convey meaning, namely, to make particular points to an audience. For whom was this story constructed and for what purpose? What particular capacities of a story does the storyteller seek to utilize? Why is the sequence of events structured that way and not another? What narrative resources from the cultural menu does the storyteller draw on, take for granted, or ignore? Where do these resources derive from and under what circumstances and conditions? Are there gaps and inconsistencies in storytelling that might suggest preferred, alternative, or counternarratives? What does the story say and do on, for, and with people? How do listeners or readers respond to a story, with what affects, and on whom?

A narrative analysis of disability and sport might therefore highlight performance stories in which winning at all costs is the dominant theme. It could illuminate stories of anxiety and choking or stories of moments when everything comes together and the athlete experiences the sensation of flow. An analysis of the stories of athletes with disabilities who have just retired could reveal that the type of story several of them get caught up in is one that structures and shapes their retirement experiences as meaningless and devoid of purpose. The story is one that enacts a past full of glory and excitement, but now a present that is empty and a future that is perceived as desolate. Such a story, therefore, can be seen as acting on these athletes in dangerous and negative ways. Alternatively, a narrative analysis might reveal a type of story that following retirement calls on metaphors associated with a journey of self-discovery, notions of being changed for the better following retiring, and time tenses that link the person to living fully and happily in the immediate present. In this story, resilience is a dominant theme. It is used as a resource that works for the athletes to positively adapt to retirement and the adversity that can ensue. In such ways, therefore, sports and exercise psychologists can generate a compelling account of how stories affect human lives and put in place practical resources for people with disabilities to live differently.

Conclusion

As we have seen, disability is a multidimensional construct that can be modeled in several different ways. Moreover, these models lead to different ways of operationalizing disability and thus will have important methodological and practical implications for sport and exercise psychologists. When considering the literature and prior to beginning a research project, it is essential for researchers to reflect on which model of disability frames their understanding, given the impact this understanding will have on the ensuing research approach and method. To develop humanistic, complex, and rich understandings of the lives of people with disabilities, researchers might also consider using narrative inquiry. Stories, after all, affect human lives.

Brett Smith and Marie-Josee Perrier

See also Disability and Exercise; Disability and Sport; Disability Coaching

Further Readings

Gainforth, H. L., & Latimer-Cheung, A. E. (2012). Getting the wheels in motion: Physical activity promotion for people with spinal cord injury. In A. A. Martin & J. E. Jones (Eds.), *Spinal cord injuries: Causes, risk factors and management.* Hauppauge, NY: Nova Science.

Hanrahan, S. J. (2007) Athletes with disabilities. In G. Tenenbaum & R. C. Eklund (Eds.), *Handbook of sport psychology* (3rd ed., pp. 845–858). Hoboken, NJ: Wiley.

Martin, J. J., & Whalen, L. (2012). Self-concept and physical activity in athletes with physical disabilities. *Disability and Health Journal, 5,* 197–200.

Perrier, M. J., Sweet, S. N., Strachan, S. M., & Latimer-Cheung, A. E. (2012). I act, therefore I am: Athletic identity and the health action process approach predict sport participation among individuals with acquired physical disabilities. *Psychology of Sport and Exercise, 13,* 713–720.

Smith, B. (2013). Disability, sport, and men's narratives of health: A qualitative study. *Health Psychology, 32,* 110–119.

Smith, B., & Sparkes, A. C. (2005). Men, sport, spinal cord injury and narratives of hope. *Social Science & Medicine, 61,* 1095–1105.

Smith, B., & Sparkes, A. C. (2008). Changing bodies, changing narratives and the consequences of tellability: A case study of becoming disabled through sport. *Sociology of Health & Illness, 30,* 217–236.

Smith, B., & Sparkes, A. C. (2009). Narrative analysis and sport and exercise psychology: Understanding lives in diverse ways. *Psychology of Sport and Exercise, 10,* 279–288.

Smith, B., & Sparkes, A. C. (2012). Disability, sport and physical activity. A critical review. In N. Watson, A. Roulstone, & C. Thomas (Eds.), *Routledge handbook of disability studies* (pp. 336–347). London: Routledge.

Trachtenberg, L. J., Perrier, M. J., Gainforth, H. L., Minnes, P., & Latimer-Cheung, A. E. (2012). Challenging stereotypes of individuals with a physical disability: The impact of Paralympic athletes in television. In A. A. Martin & J. E. Jones (Eds.), *Spinal cord injuries: Causes, risk factors and management.* Hauppauge, NY: Nova Science.

DISABILITY AND EXERCISE

Appropriate physical activity engagement promotes a host of psychosocial benefits. These benefits are especially valuable for individuals with disabilities because they have high rates of overweight and obesity. Additionally, because people with disabilities often have associated secondary conditions (e.g., pressure sores, diabetes) physical activity is particularly important as a mechanism to prevent or attenuate secondary conditions. Unfortunately, most individuals with disabilities are sedentary or get limited physical activity. Low levels of physical activity among people with disabilities have been documented in North America, Europe, Asia, and Africa. Minimal physical activity is evident irrespective of age, gender, the setting (physical education vs. leisure), disability type (spinal cord injury vs. visual impairment), or assessment method (pedometers vs. self-report). Older females with severe disabilities from low socioeconomic-status groups are most at risk for low physical activity engagement. In this entry, the various psychosocial benefits of physical activity are highlighted, followed by a discussion of the barriers to physical activity.

Benefits

Increases in strength and endurance typically contribute to enhanced perceptions of competence. Mastery experiences and social influences both serve to contribute to enhanced competence perceptions. Competence benefits have been derived from activities as varied as lifestyle leisure activity, martial arts, youth sport, fitness training, and horseback riding. Most people also derive social benefits such as self-esteem enhancement stemming from being physically active with friends. Children in adapted sport programs find that they can more easily be themselves. Participation in physical activity also leads to increased social integration and reduces feelings of loneliness and isolation.

However, being physically active does not automatically confer social benefits upon participants. For example, it is not unusual for children to be excluded from physical education classes, ignored when sport teams are selected, and teased at recess, for looking different. Adults with disabilities (e.g., spina bifida) participating in inclusive recreation programs report both positive and negative reactions and experiences. In one study, participants with disabilities reported having difficulty ascertaining whether able-bodied participants disliked them or were simply ambivalent toward them. Other times, adult participants perceived that able-bodied exercisers treated them like children. Despite these reports, physical activity involvement helps minimize the negative influence of a disability on self-perceptions. A participant in one study reported that she felt "normal" when being physically active. Other individuals with disabilities have experienced less stigmatization which they attributed to their physical activity involvement. Researchers have also found that able-bodied people tend to evaluate people with physical disabilities more positively if they perceive them as being physically active. Two other benefits expressed by people with disabilities are greater feelings of independence from being physically active, and more opportunities to travel away from home on a sport team.

In addition to competence and social benefits, engaging in physical activity is simply enjoyable, and such experiences are valuable for quality-of-life reasons. In addition to the momentary value of increased positive affect, physical activity can also help in mood management when individuals do not have good days. For example, individuals with spinal cord injury (SCI) reported increased positive affect and decreased negative affect after exercising irrespective of whether participants had positive or negative life events that day. There is also preliminary evidence that individuals with neurotic tendencies benefit the most from the mood enhancing benefits of physical activity. In a recent study, virtually half the respondents noted enhanced emotional functioning that they viewed as stemming from their physical activity involvement. Many male adults with SCI have also experienced reduced stress, depression, pain, increased life satisfaction, and subjective well-being as a result of exercise. In brief, much research has supported physical activity as an important vehicle for quality-of-life enhancement by reducing negative emotional states and increasing positive affective states.

A growing body of research has also documented the relational benefits experienced by families who are physically active. Researchers examining family recreation and leisure experiences show that such involvement enhances family quality of life. A small body of research pertained to the family as a unit and to how physical activity experiences impact children, siblings, and parents. Adolescent participants were asked to describe how their adaptive skiing or horseback riding experiences influenced the quality of their family life. Virtually 70% agreed or strongly agreed that their experiences in these two activities enhanced their family life. Additionally, almost 80% of the participants agreed, or strongly agreed, that skiing or riding with family members contributed to the meaning of the activity. This finding has also been supported by scientists who have found that parents, particularly mothers, in families that have children with disabilities often engaged in activities like bike riding with their children in order to enhance family relationships.

Unique experiences, such as outdoor skill training programs and outdoor adventure trips including both parents and children with disabilities, are promising. Parents, for instance, have reported that their experience helped them overcome or eliminate constraints to being physically active. Both qualitative and quantitative results indicated that parents believed the experience enhanced family interactions, and promoted greater cohesion. Swedish families involved in orienteering, golf, and archery found that their children believed their participation helped the family experience "a feeling of togetherness." In brief, physical activity–oriented experiences are vehicles that enhance the psychosocial functioning of families.

Parents also benefit from their children's involvement in physical activities. Fifteen families with children with disabilities, who participated in adapted baseball, found parents derived mutual support from each. In particular, the shared social reality nature of the support was particularly meaningful. In summary, physical activity engagement results in a plethora of benefits to participants although sometimes participants report negative experiences. Individuals participating with or supporting the physical activity experiences of people with disabilities can detract from or enhance the physical activity experience.

Barriers

The benefits of being physically active are often difficult to obtain because of a multitude of barriers to physical activity. Individual based barriers include disability type. For instance, leg amputees cannot of course run or walk, although they can use crutches and wheels. Pain or discomfort is also a major barrier to being physically active. People with cerebral palsy (CP) and SCI list pain as frequently interrupting and preventing physical activity engagement. The physical discomfort of exercise is also viewed as a barrier by some individuals. In addition to pain, people with disabilities also note that fatigue, a lack of energy, disease,

injury, and poor health prevent them from being physically active.

Not knowing where exercise facilities are located or how to start and develop an exercise program also inhibits physical activity. A lack of time for physical activity is also reported by adults because of work and family responsibilities. Limited financial resources reduce or prevent travelling to exercise clubs, buying exercise equipment for the home, or purchasing exercise club memberships. A fear of developing tight muscles and joints from exercising has also been reported. Finally, inner city residents are often afraid to leave their homes for fear of crime or fear of falling.

Barriers that are more social in nature are also common. For instance, most children need their parents to transport, pay for, and facilitate their physical activity involvement. At the same time, parents are often fearful that their children might get teased by their peers for looking different. Parents also fear for their children's physical health if they engage in sports viewed as dangerous by their parents (e.g., basketball for a blind child). Parents, in turn, criticize community recreation personnel for not knowing enough about adapted sport programming principles and various disability conditions. Physical education teachers are also seen as lacking appropriate training in disability conditions and adapted physical education. Physical education teachers themselves confirm this view by indicating that they often lack adequate professional preparation in their teacher education programs. It is not unusual for physical education to be replaced by therapy or mobility training or canceled because of blanket medical excuses from doctors. Caregivers of adults with CP have asserted that they did not believe an exercise program was of value for their residents, and about a third of them believed exercise would not help their client's CP. Some caregivers even believed, contrary to research, that exercise would worsen CP.

In addition to individual and social barriers, the environment can also hamper physical activity engagement. For instance, children with disabilities often note that there are very few places to be active and rarely are facilities conveniently located. As children get older, their limited physical activity opportunities tend to diminish. Opportunities can also be illusionary, as wheelchair basketball league officials sometimes ban motorized wheelchairs and swimming pools are viewed as too cold by some swimmers with disabilities. Built environmental barriers, such as a lack of a curb cut or crosswalks without auditory signals, can prevent individuals with disabilities from crossing the street. Ramps that are ostensibly designed to facilitate access are often built too steep and cannot be used.

Barriers are also subtle. For example, although wheelchairs help people with disabilities to move, many individuals with SCI view their wheelchair as the number one barrier to physical activity. In one study, participants rated their wheelchairs as bigger barriers to physical activity than their disability. Most medical personnel and clinicians have only limited training in prescribing wheelchairs, which might explain why some individuals with SCI find manual wheelchairs uncomfortable, too wide and heavy, and therefore hard to move.

Researchers such as James Rimmer, Barth Riley, Edward Wang, Amy Rauworth, and Janine Jurkowski have examined the accessibility of health clubs and found that many (over 50%) clubs do not have curb cuts for easy access or clear paths to lockers. Most weight rooms do not have enough room for exercisers to move their wheelchairs around the exercise floor. Inadequately lighted biking and running paths and wooded walking trails with exposed tree roots can be barriers to individuals with vision loss.

In summary, physical activities ranging from formal exercise and sport opportunities to recreation and leisure lifestyle activities can all provide a wide ranging set of psychosocial benefits to participants. However, many physical activity barriers organized across individual, social, and environmental categories limit how physically active people with disabilities are, and thus, the benefits they accrue.

Jeffrey J. Martin and Laurel Whalen

See also Adapted Physical Education; Disability; Disability and Sport; Disability Coaching

Further Readings

Goodwin, D. L., & Compton, S. G. (2004). Physical activity experiences of women aging with disabilities. *Adapted Physical Activity Quarterly, 21*, 122–138.

Henderson, K. A., & Bedini, L. A. (1995). "I have a soul that dances like Tina Turner but my body can't": Physical activity and women with mobility impairments. *Research Quarterly for Exercise and Sport, 66*(2), 151–161.

Martin, J. J. (2006). The self in disability sport and physical activity. In A. P. Prescott (Ed.), *The concept of self in education, family and sports* (pp. 75–90). London: Nova Science.

Martin, J. J. (2007). Physical activity and physical self-concept of individuals with disabilities: An exploratory study. *Journal of Human Movement Studies, 52*, 37–48.

Martin, J. J. (2012). Exercise psychology for people with disabilities. In E. O. Acevedo (Ed.), *Oxford handbook of exercise psychology*. New York: Oxford University Press.

Rimmer, J. H., Riley, B., Wang, E., Rauworth, A., & Jurkowski, J. (2004). Physical activity participation among persons with disabilities. *American Journal of Preventive Medicine, 26*(5), 419–425.

DISABILITY AND SPORT

This entry presents an overview of the psychosocial research conducted at both ends of the spectrum of sport engagement. First, we examine the psychosocial benefits of recreational youth sport involvement for adolescents with disabilities. The next section discusses the psychological challenges and mental preparation at the highest levels of sport involvement for athletes with disabilities: the Paralympics.

Youth Sport Participation

This section will report on two areas within the area of youth sport. First, the research on common sport self-perceptions, such as physical self-concept, thought to be influenced by sport, is examined. Second, the sport as a setting where children can develop social connectedness and reduce loneliness is discussed. It is commonly thought that individuals with disabilities may experience low self-esteem because their disability may limit their ability to experience sport success. At the same time, sport can be a vehicle that increases competence if children participate and improve their abilities. Unfortunately, researchers have shown that poorly coordinated children are less active at play, spending more time watching other children play than better coordinated children do, thus limiting their opportunities to improve. Additionally, researchers have shown that children with movement difficulties may fail more in sport relative to children without movement difficulties and as a result have lower perceptions of athletic competence compared to children without developmental coordination disorder (DCD).

In addition to reduced feelings of pride and satisfaction from limited mastery experiences, significant others may withhold positive feedback and be critical. Children with DCD have reported feeling anxious and humiliated because they were teased. Although accomplished youth athletes with disabilities view themselves as serious athletes, they often perceive that others do not.

In contrast to the above findings, other researchers examining the self-esteem of children with disabilities have found self-esteem scores comparable to that of able-bodied athletes. In a rare intervention study, children participating in a 4-week wheelchair tennis program enhanced their general perceived and tennis competence but did not increase overall self-esteem. In a second intervention study, the impact of a 12-week sport intervention on motor skill development was examined. Students with and without disabilities were randomized into intervention and comparison groups and the intervention group participants showed increases in object control and locomotor skills compared to the comparison group. Other researchers examining both wheelchair sport and wheelchair dance have reported favorable increases in self-perceptions ranging from global self-esteem to self-confidence and control.

The motivational climate that youth sport athletes perceive can also have an important influence on perceived competence. For example, children with disabilities who perceived a strong mastery climate in physical education had higher levels of competence compared to children who viewed the climate as less mastery oriented. Social support by significant others is also important as adolescent athletes' self-efficacy is positively related to three different types of social support: listening, emotional challenge, and technical challenge support provided by friends, parents, and coaches. These findings suggest that sport self-efficacy may partly be the result of encouragement and social support coming from diverse relationships.

The social nature of sport makes it a potentially important vehicle for psychosocial development. For example, adolescents perceive that their involvement in sport increased the favorable impressions able-bodied others had of them. Given that children with disabilities have fewer friends and are lonelier than children without disabilities,

sport offers a tremendous opportunity to promote social connectedness while simultaneously enhancing health outcomes. Jeffrey Martin and colleagues have found that youth athletes with disabilities derived a variety of social benefits from having a best friend on their sport team. Gender differences were apparent with girls, compared to boys, indicating that their best friend looked out more for them, they had more common interests, stuck up for each other more, and were more encouraging after mistakes. Girls involved in formal disability sport receive more social support for their sport engagement compared to girls participating in more informal sport. Girls engaged in more serious high-level formal sport had role models who provided shared social reality support, emotional support and challenge, and technical support and challenge.

Parental encouragement has also been related to physical ability perceptions and sport commitment among international level adolescent athletes with disabilities. Athletes reporting more encouragement from their parents reported stronger perceived physical ability and a greater commitment to sport, compared with athletes reporting less parental encouragement. In contrast, children in a therapeutic martial arts program received lots of parental encouragement, but it was unrelated to their perceived physical ability. Because mean levels of support were high, the researchers interpreted their findings positively as parents did not limit their support to higher skilled children and ignore less-skilled children.

Youth with disabilities who played in an after-school disability sport program mentioned the importance of connecting with other youth who had disabilities. This sense of connectedness helped them feel more authentic. The researchers conducting the study speculated that the specific adapted nature of the sport program versus a nonadapted sport program was instrumental in creating a climate that allowed the participants to be personally expressive. Other sport psychology researchers have reported on enhanced social integration during sport because of increased opportunities for children to interact with their teammates. A benefit of this increased interaction is greater social bonding and a broadening of children's social networks.

Interviewers of 20 Swedish children participating in disability sports programs have also concluded that sport provides a means for the development of new friendships. The 36 adolescents participating in an adapted sport program who had the highest positive affect also reported the strongest peer relationships. Thus, a potential outcome of positive peer relations in a sport context is enhanced quality of life (positive mood states).

Some research suggests, however, that the experiences of children with disabilities in sport are sometimes less than positive. For instance, some individuals feel as if their physical abilities are denigrated and their sport participation trivialized. Even good intentions can go awry. For example, children with disabilities sometimes see offers of assistance in sport settings from able-bodied children as a negative assessment of their ability. Their self-esteem is threatened when they perceive that help is offered based on a negative assessment of their ability. Sport participants also report feelings of frustration and inadequacy when attempting to accomplish activities that they are inexperienced in or lack the skills to be successful in.

In summary, it should be clear that the sport setting is not inherently a context that promotes well-being among all participants all the time. As such, sport settings cannot be labeled as exclusively positive or negative. Adults, youth without disabilities, and youth with disabilities themselves, exert influence on the outcomes they experience in sport. The potential for positive experiences is greater when adults with emotional attachments (parents) or with sport expertise like coaches are actively engaged with the children in ways that are supportive and promote skill development. The potential for negative outcomes is reduced if peers are not allowed to engage in discriminatory and unkind behavior.

Elite Sport Participation

The Paralympics, like the Olympics, are considered the highest level of competition that an athlete with a disability can aspire to. The increased attention that the Paralympics get and the importance that governments, coaches, and support staff attach to Paralympic performance have the potential to make the Paralympic experience both exciting and stressful. Research with U.S. Paralympic coaches reveals that they believe athletes encounter pressure to perform well and win. Coaches also believe that the increased media and family attention increases stress.

Many researchers have substantiated the value of athlete's feeling confident, developing optimal mood states, and employing psychological skills. Researchers examining elite amputee soccer players, Paralympic wheelchair basketball players, international-level wheelchair road racers, and swimmers have all supported the value of psychological skills. Well-developed psychological skills help athletes manage and cope with stress. Sources of stress among athletes with disabilities reflect common sport sources of worry (e.g., lack of fitness), sources of stress unique to disability sport (e.g., wheelchair or prosthetic concerns), disability (e.g., pressure sores), and the nature of the Paralympic experience. We next focus on the unique challenges presented by the Paralympics.

British elite Paralympians have reported that traveling to major international competitions is stressful and noted specific factors such as having to get onto the plane first and off last as adding to their stress. A sport psychologist working with one Paralympian reported that his client's biggest source of stress was managing the 26-hour flight to the Paralympics. Getting on and off the plane, transfers from seat to wheelchair to toilet and back as well as personal care in general during the flight were all worrisome. Skiers in the 2014 Winter Paralympics will compete 60 kilometers from the Paralympic village. As a result, athletes will have extensive travel arrangements or have to stay off site and miss part of the Paralympic experience. Para-equestrian dressage riders at the 2008 Beijing Paralympics competed off site in Hong Kong. All the riders reported that they missed the main Paralympic experience. Hence, it seems wise that Paralympians psychologically prepare for either extensive travel, depending on their event, or prepare to not spend all of their time in the Paralympic village. According to British Paralympians, being away from home for a long time period is stressful. Athletes miss their significant others and the social support they receive from them.

Paralympians spend a substantial amount of time in the Paralympic village. For athletes who compete at the end of the games, they must spend a critical amount of time in an unfamiliar setting and sleep in a bed they are not accustomed to. In a study of Brazilian Paralympic athletes participating in the Beijing Paralympics, a majority of them had poor sleep quality during the games. Anxiety was linked to poor sleep as 72% of the athletes exhibiting poor sleep quality had medium levels of anxiety, whereas only 28% of the athletes who had good sleep were anxious. British National team members have also reported that they were concerned with whom they would share a room and how well they would be able to compete after a poor night of sleep.

Paralympic support staff need credentials to access the Paralympic village but these credentials are limited. As a result, compared to non-Paralympic competition, athletes may have less access to their sport psychologists and coaches. When available, coaches and support staff are often overworked and tired. The ability to see doctors, therapists, masseurs, and athletic trainers is similarly constrained.

Athletes with disabilities are functionally classified, which determines who they compete against. Being classified, which occurs prior to competition, can be stressful because athletes may anticipate being reclassified at a different level than they were previously. If athletes are reclassified, they may have to compete against better athletes. Clearly such a scenario can reduce confidence and increase anxiety at a crucial time.

Drug testing occurs at the Paralympics and may be a new, and therefore stressful, experience. Testing at the Paralympics can potentially be more involved and complicated compared with the testing done by able-bodied Olympians. For instance, many athletes urinate via catheters. Other Paralympians may have to file exemptions because of the medications they consume related to their disability. Some Paralympians endure chronic pain and may manage it with medical marijuana, which, although legal at home, is a banned substance at the Paralympics.

In summary, most elite athletes are affected by the events and conditions of their sport world. However, Paralympians have to deal with many unique conditions and challenges that can be barriers to optimal performance.

Jeffrey J. Martin and Francesca Vitali

See also Adapted Physical Education; Disability; Disability and Exercise; Disability Coaching

Further Readings

Goodwin, D. L. (2001). The meaning of help in PE: Perceptions of students with physical disabilities. *Adapted Physical Activity Quarterly, 18,* 289–303.

Hedrick, B. N. (1985). The effect of wheelchair tennis participation and mainstreaming upon the perceptions of competence of physically disabled adolescents. *Therapeutic Recreation Journal, 19*(2), 34–46.

Martin, J. J. (1999). A personal development model of sport psychology for athletes with disabilities. *Journal of Applied Sport Psychology, 11,* 181–193.

Martin, J. J. (2005). Sport psychology consulting with athletes with disabilities. *Sport & Exercise Psychology Review, 1,* 33–39.

Martin, J. J. (2006). Psychosocial aspects of youth disability sport. *Adapted Physical Activity Quarterly, 23,* 65–77.

Martin, J. J., & Smith, K. (2002). Friendship quality in youth disability sport: Perceptions of a best friend. *Adapted Physical Activity Quarterly, 19,* 472–482.

Martin, J. J., & Wheeler, G. (2011). Psychology. In Y. Vanlandewijck & W. Thompson (Eds.), *The Paralympic athlete* (pp. 116–136). London: International Olympic Committee.

DISABILITY COACHING

Optimal athletic development and sport success is almost always the product of multiple factors. Genetics, opportunity, effort, and consistent training over many years are critical. However, quality coaching is also recognized as an important influence on athletic success. This entry discusses the history and current status of coaching in disability sport, the importance of quality coaching from a psychological perspective, and unique disability sport coaching challenges.

Historically, many disability sport athletes have had to coach themselves. For example, in a survey conducted almost 15 years ago by Michael Ferrara and William E. Buckley, it was reported that only 58% of 319 elite adult athletes from the United States and only 33% of a diverse group of international athletes from Australia, Japan, and the Netherlands had coaches. Hence, it is understandable that many disability sport athletes have been known to overtrain, train inconsistently, train in nonsport-specific ways, fail to taper for major competitions, and fail to rest after major performance efforts. Consequently, wheelchair road-racing athletes often develop upper respiratory illnesses after marathons, and experience inadequate postrace rest, both of which exacerbate their difficulties. For athletes who self-coach, appropriate disability sport specific information is often hard to locate.

In recent years, athletes from wealthy countries have been supported by high-quality coaching.

Canadian Paralympic swimmers, for instance, have access to the same high-level coaches as able-bodied swimmers. However, Paralympians from other countries are deprived of professional coaching support. Many athletes are still self-coached or receive less than optimal coaching as coaches may not have the appropriate sport science or adapted physical activity education. However, the need for increased coaching quality has been recognized by national organizations. For instance, the American Association of Adapted Sports Programs offers an 8-hour coaching certification course that covers diverse topics such as sport psychology, physiology, management, and philosophy. It should be acknowledged that some athletes prefer not to have coaches.

Although the research on disability sport and coaching is limited, sufficient research allows sketching out a portrayal of the value of good coaching in disability sport. Disability sport athletes who view their coaches as supporting their autonomy express a strong sense of control over their sport involvement and have positive relationships with their teammates. Also, athletes who view their coaches as supporting their desire to be independent have higher levels of intrinsic motivation relative to athletes who perceive their coaches as less supportive. Disability sport coaches influence critical competitive psychological states in their athletes, in particular, confidence and anxiety, which play an important role in athlete's sport performances. For example, coaches who simultaneously support and challenge their athletes to become better are more likely to develop confident athletes. Coach influence on team cohesion is particularly important especially for sports where strategic and set plays are common, as in wheelchair rugby and basketball, and need to be learned in a short time span. National team athletes often live in different parts of the country, making the development of team cohesion difficult. Hence, coach influence on team task and social cohesion at national team camps is critical.

Coaching disability sport is challenging. Coach's prior experiences are usually with able-bodied athletes, heightening the importance of finding good disability sport specific coaching literature. Historically, coaches have reported having a hard time finding disability sport specific coaching material. However, a recent increase in research and disability sport literature, such as Vicky Goosey-Tolfrey's *Wheelchair Sport: A Complete Guide for Athletes, Coaches, and Teachers,* has made finding coaching material easier.

In addition to understanding their athlete's sport, coaches must gain knowledge on their athlete's disability condition. Because most coaches lack the life experience of living with a disability, specific knowledge must be learned. For coaches of youth athletes, developing sound relationships with the athlete's parents and their physical therapists helps capture their individual athlete's unique needs. In the case of athletes who are deaf, coaches without hearing impairments have additional communication challenges. Coaches also must consider the competition facility's accessibility for all of their athletes. Finally, coaches of high performance sport athletes (e.g., Paralympians) must support their athletes with issues related to traveling. Having to get on the plane first and off last can result in stress and pressure sores. Flying can promote dehydration, which necessitates the access to safe water (bottled water). Prior to travelling, and depending on the country, issues such as travel insurance, immunization, passports, and visas must be considered.

Unique to disability sport is the classification process where athletes are classified for competition depending on the severity of their disabilities. Some athletes have been known to *sandbag*, which means purposely underperforming at classification in order to be slotted into a lower classification where they will encounter inferior competition. Certainly coaches should be cognizant of this practice and insure their athletes do not engage in it. In summary, athletes with disabilities often lack coaching. Research on disability sport indicates that coaches often face challenges that are quite unique compared to the challenges of coaching able-bodied athletes. However, the limited research on disability sport coaching practices suggests that coaches can be quite influential on their athlete's motivation and confidence.

Jeffrey J. Martin

See also Coaching Efficacy; Disability; Disability and Sport

Further Readings

Banack, H. R., Sabiston, C. M., & Bloom, G. A. (2011). Coach autonomy support, basic need satisfaction, and intrinsic motivation of Paralympic athletes. *Research Quarterly for Exercise and Sport, 82,* 722–730.

Cregan, K., Bloom, G. A., & Reid, G. (2007). Career evolution and knowledge of elite coaches of swimmers with a physical disability. *Research Quarterly for Exercise and Sport, 78,* 339–350.

Goosey-Tolfrey, V. (2010). Wheelchair sport: A complete guide for athletes, coaches, and teachers. Champaign, IL: Human Kinetics.

Martin, J. J. (2011). Disability and sport psychology. In T. Morris & P. Terry (Eds.), *Sport and exercise psychology: The cutting edge* (pp. 609–623). Morgantown, WV: Fitness Information Technology.

Martin, J. J., & Mushett, C. A. (1996). Social support mechanisms among athletes with disabilities. *Adapted Physical Activity Quarterly, 13,* 74–83.

Martin, J. J., & Wheeler, G. (2011). Psychology. In Y. Vanlandewijck & W. Thompson (Eds.), *The Paralympic athlete* (pp. 113–136). London: International Olympic Committee.

DISTRACTION THEORY

See Attention–Performance Relationships

DIVERSITY

The concept of diversity encompasses a broad range of qualities and characteristics that distinguish people from one another. Diversity is used broadly to refer to demographic characteristics including, but not limited to, *sex, race, ethnicity, sexual orientation, class, ability status, age, national origin, religious beliefs,* and *education.* Diversity is important for a number of reasons. It allows a person to view issues and problems from multiple standpoints, drawing from different experiences, perspectives, knowledge, and connections. Rather than viewing the world from a single-focus lens, a person is able to expand views and consider multiple options. Diversity moves people beyond their ethnocentric and egocentric viewpoints, allowing them to not only learn about others' experiences and backgrounds but also more about themselves.

Sport is a diverse environment that includes individuals from different cultural and racial backgrounds. Sport and exercise psychology professionals work with and study these diverse groups of athletes, exercisers, and coaches. The Association for Applied Sport Psychology (AASP), an international, multidisciplinary, professional organization that offers certification to qualified professionals in the field of sport, exercise, and health psychology, outlines seven ways in which AASP actively promotes the respect and value of human diversity within its members and through professional actions. AASP members (1) do not discriminate; (2) do not tolerate remarks that reflect disrespect for individuals based on physical or cultural bias; (3) promote human diversity in research; (4) promote individuals with different backgrounds to join and participate in the organization; (5) seek education and training in multicultural methods to best serve the diverse clientele in sport and exercise psychology consulting; (6) promote equity and multicultural representation in AASP publications, conference presentations, and professional activities; and (7) demonstrate attitudes of respect and positive regard toward all colleagues, students, and clients.

Given the diversity among sport and exercise participants, it is surprising that until recently, diversity and multicultural perspectives have received only minimal consideration in the field of sport and exercise psychology. Much of the scholarly attention has focused on race or ethnicity and gender, with little attention devoted to other identities or the intersection of the varied identities. Sport and exercise psychology has traditionally been practiced from an ethnocentric, white male perspective. It is only recently that researchers have begun to seriously address diversity issues. For professionals and students in the field, it is imperative that there is an understanding of the histories and social experiences of the various cultural and identity groups with which we work or will work with in the future; the delivery, implementation and monitoring of sport and exercise psychology skills and interventions requires an understanding of cultural diversity.

Some research has addressed information about different cultural groups in relation to sport psychology consulting. Much of the earlier work in this area, however, relied on stereotypes of racial and ethnic groups and offered rudimentary recommendations of how to work with athletes of color. The early work in this area also treated athletes of color as exotic *others,* placing whiteness as the normative, privileged position. This work, however, served as the foundation for much of the recent discussion and work in this area. Recent research in this area, and in particular the work in cultural sport psychology, has begun to explore the issues pertinent to cultural and racial or ethnic diversity among athletes and multicultural approaches to sport psychology interventions. Research has also examined white racial identity and privilege in sport psychology consulting. Several researchers have noted the need for consultants to confront their personal feelings, experiences, and attitudes toward race by critically examine how their biases and assumptions influence their interactions with athletes of color.

In line with traditional psychology, gender research in sport and exercise psychology has historically focused on biologically based sex differences and neglected the study of complex gender issues and relations. More recently, researchers have stressed the need to consider athletes, exercisers, and coaches in the social context and work to understand the complexities of gender in sport and exercise.

In order to provide appropriate services to all individuals, as recommended by AASP and the American Psychological Association, Division 47, students and professionals in sport and exercise psychology should have training in issues that relate to diversity, culture, and identity. This training typically occurs in a student's graduate program in sport and exercise psychology, and requires that students take at least one course related to multiculturalism or social basis of behavior. Many have argued that multicultural training will enhance sport and exercise psychology effectiveness. Sport and exercise psychology consultants would benefit from an understanding of people of different cultures from their own. However, multicultural competency requires a heightened awareness of cultural influences in society, an ability to work with individuals from different cultural and racial backgrounds, content knowledge and intervention skills that are relevant to cultural groups, and skills to communicate across cultures. Such competencies will most likely not occur from one graduate course related to the social basis of behavior. Rather, an integrated model of multicultural training is recommended which involves integration and application of multicultural issues within each course in the curriculum. There is a need to move beyond delineating diversity as a special topic or special population toward integration of the social aspects of sport into all areas of sport and exercise psychology, including anxiety, motivation, personality, injury, and group dynamics.

Emily A. Roper

See also Cultural Competence; Gender; Multiculturalism; Race; Racism/Whiteness

Further Readings

Butryn, T. M. (2002). Critically examining white racial identity and privilege in sport psychology consulting. *The Sport Psychologist, 16,* 316–336.

Gill, D. L., & Kamphoff, C. S. (2010). Gender and cultural diversity. In J. M. Williams (Ed.), *Applied sport psychology* (6th ed., pp. 417–439). New York: McGraw-Hill.

Kontos, A. P., & Arguello, E. (2005). Sport psychology consulting with Latin American athletes. *Athletic Insight: The Online Journal of Sport Psychology, 17*(3). Retrieved from http://www.athleticinsight.com/Vol7Iss3/LatinAmerican.htm

Kontos, A. P., & Breland-Noble, A. M. (2002). Racial/ethnic diversity in applied sport psychology: A multicultural introduction to working with athletes of color. *The Sport Psychologist, 16,* 296–315.

Schinke, R. J. (Ed.). (2009). *Contemporary sport psychology.* New York: Nova Science.

Schinke, R. J., & Hanrahan, S. J. (Eds.). (2009). *Cultural sport psychology.* Champaign, IL: Human Kinetics.

DROP-OUT

The term *drop-out* has two meanings. In elite sport, drop-out refers to a premature termination of a sport career before the athlete could reach individual peak performance level. Drop-out is a typical phenomenon among athletes in childhood and adolescence. Therefore, the (young) age of the athlete may be regarded as an important evidence for premature drop-out. In contrast, career termination after reaching peak performance is called retirement. Typically retired athletes are older than drop-outs in the same sport.

In recreation and sport, drop-out means ending one's participation, for example in a club or a fitness center. In health-related sport, drop-out means leaving an exercise or rehab program before the end of that program—for whatever reason. In this sense, drop-out may happen at every age and is characterized by concluding any supervised physical activity. Different from elite sport, participants are not pursuing a sport career with the goal of peak performance. In this entry, the focus will be on the first meaning.

Drop-out can be considered from the viewpoint of the sport system and the athlete. From the viewpoint of the sport system, drop-out may be regarded as a nonnormative transition that could be avoided if only the athlete had been more motivated and had been better supported by the environment. Therefore, drop-out is considered a loss of talents and, economically speaking, a lost investment. From the viewpoint of the athlete, drop-out may be a source of regret and negative feelings, which would then accompany the transition to a career outside elite sport. Therefore, research studies and applied sport psychology alike are concerned with the reasons for drop-out, its prevention, and athletes' coping efforts. Drop-out is regarded as a complex phenomenon with a multicausal history. It may result from a deliberate decision of the athlete, for example, after seeing no future in sport due to no performance increases. But on the other hand, it may result from a forced decision because of a career-ending injury. Research shows that it makes a difference for an athlete if the decision for drop-out happens to be voluntary or involuntary. Very often, athletes make an easier transition to the postcareer if they see it as the result of a voluntary retreat that they had planned for.

Which are the most often mentioned reasons for drop-out in elite sport? As noted earlier, there is always a multitude of reasons. Most often, young athletes feel no longer able to combine school education with the high demands of sport training and competitions. They therefore finish their career in order to give priority to their education. Also, young athletes may realize that they lack the potential to make it to the top and perceive any further investment into their career as a waste of time. This feeling may be heightened by performance slumps—particularly during or after puberty—and by motivational crises, particularly after injuries. In addition, coaches may be regarded as being no longer supportive, and athletes would feel forced to leave the training group on the whole. And last, but not least, financial support—particularly from the sport system—may be withdrawn.

There exists not only a multitude of reasons for drop-out but also a multitude of reactions. Athletes who plan their postcareer tend to make a smooth transition and to feel happy with their new life. They see the end of their sport career as a necessary and even positive consequence for their further development. In these cases, drop-out can lead to positive feelings like relief and happiness, which are helpful for leading a new life. But

if athletes perceive their drop-out as a critical life event this may cause problems, which the athletes have to cope with. This feeling results more often from involuntary than voluntary drop-out. In these cases, drop-out can lead to negative feelings and even a crisis.

Apart from the reasons for drop-out mentioned above, former athletes who terminated their career prematurely seem to lack volitional and motivational qualities and they often perceive less social support or too much pressure from parents and coaches than active athletes. Some authors even speculate that coaches play a decisive role in the drop-out decision process.

Athletes thus could be better prepared against drop-out by their being helped to cope with the dual demands of sport and school or education. Special sport schools can be a solution, but also any other systematic support system. Also, coaches should have a positive attitude toward the athlete's pursuing a dual career. If athletes have problems in handling the consequences of drop-out, it would be helpful to have sport psychologists and mentors—former elite athletes in particular—teach the drop-outs how to overcome sadness and regrets and how to cope with the new demands of the postcareer.

Dorothee Alfermann

See also Burnout; Career Transitions; Talent Development

Further Readings

Alfermann, D. (2000). Causes and consequences of sport career termination. In D. Lavallee & P. Wylleman (Eds.), *Career transitions in sport: International perspectives* (pp. 45–58). Morgantown, WV: Fitness Information Technology.

Bussmann, G., & Alfermann, D. (1994). Drop-out and the female athlete. In D. Hackfort (Ed.), *Psycho-social issues and interventions in elite sport* (pp. 90–128). Frankfurt, Germany: Lang.

Butcher, J., Lindner, K. J., Koenraad, J., & Johns, D. P. (2002). Withdrawal from competitive youth sport: A retrospective ten-year study. *Journal of Sport Behavior, 25,* 145–163.

Fraser-Thomas, J., Côté, J., & Deakin, J. (2008). Understanding dropout and prolonged engagement in adolescent competitive sport. *Psychology of Sport and Exercise, 9,* 645–662. doi: 10.1016/j.psychsport.2007 .08.003

Drug Use and Control

Drugs are used for performance enhancement purposes in elite, competitive, and amateur sports. Unlike heroin, barbiturates, hallucinogens, and substances used for recreational purposes in other subcultures, athletes use and abuse drugs presumed to enhance athletic ability and performance, known as *ergogenic substances*. The most common performance-enhancing drugs include amphetamines and a range of substances thought to increase strength and muscle mass like anabolic steroids. The use of performance enhancing drugs is considered doping practice (see note at end of entry) and is therefore prohibited by the World Anti-Doping Agency (WADA), National Anti-Doping Organizations (NADOs), and sports-governing organizations. However, because athletes may face illnesses or health conditions that require medication, the use of certain prohibited substances is allowed for therapeutic purposes (known as therapeutic use exemptions). This process is regulated by the WADA's International Standard for Therapeutic Use Exemptions (ISTUE).

Health Consequences of Drug Use

Small or moderate dosages of performance-enhancing drugs are unlikely to result in noticeable changes in athletic performance. Therefore, athletes aiming to significantly improve their performance tend to engage in systematic and excessive use of drugs, especially during periods of intensive training. In fact, athletes typically self-administer drugs at much greater dosages than those prescribed for the treatment of medical conditions. However, abusing large doses of performance-enhancing drugs is associated with a wide range of side effects, including possible death. One notable example is the death of cyclist Tom Simpson in the Tour de France in 1967 as a result of amphetamine abuse. Furthermore, the abuse of anabolic steroids has been associated with various physical and psychological side effects, including but not limited to, liver toxicity, hormonal imbalance, irritability, increased aggressiveness (known also as steroid or roid rage), mania, major depression, and psychotic symptoms. Some studies have also noted that anabolic steroids can be potentially addictive, leading to withdrawal and dependence symptoms.

The Ethics of Drug Use

The spirit of sports is characterized by a range of ethical principles, such as fair play, ethics, honesty, health, character and education, respect for the self and other participants, to name just a few. Using prohibited drugs to increase athletic performance defies those principles, and, consequently hurts the image and integrity of sports. Furthermore, drug use gives an unfair competitive advantage to athletes who have the resources to secure drug supplementation, as compared to athletes without access to drugs, or who lack the financial resources needed to support drug supplementation.

Availability and Drug Use Patterns

Drugs can be supplied through drug trafficking networks either face-to-face or online. In many countries, the supplementation, possession, and trafficking of performance-enhancement drugs, and even encouraging someone to purchase prohibited ergogenic drugs, is penalized via legal sanctions. Common patterns of drug use include cycling, stacking, array, and pyramiding. *Cycling* refers to the use of drugs for periods between 8 and 12 weeks, or even longer. *Stacking* describes the concurrent use of several types of drugs to achieve greater performance effects, whereas *array* refers to using other drugs to counter the side effects of steroids, including estrogen blockers, masking agents, and diuretics. Finally, *pyramiding* is the gradual increase of dosages, from relatively low doses of drugs at the beginning of the cycling period, to higher doses toward the end of the cycle. Some athletes may also start with lower doses, move on to higher doses, and then return to lower doses of drug use at the end of the cycle. In many cases, the patterns of cycling, stacking, or pyramiding are based on arbitrary criteria and are not accompanied by the strict medical supervision that oversees therapeutic drug use. This is even more so in amateur sports and fitness, where users base their drug use patterns on word-of-mouth, or on information provided by informal channels such as drug-related websites.

Social and Psychological Predictors of Drug Use

There have been several attempts to identify the psychological drivers of drug use in sports. Relevant studies were initiated as early as the

1980s and centered on athletes' KAB (knowledge-attitudes-behavior). Over the last decade, research on drug use expanded considerably and has moved from mere KAB surveys to studying deeper psychological processes involving the interplay between personal traits and dispositions, motivational variables, cognitions and normative pressures, and behavioral intentions. Some scientists also focus on novel ways to assess social desirability, or capture the implicit beliefs and attitudes of athletes and exercisers toward performance enhancing drugs. Such research is based on the premise that athletes may be reluctant to disclose their preferences and beliefs toward prohibited drugs; therefore, studying their mental representations about the issue with unobtrusive and indirect methods can yield more reliable findings. Other researchers argue that a narrow focus on decision-making processes and cognitive functions may undermine broader cultural and social influences on drug use, such as the effects of use-reduction or harm-minimization policies, and macrolevel normative influences. It is noteworthy that social science research on performance-enhancing drugs has been supported by official antidoping organizations like WADA's Social Science Research Program, which was launched in 2005, and stimulated research on the psychological, behavioral, and social factors associated with drug use. The available studies suggest that doping is a deliberate process that requires decision making and intention formation. Doping intentions are likely to be influenced by doping-related attitudes, goal orientations, motivational variables, and social influences.

Drug Control

A commonplace drug control method is urine testing. This approach is based on a detect-and-punish premise and assumes that drug traces may be present in an athlete's urine during drug use and remain for some time after. Nevertheless, athletes can evade drug controls or tamper with their results by refusing to participate in drug testing, failing to declare whereabouts (a requirement for elite athletes to state their location to official sporting associations and NADOs in order to facilitate unexpected drug controls), discontinuing drug use before competition so that the drug is cleared from the body, drinking excessive amounts of water, or taking masking agents in order to tamper with

or invalidate urine tests. Another problem with existing doping control methods is that drug testing cannot be applied to the entire population of professional and junior athletes, mainly because of the high administrative and financial costs involved. Also, drug controls often fail to detect new substances and are even less effective in capturing gene doping. Finally, the detect-and-punish approach does not prevent the onset of drug use among young people and early-career professional athletes.

Athletes' Beliefs Toward Drug Control

Research on athletes' beliefs toward drug control and testing is still limited. Some of the available studies have shown that collegiate athletes in the United States were in favor of mandatory drug control if it was followed by systematic efforts and education programs aiming to increase awareness about the side effects of drug use. Other studies have shown that collegiate athletes lacked knowledge and awareness of the standard procedures involved in drug controls and displayed little awareness of the side effects of prohibited performance enhancement drugs. On the other hand, evidence from elite athletes is controversial; some athletes appear supportive of rigorous drug testing, whereas others are less in favor of drug controls, and even believe that existing procedures (e.g., urinating in public to supply a sample for analysis) hurts their dignity and personal privacy.

Education and Prevention

An alternative approach to drug control in sports that has gained momentum in the recent years is concerned with the investigation of psychological and social risk factors. This approach suggests that drug use can be explained by the interplay between a person's motivations, cognitions and beliefs, and normative influences. Knowledge about these processes can be used to inform subsequent, evidence-based preventive strategies that focus on education, awareness, and behavior modification interventions.

The ATLAS (Adolescents Training and Learning to Avoid Steroids) and ATHENA (Athletes Targeting Healthy Exercise and Nutrition Alternatives) projects are based on these principles, and are used to train adolescent and junior athletes, trainers and coaches, and team leaders about the effects of drug use. ATLAS and ATHENA provide knowledge about the side effects of drug use, build refusal efficacy skills, and inform athletes about alternative and safer performance enhancement methods. Empirical studies have shown that both ATLAS and ATHENA are effective in significantly reducing future use of steroids and related performance enhancement drugs among young athletes in both the short and long term.

Conclusion

Drug use is an ongoing issue in both competitive and elite sports and in amateur, nonprofessional sports and leisure time exercise. Anabolic steroids, amphetamines and stimulants, and other anabolic agents are used by athletes to enhance performance. Users tend to self-administer high dosages of drugs and engage in unregulated and unsupervised drug use patterns, thus endangering their physical and mental health. Research on drug use in sports has shown that athletes engage in this practice for various reasons, including motivational and dispositional variables, as well as normative influences. Recent research trends focus on unobtrusive methods to capture athletes' beliefs toward drugs, whereas other researchers call for studies that address broader sociocultural influences such as policy making. So far, drug control approaches have focused largely on punitive methods, but more recent trends support education and awareness-raising campaigns that tackle the psychosocial processes underlying drug use in sports and exercise and contexts and prevent future use by young athletes. Still, it appears that the road to drug-free sports is still long, and much work has to be done in order to eradicate the seemingly well-established drug-based performance enhancement mentality.

Lambros Lazura and Vassilis Barkoukis

Note: The World Anti-Doping Agency prohibits the use of anabolic steroid agents and other ergogenic substances, such as stimulants and amphetamines. Nevertheless, as described in the entry "Performance-Enhancing Drugs" in this encyclopedia, athletes may use nutritional supplements and herbal products to enhance their performance. These substances are considered legal and are not prohibited by WADA or related organizations, and their use is still unregulated. Nevertheless, for reasons of clarity and to avoid overlap with other entries in this encyclopedia, the present entry discusses only prohibited performance-enhancing drugs.

See also Diet Drugs; Narcotic Analgesics; Performance-Enhancing Drugs; Psychopharmacology

Further Readings

Elliot, D. L., Goldberg, L., Moe, E. L., De Francesco, C. A., Durham, M. B., McGinnis, W., et al. (2008). Long-term outcomes of the ATHENA (Athletes targeting healthy exercise & nutrition alternatives) program for female high school athletes. *Journal of Alcohol & Drug Education, 52,* 73–92.

Goulet, C., Valois, P., Buist, A., & Côté, M. (2010). Predictors of the use of performance-enhancing substances by young athletes. *Clinical Journal of Sport Medicine, 20,* 243–248.

Hanson, G. R., Venturelli, P. J., & Fleckenstein, A. E. (2004). *Drugs and society* (8th ed.). Mississauga, ON: Jones & Bartlett.

Harmer, P. A. (2010). Anabolic-androgenic steroid use among young male and female athletes: Is the game to blame? *British Journal of Sports Medicine, 44,* 26–31.

Kafrouni, M. I., Anders, R. A., & Verma, S. (2007). Hepatotoxicity associated with dietary supplements containing anabolic steroids. *Clinical Gastroenterology and Hepatology, 5,* 809–812.

Laure, P., & Bisinger, C. (2007). Doping prevalence among preadolescent athletes: A 4-year follow-up. *British Journal of Sports Medicine, 41,* 660–663.

Lucidi, F., Zelli, A., Luca, M., Russo, P. M., & Violani, C. (2008). The social-cognitive mechanisms regulating adolescents' use of doping substances. *Journal of Sports Sciences, 26,* 447–456.

Petróczi, A., & Aidman, E. (2008). Psychological drivers in doping: The life-cycle model of performance enhancement. *Substance Abuse Treatment, Prevention, and Policy, 3.*

Simon, P., Striegel, H., Aust, F., Dietz, K., & Ulrich, R. (2006). Doping in fitness sports: Estimated number of unreported cases and individual probability of doping. *Addiction, 101,* 1640–1644.

Wiefferink, C. H., Detmar, S. B., Coumans, B., Vogels, T., & Paulussen, T. G. W. (2008). Social psychological determinants of the use of performance-enhancing drugs by gym users. *Health Education Research, 23,* 70–80.

DUAL-PROCESS THEORY

Although dual-process theories have become popular over the last few decades, ideas about mental division have existed for centuries. Significant philosophers and psychologists, such as Plato and

Sigmund Freud, believed that the mind was partitioned, and the early work in this area has contributed much to modern dual-process theories. These theories, which have recently become popular in a variety of psychologies, share the notion that humans possess two distinct modes of information processing. One, which is commonly called System 1, the *impulsive system*, or the *automatic system*, is often characterized as fast, effortless, automatic, nonconscious, and it places little demand on working memory. It is a form of universal cognition that humans share with animals. System 2, sometimes referred to as the *reflective system* or *controlled system*, is commonly described as slow, effortful, controlled, conscious, and it is demanding on working memory. It permits abstract reasoning and hypothetical thought, and it is uniquely human. Early evidence for these two information processing systems was obtained from research in which participants were asked to respond to vignettes from three perspectives: how they believed most people would behave in the situation described, how they themselves would behave, and how a logical person would behave. Participants tended to indicate that people, including themselves, would often not act in accordance with logic.

Many dual-process theorists contend that processing in System 1 relates to the automatic access of knowledge or affective reactions that have become associated with a cue. The repeated pairing of a stereotype (slow) to a social group (elderly), for example, can lead to automatic access to the stereotype after perception of the group. Behavior and judgments can then align (or, in some cases, conflict) with the primed stimulus. Although this associative system operates fast, it is built via a slow conditioning process. Processing in System 2 is often discussed as analytical and rule based, and one which can draw from both slow-learning and fast-learning memory systems. The actual operation of System 2 is significantly slower than that of System 1.

Factors That Influence People's Reliance on Systems 1 or 2

Motivation

System 1 and System 2 compete for control of our inferences and actions. System 1 is generally more influential under conditions of low motivation, whereas System 2 can override the impulses of System 1 when motivation is available. The rule-based system that System 2 operates under is subjectively effortful and requires attentional resources. Thus, if people are not motivated to engage in this form of processing, responses will be governed by the effortless operation of System 1.

Cognitive Capacity

Cognitive capacity, as well as motivation, is important in determining the contributions of System 1 and System 2. Capacity refers to available processing time as well as attentional resources. Thus, responses that are made quickly or when the perceiver is busy or distracted will be governed by the associative processing of System 1. Alternatively, if an individual is given adequate time and is not distracted, System 2 may override the operations of System 1.

Type of Judgment

Motivation and cognitive capacity are perhaps the two most widely recognized factors that impact the utility of Systems 1 and 2. Nevertheless, other factors, including type of judgment, have also been proposed to influence people's reliance on the two systems. Those judgments that are more intuitive and affective, for example, "How would you feel if an opponent injured you behind play?" seem to be more influenced by System 1 than more rational judgments that are governed primarily by System 2 like "Why did the player injure you behind play?"

Generality of Stimuli or Judgment

The average of a collection of attitudes toward individual members of a team might be quite disparate from an overall attitude of the team. One reason for this is that the associative processing of System 1 seems to prefer specific, concrete stimuli, whereas general and abstract stimuli are better processed by symbolic rules (System 2). Thus, the systems are likely to contribute differently to questions or responses that vary in generality.

Mood

The associative system (System 1) is more often relied upon when positive mood is experienced, whereas negative mood promotes rule-based processing (System 2). Evolutionary reasons have been proposed to cause this effect, such as that consciousness is employed to direct individuals away from the aversive stimuli causing the negative mood.

A positive mood implicitly indicates that all is well, and the effortless System 1 is more likely to be allowed control in these circumstances.

An Example of the Effects of Systems 1 and 2 in Exercise

The motivation of an individual to attend an exercise class might be primarily a function of System 1, System 2, or a combination of both. A person for whom exercise is habitual will rely on System 1; motivation (and behavior) for the class will be activated automatically, and they will begin the session without much conscious effort. Alternatively, a new exerciser might contemplate attendance at an exercise class, and will therefore engage System 2. As a final alternative, both systems might be operational. A person's conscious thoughts about the benefits of an exercise class (System 2), for example, might be biased according to the operation of System 1.

James Dimmock

See also Automaticity; Automaticity: Evaluative Priming; Automaticity: Implicit Attitudes; Decision Making; Habit; Information Processing; Mindfulness; Priming

Further Readings

Chaiken, S., & Trope, Y. (Eds.). (1999). *Dual-process theories in social psychology.* New York: Guilford Press.

Evans, J. St. B. T. (2003). In two minds: Dual-process accounts of reasoning. *Trends in Cognitive Sciences, 7,* 454–459.

Evans, J. St. B. T., & Frankish, K. (2009). *In two minds: Dual processes and beyond.* Oxford, UK: Oxford University Press.

DUAL-TASK PARADIGM

It has been known for a long time that there are significant limitations in the human capability to attend to and perform two or more tasks concurrently. Observations of the performance errors arising from the simultaneous performance of multiple tasks date back at least to the late 19th century and form the basis for cognitive theories that regard attention as a limited capacity or resource. When attention is divided between tasks in a way that exceeds the available capacity or resources,

suboptimal performance in the form of increased errors or delayed responding becomes evident on one or more of the tasks. The dual-task paradigm is an established methodology to measure performance capability under these conditions where attention must be divided between two concurrently performed tasks. This entry first outlines the basic rationale and assumptions underlying the dual-task paradigm before describing some of the key factors that affect dual-task performance and some of the existing and prospective uses of the paradigm within the sport domain.

Basics of the Dual-Task Paradigm

As the name implies, the dual-task paradigm involves the simultaneous performance of two tasks—a primary task and a secondary task. In the simplest application of the method, participants are required to assign priority to the primary task (so that performance on this task remains at a comparable level in the dual situation as when the task is performed alone), and then changes in performance of the secondary task are used to provide a measure of the attentional requirements of the primary task. The primary task is generally the task that the researcher is most interested in understanding, whereas the secondary task is simply a tool used to help assess the attentional demands of primary task performance. For example, in research examining the attentional demands of walking control in the elderly, the walking task is the primary task while there is a wide range of possible secondary tasks available, including continuous tasks (such as counting backwards from 100 in 3s) or discrete tasks (such as a reaction time task with an auditory stimulus and a vocal response).

The extent of the deterioration in secondary task performance between the condition in which it is performed concurrently with the primary task compared to when it is performed alone provides a measure of the attentional demands of the primary task. Poor secondary task performance accompanies primary tasks that are extremely difficult and require many of the participant's information processing resources, whereas secondary task performance that remains unchanged from the solitary performance condition to the dual performance condition suggests a primary task that can be performed essentially automatically, requiring no processing resources.

An alternative instructional set that is sometimes used is to ask participants to assign equal priority to both tasks. This particular approach is used if the interest is less in quantifying the attentional requirements of one of the tasks and more in ascertaining the general time-sharing and attention-switching capabilities of the participants. In all applications of the dual-task paradigm, the selection of the secondary task, the monitoring of adherence to the instructional set, and the careful measurement of the performance on both tasks in isolation as well as contemporaneously is pivotal to the generation of interpretable data.

Factors Affecting Dual-Task Performance

Although there is some indication that the total available attentional resources (or processing capacity) available at any given instant may vary with factors such as arousal—being theoretically maximal when arousal is optimal—by far the biggest factor influencing dual-task performance is the complexity and attentional demand of the primary task. The proportion of the available processing capacity that is consumed by the primary task depends on the extent to which the primary task can be controlled by automatic processes and this, in turn, is dependent on the extent to which the skill has been learned. Primary tasks that are intrinsically simple or that are effectively made simple as a consequence of extensive amounts of practice and skill learning require relatively little central processing capacity and can be performed concurrently with only limited impact on secondary task performance. A large number of studies from different domains including aviation, transport, rehabilitation, and sport have consistently demonstrated that the ability to perform two (or even more) tasks simultaneously improves with practice of the primary task and is superior for experts than novices in the task domain. The improvements that occur with skill development are likely attributable to both a transition of at least some of the control of the primary task from deliberate processing to automatic processing and the development of effective time-sharing and attention-switching strategies that help minimize interference between the concurrently performed tasks.

Uses of the Dual-Task Paradigm in Sport

Because many sports activities necessitate the dividing of attention between two or more concurrent tasks (e.g., the basketball player dribbling the ball while scanning around for a suitable teammate to whom to pass), the dual-task paradigm is ready made for the study of skill in sport. The main use of the paradigm to date has been in assessing the skill level of individual athletes and in this respect the dual-task method is advantageous in that it offers a means of assessing the extent to which primary skills are automated and a means of revealing individual differences that are not apparent from simply observing the primary skill performed by itself. A fundamental premise is that athletes whose primary skills are well automated are more likely to be able to cope with competitive pressure and the time constraints of high-level competition than are athletes who need to devote a considerable proportion of their available attention to their basic skills in order to perform these to an acceptable level. In a recent study in rugby league, it was demonstrated that performance on a dual-task test of 2-on-1 passing skills was predictive of match performance of the same skill. Other potential, but as yet largely untapped, uses of the dual-task paradigm in sport include (1) using comparisons of the secondary task performance under match and simulation conditions to ascertain the effectiveness of simulation drills, (2) making objective assessment of the relative demands of different skill learning drills in order to introduce them in appropriate order of increasing complexity, and (3) exploiting the attentional overload available through dual task methods to attempt to further stimulate the automation of key skills or encourage the learning of skills via a form of control that is below the level of consciousness.

Conclusion

The dual-task paradigm offers a simple but potentially powerful approach for the assessment of the attentional demands of skills and tasks that are fundamental to successful performance in many domains. Although the paradigm has a long history of use in cognitive psychology, especially in the testing of different theories of attention, it has thus far been underutilized in the understanding and enhancement of the skills for sport.

Bruce Abernethy

See also Attention Theory; Attentional Focus; Automaticity; Expertise; Motor Control

Further Readings

Abernethy, B. (1988). Dual-task methodology and motor skills research: Some applications and methodological constraints. *Journal of Human Movement Studies, 14,* 101–132.

Abernethy, B. (2001). Attention. In R. N. Singer, H. A. Hausenblas, & C. Janelle (Eds.), *Handbook of research on sport psychology* (2nd ed., pp. 53–85). New York: Wiley.

Gabbett, T. J., & Abernethy, B. (2012). Dual-task assessment of a sporting skill: Influence of task complexity and relationship with competitive performances. *Journal of Sports Sciences, 30*(16), 1735–1745. doi: 10.1080/02640414.2012.713979

Taylor, M. E., Delbaere, K., Mikolaizak, A. S., Lord, S. R., & Close, J. C. (2013). Gait parameter risk factors for falls under simple and dual task conditions in cognitively impaired older people. *Gait and Posture, 37*(1), 126–130. doi: 10.1016/j.gaitpost.2012.06.024

DYNAMICAL SYSTEMS

Every biological system—microbe, athlete, or team—can be described formally in terms of its time evolution or dynamics. This becomes feasible if one capitalizes on a crucial characteristic of biological systems, namely that they exchange energy and matter, and in some cases also information, with their surroundings. In statistical physics, such systems are called open systems, as opposed to closed systems without environmental contact. Certain classes of open systems may self-organize and form coherent macroscopic patterns due to interactions between their constituent subsystems. When applied to sports behavior, the term *subsystems* may refer to the neurons, muscles, organs, and limbs of an individual athlete, but also to the individual athletes themselves, for instance when in combat with an opponent, be it one on one (boxing), one against many (cycling), or in teams (football). Furthermore, the term *system* may refer to virtually any aspect of sports behavior, including action, perception, emotion, and cognition, as well as their physiological underpinnings. Finally, each of these behaviors may change as a function of development and learning, which introduces an extra layer of dynamics. All of this implies that the opportunities for applying the concepts and methods of dynamical systems theory in sports science are virtually boundless and that any attempt at a priori demarcation is futile. This entry first provides an intuitive, yet necessarily abstract, introduction to the main concepts of dynamical systems theory, which are then brought alive by a collection of examples that highlight their relevance to sports science.

Concepts: A Fling With Physics and Mathematics

An important feature of open systems consisting of many interacting subsystems is that they form spatial, temporal, or functional behavioral patterns. Such coherent macroscopic patterns may be described by a small number of collective variables, called *order parameters.* Spontaneous switches between macroscopic patterns are termed *non-equilibrium phase transitions*[1] in equivalence with similar qualitative, structural changes studied in statistical physics. Phase transitions may be induced by continuous, gradual changes in relevant system parameters that do not specify the macroscopic patterns and are called control parameters. In what follows, it will be argued that, in the vicinity of these phase transitions, any system can, to a good approximation, be described as a low-dimensional dynamical system. The art of dynamical systems modeling is to find appropriate low-dimensional descriptors—that is, the order parameters—and to derive dynamical equations that describe their time-evolution and nonlinear dependence on control parameters. Such equations provide formal analogies of the macroscopic patterns and phase transitions exhibited by the system under study.

Steady States: Fixed Points, Limit Cycles, and More

Like macroscopic behaviors, dynamical equations often show steady-state behavior. That is, as time goes to infinity, they will settle asymptotically on a steady-state solution, which is often an attractor (a subspace of the state space to which trajectories are attracted). Dynamical systems theory may display four types of attractors: fixed points, limit cycles, limit tori, and chaotic attractors. Fixed points and limit cycles are the simplest attractors: a single point or a series of connected points that are visited at certain intervals, respectively. Some attractors are governed by more than one frequency. If these frequencies stand in rational relation to one another (are commensurate), the resulting behavior will still be a limit cycle. However, if these frequencies stand in irrational relation to one another (are incommensurate), the resulting trajectory is no longer closed, and the limit cycle becomes a limit torus. In this case, the resulting behavior is called *quasiperiodic*, implying that the trajectory passes arbitrarily close to every point on the torus without ever revisiting precisely the same point. A chaotic attractor is no longer a simple geometrical object like a point, cycle, or torus and thus defies precise definition. The outstanding property of chaotic systems is that they are sensitively dependent on initial conditions: trajectories that emanate from two arbitrarily close starting positions diverge at a characteristic rate. Hence, chaotic behavior, although entirely deterministic, is inherently unpredictable.[2]

Instabilities and Phase Transitions: Isolated Switches in Behavior

Phase transitions are accompanied by a colossal separation of time scales between different system components. Consider the case in which a certain macroscopic pattern is being replaced by another one. In dynamics terms, the first one becomes unstable and the second one becomes stable. Being close to an instability, however, implies that it takes a long time for a system to return to its steady state after a perturbation.[3] The order parameters hence evolve arbitrarily slowly, whereas the underlying (real) subsystems maintain their individual, finite time scales. From the viewpoint of the order parameters, all the subsystems become arbitrarily quick so that they can adapt instantaneously to changes in the order parameters. The system dynamics thus amount to that of the order parameters, implying the ordered states can always be described by a very few variables if in the vicinity of behavioral changes. Put differently, the state of the originally high-dimensional system can be summarized by a few variables or even a single collective variable, the order parameter(s). The relationship between the subsystems and the macroscopic structure, in which the subsystems generate the macroscopic structure and the macroscopic structures enslaves the subsystems, implies a circular causality. This effectively allows for a low-dimensional description of the dynamical properties of the system of interest.

Complexity: Ongoing Switches in Behavior

The merger of dynamical systems with concepts of statistical physics has provided a thorough understanding of nonequilibrium phase transitions and hence of self-organized pattern formation. One can go a step further and investigate the case in which the system under study remains in a critical state, a phenomenon called *self-organized criticality*. Self-organized critical systems have a critical point as an attractor. Consequently, their macroscopic behavior resembles the temporal scale-invariance characteristic of the critical point, which often includes fractal dynamics (as in chaotic systems) and power laws for, for example, the system's temporal correlations or spectral distribution (long-term correlations and $1/f$-spectra).

Complex Networks

Macroscopic, scale-free behavior of complex systems may not only emerge as a result of self-organized criticality. More recent studies on complex networks[4] have revealed that certain forms of network growth yield scale-free networks; that is, the distribution of connections per node in the networks obeys a power law. The mechanism is that of preferential attachment: The likelihood that a new connection will formed with a node depends on the number of connections of this node. Thus, nodes that already have a large number of connections are more likely to get even more connections ("the rich getting richer"). Many real networks such as the World Wide Web, collaboration networks of scientists, and brain networks are probably scale-free.

Examples: From Physiological Rhythms to Match Play

Entrainment of Respiration and Locomotion: A Matter of Efficiency?

A scenario germane to dynamical systems theory is the spontaneous entrainment of respiration and locomotion cycles in mammals, also known as locomotion–respiration coupling (LRC). During walking or running, particular integer frequency ratios are adopted between cadence and respiration (e.g., 2:1, 3:1, 3:2, and so on). Recall the multifrequency attractors with commensurate frequencies explained above. Top athletes explicitly train their optimal frequency ratio and learn to flexibly switch between different ratios as a function of demand and strategy. Why would LRC be beneficial? For years, it has been hypothesized that it serves to enhance performance efficiency. More recently, this notion has been linked to optimization of the effective oxygen volume in the lungs. In brief, the cyclical abdominal pressure modulates self-sustained breathing and causes maximum oxygen concentrations at integer frequency ratios between cadence and respiration.

Over the years, it has become evident that LRC is not simply a result of (bio-)mechanical constraints, such as the vertical impulse arising from the footfalls, as entrainment of breathing has been reported for a wide variety of daily activities with markedly different mechanical constraints, including cycling, wheelchair propulsion, and rowing. In general, the degree of coupling and the resulting frequency ratios depend on a variety of factors associated with task, environment, and athlete. Theoretically, this implies that respiration–locomotion entrainment is a generic phenomenon that is instantiated by, but cannot be reduced to, specific mechanisms or processes. Practically, the finding that greater expertise is associated with a broader range of solutions renders this dynamic phenomenon intrinsically relevant to training and performance enhancement in all cyclical endurance sports.

Dimensionality Reduction: A Way to Understand Coordination and Perception

An expedient tool for studying complex patterns of coordinated behavior is principal component analysis (PCA), a statistical technique for identifying reduced dimensionality in multivariate time series. The dimensions or principal components that account for the most variance in the original data set may be interpreted as the degrees of freedom, or alternatively as the order parameters of the system under study. PCA has found wide application in the study of movement coordination, also in relation to sports, and appealing examples may be found throughout the literature.

PCA revealed how (bio-)mechanical constraints lead to a considerable reduction in the number of components required to describe human walking. Only four components proved to be sufficient for this purpose. Coordination patterns were found to change markedly from walking to running, and PCA revealed a profound reduction of dimensionality during speed-induced gait transitions, as discussed earlier. Importantly, the evidence for phase transitions was prominent in the coordination patterns but not in the stride parameters. This approach may be readily extended to gait patterns in competitive running, as well as other sports behaviors like catching, throwing, and hitting, as exemplified by several recent studies.

Quite a different application of PCA can be found in the study of visual anticipation skills in tennis, in particular shots in different directions (left, right) and to different distances (long, short). A few components appeared sufficient to capture most of the variance in the shots, but they differed across shots, and tennis players could predict shot direction based on these components alone. This suggests that visual anticipation skill in tennis, and most likely also in other sports, involves the extraction of low-dimensional dynamic information from high-dimensional displays.

This series of examples highlights the fact that (physical theories of) emerging patterns (order or disorder) can be utilized for decomposing complex movement patterns. Ultimately, a better understanding of the principles that govern the complementary processes—pattern formation and pattern decomposition—will help advance perceptual and motor skill training in sports.

Temporal and Spatial Correlations: From Individuals to Teams

Heart rate variability is a measure that is often used in sports practice to individualize training intensity and recovery. But how should it be understood form a dynamical systems perspective? Considering the complexity of the mechanisms regulating heart rate, it is reasonable to assume that its dynamics are nonlinear, although no firm evidence for this could be found. Instead, it appeared that the heart rate time series of athletes is characterized by long-term correlations with a fractal signature. In particular, scaling analysis (detrended fluctuation analysis or DFA) of heart rate time series revealed scale invariance in distinct regions, corresponding to well-known frequency bands in the power spectra of heart rate variability. Furthermore, during training, marked changes were found in the scaling exponents of the scale-invariant regions in question, as well as during recovery after heavy exercise. These findings suggest that (also) the scaling characteristics of heart rate variability might be used to monitor the training status of athletes.

Dynamics of Team Sports

Matches among sports teams represent highly complex dynamical events. The positions of the players on the field evolve over time and may be described in terms of their spatial, directional, and temporal characteristics. Although this is already a rather laborious exercise, it is not sufficient for an adequate understanding. The reason is that the actions of the players on the field only make sense in light of specific, yet not necessarily known, individual and collective objectives and strategies. In any situation, players have a multitude of solutions at their disposal to pursue their strategic objectives, while actions unfold in parallel. As a result, the dynamics of match play represent a notoriously difficult area of investigation. Nevertheless, although still in its infancy, the analysis of match play is on its rise due to both technological and conceptual advances. Notable among the latter is the advent of network theory, which concerns itself with the study of graphs as a representation of connections between discrete objects (nodes).

As a case in point, a network analysis of passes among the players of the Spanish team during the FIFA World Cup 2010 was performed, where the team was considered a network with players as nodes and passes as (directed) connections. This revealed the effectiveness of the Spanish game in terms of several network measures over time, most importantly the clustering coefficient and passing length and speed. Likewise, in searching for the *greatest* team in cricket, matches played from the late 19th century onward were analyzed as networks using a page–rank algorithm to assess the importance of the wins and the rank of teams and captains; the same approach is used, for example, by Google to rank websites by keywords.

Team sports do not only form a network as players interact during team play but also sociologically in that players of the same club are linked. The latter relations have been analyzed in soccer using bipartite networks with nodes being players and clubs. The probability that a player has worked at n clubs or played m games shows an exponential decay, whereas the probability that he has scored g goals represents a power law. If two players who have played simultaneously for the same club are connected by an edge, then a new network arises with an exponentially decaying degree distribution. Of course, performance (scoring) and social interaction (club sharing) influence each other.

Conclusion

The study of a system's dynamics comes with a rich and sophisticated conceptual framework to address the complexity of sports behaviors. This is true for both the research questions that may be addressed and the methods used for that purpose. Absolute guidelines do not exist for this, only reasonable assumptions. Theoretical concepts may serve as sources of inspiration when linked to real-life phenomena and pertinent questions; conversely, the specifics of those phenomena and questions require an adequate conceptual and methodological approach. The focus on dynamical systems in sports science is still in its infancy but—given its marvels and intricacies—holds great promise for the future.

Peter J. Beek and Andreas Daffertshofer

See also Anticipation; Coordination; Freezing; Modeling; Motor Control; Motor Development; Motor Learning; Movement; Perception

Notes

1. The term *phase* refers to a system's state, a term that will be used throughout this article. Switches in macroscopic patterns are seminal for self-organizing systems, as they involve no external agents imposing order from the outside.

2. Chaotic systems exhibit a random-like behavior that is not readily distinguishable from real random behavior originating from a stochastic process based on chance events, that is, the probabilistic counterpart to a deterministic process. In order to do so, special mathematical techniques are required that only work well when specific conditions are met. Unfortunately, when studying dynamical systems in the real world, their behavior will typically result from a combination of both deterministic and stochastic processes that are unknown beforehand. This turns the identification and modeling of the behavior of interest into a formidable problem.

3. At precisely the critical point the dynamics of the order parameter is scale-invariant, that is, it does not change if its time scale is multiplied by a common factor.

4. The theory of networks has its roots in both mathematics and sociology. In 1736, Leonard Euler (1707–1783) solved the "bridges of Königsberg" problem: Is it possible to take a walk crossing exactly

one time each of the seven bridges connecting the two islands in the river Pregel and its shores? Euler proved that this is not possible by representing the problem as an abstract network: a "graph." This is often considered the first rigorous proof in graph theory.

Further Readings

Bak, P. (1996). *How nature works: The science of self-organized criticality.* New York: Copernicus.

Baumert, M., Brechtel, L., Lock, J., & Voss, A. (2006). Changes in heart rate variability of athletes during a training camp. *Biomedizinische Technik, 51*(4), 201–204. doi: 10.1515/Bmt.2006.037

Bernasconi, P., & Kohl, J. (1993). Analysis of coordination between breathing and exercise rhythms in man. *Journal of Physiology-London, 471,* 693–706.

Bramble, D. M., & Carrier, D. R. (1983). Running and breathing in mammals [Comparative Study]. *Science, 219*(4582), 251–256.

Cotta, C., Mora, A. M., Merelo, J. J., & Merelo-Molina, C. (2013). A network analysis of the 2010 FIFA world cup champion team play. *Journal of Systems Science & Complexity, 26*(1), 21–42. doi: 10.1007/S11424-013-2291-2

Daffertshofer, A., Huys, R., & Beek, P. J. (2004). Dynamical coupling between locomotion and respiration. *Biological Cybernetics, 90*(3), 157–164.

Daffertshofer, A., Lamoth, C. J. C., Meijer, O. G., & Beek, P. J. (2004). PCA in studying coordination and variability: A tutorial. *Clinical Biomechanics, 19*(4), 415–428. doi: 10.1016/J.Clinbiomech.2004.01.005

Haken, H. (1977). *Synergetics—An introduction.* New York: Springer-Verlag.

Huys, R., Daffertshofer, A., Beek, P. J., Sanderson, D., & Siegmund, G. (2004). Locomotion-respiration coupling: An account of the underlying dynamics. *Journal of Applied Physiology, 96*(6), 2341–2342. doi: 10.1152/japplphysiol.01341.2003

Huys, R., Smeeton, N. J., Hodges, N. J., Beek, P. J., & Williams, A. M. (2008). On the dynamic information underlying visual anticipation skill. *Perception & Psychophysics, 70*(7), 1217–1234. doi: 10.3758/Pp.70.7.1217

Mukherjee, S. (2012). Identifying the greatest team and captain-A complex network approach to cricket matches. *Physica A: Statistical Mechanics and Its Applications, 391*(23), 6066–6076. doi: 10.1016/J.Physa.2012.06.052

Onody, R. N., & de Castro, P. A. (2004). Complex network study of Brazilian soccer players. *Physical Review E, 70*(3 Pt 2), 037103.

Siegmund, G. P., Edwards, M. R., Moore, K. S., Tiessen, D. A., Sanderson, D. J., & McKenzie, D. C. (1999). Ventilation and locomotion coupling in varsity male rowers. *Journal of Applied Physiology, 87*(1), 233–242.

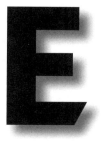

EATING DISORDERS

The eating disorders of anorexia nervosa and bulimia nervosa are characterized by severe disturbances in body image, eating, and engaging in compensatory behaviors that result in serious medical, psychological, and social problems. For example, eating disorders increase the risk of obesity, nutritional deficiencies, depression and anxiety disorders, chronic pain, osteoporosis, insomnia, neurological symptoms, cardiovascular problems, substance abuse, and death. The criteria for anorexia nervosa include an intense and unrealistic fear of becoming fat, engaging in behaviors intended to produce distinct weight loss, and amenorrhea resulting from the refusal to maintain a healthy weight. The body-image disturbance and consequential denial of the negative health effects of one's low weight are defined as maintaining a weight that is less than 85% of what is considered an ideal body weight for the individual's age, gender, and height. This denial is evident by a physiological criterion of *amenorrhea* that is defined as the absence of at least three consecutive menstrual cycles for women.

Two specific types of anorexia nervosa, restricting type and binge-eating–purging type, are based on how the extreme low weight is reached and maintained. The *restricting type* is defined as the absence of bingeing and purging behaviors. The *binge-eating–purging* type states that during the current episode of anorexia nervosa, the individual also engages in binges (eating inappropriately massive amounts of food in one set period of time) or purging behavior (self-induced vomiting, misuse of laxatives, diuretics, or enemas). While anorexia nervosa can affect men and women of any age, race, and socioeconomic and cultural background, the occurrence of anorexia nervosa is 10 times higher in the female population than among males.

The criteria for bulimia nervosa are similar to that of anorexia in that they also outline an intense fear of becoming fat, but they differ by including the requirements of powerful urges to overeat and subsequent binges that are followed by engaging in some sort of compensatory behavior in an attempt to avoid the weight gain effects of excessive caloric intake. The fear experienced by an individual with bulimia nervosa is also in regard to body-image disturbance. The paradox is the presence of the uncontrollable urges to overeat, resulting in binges. These binges are defined as occurring within 2 hours and eating an amount of food that is larger than most people would consume in a similar time and setting coupled with a sense of lack of control (inability to stop eating) during the binge. Both the body-image disturbance and binges result in engaging in compensatory behaviors to evade weight gain. Compensatory behaviors are separated into purging and nonpurging types. Purging behaviors include self-induced vomiting, use of laxatives, diuretics, enemas, or medication abuse. In comparison, nonpurging behaviors include fasting or excessive exercising. A qualification for a diagnosis of bulimia nervosa is that the binge eating and inappropriate compensatory behaviors must occur, on average, at least twice a week for 3 months. In contrast to those with anorexia nervosa, people with bulimia nervosa are able to maintain body weight at or above a minimal normal level.

Bulimia nervosa is considered to be less life threatening than anorexia nervosa; however, the incidence of bulimia nervosa is higher. Bulimia nervosa is nine times more likely to occur in women than men. The vast majority of those with bulimia nervosa are at normal weight. Antidepressants are widely used in the treatment of bulimia nervosa. Patients who have bulimia nervosa are often linked with having impulsive behaviors involving overspending and sexual activity, as well as having family histories of alcohol and substance abuse and mood and eating disorders.

Eating disorders exist and develop on a continuum with health detriment occurring throughout the entire span of the development and maintenance of the disorder. That is, cognitions and behaviors seen in full-blown disorders begin with less frequency or intensity and subsequently increase as the disorder develops. While the antecedents and causes of eating disorders are myriad and complex, excessive exercise has been the focus of much research and clinical attention. Although study design and quality have varied greatly, researchers typically find that a large percentage of individuals with eating disorders engage in excessive exercise. Thus, this entry will primarily focus on the relationship between excessive exercise behavior (exercise dependence) and eating disorders. Note that the entry on the female athlete triad focuses on eating disorders and athletes.

Of importance, according to the *Diagnostic and Statistical Manual of Mental Disorders, 4th Edition, Text Revision (DSM-IV-TR)*, exercise becomes excessive when "it significantly interferes with important activities, when it occurs at inappropriate times or in inappropriate settings, or when the individual continues to exercise despite injury or other medical complications" (American Psychiatric Association, 2000, pp. 590–591). This definition, however, fails to quantify the amount needed to determine if exercise is excessive. Because excessive exercise and its negative health outcomes have been studied far less than the other diagnostic symptoms, more research is needed to better understand excessive exercise and eating disorders. In an attempt to provide clarity to the excessive exercise construct, researchers advocate for either revising the diagnostic criteria

with regard to excessive exercise, or eliminating excessive exercise as a diagnostic criterion because of lack of empirical support for it. In short, considerable debate exists regarding eating disorder classification in general, and in particular with excessive exercise, regarding how best to define it, or even whether to include excessive exercise as a compensatory behavior for bulimia nervosa.

Relationship Between Excessive Exercise and Eating Disorders

Current exercise guidelines identify the minimum amount of exercise needed to experience health benefits. The guidelines also recommend that an increased amount of exercise is associated with additional benefits. Although increases above the minimum guidelines are encouraged, no consensus exists on *how much is too much*, that is, at what point any further increase in exercise may have a negative effect on one's health.

By definition, a regimen of exercise that has become detrimental to an individual's physical and psychological health constitutes *excessive exercise* or *exercise dependence*. Simply stated, exercise dependence is a craving for leisure-time physical activity, resulting in uncontrollably excessive exercise behavior that manifests itself in physiological (e.g., tolerance) or psychological (e.g., withdrawal) symptoms. Characteristics of exercise dependence include exercising despite either injury or illness; experiencing withdrawal effects when an exercise session is missed; and giving up social, occupational, and family obligations to exercise. Exercise dependence may also play a pivotal role in explaining the function of exercise behavior in the development and maintenance of eating disorders.

The relationship between exercise and eating pathology, however, is complex and controversial. Diagnostic criteria, correlational research, and clinical observation show a higher prevalence of exercise in individuals with bulimia nervosa and anorexia nervosa than in non-eating-disordered samples. This is in part because of exercise's ability to offset caloric intake, resulting in weight loss. For many individuals beginning to experience an eating disorder, diet and compensatory behaviors, such as picky eating, skipping meals, and fasting, may only reduce the number of calories consumed. Consequently, weight loss is slowed and the individual may seek complementary methods to accelerate weight loss. If progress with weight loss seems slow, compulsive exercise may be added in an attempt to increase weight loss. While this seems reasonable and sufficient to explain the role of exercise in eating disorders, simply examining the amount of exercise does not explain either why or to whom excessive exercise may become problematic. Thus, more recent investigations reveal that psychological factors such as exercise dependence may better explain the role of exercise in eating disorders. Therefore, a closer examination of prevalence rates and psychological factors indicates a much more complicated relationship between exercise and eating disorders.

The belief that exercise is associated with the development and maintenance of eating disorders is based largely on cross-sectional, retrospective, and case study designs that fail to adequately assess and quantify excessive exercise. For example, there is a long standing clinical observation that most hospitalized inpatients receiving treatment for anorexia nervosa engage in excessive amounts of exercise during the development or maintenance of their eating disorder. However, no definition is provided for what is considered excessive exercise. Similarly, recent studies have correlated participation in athletics (populations that engage in large amounts of physical activity) with deleterious eating attitudes related to eating disorders. Thus, researchers have focused on exercise amount contributing to the development and maintenance of eating disorders. However, focusing on exercise amount may be misleading because much of the research examining *excessive* exercise has relied on biased sampling methods using unvalidated self-report exercise measures that lack a clear, concise, and consistent definition of how much exercise is excessive. Furthermore, many of the operational definitions used for excessive exercise fail to meet the minimum amount of exercise needed to achieve the health-related benefits of physical activity.

Primary Versus Secondary Dependence and Eating Disorders

Most of the research examining the relationship between excessive exercise and eating disorders has focused on the amount of exercise contributing to the development of eating disorders but has overlooked psychological variables that may mediate such a relationship. Understanding the psychological antecedents of exercise may help clarify the relationship between eating disorders and excessive exercise by offering insight into the distinction between primary versus secondary exercise dependence. *Primary exercise dependence* occurs when the individual meets criteria for exercise dependence and continually exercises solely for the psychological gratification resulting from the exercise behavior. *Secondary exercise dependence* occurs when an exercise dependent individual uses increased amounts of exercise to accomplish some other end, such as weight management or body composition manipulation.

Simply stated, it is important to distinguish whether the individual is exercising excessively to satisfy the need to exercise (primary dependence) or if they are engaging in increased amounts of exercise as a compensatory behavior that is secondary to other pathology, such as an eating disorder (secondary dependence). Because exercise can be used as a compensatory behavior to prevent or reverse weight gain, secondary exercise dependence in the context of eating disorders occurs when individuals meet the criteria for exercise dependence and continually exercises to manipulate and control their own body; thus, exercise dependence is secondary to an eating disorder. Recently, researchers have found that exercise dependence symptoms, not exercise behavior, mediate the relationship between exercise and eating pathology. Thus, psychological factors, not the amount of exercise, may better explain why the exercise dependence–eating disorder relationship exists.

The Exercise and Eating Disorders Model

The limitations of biased clinical observations, retrospective research designs, vague operational definitions of excessive exercise, inconclusive animal research, and overlooking potential mediating psychological variables support the need for theoretically driven models that explain the relationship between eating disorders and the psychological motivation as well as the physical effects of exercise.

Previous models have been advanced that postulate how and why obligatory attitudes toward exercise may influence the development and maintenance of eating pathology and disorders. However, these models offer limited insight into why the benefits typically experienced as a result of regular exercise do not occur in eating disorders. For example, exercise may impart positive improvements on the eating disorder risk factors of anxiety, body image, depression, stress reactivity, and self-esteem in non-eating-disordered populations. Similarly, cardiovascular benefits, such as increased cardiac mass, increased stroke volume and cardiac output at rest and during exercise, lower resting heart rate and blood pressure, and a decreased tendency for blood clotting are pertinent to eating disorder research because cardiac damage can occur early during eating disorder development. Exercise also has the ability to reduce adiposity, thus contributing to a leaner, more fit, and culturally ideal body type. Moreover, sociocultural pressures to be thin and social comparison are risk factors for the development of eating disorders. Furthermore, the metabolic benefits of exercise include decreased triglycerides and increased high-density cholesterol, increased insulin mediated glucose uptake, and a possible increase in resting metabolism. Finally, exercise increases skeletal muscle mass and bone density in youth and it is related to the retention of bone mineral density in older adults. This has implications in the development of osteoporosis, a common consequence of prolonged eating disorder behaviors. Thus, exercise is an effective intervention for many physical and psychological health issues, and yet recent recommendations for research to reexamine the role of exercise in eating disorders have been largely overlooked.

Heather Hausenblas, Brian Cook, and Nickles Chittester presented a conceptual model examining such aforementioned relationships (see Figure 1). Their Exercise and Eating Disorders Model states that regular exercise is associated with improvements in several physical (cardiovascular, metabolic benefits, decreased adiposity, and increases in bone density), psychological (body image, depression, anxiety, stress reactivity, and self-esteem), and social benefits that are also risk factors, maintenance factors, outcomes, or diagnostic criteria for eating disorders. Hence, this exercise and eating disorders model has consolidated and supported several narrative and meta-analytic reviews that have shown exercise's ability to impart positive improvements on eating disorder risk, development, and maintenance factors. The model also extends our current understanding of the relationship of exercise and health status by including exercise dependence. That is, exercise dependence may explain why the development of eating disorders may supersede the expected benefits of exercise. Simply stated, this model posits that in the absence of pathological psychological factors such as exercise dependence, the benefits conveyed by regular exercise—improvements in depression, anxiety, stress reactivity, self-esteem, and body composition—may counteract the risk factors for eating disorders like body dissatisfaction, depression, anxiety, and increased body mass.

Recent research by Cook and colleagues, Hausenblas, Daniel Tuccitto, and Peter Giacobbi, has provided initial support for this exercise and eating disorder model, revealing that the psychological health benefits, conveyed by exercise can reduce the risk of eating disorders.

First, university students completed self-report measures of physical and psychological quality of life, exercise behavior, eating disorder risk, and exercise dependence symptoms. Structural equation modeling analysis found support for the mediation effect of exercise dependence on eating disorders as well as the effect of psychological well-being on eating disorders. Together, exercise behavior, psychological well-being, and exercise dependence symptoms predicted 22.9% of the variation in eating disorders. Thus, these results indicated that the psychological health benefits conveyed by exercise reduced eating disorders. These results were replicated in a more diverse sample of college students in another study by Cook and various colleagues in 2011.

Exercise Interventions and Eating Disorders

The initial tests of the Exercise and Eating Disorders Model suggest that the model may synthesize two divergent lines of research. That is, exercise may play a role in the development of eating disorders when exercise dependence is simultaneously present. Similarly, the psychological health benefits of exercise may also reduce eating disorder risk for individuals without exercise dependence.

Conclusion

Preliminary research has found that mild to moderate exercise appears to attenuate eating disorder symptoms in patients suffering with anorexia or bulimia nervosa. However, before exercise interventions are considered mainstream, future randomized controlled trials are needed to establish a dose–response relationship for exercise and identify the conditions (e.g., type or severity of eating

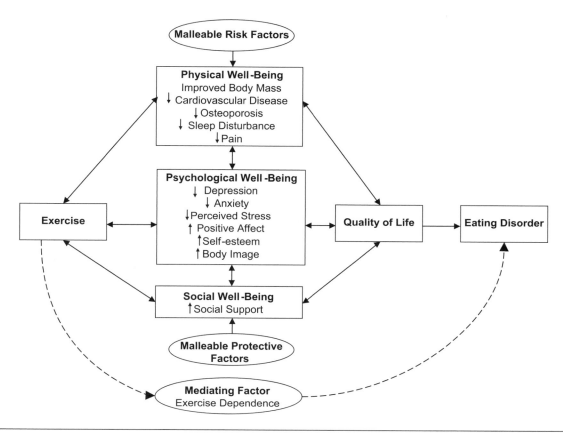

Figure 1   The Exercise and Eating Disorder Model

Source: Hausenblas, H. A., Cook, B. J., & Chittester, N. I. (2008). Can exercise treat eating disorders? *Exercise and Sport Sciences Reviews, 36,* 43–47. Copyright © Wolters Kluwer Health. Reprinted by permission.

disorder, minimum weight level, and exercise environment) under which an exercise intervention may be undertaken. Interest in exercise dependence and eating disorders is recent but provides a context as to why the relationship between exercise and other pathologies, such as body-image disturbance and eating disorders, exists.

Heather Hausenblas and Brian Cook

See also Body Dissatisfaction; Body Image; Exercise Dependence; Female Athlete Triad; Psychological Well-Being

Further Readings

Adkins, C. E., & Keel, P. K. (2005). Does "excessive" or "compulsive" best describe exercise as a symptom of bulimia nervosa? *International Journal of Eating Disorders, 38,* 24–29.

American Psychiatric Association. (2000). *Diagnostic and statistical manual of mental disorders* (4th ed., text revision). Washington, DC: Author.

Cook, B. J., & Hausenblas, H. A. (2008). The role of exercise dependence for the relationship between exercise behavior and eating pathology: Mediator or moderator? *Journal of Health Psychology, 13,* 495–502.

Cook, B. J., & Hausenblas, H. A. (2011). Eating disorder specific health-related quality of life and exercise in college females. *Quality of Life Research, 20*(9), 1385–1390. doi: 10.1007/s11136-011-9879-6

Cook, B. J., Hausenblas, H. A., Tuccitto, D., & Giacobbi, P. (2011). Eating disorders and exercise: A structural equation modeling analysis of a conceptual model. *European Eating Disorders Review, 19,* 216–225.

Dalle Grave, R., Calugi, S., & Marchesini, G. (2008). Compulsive exercise to control shape or weight in eating disorders: Prevalence, associated features, and treatment outcome. *Comprehensive Psychiatry, 49,* 346–352.

Hausenblas, H. A., & Fallon, E. A. (2006). Exercise and body image: A meta-analysis. *Psychology and Health, 21,* 33–47.

Hausenblas, H. A., Cook, B. J., & Chittester, N. I. (2008). Can exercise treat eating disorders? *Exercise and Sport Sciences Reviews, 36,* 43–47.

Hausenblas, H. A., & Symons Downs, D. (2002). Exercise dependence: A systematic review. *Psychology of Sport and Exercise, 3,* 89–123.

Holm-Denoma, J. M., Scaringi, V., Gordon, K. H., Van Orden, K. A., & Joiner, T. E. (2009). Eating disorder symptoms among undergraduate varsity athletes, club athletes, independent exercisers, and nonexercisers. *International Journal of Eating Disorders, 42,* 47–53.

Meyer, C., Taranis, L., & Touyz, S. (2008). Excessive exercise in the eating disorders: A need for less activity from patients and more from researchers. *European Eating Disorders Review, 16,* 81–83.

ECOLOGICAL THEORY

Ecological theory is a global perspective or metatheory, because the broad heading represents several scientific approaches that view human behavior as the result of the relationship between individuals and their environments. Ernest Haeckel, German zoologist and evolutionist, coined the term *oekology* in 1866 to define a field of study that examined organisms in their living environments. Ellen Swallow Richards, chemist and founder of the field of home economics, brought the term to English-language use in 1907. She described human ecology as the study of the influence of the surroundings of human beings on their lives. Swallow Richards provided an example of the application of ecological theory to physical activity with several observations about the interactions between individuals and their environments to promote healthy lifestyle behaviors. For example, in her 1904 publication *The Art of Right Living*, she noted that there is no better way to raise a child to perform healthy habits than to expose a child to environments that utilize the natural desire for effective movements. She recommended giving a child a garden because the care of a garden bed combines exercise, enjoyment, and adds indirect instruction on attaining satisfaction through work. Since the early 1900s, the study of human ecology has been fragmented, with work occurring in a range of disciplines, such as anthropology, geography, sociology, psychology, and kinesiology. The focus here is on describing several ecological perspectives that fall under the heading of ecological theory and illustrating their influence on sport and exercise psychology. By illuminating the influence of ecological perspectives on sport and exercise psychology, this entry offers a description of an ecological metatheoretical approach. The ecological perspectives described include Kurt Lewin's ecological psychology, Roger Barker's ecological psychology, James Gibson's ecological approach to human perception, Uri Brofennbrenner's ecological systems theory, and recent application of these ecological perspectives to inform physical activity promotion.

Kurt Lewin's Psychological Ecology

In 1943, Kurt Lewin used the term *psychological ecology* to propose that, for an understanding of individual and group behavior, it was necessary to study the opportunities and constraints of environments. But Lewin did not focus on studying environmental opportunities and constraints. Rather his major influence on sport and exercise psychology was his well-known equation $B = f(P,E)$, which stated that behavior is a function of the person and one's environment. While the person–environment interaction concept is adopted by social cognitive approaches, it is a central focus of ecological theory. Lewin viewed individual behavior as a function of the immediate social environment and believed that the social group to which individuals belong was the basis for individual psychological processes. The ecological perspective of Lewin's work departs somewhat from most contemporary ecological theories in that he considered the environment to only have an indirect influence on people's behavior and it was people's subjective perception of the environment that should be the central focus of study and intervention. In contrast, ecological theories place greater emphasis on the study of and intervention on actual, rather than perceived, features of the environment.

James Gibson's Ecological Approach to Perception

James Gibson rejected the premise that perception is part subjective and part objective. He argued that there is a subjective aspect and an objective aspect to every experience, but this does not mean that there is subjective determination of perception. Gibson's approach differed from Lewin's because the target of study and intervention began with environmental features. Because perception was described as a direct process of extracting information from the environment, the differences among individuals in perception were largely attributed to attention to environmental features. Gibson introduced the concept of affordances. An *affordance* was defined as a latent feature of the environment that provides action possibilities. An affordance was viewed as ecological (person–environment interaction), because an object's use is always dependent on individual capabilities. For example, a 7-foot-tall individual may not perceive a small chair as affording the opportunity to sit, while a 5-foot-tall individual perceives the same objective features and sits down. Much of the influence of Gibson's ecological approach within sport and exercise psychology has been in the area of motor skill learning and performance.

Roger Barker's Ecological Psychology

The study of objective features of the environment in the daily lives of individuals was the center of the work of Roger Barker from the late 1940s to the early 1970s. Although Barker spent 2 years as a postdoctoral fellow with Kurt Lewin and was strongly influenced by him, he shifted his path of research from a focus on the subjective perception of the environment to conduct studies of human behavior within natural environments. He set up the Midwest Psychological Field Station in the small town of Oskaloosa, Kansas, developed empirical methods for observing the activities of individuals in their everyday settings, and did copious measurements of daily life.

Barker's *ecological psychology* focused on person–environment interaction within the immediate environmental experience, which he labeled a *behavior setting*. Behavior settings were defined as the social and physical environments where behavior takes place. Behavior settings are a natural phenomenon that is bounded by time and place, a specific measurable unit, and recognized by people going about their daily lives. A school, for example, is not a behavior setting. But a basketball game at a school could be a behavior setting. It has a standing pattern of behavior, is not only a characteristic of the individuals involved but can function with different individuals, and is tied to a time and place.

Barker established that the strongest influence on behavior was not personality or global social inputs but rather the places in which people live their lives. For example, when a young girl entered a worship service, she behaved "worship service." If she left the worship service, and then went to a basketball game, she behaved "basketball game." After identifying the behavior setting as the unit of study, Barker shifted his focus from studying individual behavior to studying the environment. Barker and his colleagues provided evidence that knowledge about the place of behavior was more important than individual differences in predicting individual behavior.

Behavior settings were shown to influence physical activity. Studies of small schools and large schools were shown to have a similar number and types of behavior settings, such as basketball games and practices. But small schools offered more behavior settings relative to the population (understaffed). For example, a basketball game requires five players plus substitutes on each team. A basketball practice requires more players, but the number involved in practice games is limited to 10 plus substitutes. Although basketball game or practice behavior settings are similar at both large and small schools, at large schools behavior setting forces eliminate individuals from participation in physical activity through a selection process because of being "overstaffed." At small schools, however, the behavior setting may foster recruitment of individuals to participation in physical activity because more players are needed for a game or practice than may initially turn out. While Barker's theoretical perspective has not had a large impact on sport and exercise psychology, many contemporary ecological perspectives have adopted the term *behavior setting* to represent a social and physical environment for physical activity.

Uri Bronfenbrenner's Ecological Systems Theory

Uri Bronfenbrenner outlined his theory of the ecology of human development beginning in 1958 and continued to develop his ecological perspective over 5 decades. Bronfenbrenner's theory was strongly influenced by Kurt Lewin, under whom he worked as a young PhD in the Office of Strategic Services of the Army during World War II. Lewin constantly reminded Bronfenbrenner that space is not physical but psychological. This focus on the perceived environment contributed to distinguish Bronfenbrenner's approach from Roger Barker's.

In addition, Bronfenbrenner's ecological systems model focused on the impact of the environment on the individual. He viewed individual development as the result of being exposed to many different environments over time.

Bronfenbrenner's largest contribution to contemporary sport and exercise psychology was the concept that the environment is a set of nested systems or multiple levels of influence, each inside the next like a set of Russian dolls. The most proximal of these systems was termed the *microsystem*. This is the immediate situation where person–environment interaction occurs. Key to the nested-system concept is the idea that the immediate microsystem environments that people encounter, while the key to behavior and development, are the outcomes of the larger systems in which they are housed. The next-level (larger) system, called the *mesosystem*, was defined as a system of microsystems. For example, a child may encounter the school bus, classroom, school lunch, recess, and home environments throughout the school day. These could all be considered microsystems. The mesosystem is the combination of exposure to all these microsystems for the developing individual. The next level of the environment is the *exosystem*, which is a microsystem that does not contain the developing person but impacts on the child's micro- and mesosystem. For the child, the exosystem may include the parent's workplace or a school district's administration. Decisions made within each of these microsystems have an influence on the microsystems that the child encounters. The next level in the multilevel system is the *macrosystem*, which was defined as the larger sociocultural context. Bronfenbrenner proposed that cultural influences filtered down to the microsystem level to influence the daily practices of individuals that create the environments with which individuals interact. Later in his work, Bronfenbrenner added the chronosystem to his theory to recognize the impact of the patterning of environmental events over time. The last development of Bronfenbrenner's ecological systems theory was to imbed it within a bioecological model that addressed the genetic influences on behavior and development within the ecological environment.

While there has been little true integration across the ecological perspectives described earlier, they share many principles that can inform sport and exercise psychology research and practice. A summary of the principles of ecological theory suggests (a) the focus of study represents person–environment interaction; (b) study and intervention begins with examining characteristics of the environment; (c) person–environment interaction leads to behavioral outcomes and proximal developmental processes; (d) behaviors and proximal developmental processes occur in environments that, when studied directly, exhibit characteristics of self-regulating behavior settings; and (e) multiple levels of influence operate to impact the quality of the person–environment interaction over time to determine physical activity and development.

Application of Ecological Theory to Physical Activity Promotion

Perhaps one of the strongest influences of ecological theory within sport and exercise psychology has been in the study of physical activity promotion. Physical activity promotion researchers have embraced the principle of multiple levels of influence, as well as the focus on environmental characteristics. The public health focus of physical activity promotion researchers directs their attention to the primary target of population health. Individually targeted behavior change interventions that do not address environmental factors have not been successful in changing the health behaviors of communities. To solve this problem, in 1988, Kenneth R. McLeroy proposed that interventions be targeted at multiple levels of influence, defined as *interpersonal, organizational, community*, and *public-policy* factors. Corresponding with physical activity being identified by the U.S. Surgeon General as a major public health problem in the late 1990s, first mention of the adoption of an ecological approach within the sport and exercise literature occurred. A few public health scientists, including David Dzewaltowski, James Sallis, and Neville Owen charged researchers to embrace an ecological perspective. While several years and significant work has been conducted, there is still no consensus on an ecological theory for physical activity promotion or on how to define the levels of influence.

Ecological principles have been applied in the design of some interventions. Physical activity interventions for diabetes management have included, in addition to individual health behavior change components, multilevel strategies targeting healthy system change and community resources for regular physical activity. Interventions targeting settings such as worksites and schools have included broad environmental and policy components. In schools, for example, students may receive curriculum on self-regulation skills, school policy change interventions to increase the amount and quality of physical education, and community outreach to increase physical activity opportunities. Comprehensive community multilevel programs may include legislation for physical environmental changes like parks and walking and bicycle paths; mass media campaigns; and targeted school, worksite, and other delivery setting programs that include building social and physical environments for physical activity and curriculum-based education on behavior-change skills.

Many community-based physical activity approaches also use participatory strategies, whereby individuals in the community are empowered to lead change. These social and physical environment change leaders become champions of physical activity initiatives. Consistent with the ecological approach, interventions are tailored to the natural environments where people live and it is the residents of these environments that are best equipped to understand these unique local variables. Since ecological–psychology perspectives focus on the multiple systems that filter down to create local environmental variables, this multiplicity presents substantial logistical challenges for study and practice.

David A. Dzewaltowski

See also Health Promotion; History of Exercise Psychology; Leadership in Sport: Social Cognitive Approaches; Motor Learning; Perception; Psychological Skills Training

Further Readings

Araújo, D., & Davids, K. (2009). Ecological approaches to cognition and action in sport and exercise: Ask not only what you do, but where you do it. *International Journal of Sport Psychology, 40,* 5–37.

Dzewaltowski, D. A. (1997). The ecology of physical activity and sport: Merging science and practice. *Journal of Applied Sport Psychology, 9,* 254–276.

Richard, L., Gauvin, L., & Raine, K. (2011). Ecological models revisited: Their uses and evolution in health promotion over two decades. *Annual Review of Public Health, 32,* 307–326.

Sallis, J. F., Owen, N., & Fisher, E. B. (2008). Ecological models of health behavior: Theory, research, and practice. In K. Glanz, B. K. Rimer, & K. Viswanath (Eds.), *Health behavior and health education: Theory, research, and practice* (4th ed., pp. 465–485). San Francisco: Jossey-Bass.

Schneider, M., & Stokols, D. (2009). Multilevel theories of behavior change: A social ecological framework. In S. A. Schumaker, J. K. Ockene, & K. A. Riekert (Eds.), *The handbook of health behavior change* (3rd ed., pp. 85–105). New York: Springer.

Spence, J. C., & Lee, R. E. (2003). Toward a comprehensive model of physical activity. *Psychology of Sport and Exercise, 4,* 7–24.

Tudge, J., Gray, J. T., & Hogan, D. M. (1997). Ecological perspectives in human development: A comparison of Gibson and Bronfenbrenner. In J. Tudge, M. J. Shanahan, & J. Valsiner (Eds.), *Comparisons in human development* (pp. 72–105). New York: Cambridge University Press.

EFFORT

Individuals possess a remarkable ability to detect and interpret sensations arising from the body during physical work. As noted by William P. Morgan, terms such as *perceived exertion, perception of effort,* and *effort sense* have been used to describe this psychophysiological phenomenon. Interest in this aspect of performance was initiated by the pioneering work of the Swedish psychophysicist Gunnar Borg in the early 1960s. He introduced the concept of perceived exertion and proposed ways by which overall exertion, breathlessness, and localized sensations of fatigue could be numerically and verbally rated. This led to the development of rating of perceived exertion (RPE) scales, the most common of which is the Borg 6–20 RPE Scale. This entry describes Borg's concept of perceived exertion and outlines its underpinning factors, methods of measurement, and how it has been used.

Effort Continua

Borg originally proposed that subjective responses to an exercise stimulus involve three main effort continua: perceptual, physiological and performance. Although a number of more complex models of perceived exertion have been developed, they are founded on the same three effort continua. Borg used the *perceptual continuum* as the initial basis from which to explore the derivations of the ratings of perceived exertion, on the premise that perception plays a fundamental role in human behavior and in how one adapts to a situation. He stressed that the perceptual continuum will be influenced by a person's subjective experience and that these experiences will be directly affected by psychological traits. The physiological continuum includes a wide variety of variables, such as heart rate, blood lactate, oxygen uptake, and ventilation, which may be characterized by different growth curves as a function of exercise intensity. For example, heart rate and oxygen uptake are characterized by a linear growth in relation to increases in intensity as measured by power output (watts), whereas blood lactate concentration and ventilatory volume are characterized by a nonlinear (positively accelerating) growth function.

The influence of the perceptual and physiological continua on RPE will also be moderated by the situational characteristics of the performance (the third continuum). In this regard, one has to take into account the nature of the performance and the social and physical environment in which it takes place. Performance may involve timed (short or long) incremental stages to exhaustion, the highest workload that can be sustained for a specific period of time, the greatest distance one can cover in a given time period or the fastest time in which one can cover a given distance. Submaximal performances may involve monitoring the time to exhaustion at a given exercise intensity (for example, at a given percentage of maximal oxygen uptake or at an intensity corresponding to a ventilatory threshold reference point). Knowledge of the duration of the task or distance to be completed is also a critical factor in gauging effort. Social environmental factors may include whether or not performance is alone or with others, whether it is competitive, the presence or absence of an audience, and how supportive the audience is. Physical environmental factors include location, ambient conditions of temperature, humidity, and altitude, and any external distractions such as music and visual stimuli.

So, effort perception involves the collective integration of afferent feedback from cardiorespiratory, metabolic and thermal stimuli and feed-forward mechanisms to enable an individual to evaluate how *hard* or *easy* an exercise task feels at any point in time. It is moderated by psychological factors, such as personality traits, cognition, memory, previous experience and understanding of the task; situational factors, such as knowledge of the end-point, duration, and temporal characteristics of the task; and social and physical environmental factors. The extent to which these factors moderate the perception of exertion has been shown to be exercise intensity dependent.

Measurement and Calibration of Effort

The most common method of measuring perceived exertion is the Borg 6–20 Category Scale followed by the Borg Category Ratio 10 (CR10) Scale. The development and correct use of these scales is described in detail by Borg. The scales are designed to assess sensations of exertion in relation to physiological markers, such as heart rate and oxygen uptake, which rise commensurately with increments in exercise intensity. In both scales, numbers are anchored to verbal expressions. For example, in the 6–20 Scale the numbers 6, 9, 11, 13, 15, 17, 19 and 20 are anchored to verbal expressions of "no exertion at all, very light, light, somewhat hard, hard, very hard, extremely hard and maximal exertion," respectively. As research questions and applications involving perceptions of exertion have developed, a number of additional scales for adults have been developed. These include Foster's 0–10 Session RPE Scale, used in the calculation of an athlete's training load, and Garcin's 1–20 Estimated Time Limit Scale, which is used in the estimation of the time remaining until volitional exhaustion.

As the antecedents of RPE include the memory of physical work experiences and the level of cognition and understanding, a number of simplified RPE scales for children have also been developed. For a child to perceive effort accurately, and then reliably produce a given intensity at a given RPE, learning must occur. Implicit in the process of learning is practice and the cognitive ability of the child. According to Jean Piaget's stages of development, children around the ages of 7 to 10 years can understand categorisation but find it easier to understand and interpret pictures and symbols rather than words and numbers. For this reason, more recent pediatric RPE scales include pictures to portray the degree of effort and acute fatigue experienced and understood by the child. These developments have also recognized the need for verbal descriptors and terminology that are more pertinent to a child's cognitive development, age, and reading ability. These scales therefore use a limited number range based around 0 to 10 or

1 to 10, pictorial descriptors, and wording that is more familiar to children (e.g., Roger Eston and colleagues' CERT, BABE, CALER, E-P Scales and Robertson's OMNI Scales).

Central and Localized RPE

Sensations of effort can be used to assess overall respiratory–metabolic (central) perceptions of exertion or they can be used to differentiate between central and peripheral (local) signals of exertion. For example, differentiated ratings of perceived exertion may be used to segregate the sensations arising from the upper body and the lower body during cycling exercise or during rowing, running, or stepping. For cycling, localized perception of exertion in the leg muscles tends to dominate the overall perceived exertion response. Consequently, the strength of the perceptual signal of exertion is greater for a given work rate for cycling compared to treadmill exercise.

Estimation and Production of Effort

The sensation of effort has been applied in a variety of ways to assess and understand performance. It is generally observed that RPE measured during an exercise bout increases as exercise intensity increases in adults and children, particularly when the exercise stimulus is presented in an incremental fashion. Such relationships have been most frequently observed using the so-called passive *estimation* paradigm. In this way, a rating of perceived exertion is given in response to a request from the exercise scientist or clinician to indicate how "hard" the exercise feels. The information can be used to assess changes in fitness using standardized submaximal exercise test procedures, such as in the Lamberts and Lambert Submaximal Cycling Test. It may also be used to assist the clinician or coach in prescribing exercise intensities. For example, an exercise intensity (e.g., heart rate, work rate or oxygen uptake), which coincides with a given RPE, may be prescribed by the coach or clinician.

Given the robust relationship between RPE and exercise intensity, particularly if known for an individual, the RPE can be used as a subjective guide to gauge exercise intensity during cardiorespiratory and resistance exercise. Thus, an active *production* paradigm can be employed whereby the individual is requested to regulate exercise intensity to match specified RPE values. A number

of studies show support for the use of the RPE in this way for both aerobic fitness training and for estimating aerobic power and fitness.

Assessment of Training Load

As optimization of training load is a key factor for peak performance, the quantification of effort is considered to be important. Recently, the session RPE method, calculated by multiplying the relative perceived exertion of the session (scale of 0–10) by the duration of the exercise (in minutes), or the number of repetitions for resistance training, has become a popular method of assessing acute and chronic training load in athletes.

Prediction of Maximal Exercise Levels

The RPE elicited from submaximal work rates can be used to provide acceptable predictions of maximal aerobic power (VO_2max) that are as good as or better than heart rate. This is true for healthy active and sedentary groups and able-bodied and paraplegic athletes. The RPE also predicts 1-RM (one repetition maximum) in adults and children and maximal intermittent vertical jump performance.

It has been noted that RPE 20 is infrequently reported at volitional exhaustion during maximal incremental exercise tests or constant-load tests to maximal volitional exhaustion. As the subjective limit of fatigue normally occurs around RPE 19 (extremely hard) on the Borg 6–20 scale, studies have shown that RPE 19 is a better predictor of VO_2max than the theoretical maximal RPE 20.

Perceptually Regulated Exercise Testing

On the basis that RPE alone may be used to regulate exercise intensity, perceptually regulated exercise testing is an alternative method of estimating maximal exercise capacity and training status. The standard procedure involves a series of short incremental stages (2, 3 or 4 min.) that are clamped to RPEs of 9, 11, 13, 15 (and sometimes 17). Extrapolation of the individual RPE: intensity relationship to a maximal RPE (19 or 20) enables VO_2max or maximal work rate to be estimated with reasonable accuracy. This method has the advantage of allowing subjects the autonomy to set the intensity of exercise to a given RPE, through changes in pace, work rate, or gradient. First applied in cardiac patients, the efficacy of this method has been confirmed across a broad range of ages, fitness levels, and levels of physical ability.

Relationship With Time or Distance Remaining to Exhaustion

When the RPE is expressed against the proportion (%) of the time or distance completed, regardless of the length of an effort, the RPE rises similarly relative to the percentage of distance or duration completed or yet to be completed. This has been observed in open-loop, fixed intensity exercise to exhaustion (in which the distance or time is unknown) and during closed-loop tasks (the duration or distance to the end point is known) despite the effects of changed environmental conditions and competitive distances. Certainty about the exact duration and end point has been shown to affect both the RPE strategy and performance, as the rate of increase in perceived exertion is not always constant in all conditions, but changes in relation to the degree of certainty about the endpoint of exercise as well as exercise duration. Disruption in the rate of RPE increase occurs when uncertainty about the anticipated end point is invoked by deception during fixed intensity cycling and treadmill exercise.

The practical implication of this knowledge is that it is theoretically possible to use the rate of increase in the RPE to estimate the exercise duration or time remaining to exhaustion at a given work rate or pace. It is postulated that athletes continually compare their *momentary* or *conscious* RPE with an expected RPE (the "template RPE") through a process of internal negotiation at a particular portion of a race, and adjust pace to match the anticipated and experienced values for RPE

Murielle Garcin and colleagues introduced the 1–20 Estimate Time Limit (ETL) scale to provide a direct measure of how the effort at any given point during exercise can be used to provide a subjective estimation of the time remaining to exhaustion. The validity and applications of the scale have been reviewed by Coquart et al. (2012). In this scale, the numbers 17, 13, 9 and 4 relate to an anticipated end time to exhaustion of 4, 15 and 60 minutes and 2 hours, as listed on the ETL Scale, respectively. The ETL scale provides further information on the psychological load (intensity and duration) of exercise and allows for a direct subjective estimation of time that can be maintained at any intensity and at any given instant. Use of the ETL, in conjunction with the RPE, provides a further method of understanding the relationship between perceived effort, exercise intensity, and the duration that remains until physical exhaustion.

Conclusion

The concept of perceived exertion is a key variable of interest in sport and exercise science. It has applications in children and adults, from sedentary through elite athletic status. Practitioners have used it successfully with paraplegic, partially sighted, obese, cardiac and other clinical populations. It can be used to predict the limits of exercise, to regulate exercise intensity, to assess training load and to compare training status. However, its utility has to be considered within the dynamic context of the fundamental continua originally identified by Borg.

Roger Eston and Gaynor Parfitt

See also Brain; Fatigue; History of Exercise Psychology; Mindfulness; Personality Traits and Exercise; Psychophysiology; Timing

Further Readings

Borg, G. (1998). *Borg's perceived exertion and pain scales*. Champaign, IL: Human Kinetics.

Coquart, J. B., Eston, R. G., Noakes, T. D., Tourny-Chollet, C., L'hermette, M., Lemaitre, F., et al. (2012). Estimated time limit: A brief review of a perceptually-based scale. *Sports Medicine, 42,* 845–855.

Eston, R. G. (2012). Use of ratings of perceived exertion in sports. *International Journal of Sports Physiology and Performance, 7,* 175–182.

Eston, R. G., & Parfitt, C. G. (2007). Effort perception. In N. Armstrong, *Paediatric exercise physiology* (pp. 275–298). London: Elsevier.

Morgan, W. P. (1994). Psychological components of effort sense. *Medicine & Science in Sports and Exercise, 26,* 1071–1077.

Noble, B. J., & Robertson, R. J. (1996). *Perceived exertion*. Champaign, IL: Human Kinetics.

Scherr, J., Wolfarth, B., Christle, J. W., Pressler, A., Wagenpfeil, S., & Halle, M. (2012). Associations between Borg's rating of perceived exertion and physiological measures of exercise intensity. *European Journal of Applied Physiology, 113,* 147–155.

Tenenbaum, G., & Hutchinson, J. C. (2007). A social-cognitive perspective of perceived and sustained effort. In G. Tenenbaum & R. C. Eklund (Eds.), *Handbook of sport psychology* (3rd ed., pp. 560–577). Hoboken, NJ: Wiley.

ELECTROENCEPHALOGRAPH (EEG)

One approach to understanding the effects of exercise on the brain and the cortical processes underlying peak performance is to measure brain activity using electroencephalography. Electroencephalography is a noninvasive technique that uses highly conductive silver or silver chloride (Ag/AgCl) electrodes to record brain activity, which is also referred to as electroencephalographic (EEG) activity.

The EEG recording is actually a measure of electrical signals that are produced by neural cells in the brain and are measurable at the scalp. Because the electrical signals must pass through the dura mater, cerebrospinal fluid, skull, and skin before reaching the electrodes, these signals are recorded in a small unit of measurement called microvolts. EEG can be measured using either single electrodes (flat metal disks) that are attached at particular locations on the head or an electrode cap that has fixed electrodes sewn into the cap. The electrodes are adhered to the scalp using a specific type of gel or paste that maximizes conductance. The electrodes are connected by wires to an amplifier and a computer that records the brain activity. The internationally standardized 10–20 system developed by Herbert Jasper in 1958 is frequently used to communicate particular scalp locations used to record EEG. The locations of the sites are judged relative to landmarks on each individual's scalp, including the bridge of the nose, the bony protuberance at the base of the skull, and the midpoints of the ears. This original system included 21 electrodes that reflect measurement at frontal (F), temporal (T), parietal (P), occipital (O), and central (C) regions of the brain (Figure 1). In this system, the odd number indicates that the locations are on the left side of the brain and the even numbers indicate that the locations are on the right side of the brain. More modern EEG systems can include electrode placements that record information from 32, 64, 128, or up to 256 sites. In addition to the electrodes that are used to record EEG from sites of interest, an additional electrode called the *reference electrode* is used to subtract out basal activity so that the resultant recording from the sites of interest is reflective only of activity at those sites. This electrode is typically placed on the bridge of the nose or on an earlobe.

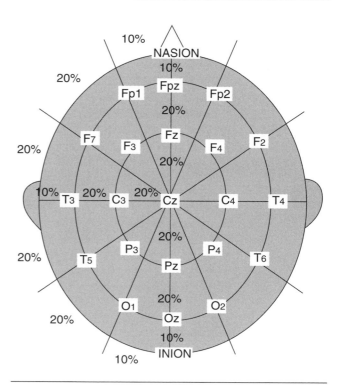

Figure 1   Jasper 10–20 System for Electrode Identification

Source: Adapted from Teplan, M. (2002). Fundamentals of EEG measurement. *Measurement Science Review, 2*(2), 1–11. Used with permission.

There are several computer software programs that can be used to record and analyze EEG data. In addition to recording EEG activity, some software programs can also be used for creating and presenting different types of visual and auditory stimuli so that EEG activity can be recorded relative to behavioral responses to those stimuli. More advanced software programs integrate EEG data with measures using other neuroimaging techniques like magnetic resonance imaging (MRI), positron emission topography (PET), and single photon emission computed tomography (SPECT) data. When collecting EEG data, there are several important things to remind participants of when preparing for the test. Participants should avoid taking certain medications that may alter the brain's electric activity, such as sedatives, muscle relaxants, and sleeping aids. Participants should also avoid caffeine and exercise within 12 hours of the test. The use of hair spray, gels, oils, or other hair chemicals should be avoided on testing day. The participant should be instructed to be as still as possible and remain quiet when assessing resting EEG. However, current EEG technology does permit EEG measures to be taken during exercise and sport performance. When the EEG data is collected, analog filters are used to limit the recording of low and high frequency signals outside the range of interest, such as low frequency signals from breathing. Nonetheless, prior to analyzing the EEG data, several steps must be taken to further ensure that the collected data is clean. Clean data most purely reflects the EEG data itself and does not include data that reflect muscle movement. Thus, in addition to the EEG electrodes, participants typically wear two electrodes placed around the outside of the eye to record eye blinks. Eye blinks and other muscle movement (e.g., from a cough, tensing muscles in the jaw) alter the EEG signal in a readily observable fashion and portions of the recording that contain these artifacts can be excluded prior to analysis using either manual or automated techniques. Once the data has been cleaned, it is then digitally filtered, which decreases extraneous data in the signal while maintaining the integrity of the EEG data. At this point, the data is ready for analysis.

Spontaneous EEG

There are four main wave forms measured by EEG: alpha, beta, theta, and delta. *Alpha activity* consists of waveforms that occur 8 to 12 times per second (Hz) and is interpreted as reflecting a relaxed state. Alpha activity tends to be low during mentally challenging situations. In sport psychology research, alpha activity has been associated with being relaxed and focused and mentally prepared for performance. EEG data has been used to distinguish mental states between novice and expert performers prior to task execution like a golf putt or free throw. Imagery training has also been linked to increased alpha activity. Biofeedback training has been used to teach participants to increase alpha activity with the expectation that this will result in better performance.

Beta waves (13–30Hz) are the most common type of EEG activity during wakefulness and are present during mental thought and activity, particularly during decision-making processes. Theta waves (4–8Hz) appear during drowsiness and light sleep. Delta waves (.5–3.5Hz) are found during periods of deep sleep and are characterized by very irregular and slow wave patterns. Delta waveforms are of particular interest to researchers exploring the effects of exercise on sleep quality.

In addition to interest in activity at a given site, there is also interest in examining hemispheric asymmetry in EEG responses. In the sport performance literature, expert performers typically display a *quieting* of left hemisphere activation, as inferred by greater EEG alpha power. This has been interpreted as being indicative of expert performers' ability to block out distractions, unwanted emotions, and negative thoughts prior to motor responses and suggests that there is a causal link between this ability and performance. Exercise psychology literature has focused on EEG asymmetry as a marker of affective changes often associated with exercise. The cerebral lateralization hypothesis suggests that anxiety reductions and enhanced affect caused by exercise are due to a decrease in right, relative to left, hemisphere activation.

Event-Related Potentials

Event-related potentials (ERPs) are time-locked waveforms that are identified after averaging the EEG response recorded relative to a particular event. The event-related portion of the name expresses that the timing of the EEG activity is directly related (time-locked) to an event; this is typically a stimulus presentation (e.g., seeing or hearing a stimulus) or a voluntary motor response that is made (e.g., pushing a button). The EEG signal is averaged using the presentation of the stimulus as the anchor so that the patterns of activity are synchronized to the same event. The potential portion of the name expresses that ERPs reflect cumulative electrical potentials generated by neurons in the brain.

There are several different kinds of ERPs. ERPs that occur in response to a stimulus are called *sensory-evoked potentials*; ERPs that occur relative to a motor response are called *motor potentials*. A common experimental paradigm that is used to assess ERPs is the *oddball paradigm*. In this paradigm, the participant is asked to watch a computer monitor on which frequent stimuli (e.g., an *X*) and infrequent stimuli (e.g., an *O*) are displayed. The participant is instructed to respond as quickly as possible to one stimulus (e.g., the *X*) by pressing a button but is asked not to respond when the other stimulus (the *O*) is displayed. The EEG signal is time-locked to the presentation of the stimulus, which allows sensory-evoked potentials to be observed. Interpretations of ERP data are based on the amplitude of the potential (the vertical distance from the baseline activity to the peak or trough of the component) and the latency of the potential (the elapsed time to the peak amplitude of the component from the time-locked event). The amplitude and latency of the sensory-evoked potential differ depending on whether the stimulus was the frequently occurring stimulus or the rarely occurring stimulus and also depending upon whether the participant responded correctly, for example, pressing the button when *X* was presented or incorrectly by pressing the button when *O* was presented to the stimulus. The motor potential is observed when the EEG signal is time-locked to the initiation of the motor response to press the button.

Two additional types of ERPs are referred to as *slow* ERPs because they occur over a relatively longer period of time than do the sensory-evoked and motor potential. Contingent negative variation (CNV) is observed when a participant is given a warning stimulus prior to presentation of a stimulus that is to be responded to, and its amplitude is increased by attention and decreased by distraction. A readiness potential is evident in the period prior to a voluntary movement and its amplitude has been shown to be related to motivation and to movement speed.

Once the data have been cleaned and averaged, the resultant waveforms are examined to identify the components of interest. The names of the components of the ERPs reflect the direction of the waveform (positive, *P*, or negative, *N*) relative to the baseline activity prior to the presentation of the stimulus and the approximate timing of the component relative to the stimulus. As previously described, components of the ERP are quantified based upon their amplitude and latency.

One ERP component that is of interest to sport and exercise psychology is the P300. The P300 is a positive waveform that occurs between 250 and 500 ms after the stimulus presentation. This component has been shown to be linked to the allocation of attention. The amplitude of the P300 is thought to be indicative of increased attention while the latency provides evidence of the time necessary to evaluate the stimulus (speed of cognitive processing). When considered simultaneously, the amplitude of the P300 is expected to be larger and the latency shorter when participants are using relatively few attentional resources to evaluate a stimulus and perform a task. The CNV (slow ERP)

occurs approximately 260 to 470 ms after a warning stimulus and is a sustained negative component of the waveform. The CNV is thought to be indicative of a participant's expectancy or anticipation of a stimulus. In the sport and exercise psychology literature, higher amplitude CNV has been linked to quicker reaction time.

Jennifer L. Etnier and Jennifer I. Gapin

See also Brain; Neuroscience, Exercise, and Cognitive Function; Psychophysiology

Further Readings

Crabbe, J. B., & Dishman, R. K. (2004). Brain electrocortical activity during and after exercise: A quantitative synthesis. *Psychophysiology, 41*(4), 563–574.

Hatfield, B. D., & Kerick, S. E. (2007). The psychology of superior sport performance: A cognitive and affective neuroscience perspective. In G. Tenenbaum & R. C. Eklund (Eds.), *Handbook of sport psychology* (3rd ed., pp. 84–112). Hoboken, NJ: Wiley.

Niedermeyer, E., & Lopes Da Silva, F. H. (2005). *Electroencephalography: Basic principles, clinical applications, and related fields.* Philadelphia: Lippincott, Williams & Wilkins.

Petruzzello, S. J., Ekkekakis, P., & Hall, E. E. (2006). Physical activity, affect, and electroencephalogram studies. In E. O. Acevedo & P. Ekkekakis (Eds.), *Psychobiology of physical activity* (pp. 111–128). Champaign, IL: Human Kinetics.

Teplan, M. (2002). Fundamentals of EEG measurement. *Measurement Science Review, 2*(2), 1–11.

Thompson, T., Steffert, T., Ros, T., Leach, J., & Gruzelier, J. (2008). EEG applications for sport and performance. *Methods, 45*(4), 279–288.

Electromyography (EMG)

Electromyography (EMG) is an electrical record of muscle activation. It is a measure that is recorded by placing sensors on the skin of a participant and monitoring changes in the electrical activity of the underlying musculature relative to movement. Greater levels of activation occur as motor unit recruitment increases in order to perform movements successfully. EMG provides a useful window into mind–body relationships, both within exercise and sport domains. While the use of EMG in sport and exercise psychology has been fairly sporadic, there are pockets of research in both exercise and sport where the use of EMG has provided valuable insights into the mind–body relationship.

One area in which EMG has been used with interesting results is in the study of the *tranquilizer effect* of exercise. More specifically, the study of the anxiolytic (anxiety-reducing) properties of exercise has been a popular topic for decades. Anxiety is a psychophysiological construct, having both psychological (e.g., feelings of worry, fear, apprehension) and physiological (e.g., increased heart rate and respiration, increased muscle tension) manifestations. As such, if one operationalizes anxiety as being reflected as increased muscle tension, EMG can be used to examine changes in that tension before and after exercise. One scientist, who made significant advances in this area, indeed coining the phrase *tranquilizer effect of exercise,* was Herbert deVries. In a series of studies beginning in 1968, deVries demonstrated that muscle tension was significantly reduced following aerobic exercise. This effect proved fairly robust, occurring for relatively brief bouts of exercise in college-age students, in older adults recruited for having elevated levels of resting muscle tension and being superior to tranquilizer medication, and at different levels of the skeletal muscular signal (innervation of muscle fiber, innervation of muscle spindle). This effect has been shown by others as well, with some finding the tension-reducing effect of leg cycling exercise to be specific to the soleus muscle and not to other muscle groupings like flexor carpi radialis. Furthermore, the tension-reducing effect has been shown to occur following both active and passive leg cycling exercise.

Relatively little work has tried to examine the relationship between the physiological reduction in muscle tension and self-reported tension, namely state anxiety (assessed via questionnaire). In one of the few studies, Robert Motl and Rod Dishman examined the effects of moderate intensity leg cycling on muscle tension in the soleus, reflected through the Hoffmann reflex (H-reflex; index of motor neuron excitability), and self-reported state anxiety. Further, using an interesting approach, they manipulated anxiety by having participants ingest a relatively large dose of caffeine (based on body weight) prior to exercise. Muscle tension was reduced following exercise regardless of whether caffeine or placebo was used, but self-reported anxiety was reduced only following the exercise

+ caffeine condition (exercise + placebo did not result in self-reported anxiety reduction). They also showed no significant relationship between changes in muscle tension (H-reflex) and changes in state anxiety. Finally, in an approach using the startle probe paradigm developed by Peter Lang and Margaret Bradley, the relationship between changes in facial muscle tension, specifically the musculature surrounding the eyes (corrugator superciilii), and different intensities of leg cycling exercise has been examined. An overall reduction in EMG activity followed both low- and moderate-intensity exercise compared to seated quiet rest. There was no relationship between the reductions following exercise and self-reported anxiety changes, as anxiety was reduced following both exercise and quiet rest. Self-reported anxiety reductions were largest following quiet rest and smallest following moderate-intensity cycling, but EMG reductions were largest following moderate-intensity cycling and smallest following quiet rest (exactly opposite of what would be expected if the two were related).

Clearly, more work is needed to better understand the relationship between muscle activity and affective responses, particularly with respect to exercise. Most of the work to date has focused only on self-reported anxiety, but other measures of affect related to anxiety, such as tension, tiredness, and calmness, should also be investigated. Furthermore, timing of measurements of both the physiological and psychological events is crucial to uncovering any relationship between the two, should they in fact exist.

The relationship between muscle tension (using EMG) and motor performance has also been a topic of interest in sport psychology. In an initial study in 1976, Robert Weinberg and Valerie Hunt measured self-reported anxiety and EMG activity during a task involving throwing a tennis ball at a target. Participants completed trials without feedback and then completed trials where they were given failure feedback meant to induce pressure. Participants who had higher levels of anxiety had EMG patterns reflecting longer contractions of both the biceps and triceps than those who had lower anxiety. This high-anxious pattern was interpreted as reflecting a reduction in muscular efficiency. Although it did not have negative influence on performance, the low-anxiety group did show performance improvement (greater accuracy) when given failure feedback, as it was thought that the high-anxiety group could have performed better if muscle tension had not increased under pressure. Subsequent work has essentially replicated these findings. More recent work, using golf putting as the motor task, has examined the effects of performance pressure on anxiety, effort, and EMG activity during the putt swing. Increasing pressure resulted in worsening performance (fewer putts made), increased anxiety, and increased sense of effort. Like the original Weinberg and Hunt study, the patterning of EMG activity was indicative of inefficient use of muscular energy.

Another area of sport and exercise psychology where EMG has shown promise is in the area of imagery, mental practice, or visualization. Whereas imagery has been shown to result in improved performance, the reason for this improvement has been elusive. One explanation for the improvement in physical performance following mental practice has been termed the *inflow explanation*. In essence, the inflow explanation, captured in psychoneuromuscular theory, proposes that EMG activity should be similar in patterning during imagined movements as it is during the actual movement as it activates the same motor structures as the actual movement. Dating back to Edmund Jacobson's pioneering work in the 1930s, researchers have sought to determine whether muscle activation (EMG) during imagery is similar to that obtained during the actual movement. This inflow explanation was supported in work by some, but not by others. More recent studies seem to suggest that the EMG activity seen during imagery is more an outcome of the imagery rather than what causes the imagery or its benefits.

It is actually rather surprising, given the results from studies like those presented, that the use of EMG as a physiological measure has not occurred more frequently. As measurement technology continues to improve, allowing more real-time assessments to take place, it would be worthwhile to see the extent to which some of the findings presented above can be replicated in more natural settings, both in the exercise and sport domains. Although it would certainly require background and training in psychophysiology, the yields of such research could be fruitful indeed.

Steven J. Petruzzello

See also Affective Responses to Exercise; Effort; Emotional Reactivity; Imagery; Mental Rehearsal; Psychophysiology; Relaxation

Further Readings

deVries, H. A. (1981). Tranquilizer effect of exercise: A critical review. *Physician & Sportsmedicine, 9,* 47–54.

Jacobson, E. (1932). Electrophysiology of mental activities. *American Journal of Psychology, 44,* 677–694.

Lang, P. J., Bradley, M. M., & Cuthbert, B. N. (1992). A motivational analysis of emotion: Reflex-cortex connections. *Psychological Science, 3,* 44–49.

Lutz, R. S. (2003). Covert muscle excitation is outflow from the central generation of motor imagery. *Behavioural Brain Research, 140,* 149–163.

Motl, R. W., & Dishman, R. K. (2004). Effects of acute exercise on the soleus H-reflex and self-reported anxiety after caffeine ingestion. *Physiology & Behavior, 80,* 577–585.

Weinberg, R. S. (1990). Anxiety and motor performance: Where to from here? *Anxiety Research, 2,* 227–242.

Weinberg, R. S., & Hunt, V. V. (1976). The interrelationships between anxiety, motor performance and electromyography. *Journal of Motor Behavior, 8,* 219–224.

EMOTIONAL REACTIVITY

Participants in sports and other performance settings routinely encounter emotionally salient cues or stimuli that can affect the quality and enjoyment of the activity. Given the emphasis placed on consistently performing at a high level, researchers, coaches, consultants, and practitioners have sought to better understand how athletes and other performers respond to various affective states. A myriad of factors contribute to successful performance, but emotional states directly influence motivation, attention, and movement execution. In some instances, emotional information must be attended to perform optimally. Other times, emotions precipitate internal and external distractions that should be ignored. In either case, the period of emotional reactivity following the onset of a stimulus is critical to performance. Information regarding emotional reactions and the ability to regulate them during competition is ultimately used to develop practice and performance recommendations that ensure peak performance. In this entry the focus is on reactivity; other entries in this encyclopedia address the ability to regulate emotions once they are elicited.

Emotion

Emotions are holistic phenomena, involving both subjective appraisals of affective stimuli and overt physiological changes that prepare the body to interact with the environment. While moods can be considered a general averaging of affective states over a period of time, emotions are comparatively brief reactions. By preparing the body to move, emotions motivate behaviors and actions toward desired goals and away from undesirable situations. In sport, these motivations can be to score a goal, win a championship, or avoid injury, among others. In exercise settings, emotions can motivate individuals to adhere to an exercise program, or to attain new personal records. Emotions can be self-initiated or externally generated. They can also exist in the period preceding a performance or spontaneously erupt during competition. Finally, emotional responses are influenced by situational demands and individual traits. Historically, self-report indices have been relied on to assess emotional reactivity in the sport psychology literature, but a more comprehensive assessment of emotional reactivity can be obtained through a conjunctive evaluation of three primary response systems: *subjective* feelings, *physiological* arousal, and *behavioral* indices.

Reactivity: Self-Reported Feelings

Self-reports assess an athlete's subjective feeling states prior to, during, or after competition. Although a wide array of emotions can be experienced in a performance scenario, anxiety is the most commonly measured emotion among sport and exercise psychologists. Anxiety can be measured at a dispositional (or trait level) and a competition (or state) level. The State-Trait Anxiety Inventory (STAI) is a popular general measure of trait and state anxiety. Sport specific measures of trait like the Sport Anxiety Scale-2 (SAS-2) and state anxiety like the Competitive State Anxiety Inventory-2 Revised (CSAI-2R) are also common. General and sport-specific self-reports differentiate anxiety into both somatic (bodily symptoms) and cognitive (worrying thoughts) components. For example, the CSAI-2R assesses the degree to which an athlete has bodily feelings of tension or *stomach sinking*. Additionally, athletes state how concerned or confident they are about performing well. Such questionnaires provide a more detailed individual profile of emotional reactivity. Sport

psychologists also study specific emotions, such as anger, joy, and multidimensional concepts such as passion. Self-reports are not the only method of determining emotional responses. Questionnaires are often used alongside physiological measures to quantify the relative pleasantness and motivational direction of perceived emotions with physiological changes in arousal.

Reactivity: Physiological Arousal

Emotions are psychophysiological phenomena, resulting from the interaction between environmental stimulation and neurochemical communication between sympathetic and parasympathetic divisions of the body, such as circulatory, respiratory, integumentary, nervous, and muscular. A limitation of self-report measures is that they only provide subjective perceptions of emotional arousal, and these perceptions do not always coincide with actual changes in arousal. Physiological measures of reactivity are aimed at quantifying those changes. Sport and exercise inherently increases physiological arousal, explaining why many athletes cannot accurately describe changes in their arousal due solely to emotional responses. The most common measure of physiological arousal is heart rate (HR), because of the ease of collection, measurement reliability, and being a noninvasive measure. Additional measures of physiological arousal, such as electrodermal activity (EDA), electromyography (EMG), and electroencephalography (EEG), use surface electrodes to assess changes in voltage across or under the skin. EDA and EMG measure changes in voltage related to skin conductivity or motor unit activation respectively, while EEG measures the frequency of cortical activity across the skull. EEG activity can be summed to relate changes in emotion with activation of brain areas known to involve arousal, attention, and cognitive processes. Finally, brain imaging techniques such as functional magnetic resonance imaging (fMRI) are emerging as viable methods to assess brain regions involved in emotional reactivity and regulation.

Reactivity: Behavioral Modification

Self-report and physiological measures can be used in conjunction to establish changes in arousal following an emotional experience, but behavioral responses are the most proximal predictors of overall performance. The most overt index of behavioral reactivity is how the emotional experience manifests in athletes' movements. From a movement perspective, emotions can impact how quickly we perform a task, the amount of muscle tension or cocontraction in agonist muscles, the smoothness of movement, and error from movement targets. Another behavioral index of emotional reactivity is gaze related behaviors (eye movements), which are linked to changes in attention and effort. In both sport and other performance environments, attention to the right situational information at the right time is crucial to performance. Emotions alter both preferences in the visual field and the length of visual fixations. In sports, where decisions and subsequent movements must be made in a quick and efficient manner, changes in gaze behaviors can have a significant impact on performance. Another important gaze behavior which is affected by emotion is the quiet eye period. Quiet eye is the duration between the last fixation to the target and the onset of movement. Longer quiet eye duration is associated with expertise and improved performance, but emotions have been shown to reduce this period, negatively impacting performance.

Conclusion

Emotions affect what we attend to and the way we move, which affects how well we are capable of playing sports and performing other physical activities. How we move can also impact the emotions we experience and our motivation to continue to participate in sport, exercise, and performance settings. Emotional reactions, therefore, play a critical role in sport performance and are a central focus of sport psychology interventions.

Christopher M. Janelle and Bradley Fawver

See also Affect; Affective Responses to Exercise; Basic Emotions in Sport; Emotional Responses; Emotional Schemas; Individual Response Stereotype; Stress Reactivity

Further Readings

Cottyn, J., De Clercq, D., Pannier, J.-L., Crombez, G., & Lenoir, M. (2006). The measurement of competitive anxiety during balance beam performance in gymnasts. *Journal of Sport Sciences, 24,* 157–164.

Cox, R. H., Martens, M. P., & Russell, W. D. (2003). Measuring anxiety in athletics: The Revised Competitive State Anxiety Inventory-2. *Journal of Sport & Exercise Psychology, 25,* 519–533.

Smith, R. E., Smoll, F. L., Cumming, S. P., & Grossbard, J. R. (2006). Measurement of multidimensional sport performance anxiety in children and adults: The Sport Anxiety Scale-2. *Journal of Sport & Exercise Psychology, 28,* 479–501.

Spielberger, C. D. (1983). *State-Trait Anxiety Inventory for adults sampler set: Manual, test, scoring key.* Redwood City, CA: Mind Garden.

Vickers, J. N., & Williams, A. M. (2007). Performing under pressure: The effects of physiological arousal, cognitive anxiety, and gaze control in biathlon. *Journal of Motor Behavior, 39,* 381–394.

EMOTIONAL RESPONSES

Regular leisure-time physical activity provides a boost to positive emotions: Individuals who exercise are routinely found to have lower levels of depression, anxiety, stress, and hostility. Moreover, programs of exercise have also been shown to be an effective treatment for depression, with similar findings emerging for anxiety disorders. This entry focuses on the nature of the link between exercise and emotion, explicating what is known about the range, limits, and mechanisms behind emotional responses to exercise.

Exercise Intensity and the Time Course of Emotional Responses

The positive emotional effects of exercise do not depend on high-intensity workouts. Positive mood benefits are routinely observed after moderate-intensity exercise, with benefits (reductions in negative emotions and enhancement of feelings of well-being) reported within 5 to 10 minutes of completing exercise. Positive emotional responses also follow high-intensity exercise, but may be delayed by almost a half hour. This delay in positive mood may be a product of the negative moods that are induced by higher intensity or emotionally taxing workouts so that the experience of positive mood benefits from exercise must await recovery from the negative mood induction brought by intense exertion. Indeed, one prominent determinant of negative moods during exercise is exertion beyond the ventilatory threshold—commonly reached when one has difficulty talking during exercise. Also, during exercise, more negative moods in response to feelings of physical exertion are reported by sedentary individuals, those who are more sensitive exercising in front of others (secondary to concerns that others may judge their appearance negatively), and those who tend to fear sensations of emotional arousal (termed *anxiety sensitivity*). Mood during exercise is of particular importance for the maintenance of leisure-time physical activity; negative mood emerging during exercise appears to be a powerful predictor of exercise adherence 6 and 12 months later. In short, more feelings of pleasure during exercise translate into higher rates of exercise over the longer term.

Changes in Depression

The beneficial mood effects of exercise are reliable enough that programmed exercise has emerged as a treatment for depression. Numerous clinical trials indicate that depressed psychiatric patients, as well as individuals depressed due to medical or other stressors, can successfully use exercise as a treatment. In these treatment trials, moderate exercise (frequently walking for 30 to 40 minutes) is prescribed 4 to 5 times a week. Results of this exercise can rival that for antidepressant medications when responses are evaluated after 3 to 4 months of treatment. Exercise also appears to offer benefit to depressed outpatients who have failed to respond to previous trials of antidepressant medication. As such, programs of regular exercise can be considered an empirically supported treatment for clinical depression, as well as a strategy for nonclinically depressed individuals to boost their mood.

Changes in Anxiety

As indicated by almost 50 studies, programs of moderate exercise can also significantly reduce anxiety and stress. This evidence comes from studies of adults challenged by medical conditions or other specific stressors, studies of the elderly, studies of adults in the general population, and studies of psychiatric samples. Again, in the context of well-controlled clinical trials, results of exercise programs for anxiety rival those found for antidepressant medications. A program of regular exercise has also been shown to extend the benefits offered by cognitive behavioral treatment for anxiety.

Type of Exercise and Mood Change

The question of whether the mood benefits of exercise depend on dose (frequency, intensity, duration) or exercise type (aerobic training vs. strength training) has been examined only in a handful of studies. These studies show that there is no reason to discourage people from focusing on activities such as weight training or calisthenics for mood improvement instead of pure aerobic activity. That is, while the evidence base is strong for aerobic training, such as walking, running, or biking, the studies that have compared aerobic training to strength training have tended not to find meaningful differences. Whether more is better is also not entirely clear in the case of exercise for mood and anxiety. Results of studies examining the effects of exercise on anxiety, for example, indicate that the amount of change in anxiety reaches a peak at a dose of exercise that is roughly 1.5 times higher than the public health recommendation for exercise, which is 30 minutes of moderate exercise on 5 days of the week. At doses higher than that, the anxiety reduction benefits of exercise tended to decrease.

Exercise, Brain Physiology, and Mood Changes

Exercise brings about a cascade of brain activity, with current research supporting a number of mechanisms behind the positive mood changes with exercise. Animal studies provide reliable evidence that exercise alters some of the same neurochemical systems presumed to underlie pharmacologic treatments for depression and anxiety. Specifically, exercise appears to modulate serotonergic and noradrenergic activity in the brain, with some emerging evidence for γ-aminobutyric acid (GABA) modulation as well.

Acute aerobic exercise has been shown to increase brain-derived neurotrophic factor (BDNF) levels in both healthy individuals as well as those with psychiatric disorders. BDNF is a neurotrophin involved in brain neuroplasticity, differentiation and survival of neurons in both the central and peripheral nervous system; adequate BDNF levels appear to be an important factor in the maintenance of normal cognitive function and mood. Low BDNF has been associated with depression and anxiety, and antidepressant medications tend to enhance BDNF levels. As such, BDNF is considered as having a potential role in antidepressant activity, perhaps including the antidepressant and antianxiety effects of aerobic exercise.

Although endorphin activity has been considered a correlate of the *runner's high* that may occur after prolonged exercise, at the present time there are several lines of evidence suggesting that endorphin activity does not explain the mood effects brought by moderate exercise.

Finally, atrial natriuretic peptide (ANP) is a peptide hormone that inhibits hypothalamic pituitary adrenocortical activity and may have anxiolytic properties. Importantly, submaximal and maximal exercise bouts significantly increase ANP concentrations, with early work linking these changes to anxiety reductions, raising the possibility that ANP changes may mediate some of the antianxiety effects of exercise.

Exercise to Buffer the Negative Effects of Stress on Mood and Anxiety

Among other biological and psychological processes, attention has been paid to reduced stress reactivity as an additional mental health benefit of exercise. The idea is that exercise may help individuals better modulate the kind of stressors that are so often the trigger for the development of mood and anxiety problems. Several studies have now shown that trained individuals show less physiological (e.g., heart rate, blood pressure, cortisol) and psychological (e.g., anxiety, tension, sadness) reactivity when exposed to psychological stressors as compared with their untrained counterparts. Importantly, research also shows that these protective effects are evident with single exercise sessions. That is, people tend to be less bothered by stressors when these stressors are preceded by exercise. In addition to getting protection against the development of chronic mood and anxiety problems, these observations suggest that people may notice meaningful immediate mood benefits with regular exercise.

Overexercise and Negative Mood

Although there are anecdotal reports of the emergence of depression-like conditions from overexercise in humans (and anxiety-like reactions from overexercise in rodents), there has not been systematic study of these effects. What is more certain is that strenuous exercise may lead to a plummeting mood during the exercise session, and that these mood changes may make adherence to exercise more difficult. Also, given the substantial delay between exercise and improvement in fitness or shape goals, the process of regular exercise in pursuit of weight reduction or shape improvement is a daunting enterprise. Attending to the emotional benefit brought by exercise offers exercisers a more contingent (tightly time-linked) positive outcome for their exercise efforts.

Conclusion

Evidence from a variety of sources provides justification for prescribing exercise as a mood and anxiety management strategy. The mood and anxiety benefits of exercise are apparent immediately following exercise bouts, particularly among individuals who experience significant distress. For these people in particular, exercise training programs that help them establish a habit of repeated (moderate intensity) exercise sessions every week can provide long-term mood benefits that rival those provided by established pharmacological and psychological treatments.

Michael W. Otto and Jasper A. J. Smits

See also Affective Disorders; Affective Responses to Exercise; Brain; Psychological Well-Being; Quality of Life; Resilience

Further Readings

DeBoer, L. D., Powers, M. B., Utschig, A. C., Otto, M. W., & Smits, J. A. J. (2012). Exploring exercise as an avenue for the treatment of anxiety disorders. *Expert Review of Neurotherapeutics, 12,* 1011–1022.

Ekkekakis, P., Parfitt, G., & Petruzzello, S. J. (2011). The pleasure and displeasure people feel when they exercise at different intensities: Decennial update and progress towards a tripartite rationale for exercise intensity prescription. *Sports Medicine, 41,* 641–671.

Herring, M. P., Puetz, T. W., O'Connor, P. J., & Dishman, R. K. (2012). Effect of exercise training on depressive symptoms among patients with a chronic illness: A systematic review and meta-analysis of randomized controlled trials. *Archives of Internal Medicine, 172,* 101–111.

Otto, M. W., & Smits, J. A. J. (2011). *Exercise for mood and anxiety: Proven strategies for overcoming depression and enhancing well-being.* New York: Oxford University Press.

Rimer, J., Dwan, K., Lawlor, D. A., Greig, C. A., McMurdo, M., Morley, W., et al. (2012). Exercise for depression. *Cochrane Database of Systematic Reviews, 7,* CD004366.

Wipfli, B. M., Rethorst, C. D., & Landers, D. M. (2008). The anxiolytic effects of exercise: A meta-analysis of randomized trials and dose-response analysis. *Journal of Sport & Exercise Psychology, 30,* 392–410.

EMOTIONAL SCHEMAS

Emotional feelings are fundamental aspects of human experience. In sport, emotions have powerful influences on athletes' thoughts and actions. The study and explanation of emotions in sport is difficult because there are many ongoing controversies and disagreements. Most theorists would agree, however, that emotions have motivational and regulatory functions, and that there is an interface of emotional feeling with cognitions and behavior in many adolescent and adult experiences. Psychologist Carroll E. Izard has forwarded a theory of emotion, called *differential emotion theory* (DET), which attempts to explain how emotional feelings and cognitions interact to influence the self-regulation of plans and actions. In DET, Izard proposed there are clear distinctions between basic or primary emotions and emotional schema. Basic emotions require only minimal lower order cognitions, whereas emotional schemas involve both emotional feelings and typically higher order cognitions in a dynamic interaction.

To understand emotional schema, which Izard believes involves most emotional experiences, it is necessary to briefly discuss emotional feeling of basic emotions. Basic emotions arise in infancy and are modified throughout childhood, adolescence, and adult development. These basic emotions, such as joy and happiness, sadness, anger, disgust, and fear, are thought to be principally a product of specific neural circuits in "old brain" systems (e.g., amygdala, basal ganglia, anterior cingulate cortex, and insula) that support a distinct feeling. These feeling states have distinct properties that serve to motivate behavior. Basic emotions occur primarily in infancy and are triggered rapidly and automatically by evolutionary meaningful stimuli.

Emotion schemas occur when the motivational and cue-producing emotion feeling interacts with cognitions to influence thought, actions, and sometimes other emotions. Emotion schemas may be triggered by simple or highly complex cognitive evaluation (appraisal) processes and always involve higher order cognitions, such as memories and thoughts connected to self-concept, values, and beliefs. As such, the developments of emotional schemas are highly influenced by the acquisition of language and social cognitive development.

Specific emotional feelings are associated with specific emotional schemas within a person. For example, feelings of fear activate fear-related cognitions and actions but not cognitions and actions related to joy. However, the actual thoughts and actions of an emotional schema in a particular context can vary widely across individuals because of individual differences in personality, culture, learning, and self-concept.

Emotional schemas help explain the great variety of emotional reactions seen within and across sport. Emotional feelings are often triggered by the athlete's appraisal of the personal and social meaningfulness of the situation. Although personal and social meaningfulness may be shared by athletes, there are differences among athletes even within a team because of their different social histories. The emotional feelings triggered within a particular context interact with higher order cognitions to produce plans and actions. The emotional feeling and associated emotional schemas can also trigger a cascade of physiological responses associated with the emotion process. However, the emotion schema can create a number of emotion-specific experiences that have the same core emotion feeling but have different thoughts and actions. Because of individual differences, culture, and learning, the same situation may activate an emotion feeling state in one athlete but not another. Even if the same emotion feeling is activated in two athletes, differences in higher order cognitions, such as evaluations of consequences, values, expectations, and coping options, will result in a qualitatively different emotional schema.

The complexity of emotional schemas is revealed in the example of a fear-related emotional schema in a high-performance gymnast attempting to perform a difficult routine on a balance beam. The routine involves two back flips on the beam followed by a double back somersault dismount. Years of skilled training has allowed the athlete to overcome the initial fear feeling state often associated with performing a potentially dangerous skilled action. High self-efficacy for the specific task allows the athlete to appraise the skill as challenging. However, a bad fall resulting in pain, but no serious injury, results in many of her teammates telling her of their surprise that she was not seriously hurt. She freezes upon mounting the beam the next time she attempts the routine, with the memory of the fall, pain, and comments of her teammates triggering a very rapid and automatic emotional feeling of fear. The emotional feeling is associated with high arousal and the urge to flee. The emotional feeling is quickly integrated with higher order cognitions, such as the importance of being a high-performance athlete, beliefs of overcoming fear, evaluations of skill, but also the consequences of falling and images of other gymnasts being seriously injured. These conflicting higher order emotions result in continuing experiences of fear and a less than desirable action plan. She begins the routine but bails out after the first back flip and dismounts. Successive attempts produce similar fear emotional schema, resulting in either freezing behavior or incomplete routines.

Sport-specific culture and social learning also help explain why some participants within a sport may share similar emotional schemas to a specific emotion-provoking situation. For example, some professional baseball managers emotionally react to perceived poor calls by umpires in a very sport-specific ritualistic manner, such as standing toe to toe and arguing with the umpire or kicking dirt over bases. These actions would seldom, if ever, be demonstrated by coaches in a sport like volleyball.

It is rare in the sport psychology literature to see any distinction between emotion and emotional schema. Many sport researchers have investigated joy, pride, interest, anger, anxiety, guilt, and shame but seldom examine the integration of emotional feeling and higher order cognitions. From a DET perspective, it is important to distinguish *basic emotions* from *emotion schemas*. Basic emotions typically only occur in infancy and motivate rapid actions that are in response to evolutionary defined survival situations. These emotions are of short duration and highly adaptive. After infancy, emotional experience is increasingly defined by emotion schemas. Schemas may have a brief duration or continue for a longer time course. Schema can continue through a long duration because of the role of higher order processes like reflection and rumination that continue to trigger emotional feelings. The interface of emotional feeling and higher order cognitions is critical to athlete functioning since the cognitive component is intimately part of the emotional experience and is involved in formulating plans and actions. From an applied perspective, understanding the interacting features of emotional feelings and higher order cognitions within an athlete will allow practitioners to develop effective emotional utilization and emotional self-regulation strategies.

Peter R. E. Crocker and Katie E. Gunnell

See also Affect; Basic Emotions in Sport; Self-Conscious Emotions; Stress Management

Further Readings

Izard, C. E. (2007). Basic emotions, natural kinds, emotion schemas, and a new paradigm. *Perspectives on Psychological Science, 2*, 260–279.

Izard, C. E. (2009). Emotion theory and research highlights, unanswered questions and emerging issues. *Annual Review of Psychology, 60*, 1–25.

Izard, C. E., Woodburn, E. M., Finlon, K. J., Krauthamer-Ewing, E. S., Grossman, S. R., & Seidenfeld, A. (2011). Emotion knowledge, emotion utilization, and emotion regulation. *Emotion Review, 3*, 44–52.

ENERGIZING (ACTIVATION) STRATEGIES

Energizing strategies, sometimes called activation strategies, are primarily designed to increase the task-specific level of performer's mental and physical activity. They are of interest to applied sport psychologists, coaches, and athletes alike as on occasion performers require strategies that help stimulate levels of physical and mental activity.

Arousal and Activation

Given their often interchangeable use by applied sport psychologists, it is important to distinguish between the concepts of arousal and activation. The critical distinguishing factor here rests with the unplanned (automatic) versus planned (prepared) nature of the two responses. *Arousal* is the mental and physiological response activity experienced in relation to an unexpected (or unplanned) input into the system like an unexpected shout from the crowd. *Activation* is the mental and physiological activity geared deliberately toward preparing a planned response to an anticipated situation or stimulus like the execution of the long-jump in track and field. Therefore, the focus in this entry is on activation states and, in particular, activation states that facilitate performance on a given sport task. This will differ from sport to sport and from task to task; for example, the activation state required by a golfer attempting to sink a 4-foot putt differs markedly from that required by an Olympic weight lifter in the clean and jerk. Therefore, in some instances athletes will be required to increase their state of mental and physical activation. The strategies outlined in this entry give some insight into how performers may induce such increased activated or energized states. These strategies are usually introduced to the athlete once they have become proficient at using strategies designed to lower their activation state, such as relaxation strategies.

Breathing Strategies Used to Energize and Increase Activation State

In addition to being used to relax performers, controlled breathing can also be used to increase levels of activation. Once athletes have attained a controlled, rhythmic, relaxed breathing pattern, they should be asked to consciously increase breathing rate. Inhaling, the athlete should purposefully try to imagine being more energized, whereas in exhalation, the performer should imagine that with each expired breath fatigue and wasted effort are removed. As the breathing rate is steadily increased, cue words can be used to supplement the energized breathing pattern. For example, "energy in" can be verbalized with each inhalation and "fatigue out" can be the self-statement used during exhalation.

Verbalization and Self-Talk Strategies Used to Energize and Increase Activation State

The use of self-talk strategies can provide performers with a route to increase their level of activation in a very efficient manner. Traditionally, the generation of self-talk statements involves athletes diarizing the type of words, statements, and feeling states they associate with an energized activated state. Examples of such words or statements include *explode*, *power*, *fast*, *hit*, and *psych up*. Once athletes have produced a bank of statements, they should select those they deem most applicable for use in their sport or for a particular task within their sport. The applied sport psychologist should ensure the self-talk statements adhere to the guidelines surrounding optimal use of self-talk—specifically, ensuring the statements are phonetically simple, positive in form, related to the activation state conducive to the action involved in the forthcoming task, and consistent with the energized state the performer is attempting to induce.

Imagery and Visualization Strategies Used to Energize and Increase Activation State

In order to create a more activated state, imagery content, such as imagining a particular situation in one's mind, can be manipulated to create high-impact visualizations that help alter the energized level of the performer. The athlete will require a high level of imagery ability to create these images, owing to the often fast-paced form of the imagery routines. As such, assessment and work on the imagery ability of the performer should be a prerequisite of such strategy use. To increase the activation state of the performer, the image should reflect fast moving, powerful, impactful, and energized content; examples include working machinery, animals, forces within nature, and the execution of explosive sporting movements. Where circumstances allow, the performer can be asked to develop images that show a progressive increase in an energized state in order to steadily increase the activation state—for example, a large boulder slowly gathering momentum as it falls downhill, gaining speed and energy as it begins to fall faster and faster before reaching full speed and power crashing through the obstacles in its path.

Combinations of Strategies Used to Energize and Increase Activation State

A combination of several of the strategies outlined is a useful approach to increasing activation states. Breathing strategies are often combined with self-talk statements to increase the efficacy of the energizing strategy. Imagery routines can often be supplemented with self-talk statements oriented around the content and desired activation state the performer is seeking to create. Further, the nature of the situation may shape the performer's choice of energizing strategies used. On occasion, the performer may not have time within the fast-paced, real-time environment of the sport to use an imagery routine. Instead, short, sharp, phonetically simple self-talk statements like "fast" might better suit the confines of such a situation. In comparison, an athlete who requires an increased activation state for a training routine might have the time to combine breathing, self-talk, and imagery strategies into one holistic energizing strategy.

Conclusion

The applied sport psychologist, coach, and performer all have a role to play in establishing the applicable activation state for the performer. The strategies outlined in this entry offer insights for increasing activation states. These strategies can either be used individually or combined to form a more holistic energizing program. However, research testing the efficacy of energizing strategies for the performer remains in its infancy within applied sport psychology literature. Very few studies have tested the efficacy of individual or combined activation strategies on performance. Those that have done so recommend that sports, or specific closed skill tasks within a sport that require high activation or energized states, do benefit from some form of energizing strategy. Clearly, further research is required to establish the potential performance enhancing effects of activation strategies and whether one strategy, or a specific combination of strategies, is more effective at raising the energized state of a performer over another. Therefore, the practitioner should teach the performers a range of strategies and allow them to explore which is most effective for them and their needs. As with the use of all new strategies or techniques, the performer needs to become proficient in the execution of these strategies before attempting to use them in competitive settings.

Owen Thomas and Richard Neil

See also Breathing; Imagery; Relaxation; Self-Talk; Stress Management

Further Readings

Hanton, S., Thomas, O., & Mellalieu, S. D. (2009). Management of competitive stress in elite sport. In B. W. Brewer (Ed.), *Handbook of sports medicine and science: Sport psychology* (pp. 30–42). Chichester, UK: Wiley-Blackwell.

Mellalieu, S. D., Hanton, S., & Shearer, D. A. (2008). Hearts in the fire, heads in the fridge: A qualitative investigation into the temporal patterning of precompetition psychological response in elite performers. *Journal of Sports Sciences, 26,* 854–967.

Williams, J. M. (2010). Relaxation and energizing techniques for regulation of arousal. In J. M. Williams (Ed.), *Applied sport psychology: Personal growth to peak performance* (6th ed., pp. 247–266). New York: McGraw-Hill.

ENERGY, EFFECTS OF EXERCISE ON

For more than 100 years, researchers have noted how exercise enhances the subjective sense of mental and physical energy. *Affect* refers to the quality of a subjective mental state along the dimensions of valence (pleasant or positive vs. unpleasant or negative) and activation (alert or activated vs. sleepy or deactivated). This entry will summarize research related to the effects of exercise on affective states having positive valence and moderately high levels of activation. This category of affective states describes a *sense of energy* and can be termed *positive activated affect* (PAA).

Improvements in postexercise self-reported PAA occur for activities such as walking, jogging, swimming, weight training, and tai chi, and a recent study provides some support for a causal effect of exercise on PAA. Published meta-analyses show medium effect sizes for aerobic exercise (0.47 for acute bouts and 0.57 for regular participation). Taken together, the meta-analytical results of acute and regular aerobic exercise indicate that self-reported PAA increases by about one half (.50) of a standard deviation from pre- to postexercise in participants who performed aerobic exercise (experimental groups) compared to those who did not (control groups). Quantified another way, the meta-analytical results indicate that a randomly chosen person from the population who recently finished an aerobic exercise session would be about 65% to 70% more likely to report higher PAA compared to a randomly selected non-exerciser.

Several variables influence the size of the effect of exercise (in particular aerobic exercise) on postexercise PAA. Participants with lower pre-exercise PAA often report greater postexercise PAA, a finding in line with the idea that exercise can be a self-regulatory strategy to improve energy. Low and moderate intensity exercise appears best for increasing postexercise PAA, although higher intensity exercise can improve postexercise PAA after a short delay, especially in fit individuals. Exercise sessions of 15 to 45 minutes improve PAA, but durations longer than 60 minutes may result in little improvement. PAA typically peaks within 5 minutes after exercise and remains elevated above baseline for 20 to 30 minutes. This pattern of postexercise PAA change applies to typical exercise sessions (low to moderate intensity, 15 to 60 minutes), but not to extreme bouts like marathon. The motivational state of the exerciser may be another variable that alters the effect of exercise on PAA. For example, participants with a goal-oriented motivational state during exercise will likely report lower postexercise PAA compared to participants in a less goal-oriented, more playful motivational state. A variable that does not appear to change the magnitude of the effect is the length of an exercise program. In other words, successive acute bouts simply restore postexercise PAA from previous sessions without producing an additive effect over time providing further support for exercise as a self-regulatory method to improve energy. Data from college students comprise the majority of the study results and more information is needed on community and clinical samples.

Affect during exercise is related to exercise self-efficacy, exercise history, hydration and blood glucose levels, postexercise affect, and exercise adherence. For example, higher PAA during exercise predicts exercise adherence. In line with pre-to-post exercise data, there is an inverse relationship between exercise intensity and affect during exercise. According to the dual-mode model, cognitive and physiological factors mutually influence affect during exercise, with cognitive factors prominent at lower intensities and physiological factors becoming more salient at high intensities. There is also evidence of a shift in attentional focus toward pleasant stimuli and away from unpleasant stimuli during moderate-intensity exercise. As a result of these interrelationships, PAA during exercise may provide a useful method of monitoring exercise intensity for the development of subjectively based exercise prescriptions. However, although the data show that exercise improves mental well-being including a sense of energy, most people underestimate how much they might enjoy exercising and are therefore physically inactive in part because they anticipate a lack of benefit. This is an interesting inconsistency worthy of further study.

Justy Reed

See also Adherence; Affective Responses to Exercise; Psychological Well-Being; Self-Regulation; Stress Management

Further Readings

Ekkekakis, P., Parfitt, G., & Petruzzello, S. J. (2011). The pleasure and displeasure people feel when they exercise at different intensities: Decennial update and progress towards a tripartite rationale for exercise intensity prescription. *Sports Medicine, 41*(8), 641–671.

Legrand, F. D., & Thatcher, J. (2011). Acute mood responses to a 15-minute long walking session at self-selected intensity: Effects of an experimentally-induced telic or paratelic state. *Emotion, 11*(5), 1040–1045.

Reed, J., & Buck, S. (2009). The effect of regular aerobic exercise on positive-activated affect: A meta-analysis. *Psychology of Sport and Exercise, 10*(6), 581–594.

Thayer, R. E. (1996). *The origin of every day moods: Managing energy, tension, and stress.* New York: Oxford University Press.

Wichers, M., Peeters, F., Rutten, B. P. F., Jacobs, N., Derom, C., Thiery, E., et al. (2012). A time-lagged momentary assessment study on daily life physical activity and affect. *Health Psychology, 31*(2), 135–144.

ENJOYMENT

Sport enjoyment, or *fun* in children's terms, is the most important and most studied positive emotion in youth, adolescent, and elite sport. Early youth sport research found that fun was one of the most important reasons given by athletes for choosing to participate in sports, and lack of fun was a prime explanation for dropping out. Consequently, to have fun in sports was one of the rights included in the "Bill of Rights for Young Athletes," written by a special task force established by the National Association for Sport and Physical Education. Subsequent research defines *sport enjoyment* as athletes' positive emotional response to their sport involvement that encompasses generalized feelings, such as fun, pleasure, liking, and love. Detailed in this entry are the research findings addressing two key questions. First, how does enjoyment affect athletes' motivation in sport? Second, what makes sport enjoyable? Importantly, the results presented on both of these issues characteristically generalize or apply to both genders, as well as to diverse sports and competitive levels.

How Does Enjoyment Affect Athletes' Motivation in Sport?

Sport enjoyment has important motivational consequences and is incorporated into many theories dealing with athletes' participation, persistence, and exertion of effort in their sport. Findings show that the higher the enjoyment experienced, the more athletes elect to participate and persist in their sport, the more they feel the desire to exert greater effort and perceive that they actually have expended more effort, and the higher their *enthusiastic sport commitment*. Enthusiastic sport commitment is a psychological state defined as athletes' enduring determination and desire to continue participating in their sport. Research focused on the sport commitment model, elaborated elsewhere in this encyclopedia, shows that sport enjoyment is the strongest and most consistent predictor of commitment to sport.

What Makes Sport Enjoyable?

Knowing that enjoyment is so crucial to positive motivation makes it important to understand what makes sport enjoyable. Knowledge of the sources of enjoyment not only allows for a more comprehensive understanding of emotion and motivation in sport from a research perspective, but it also tells us the ways to make sport enjoyable for athletes from an applied point of view. In effect, the sources of enjoyment are the buttons that can be pushed to create the enjoyment that kindles positive motivation. Extensive study reveals that there are many potential sources of enjoyment inherent in sport and that they are diverse.

Sources of enjoyment fall under three broad categories: *intrapersonal sources* that emanate from the person; *situational sources* that are inherent to the sport context; and *significant other sources* that are influences from important people to the athlete such as parents, coaches, and teammates. Specific examples of sources of enjoyment will be presented under these three classifications.

Intrapersonal Enjoyment Sources

Athletes' perceptions of high personal competence in their sport, and a number of achievement factors related to these ability perceptions, make sport enjoyable. These sources reflect the positive processes and outcomes of engaging in mastery—including exerting effort, learning, practicing, improving, and perfecting challenging athletic skills—and achieving mastery of these skills.

Athletes' own motivational goal orientation is also a source of enjoyment. Greater enjoyment is experienced by high-task-oriented athletes who define success in a self-referenced manner with criteria like successful skill mastery and high effort expenditure.

Personal movement experiences emanating from the movement and execution of sport skills are enjoyable. These sources include feeling athletic; experiencing movement sensations, such as freedom and exhilaration; and being able to creatively express one's self through movement.

Situational Enjoyment Sources

Both the process and outcomes of competition are sources of enjoyment. In terms of process, enjoyment is experienced from engaging in competition and comparing one's skill against a competitor. Winning a game and having a winning season are enjoyable outcomes.

Receiving recognition from other people for successful performance is also enjoyable. This recognition includes such specific sources as being in the newspaper, yearbook, or record books of one's sport and receiving medals, trophies, and standing ovations.

Significant Other Enjoyment Sources

There are two sets of significant other sources of enjoyment: those that come from adults, and those that stem from teammates. With respect to parental and coach sources, enjoyment is experienced when athletes perceive that these adults are supportive and highly involved in their sport experience, and are satisfied with their performance. Elite athletes find it enjoyable to bring pleasure and pride to these adults through demonstrating their talent. Sources specific to parents involve athlete perceptions of realistic parental performance expectations and lack of pressure to participate in sport. Finally, sources of enjoyment come from being on a team with peers, including positive interactions with teammates, building friendships, and supporting each other. And so we see that there are numerous and many different types of sources or buttons that can be pushed in sport to create the enjoyment that increases and maintains positive motivation.

Tara K. Scanlan, Graig M. Chow,
and Lawrence A. Scanlan

See also Affect; Basic Emotions in Sport; Commitment; Emotional Responses; Passion

Further Readings

Martens, R., & Seefeldt, V. (Eds.). (1979). *Guidelines for children's sports*. Washington, DC: American Alliance for Health, Physical Education, Recreation and Dance.

Scanlan, T. K., Babkes, M. L., & Scanlan, L. A. (2005). Participation in sport: A developmental glimpse at emotion. In J. L. Mahoney, R. W. Larson, & J. S. Eccles (Eds.), *Organized activities as contexts of development: Extracurricular activities, after-school and community programs* (pp. 275–309). Mahwah, NJ: Lawrence Erlbaum.

Scanlan, T. K., Russell, D. G., Magyar, T. M., & Scanlan, L. A. (2009). Project on elite athlete commitment (PEAK): III. An examination of the external validity across gender, and the expansion and clarification of the sport commitment model. *Journal of Sport & Exercise Psychology, 31,* 685–705.

ENJOYMENT, AS MEDIATOR OF EXERCISE BEHAVIOR CHANGE

To enjoy means to take pleasure or satisfaction from something; *enjoyment* is the act or condition of enjoying. Thus, enjoyment of physical activity is the act or condition of taking pleasure or satisfaction from physical activity. This entry discusses the conceptualization and assessment of enjoyment, as well as the role of enjoyment as a predictor of physical activity behavior and a mediator of the effects of physical activity promotion interventions on adherence to physical activity programs.

Enjoyment is a broad concept encompassing both pleasure and satisfaction. Pleasure is typically conceptualized as the subjective experience of positive hedonic tone and can occur in the absence of higher cognitive processing regarding the meaning of a stimulus—in this case, physical activity. Satisfaction occurs following the fulfillment of a need or goal and thus, relative to pleasure, typically entails more cognitive mediation to ascertain the meaning of the triggering stimulus. Thus, one may report enjoyment of physical activity like a walk in the park because of the immediate pleasure experienced during the activity or because of thoughts about having accomplished one's daily physical activity or how it might benefit health.

In research on physical activity enjoyment, the concept is most often assessed by the Physical Activity Enjoyment Scale (PACES) developed by Deborah Kendzierski and Kenneth J. DeCarlo. The PACES includes 18 semantic differential items, which require respondents to select a point along a 7-point continuum between two opposite descriptors relevant to enjoyment of physical activity (e.g., I enjoy it . . . I hate it; I dislike it . . . I like it; I find it pleasurable . . . I find it unpleasurable). While separate measures have been used to independently assess pleasure and satisfaction in response to physical activity, the PACES remains the most popular measure of the global concept of enjoyment.

Enjoyment of physical activity, as measured by the PACES, is a robust correlate and predictor of physical activity behavior in youth, as well as younger and older adults. This correlation between physical activity enjoyment and physical activity behavior simply means that people who enjoy physical activity are more likely to engage in it.

Considerably less research has examined whether enjoyment of physical activity can act as a mediator between physical activity promotion interventions and increases in physical activity behavior. That is, few studies have examined the effects of public health interventions on people's enjoyment of physical activity, and, in turn, increases in physical activity behavior. Thus, it remains unclear as to whether enjoyment of physical activity is malleable through intervention or whether certain people are—because of biological predispositions or early childhood experiences—more likely to enjoy physical activity and more likely to engage in it. More research is needed to investigate whether, how, when, and for whom physical activity enjoyment can be increased through public health interventions or individual efforts.

David M. Williams

See also Affect; Affective Responses to Exercise; Basic Emotions in Sport; Emotional Responses; Hedonic Theory; Intrinsic/Extrinsic Motivation, Hierarchical Model of; Models of Emotion–Performance; Pleasure

Further Readings

Kendzierski, D., & DeCarlo, K. J. (1991). Physical activity enjoyment scale: Two validation studies. *Journal of Sport & Exercise Psychology, 13,* 50–64.

Mullen, S. P., Olson, E. A., Phillips, S. M., Szabo, A. N., Wójcicki, T. R., Mailey, E. L., et al. (2011). Measuring enjoyment of physical activity in older adults: Invariance of the physical activity enjoyment scale (paces) across groups and time. *International Journal of Behavioral Nutrition and Physical Activity, 8,* 103.

Rhodes, R. E., Fiala, B., & Conner, M. (2009). A review and meta-analysis of affective judgments and physical activity in adult populations. *Annals of Behavioral Medicine, 38,* 180–204.

ERRORS

Biological organisms cannot repeat a movement exactly the same way across practice trials or attempts. In other words, there is an inherent amount of imprecision in the motor systems of animals, including humans. This variability can be considered a source of error. Second, in any attempt to solve a new motor problem, whether a young athlete pole vaulting or a dog attempting to catch a tennis ball for the first time, there is inaccuracy—in other words, error—as the organism figures out how to solve these motor problems.

Definition and Measurement

Error is defined as the difference between an observable behavior and a desired behavior. More formally, error is the difference between an observed score and a desired score, called a target:

$$e_i = X_i - T$$

where e is the error, X is the score on trial i, and T is the target score. Traditionally error has been classified as bias, precision, and accuracy.

Bias means that a set of scores tends to produce either a negative or a positive error. Bias is also called *algebraic error*, as it has a magnitude and a direction (positive or negative) on each and every trial. The average algebraic error, or bias, over a series of trials has been called *constant error*.

Precision is a measure of response consistency. In other words, does the individual perform identically every time? *Variability* is the usual measure of imprecision. Variability is considered the average distance a set of scores is from the mean score. Typically, the measure of precision is just the standard deviation of the set of scores. Thus, a smaller standard deviation means an increase in consistency (precision) compared to a larger standard deviation. Historically, *variable error* is the name of this error score.

Accuracy, the most commonly used and important measure of error, is defined as the average *distance* a set of scores is from a target value. Traditionally, *absolute error,* defined as the average absolute difference (computed on a trial by trial basis, and then averaged) between a score and a target, was the accuracy measure of choice. Absolute error has several statistical issues that have resulted in researchers abandoning this measure. A much better measure of accuracy is root mean squared error (RMSE). This measure uses the one-dimensional distance formula and then takes the average of the set of distances. RMSE is a combination of bias and variability.

So far in this discussion of error, we have focused on measuring performance as the outcome of a single trial and then describing the average of a set of trials. In other words, these measures are *outcome* scores. Error also can be used to capture the *process* of movement. The movement of the effector over time (a trajectory) provides a rich source of information concerning the underlying movement control processes. For example, a movement trajectory can be compared to an ideal movement trajectory and deviations from the ideal would be considered an error. The standard measure of error for a continuous trajectory is RMSE. The error is summed up across samples across a single trajectory. The larger the RMSE, the less *accurate* the trajectory is to the template or standard.

The trajectory RMSE measure can be slightly altered to ask an important theoretical question in motor control. Are trajectories scalable in space and time? In other words, does the production of a skilled action show evidence for an ideal template that might exhibit spatial variability and temporal variability, while the movement appears to be derived from a common invariant trajectory? In speech motor control, Anne Smith, Lisa Goffman, Howard Zelaznik, Goangshiuan Ying, and Clare McGillem developed a measure known as the *spatial–temporal index* (STI). First, the trajectory time base is changed to a percentage. Therefore, all movements have a temporal scale from 0 to 100. Second, the displacement values are placed on a normal scale (they usually range from –1.5 to +1.5). At each 2-percentage interval, the standard deviation of the normalized displacements is computed. The 50 standard deviations are either summed or averaged. The STI captures how closely a set of trajectories follows the average spatial–temporal trajectory. The average normalized trajectory purportedly represents the invariant template. The STI measure does not make any theoretical statements about the cause of any spatial–temporal invariance. The measure has been shown to capture development of speech motor patterns and the effects of practice on speech learning. Although the assumptions of linear scaling might not be fully justified, the measure appears to be fairly robust in spite of these issues.

The Value of Errors

The previous section presented the descriptive aspects of error. Now, attention is focused on whether errors are good, bad, or indifferent. Obviously, at high levels of performance errors generally are considered *bad*. Missing the putt to lose the championship is not a good thing. In competition, errors might seem to always be bad. But, that clearly does not have to be the case. A good baseball pitcher deliberately may throw a bad pitch so that the batter might swing and miss, or the batter might be expecting a pitch in the future series of pitches. Is home plate the target on every pitch? No! Thus, errors in pitching are difficult to measure. However, errors in pitching can be measured in practice. The target changes, but during the game, error in pitching can only be measured if we know the goal of the pitcher.

What about errors during practice? For high-level performers errors might be necessary for an expert to figure out the nuances of a difficult task. For example, when concert pianists need to learn a new fingering sequence, they experiment with the best method to get it done. In other words, they are making deliberate errors to help them search for the solution to this new problem. New learners need and use errors to guide the learning process. James A. Adams, one of the first, if not the first, to propose a major role of errors in learning, believed that errors provided motivation and information that learners use to change their attempt on the next trial. Ann Gentile, although not explicit on this matter, believes that learning is a search process. The learner is attempting to find a reasonable solution to the motor learning problem. She calls this *getting the idea* of the movement. After this approximate solution, the learning then works at refining the solution. One can define getting the idea when the learner is consistently producing an acceptable level of error and then moves to a deliberate attempt to reduce error. What would be the consequences of a performer not being able to control and produce error? One would be an inflexible robot. Errors provide the flexibility for individuals to respond to their environment.

Human beings would not be functional if they only possessed fixed action patterns, such as stereotypical reflexes.

Errors also are organized. Robert Sessions Woodworth in 1899, Paul M. Fitts in 1954, and more recently Richard A. Schmidt, Howard Zelaznik, Brian Hawkins, James S. Frank, and John T. Quinn in 1979 described this organization. The organization is called the speed-accuracy trade-off. With some exceptions the cost of increasing movement speed (decreasing duration, increasing distance, or the combination of the two) is a decrease in movement accuracy in the spatial dimension. Home run hitters tend to strike out more often than singles hitters. Why? A home run in baseball requires increased bat speed. The cost of that increase is paid in the currency of an increase in spatial variability. There is a clear exception to this speed–accuracy trade-off in the temporal domain. Temporal variability decreases as the timed interval decreases (in other words, doing the task faster). Therefore, in tasks that require both spatial as well as temporal accuracy performers need to learn the optimal movement speed to minimize spatial error but maximize temporal accuracy.

What is the source of error and variability? One way to view errors and variability in performance is via the classic view of test theory. A performance score is composed of two components, the *true* score and a source of random variations called an *error*. The true score represents the mean of an infinite number of trials. In other words, the true score is a construct, and thus it represents the individual's level of performance.

Recently, scholars in motor behavior have begun to discover that error over a series of trials does have a random component. However, error also has a predictive component. In other words, a performance score in series predicts a performance score in later in the time series. These relations are called *long-term correlations,* and are thought to be the results of the underlying nonlinear dynamics of human performance. These long-term correlations are shown in fluctuations of step–cycle duration, reaction time, and cycle duration in repetitive timing tasks. There are some very exciting hints that these long-term fluctuations are crucial to healthy behavior, and the lack of these correlations might be the signature of diseased states. Fluctuations, which are not random, but structured, are a reliable signature of normal biological function.

The observation that errors have a nonrandom component might be the reason for the success of sport psychologists working with high-level performers. Obviously if errors in performance were solely random, the only way to improve performance would be to dramatically increase the amount of deliberate practice. However, most high-level performers already practice many hours per day. If performers acquire techniques to control the nonrandom component of performance fluctuations, performance will improve.

Howard Zelaznik

See also Coordination; Motor Commands; Motor Control; Motor Learning; Sensorimotor Representations; Skill Acquisition

Further Readings

Adams, J. A. (1971). A closed loop theory of motor learning. *Journal of Motor Behavior, 3,* 111–150.

Fitts, P. M. (1954). The information capacity of the human motor system in controlling the amplitude of movement. *Journal of Experimental Psychology, 47,* 381–391.

Gentile, A. (1972). A working model of skill acquisition with application to teaching. *Quest, 17,* 3–23.

Schmidt, R. A., Zelaznik, H. N., Hawkins, B., Frank, J. S., & Quinn, J. T. J. (1979). Motor-output variability: A theory for the accuracy of rapid motor acts. *Psychological Review, 86,* 415–451.

Schutz, R. W., & Roy, E. A. (1973). Absolute error—devil in disguise. *Journal of Motor Behavior, 5,* 141–153.

Smith, A., Goffman, L., Zelaznik, H. N., Ying, G. S., & McGillem, C. (1995). Spatiotemporal stability and patterning of speech movement sequences. *Experimental Brain Research, 104,* 493–501.

Woodworth, R. S. (1899). The accuracy of voluntary movement. *Psychological Review, 3,* 1–114.

ESPECIAL SKILLS

An *especial skill* is a unique case where one very specific variation of a motor skill exhibits a markedly superior task performance in comparison to performances on all other variations within the same skill class. This effect has been clearly demonstrated with basketball set shots from the regulation free-throw (foul) line, as well as with baseball pitches over the regulation pitching distance. To illustrate, as one moves closer to or farther from the basketball goal there is typically a consistent change in the percentage of shots made, with accuracy decreasing linearly as the distance to the target is increased. However, for highly practiced players, the shooting percentage is significantly better than expected at exactly 15 feet (4.57 meters) straight out from the basket—precisely at the foul line. It is reasoned that the especial skill effect emerges due to the massive amount of practice at that one variation of the skill relative to any other variant. The free-throw line is the only distance from which basketball players regularly and consistently practice set shots. This phenomenon is an example of the specificity principle of practice taking precedence over the generality principle of motor skill development. It is of particular interest because no current theories of motor control have been able to satisfactorily explain the intricacies of the especial skill phenomenon.

Specificity and Generality of Motor Skills

The notion of specificity of training in motor skill learning and performance is well established. The more that conditions of the performance task match those that were present during practice, the greater the transfer of benefits from training to test performance. The same shot from the same distance, with the same ball, under the same environmental conditions would be a classic example. The more those conditions are dissimilar, the less transfer is seen from training to test performance. It is reasoned that repeated training of the same skill under the same conditions builds up a strong memory representation for the correct motor action. Such a representation would be at best only partially correct if any condition for performing the skill was changed.

Specificity, therefore, poses theoretical problems because it would be essentially impossible for even an expert to practice every possible variation that they might encounter during motor skill challenges. Under most normal situations, every motor skill execution is subject to differing sensorimotor, contextual, or processing demands. To explain flexibility in performance, theories of generality (most prominently, Schmidt's schema theory of motor skill learning) suggest that performers build up general representations for each class of movement skill. Through practice the skill is increasingly capable of being altered to match the demands of the task at any particular moment. The performer learns the common coordination pattern for the skill class, and then learns the rules by which forces and timing might be adjusted to create the skilled action for that situation. As the performer adds experience and practice, improvement is seen across the whole skill class. General motor program concepts can be used to explain, for example, how a basketball player can be accurate at jump shots from any one of numerous court positions under continuously changing dynamics of game play.

The most interesting feature of especial skills is that they seem to be an example of specificity emerging within a landscape of generality. All basketball players can shoot set shots (a shot where the feet do not leave the ground) with a general level of accuracy commensurate with their experience and the physical difficulty of the shot. All baseball pitchers can throw a straight fast-ball-style throw to a target of varying distances, again with accuracy varying according to experience and the physical demands of the throw. When the range of those variations is examined for patterns, theories of generality accurately account for performance outcomes. However, in the particular instance of a case that is special to that sport—the one that is practiced far beyond all others—the principle of specificity appears to take precedence.

Explanations

Several theoretical explanations have been offered for the especial skill effect. The *visual context hypothesis* posits that certain consistent visual information, such as the particular angle of viewing, may enhance perception–action coordination under the one special condition. This concept received some support from research showing that 15-foot set shots at angles different than straight out from the basket did not produce the effect. However, other studies where the visual context was significantly altered have nonetheless demonstrated especial skills. The *learned parameters explanation* suggests that repeated practice of one variation of a skill leads to optimization of movement parameters, such as force, speed, or release angle, for that specific instance. This hypothesis has received some research support when weight of the ball was altered, but not supported in other research when the ball and distance were constant but changing the visual angle eliminated the

effect (different viewpoint, but identical movement parameters). Another hypothesis is that experienced performers might develop a special general motor program used solely for the one massively practiced variation of the task. Hypothetically, this would be evidenced by kinematic information (relative angles, velocities, or accelerations of the involved joints and limbs) that shows unique coordination patterns for the especial skill in comparison to those common to the rest of the skill class. Yet, such kinematic analysis has failed to support this explanation with basketball shooting. Lastly, it has been suggested that the phenomenon might be simply a matter of confidence, rather than some difference in motor control per se. However, research has shown measures of performance efficacy to vary independently of the especial skill effect. In fact, such psychological measures call into question any cognitive (conscious processing) explanations. In sum, the phenomenon has yet to receive a fully satisfactory theoretical explanation.

Conclusion

The especial skill effect is interesting because it reflects high levels of practice or expertise, it may serve as a marker in the development of motor skill expertise, and it may highlight noncognitive aspects of human motor control.

Jeffery P. Simons

See also Expertise; Generalized Motor Program; Laws of Movement Learning and Control; Transfer

Further Readings

Breslin, G., Hodges, N. J., Kennedy, R., Hanlon, M., & Williams, A. M. (2010). An especial skill: Support for a learned parameters hypothesis. *Acta Psychologica, 134,* 55–60.

Keetch, K. M., Lee, T. D., & Schmidt, R. A. (2008). Especial skills: Specificity embedded within generality. *Journal of Sport & Exercise Psychology, 30*(6), 723–736.

Keetch, K. M., Schmidt, R. A., Lee, T. D., & Young, D. E. (2005). Especial skills: Their emergence with massive amounts of practice. *Journal of Experimental Psychology: Human Perception and Performance, 31,* 970–978.

Simons, J. P., Wilson, J., Wilson, G., & Theall, S. (2009). Challenges to cognitive bases for an especial motor skill at the regulation baseball pitching distance. *Research Quarterly for Exercise and Sport, 80*(3), 469–479.

ETHICS

Ethics is the investigation of the primary moral assumptions held by individuals, organizations, or professions that are used to help members make sound decisions about what is right and wrong. To expand on this definition, ethics refers to an organization's attempts to protect the welfare of clients by developing, adopting, and enforcing guidelines that regulate member conduct in professional and scientific settings. These ethical guidelines are essentially a set of values that have been agreed upon by the members of an organization or profession. By developing ethical guidelines, the organization or profession is protecting the welfare of those they serve but also communicating their values to society. Ethics in sport psychology have been an area of concern, as the discipline grows in research, education, and practice. While psychologists are encouraged to behave in socially acceptable ways within their personal lives, the ethics codes are only designed to govern their actions in professional settings (research, education, and practice) in their work as psychologists.

Many consistencies exist in the codes of ethics between general psychology and the field of sport and exercise psychology. In fact, as a subset of psychology, many of the sport and exercise psychology codes of ethics are closely based upon those previously written in psychology.

Ethical practice can be considered to be the *coin of the realm* for psychology and sport and exercise psychology practitioners. It is through ethical behavior that professionals take steps to protect their clients from harm. Ethical guidelines of ethical behavior are aimed at helping practitioners make decisions in difficult situations that could prove to be harmful to the client or related person.

Components of Codes of Ethics

It is common for ethical codes to have several sections to them, each serving its own purpose. These sections often include an introduction, preamble, principles, and standards. The purpose of an introduction is to discuss issues such as the intent of the code of ethics, as well as to provide procedural and organizational clarity about the codes and their use. The purpose of a preamble is to outline the value structure of the organization and to encourage practitioners to meet the highest possible ideals set by the organization and outlined within the code.

Principles are commonly seen as general statements about the codes of ethics that give background context into the rationale for the development of the specific standards and guide practitioners toward the highest ideals for practice. In essence, the principles are aspiration and unenforceable value-driven statements designed to provide guidance to individuals who are faced with ethical decisions. While principles may change from ethics code to ethics code, the most common psychology based principles involve such things as

- Do no harm (nonmaleficence)
- Help others (beneficence)
- Respect and promote autonomy
- Treat others fairly and equitably
- Be trustworthy
- Respect dignity

Ethical standards are the enforceable and more specific portion of the ethics code. These aim to influence the conduct of psychologists in professional settings. While ethical standards are more specific than principles in terms of directing behavior, they are often written somewhat broadly to help psychologists make difficult decisions across a broad array of situations. Because of the many different settings in which psychologists practice, general standards help them make difficult decisions which vary in their working.

Role of Ethics Codes

Students and professionals generally understand and appreciate the usefulness of codes of ethics, but that is not always sufficient to keep individuals behaving ethically. To consistently behave in an ethical manner requires practitioners to possess a number of skills and attributes. While knowledge of and familiarity with the appropriate codes of ethics and a sincere desire to act ethically are a good starting point to help people behave ethically, this step in and of itself is not enough to ensure that professionals will behave ethically when faced with challenging and complicated scenarios. Other factors that help practitioners behave ethically include the following:

- Being able to recognize when challenging ethical situations arise

- Having and using maturity, judgment, discretion, and wisdom in one's decision making
- Understanding the competing influences affecting one's judgment
- Thoroughly considering the consequences of one's actions
- Having a clear understanding of the principles behind the code and using them during the decision-making process
- Understanding and utilizing problem-solving models
- Developing and using a professional consultation network

Important Ethical Issues in Sport and Exercise Psychology

While many codes of ethics for sport and exercise psychology organizations may closely resemble codes of ethics from general psychology organizations, differences do exist. These differences, some stated and some implied, are important to consider, as they are often created or maintained to help deal with the unique field and setting of competitive sport. Further, there are many ethical situations or dilemmas that are unique to specific sport and exercise psychology settings.

Confidentiality

Confidentiality is probably the most commonly cited ethical concern within the field of sport and exercise psychology and is commonly identified as the most important ethical standard. Confidentiality relates to practitioners not allowing others to know their client's identity, as well as not letting others know the client's concerns or related treatment. There are some common limits to the confidentiality that are commonly addressed with a client at the beginning of the service delivery via a consent form.

While confidentiality is important in sport and exercise psychology, the guidelines by which it is judged are different from those in traditional psychology. Because of their high-profile status on campus and in the community, athletes are often more identifiable than other individuals when they enter an office. Further, because of their time commitments, travel schedules, and performance requirements, it is not uncommon for a practitioner to work with a client out in the open where others can see them talking with each other. This may happen on a pool deck, in a gym, or on the side of a field. Under these circumstances, the goal changes from not allowing others to know that the practitioner is working with a client to not allowing others to know what is being said.

Multiple Roles

A multiple-role relationship can be described as having a professional relationship with a client and at the same time interacting with the client or a close friend or family member of the client in another role. Multiple-role relationships are not necessarily unethical if handled properly. However, practitioners should avoid entering into multiple-role relationships that could cause harm to the consulting process by affecting objectivity or causing exploitation. If a multiple-role relationship is entered into, the consultant needs to be mindful of the potential problems and be willing to stop the consultation process if any are perceived.

Multiple-role relationships may be more common within the field of sport and psychology than in the general psychology. This may be due to the limited number of sport and exercise psychology practitioners. For instance, on many college campuses, sport and exercise psychology professionals often serve in other roles. A practitioner may consult with individuals and teams as well as teach classes and advise students. With such a multitude of responsibilities, practitioners are likely to have contact with clients in more than one setting. Therefore, it is essential that practitioners discuss possible multiple-role relationships with athletes at the outset of services.

Competency

The ethical issue of competency relates to the necessity for practitioners to practice only in areas and with people whom they have the requisite knowledge, skills, and abilities to provide quality services. To be viewed as competent, an individual must understand the domain-specific issues, demonstrate skills for interventions, and be able to assess their outcomes. Common forms of competence include (a) intellectual competence, which is gained from formal education; (b) emotional competence—the ability to emotionally deal with clients and limit personal biases; and (c) experiential competence or the wisdom gained from previous professional experiences.

It is difficult to identify the distinction between competence and incompetence with a given client or presenting concern. For the most part, competence is determined by ones knowledge and experience that is generated through education, training, supervised experience, and professional experience. However, competence does not last forever, and to remain competent in a particular area, practitioners must update their knowledge through continuing education, consultation, study, or additional education.

Individuals who are licensed psychologists, but receive little training in the sport sciences, must take steps to gain the sport science training necessary to understand the athletic context. Sports science trained practitioners who are not licensed need to understand the limitations of their training and their inability to provide therapy to clients. It is essential that practitioners understand their training and only provide services that are in line with their competency.

Teletherapy

Teletherapy can be described as the use of technology to deliver services to clients from a distance. Teletherapy services can be delivered asynchronously via text or e-mail platforms but can also be delivered synchronously via phone and video conferencing platforms. There are both strengths (e.g., service availability for remote, disabled and traveling clients; cost effectiveness; access to self-help resources; client disclosure and anonymity) and limitations (e.g., concerns about confidentiality, relationship development, limited accessibility, credentialing across state and provincial lines) to the use of teletherapy.

Clients are some of the primary driving forces behind the use of teletherapy. Because of their age, comfort level with technology, busy training schedules, and constant travel, athletes often feel comfortable with the use of technology in their consultation sessions. However, practitioners need to be aware of several issues before agreeing to provide teletherapy services: (1) legal issues for those who provide psychological services across state, provincial, or national lines; (2) malpractice insurance for such services; (3) personal competency in the use of technology; (4) maintenance of confidentiality; and (5) appropriateness of teletherapy for client's presenting concern.

Overidentification

Sports are often perceived by people and the public at large as very prestigious, and thus many wish to be associated with it. As such, it is not uncommon for individuals with only a peripheral connection to teams, to identify themselves closely with those teams. This is also true of practitioners who consult with teams. While overidentification with a team does not always cause problems, it has the potential to cause bias and the loss of objectivity in the practitioner.

Identifying the Client

An ethical situation that commonly occurs in sport and exercise psychology is the identification of the client (Who is the client?). In an athletic setting, one may question if the client is the athlete who has been referred for help, the coach, or the athletic department who is paying for the services. While this answer may seem simple, it becomes less clear when the practitioner is employed by the athletic department. In such cases, employees of the athletic department may question how much information they have a right to know. Such situations arise more often when the practitioner is an employee of a referring agency or is receiving payment from a third party.

Ethical Decision Making

The principles and standards identified within an organization's code of ethics are intended to support and guide professionals in the process of making ethical decisions. However, making sound ethical decisions can be complicated since ethical principles and standards oftentimes contain gaps, contradictions, and grey areas because of the multiple considerations that must be addressed. To help combat these concerns, ethical decision-making models can serve as a practical framework that professionals can use to resolve these situations.

Theoretical perspectives serve as the foundation for ethical conduct in each of us and influence how we interpret situations and potential outcomes, as well as how we use the decision-making models.

Teleology

Teleology is an ends-oriented approach that evaluates actions based upon the consequences of those actions, regardless of the intended consequences or the means used to achieve those ends. From this perspective, actions that lead to the most good for the most number of people are deemed to be ethical, with the opposite being perceived as unethical. Teleology can be viewed from both an act and a rule perspective. *Act-Utilitarianism* is a perspective that focuses on the ends, achieving the greatest good for the most people, with no regard for the means of achieving this result. *Rule-Utilitarianism* is a perspective that encourages focusing on the ends, while following previously established rules to achieve those ends.

Deontology

Deontology can be defined as a means or principled approach to ethical decision making. From this perspective, behaviors are evaluated as ethical or unethical based upon the intentions and quality of the actions rather than the outcomes produced by those actions. From this perspective, ethical behavior should be grounded in principles that would be applicable in different settings.

Models of Ethical Decision Making

While there are similarities and differences to each decision making, there are components to them that are consistent. Ethical decision-making models often include the following suggestions or steps:

- Identify and prioritize the relevant ethical issues, practices, and values.
- Identify the people affected by this situation.
- Identify the relevant ethical principles and cultural issues underlying the situation.
- Consult with other professionals about the situation.
- Identify personal factors that may distort ones perspective of the situation.
- Brainstorm alternative courses of action.
- Analyze the short- and long-term risks and benefits of each course of action.
- Choose a course of action and inform the stakeholders of the decision.
- Act on the situation and assume responsibility for the consequences.
- Evaluate the results and make changes if necessary.
- Document decisions and the decision-making process.

Common Factors That Influence Ethical Decision Making

When making ethical decisions, it is important for practitioners to understand and take into consideration the environmental influences that may affect their decisions. Ethical decisions do not happen in vacuums, and making decisions without taking external influences into consideration may risk these factors unconsciously influencing one's decisions. The primary environmental factors influencing professionals in sport and exercise psychology are likely (1) individual influences, such as moral and cognitive development and world view; (2) situational influences like the culture related to this issue in one's workplace; (3) external influences, such as politics, economy, social issues; and (4) significant other influences, such as how will others perceive one's decisions and how have they influenced one's beliefs about this situation.

Jack C. Watson

See also Character Development; Consultant Effectiveness, Assessment of; Moral Development; Moral Reasoning; Training, Professional

Further Readings

American Psychological Association. (2010). *Ethical principles of psychologists and code of conduct: Including 2010 amendments.* Retrieved from http://www.apa.org/ethics/code/index.aspx

Aoyagi, M. W., & Portenga, S. T. (2010). The role of positive ethics and virtues in the context of sport and performance psychology service delivery. *Professional Psychology: Research and Practice, 41,* 253–259.

Association for Applied Sport Psychology. (1994). *Ethics code: AASP ethical principles and standards.* Retrieved from http://www.appliedsportpsych.org/about/ethics/code

Etzel, E., & Watson, J. C., II. (2007). Ethical challenges for psychological consultants in intercollegiate athletics. *Journal of Clinical Sport Psychology, 1,* 304–317.

Etzel, E., Watson, J. C., II, & Zizzi, S. (2004). A web based survey of AAASP member ethical beliefs and behaviors in the new millennium. *Journal of Applied Sport Psychology, 16,* 236–250.

Stapleton, A. B., Hankes, D. M., Hays, K. F., & Parham, W. D. (2010). Ethical dilemmas in sport psychology: A dialogue on the unique aspects impacting practice. *Professional Psychology: Research and Practice, 41,* 143–152.

ETHNICITY

Ethnicity refers to shared cultural traditions and history of a group or population. The collection of people who share an ethnicity is often called an *ethnic group*. An ethnic group shares a common culture that is reflected in language or dialect, religion, customs, clothing, food, and music, literature, or art. Ethnic groups are often associated with nationality, geographic region, or country of origin. For example, in the United States, African Americans, Italian Americans, and Mexican Americans are examples of ethnic groups. Other countries would have different ethnic groups, based on different cultural traditions, such as religion or language.

The term *race* and *ethnicity* are often confused, but these terms are not identical. Race is based on meanings given to biological features, particularly skin color, as well as other physical traits as hair and eyes. Ethnicity is based on a shared culture and claimed identity associated with a sense of belonging and pride. As scholars have noted, ethnicity and race are dynamic, historically derived and institutionalized ideas and practices.

Economic power tends to be unequally distributed among ethnic groups. The dominant ethnic groups have power, also termed *privilege*, whereas nondominant groups often experience oppression or discrimination. Power—or the ability to get what one wants—is held by the majority group when they establish a system based on their own cultural values. Less powerful groups, such as ethnic minorities, occupy a lower status in society because of power relations.

Ethnicity is important in sport and exercise psychology because it impacts sport and physical activity patterns. Sport participation among ethnic groups varies by group, tradition, and rituals. In general, ethnic minorities have experienced a long history of being excluded from participation and leadership from organized sport, competition, and physical activity programs. Today, a few popular sports have a higher percentage of ethnic minorities, but in many sports, ethnic minorities are almost completely absent. Even when participation rates are high, ethnic minorities have been excluded from positions of power in sport, including coaching and management at the youth, collegiate, and professional levels.

Research within sport psychology indicates that negative stereotypes related to ethnicity and other social categorizations are common in sport and lead to performance decrements. Stereotype threat, which has been found to occur in sport, refers to being at risk for confirming a negative stereotype of one's group. Stereotype threat has been found to lower the performance of African Americans in academic situations because of the negative stereotype that African Americans are less intelligent then other groups. For example, members of a racial or ethnic group believed to be academically inferior score much lower on tests when reminded of their race or ethnicity beforehand.

Scholars have suggested that sport psychology professionals are often oblivious to their own beliefs about athletes from different ethnic groups. In fact, sport psychology professionals' beliefs often are based on a Eurocentric worldview due to the lack of research and discussion related to cultural diversity in sport psychology. Furthermore, cultural diversity training in sport psychology is almost completely absent, which likely contributes to many professionals' lack of understanding of ethnicity. To expand our worldview, sport and exercise psychology professionals need to conduct more research on ethnicity. Those practicing in sport psychology are encouraged to be aware of their own biases related to ethnicity and to develop appropriate skills to work with members of ethnic minorities.

Cindra S. Kamphoff

See also Race

Further Readings

Beilock, S. L., & McConnell, A. R. (2004). Stereotype threat and sport: Can athletic performance be threatened? *Journal of Sport & Exercise Psychology, 26*, 597–609.

Gill, D., & Kamphoff, C. S. (2009). Cultural diversity in applied sport psychology. In R. J. Schinke & S. J. Hanrahan (Eds.), *Cultural sport psychology* (pp. 45–56). Champaign, IL: Human Kinetics.

Lapchick, R. E., Bartter, J., Diaz-Calderon, A., Hanson, J., Harless, C. Johnson, W., et al. (2009). *2009 racial and gender report card*. Retrieved from http://www.tidesport.org/RGRC/2009/2009_MLB_RGRC_PR_Final_rev.pdf

Markus, H. R., & Mova, R. M. L. (2010). *Doing race: 21 essays for the 21st century*. New York: W. W. Norton.

Schinke, R. J., & Hanrahan, S. J. (Eds.). (2009). *Cultural sport psychology*. Champaign, IL: Human Kinetics.

Steele, C. M. (1997). A threat in the air: How stereotypes shape intellectual identity and performance. *American Psychologist, 52,* 613–629.

EXERCISE DEPENDENCE

Many people become physically active to improve their health and to look and feel better. But physical activity may become addictive for a small proportion (3%–5%) of the population. It is important to emphasize that while exercise may represent an addictive behavior for some people who engage in it to an extreme and unhealthy level, habitual exercise itself is not inherently abusive and people should be active to meet guidelines (e.g., 150 minutes of moderate-intensity physical activity per week) to experience its numerous health benefits.

Exercise Dependence Defined

When the desire to exercise becomes an obsession and it negatively impacts a person's physical and psychological health, it is considered a serious problem known as *exercise dependence*. Simply stated, exercise dependence is a craving for leisure-time physical activity that results in uncontrollable and excessive exercise behavior that manifests in physiological (e.g., tolerance) or psychological (e.g., withdrawal) symptoms. Other general terms for exercise dependence include *exercise addiction, overexercising, obligatory exercise, compulsive exercise,* and *exercise fanaticism.* Common characteristics of exercise dependence are continuing to exercise despite having an injury or illness; giving up social, occupational, and family obligations for exercise; and experiencing withdrawal effects, such as anxiety and tension when not able to exercise.

The growing consensus in recent years is that exercise dependence is similar to other substance dependence disorders and should be defined within a cluster of cognitive, behavioral, and physiological symptoms. Researchers have thus defined exercise dependence as a maladaptive pattern of exercise, leading to clinically significant impairment or distress, as manifested by three (or more) of the criteria listed in Table 1, occurring at any time in the same 12-month period.

Exercise dependence may also play a pivotal role in explaining the function of exercise behavior in the development and maintenance of eating disorders. To this end, it is necessary to distinguish the etiology of the exercise dependence symptoms. Understanding the psychological antecedents of exercise may help clarify the relationship between eating disorders and excessive exercise by offering insight into the distinction between primary versus secondary exercise dependence. *Primary exercise dependence* occurs when the individual meets criteria for exercise dependence and continually exercises solely for the psychological gratification resulting from the exercise behavior—for example, a runner who continually increases distance and speed to facilitate the enjoyment that is experienced from the running itself. *Secondary exercise dependence* occurs when an exercise-dependent individual uses increased amounts of exercise to accomplish some other end, such as weight management or body composition manipulation—for example, a runner who continually increases distance and speed to burn calories and facilitate weight loss. Because exercise can be used as a compensatory behavior to either prevent or reverse weight gain, secondary exercise dependence in the context of eating disorders occurs when an individual meets the criteria for exercise dependence and continually exercises to manipulate and control one's own body; thus, exercise dependence is secondary to an eating disorder. Recently, researchers have found that exercise dependence symptoms, not exercise behavior, mediate the relationship between exercise and eating pathology. That is, psychological factors, rather than the amount of exercise itself, may better explain why the exercise dependence–eating disorder relationship exists.

Prevalence and Societal Importance of Exercise Dependence

Despite the worldwide increase in obesity over the past several decades, there is nevertheless a growing rate of excessive behavioral addictions, such as gambling; Internet use; and exercise dependence that can result in poor psychological and physiological health outcomes, including increased risk for illness, stress, depression, and injury. Recent evidence suggests the estimated prevalence of exercise dependence in the general adult population is 3% to 5%. Among particular subgroups of adult exercisers, for example marathoners and sport science students, the prevalence of exercise dependence is even higher. In general,

Table 1 Exercise Dependence Criteria

Criteria	Description	Example
Tolerance	Need for increased exercise levels to achieve the desired effect, or diminished effects experienced from the same exercise level	Running 5 miles no longer results in improved mood
Withdrawal	Negative symptoms are evidenced with cessation of exercise, or exercise is used to relieve or forestall the onset of these symptoms	Anxiety, depression, or fatigue experienced when unable to exercise
Intention	Exercise is undertaken with greater intensity, frequency, or duration than was intended	Intended to run for 5 miles but ran for 7 miles instead
Lack of Control	Exercise is maintained despite a persistent desire to cut down or control it	Ran during lunch break despite trying to not exercise during work hours
Time	Considerable time is spent in activities essential to exercise maintenance	Vacations are exercise related, such as skiing and hiking trips
Reduction in Other Activities	Social, occupational, or recreational pursuits are reduced or dropped because of exercise	Running rather than going out with friends for dinner
Continuance	Exercise is maintained despite the awareness of a persistent physical or psychological problem	Running despite shin splints

Source: Heather Hausenblas and Danielle Symons Downs.

men present higher rates of exercise dependence symptoms, which parallels the higher rates of physical activity participation among men than women. The prevalence rate is about 10% for at risk for exercise dependence among regular adult exercisers. Even more concerning is the recent evidence that youth may also be at risk for exercise dependence symptoms. One study found that 6% of youth ages 14 to 16 years were classified as at risk for exercise dependence and an additional 65% were classified as nondependent but with some symptoms. Compared to the girls, the boys reported more overall exercise behavior and exercise dependence symptoms. While it has historically been thought that men develop exercise dependence symptoms in early adulthood as they hit their peak fitness level, this recent evidence suggests that boys may be more at risk for developing exercise dependence symptoms at an earlier age in the developmental timeline—possibly due to their greater involvement in leisure-time play, youth sports, and the types of vigorous activities like running and weight lifting that can perpetuate overexercising. This is problematic because it increases the chances for long-term chronic health problems (injury, illness).

There is also a growing body of research beginning to quantify the exact aspects of health that are affected by exercise dependence. Specifically, compared with nondependent controls, individuals with exercise dependence often experience an increased amount of overuse injuries like tendinitis and muscle injuries, negative affect (particularly during exercise cessation), anxiety about the shape of one's body, neuroticism, hypochondria, and compulsive shopping or buying. Unfortunately, exercise dependence tends to be overlooked because it represents a socially acceptable (or socially tolerated) addiction that appears to be a reasonable form of dependence.

Measurement of Exercise Dependence

Measurement of exercise dependence relies primarily on self-report assessments due to the manifestation of psychological, behavioral, and cognitive symptoms. Assessing the frequency, duration, and intensity of physical activity alone does not provide an accurate estimate of the underlying psychological factors that drive the symptomatology. Although there are several unidimensional measures of excessive exercise (e.g., Negative Addiction Scale, Commitment to Running Scale, and Obligatory Exercise Questionnaire), these measures have been criticized for not providing a complete assessment of the construct of exercise dependence.

The growing consensus among researchers and practitioners is that exercise dependence is better conceptualized as a multidimensional construct that parallels behavioral addiction, and therefore, is more appropriately measured by multidimensional assessments that take into account the theoretical underpinnings of addiction. Researchers have posited that behavioral addictions manifest when a behavior can provide either pleasure or relief from internal discomfort of anxiety or stress, and the behavior is characterized by feelings of powerlessness or loss of control, and is maintained despite serious physical or psychological consequences. It is now accepted that addictions are a part of a biopsychosocial process that share a set of common symptoms, such as tolerance, withdrawal, mood modification, conflict, and relapse.

One validated self-report measure that falls within this categorization of addiction is the Exercise Addiction Inventory (EAI) developed by Annabel Terry, Attila Szabo, and Mark Griffiths. The EAI assesses six components of exercise addiction: salience, mood modification, tolerance, withdrawal, conflict, and relapse. Another psychometrically validated measure to assess exercise dependence is the Exercise Dependence Scale-Revised (EDS-R) developed by Heather Hausenblas and Danielle Symons Downs and is based on the *Diagnostic and Statistical Manual of Mental Disorders, 4th Edition, Text Revision (DSM-IV)* criteria for substance dependence. This 21-item measure assesses symptoms across seven criteria (tolerance, withdrawal, intention effects, loss of control, time, reduction in other activities, and continuance). The EAI and EDS-R are easy to administer and offer researchers and practitioners useful tools for assessing exercise dependence symptoms.

Exercise Dependence Diagnosis and Treatment

Currently there are no formal diagnostic criteria for exercise dependence. However, the *DSM-IV* now includes behavioral addictions (although gambling is the only designated behavioral addiction in this category). A key factor in identifying a person with exercise dependence symptoms is distinguishing between the excessive exercise behavior and eating pathology. As noted above, primary exercise dependence occurs in the absence of an eating disorder, whereas secondary exercise dependence co-occurs with eating pathology. Thus, a diagnostic hierarchy is required whereby a person should be first evaluated for an eating disorder such as anorexia nervosa or bulimia nervosa. If the exercise behavior is secondary to the eating pathology, then referral and treatment for an eating disorder should be the priority. If eating pathology is ruled out, the individual may meet the criteria for primary exercise dependence. However, focusing only on the excessive exercise behavior in terms of frequency and intensity of exercise patterns fails to take into account the criteria that are unique to substance dependence, such as tolerance and withdrawal. Thus, determining if a person meets the aforementioned criteria for exercise dependence may provide insight to the excessive exercise. Both the EAI and EDS-R are reliable and useful tools that may assist clinicians in assessing exercise dependence. Also considering other coexisting addictions, such as alcohol or drugs or behavioral addictions like gambling, spending, or Internet use, can provide additional context to whether the person has an addictive personality disorder. Identifying individuals who are at risk for exercise dependence is a major challenge because exercise is considered a positive health behavior. Thus, excessive exercise often goes unnoticed as a negative health behavior until it has reached an extreme form. A key warning sign to distinguish between healthy and dependent exercise is that healthy exercisers organize their exercise around their *lives*, whereas dependents organize their lives around their *exercise*.

Danielle Symons Downs and
Heather Hausenblas

See also Adherence; Body Dissatisfaction; Body Dysmorphic Disorder, Muscle Dysmorphia; Eating Disorders

Further Readings

American Psychiatric Association. (2000). *Diagnostic and statistical manual of mental disorders* (4th ed., text revision). Washington, DC: Author.

Cook, B. J., & Hausenblas, H. A. (2008). The role of exercise dependence for the relationship between exercise behavior and eating pathology: Mediator or moderator? *Journal of Health Psychology, 13,* 495–502.

Griffiths, M. D. (2005). A "components" model of addiction within a biopsychosocial framework. *Journal of Substance Use, 10,* 191–197.

Hausenblas, H. A., & Symons Downs, D. (2002). Exercise dependence: A systematic review. *Psychology of Sport and Exercise, 3,* 89–123.

Hausenblas, H. A., & Symons Downs, D. (2002). How much is too much? The development and validation of the exercise dependence scale. *Psychology & Health, 17,* 387–404.

Monok, K., Berczik, K., Urban, R., Szabo, A., Griffiths, M. D., Farkas, J., et al. (2012). Psychometric properties and concurrent validity of two exercise addiction measures: A population wide study. *Psychology of Sport and Exercise.* Retrieved from http://dx.doi.org/10.1016/j.psychsport.2012.06.003

Symons Downs, D., DiNallo, J. M., & Savage, J. S. (2013). Self-determined to exercise: Leisure-time exercise behavior, exercise motivation, and exercise dependence symptoms in youth. *Journal of Physical Activity and Health, 10,* 176–184.

Symons Downs, D., Hausenblas, H. A., & Nigg, C. R. (2004). Factorial validity and psychometric examination of the Exercise Dependence Scale-Revised. *Measurement in Physical Education and Exercise Science, 8,* 183–201.

Terry, A., Szabo, A., & Griffiths, M. D. (2004). The exercise addiction inventory: A new brief screening tool. *Addiction Research and Theory, 12,* 489–499.

EXPECTANCY-VALUE THEORY

Why do some individuals participate intensely in sport activities over many years while others never get actively involved in sport or exercise? What influences initial participation in sport or exercise? What influences continued participation? What influences the intensity of participation? How do we explain drop-out from sport and exercise engagement? How do we explain both individual and group differences in sport and exercise engagement? Questions such as these have driven work in the area of motivation and sport and exercise for at least the last 50 years. Two main theoretical perspectives have emerged to address these types of questions: expectancy-value theory and self-determination theory. This entry focuses on one particular version of expectancy-value theory: Eccles and colleagues' Expectancy-Value Theory of Achievement-Related Behavioral Choices. This theoretical model has two components: a psychological component, illustrated in Figures 1 and 2, and a socialization component, illustrated in Figure 3. The following sections provide a brief description of each of these components and a summary of related empirical research.

Psychological Influences on Sport and Exercise Participation

Building on the work of Norman T. Feather, Victor Vroom, Albert Bandura, and John W. Atkinson, Jacquelynne Eccles and colleagues developed a comprehensive theoretical model of achievement-related choices, first published in 1983 (see Figure 1) and first directly applied to sport by Eccles and Rena D. Harold in 1991. It is henceforth referred to as the Eccles Expectancy-Value Model (EEVM). Eccles and colleagues hypothesized that both individual and group, for example gender or race or ethnic group, differences would be most directly influenced by individuals' expectations for success and the relative importance or value individuals attached to sport or exercise activities compared to other activity options (see Figure 2). They then hypothesized how these quite domain specific self- and task- related beliefs are influenced by cultural norms and stereotypes, experiences, aptitudes, and more general personal beliefs. In 1993, they specified a model of parental influences on the development of the psychological components of EEVT (see Figure 3).

According to the EEVM, people will be most likely to participate in those activities that they think they can master and that have high subjective task value for them. Expectations for success (domain-specific beliefs about one's personal efficacy to master the task), in turn, depend on both the confidence that individuals have in their various abilities and the individuals' estimations of

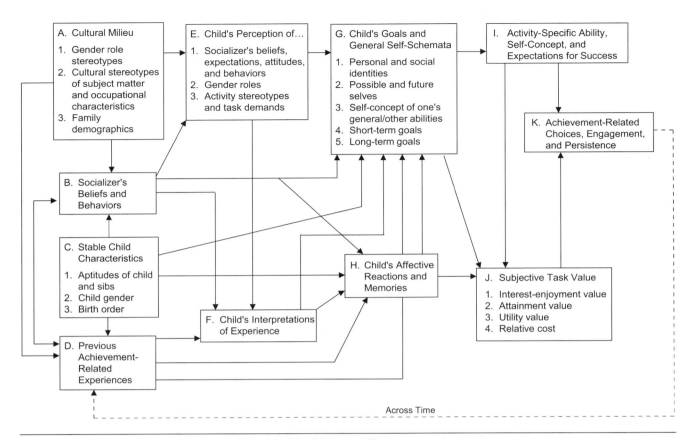

Figure I   General Eccles Expectancy-Value Model of Activity Choices

Source: Copyright © Jacquelynne S. Eccles.

Note: Since we are not assessing F, we have removed most of the arrows to and from this box.

the difficulty of the various options they are considering. Eccles and associates also predicted that these self- and task-related beliefs were shaped over time both by experiences with the related activities, and by individuals' subjective interpretation of these experiences. For example, does the individual think that personal prior and current successes reflect high ability or lots of hard work? And if the latter, will it take even more work to continue to be successful? Conversely do personal failures or difficulties reflect lack of *natural talent* or deficits in current abilities? Can the current ability level be changed through practice and instruction or does it reflect a stable entity linked to genetic or other stable biological influences—that is does it reflect natural talents? Are these natural talents believed to be linked to gender or other group characteristics? The latter interpretative questions are particularly important for explaining gender and other group differences in participation in sports and exercise. It is likely,

for example, that females in many cultures receive less support for developing a strong sense of their talent for sport from their parents, teachers, and peers than males and are more likely to attribute their difficulties in mastering sports to insufficient natural talent than males. Research has supported this prediction.

Likewise, the EEVM model specifies that the subjective task value of various activities is influenced by several factors. For example, how much does the person enjoy doing sport compared to other activities (referred to as intrinsic interest in the model)? Is participation in sport or exercise seen as instrumental in meeting the individual's long- or short-range goals (referred to as utility value)? Is being good at sport or exercise a critical part of the individual's identity (referred to as attainment value)? Does participating in sport or exercise interfere with other more valued options because of the amount of work needed to be successful either in the major or in the future

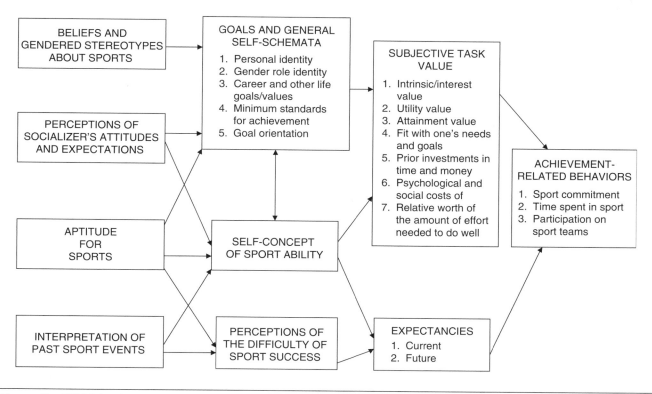

Figure 2 EEVM for Sport Participation
Source: Copyright © Jacquelynne S. Eccles.

professions linked to the major (referred to as cost)? The answers to these kinds of questions have proved critical for explaining both individual and groups differences in sport and exercise participation.

As the model was developed in the mid-1970s, it was clear that the theoretical grounding for understanding the nature of subjective task value was much less well developed than the theoretical grounding for understanding the nature of expectations for success. Consequently, Eccles and associates elaborated their notion of subjective task value to help fill this void. Drawing upon work associated with achievement motivation, intrinsic versus extrinsic motivation, self-psychology, identity formation, economics, and organization psychology, they hypothesized that subjective task value was composed of at least four components:

1. Interest value (the enjoyment one gets from engaging in the task or activity)

2. Utility value (the instrumental value of the task or activity for helping fulfill another short- or long-range goal)

3. Attainment value (the link between the task and one's sense of self and identity

4. Cost (defined in terms of either what may be given up by making a specific choice or the negative experiences associated with a particular choice)

It is the belief of Eccles and colleagues that the last three of these are particularly relevant for understanding gender and other group differences in activity choices. By and large, research has supported these predictions.

Furthermore, Eccles and colleagues believe that both individual and group differences in these aspects of subjective task value are heavily influenced by social forces and socialization, which themselves are influenced by cultural norms and stereotypes. For example, have the individual's parents, counselors, friends, or romantic partners encouraged or discouraged the individual from participating in sport or exercise? More specifically with regard to gender, for example, Eccles and colleagues argued that the socialization processes linked to gender roles are likely to influence

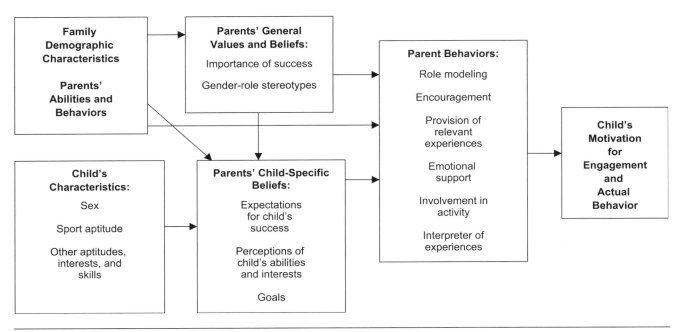

Figure 3   Eccles Parent Socialization Model
Source: Copyright © Jacquelynne S. Eccles.

both short- and long-term goals and the characteristics and values most closely linked to core identities. They predicted that males would receive more support for developing a strong interest in sport from their parents, teachers, and peers than females; research has supported this prediction. For example, gender-role socialization has been shown to lead to gender differences in adolescents' sport ability self-concepts, the subjective task value of sport, and actual engagement in sport activities. These outcomes, in turn, have been shown to predict adult involvement in sport and exercise activities.

In summary, Eccles and colleagues assume that activity choices, such as participating in sport and exercise, are guided by (a) individuals' expectations for success (sense of personal efficacy) regarding the various options, as well as their sense of competence for various tasks; (b) the relation of the options to their short- and long-range goals, to their core personal and social identities, and to their basic psychological needs; (c) individuals' culturally-based role schemas linked to gender, social class, and ethnic group; and (d) the potential cost of investing time in one activity rather than another. They further assume that all of these psychological variables are influenced by individuals' histories as mediated by their interpretation of

these experiences, by cultural norms, and by the behaviors and goals of one's socializers and peers.

Eccles and her associates have spent the last 40 years amassing evidence to support each of these hypotheses. The findings related to gender differences participation in sport and exercise are quite robust. Here are just a few examples of both the psychological and socialization models. (All of the survey instruments, details on the studies, and the publications themselves are available at www.rcgd.isr.umich.edu/garp.)

First, the researchers looked at the psychological predictors of participation in sport in high school. They used path analysis to determine whether the gender difference in sport participation was mediated by constructs directly linked to expectations for success (specifically the students' self-concept of their sport ability) and subjective task value (specifically, how much they enjoyed sport), the subjective importance of doing well in sport, and the usefulness of sport while controlling for the students' scores on. As predicted, the gender difference in participating in sport was mediated by the gender differences in these beliefs.

The second part of the research has focused on the role of experiences in the home in shaping both individual and group differences in the self- and task-related beliefs just discussed, as well as such differences in sport and exercise participation. First, using a variety of longitudinal modeling techniques, Eccles and colleagues were able to confirm most of the basic links summarized in Figure 3. Many parents do endorse gender stereotypic beliefs about general gender differences in abilities and interest in many and parents' gender-role stereotypes predict their perceptions of their own children's math, sport, and English abilities and interests even after independent assessments of their children's actual abilities in these three domains have been controlled, leading them on average to underestimate their daughters' athletic abilities. In turn, parents' estimates of their children's abilities in different skills predict developmental changes in their children's own estimates of their abilities in these skills, as well as the children's expectations for success in these different skill areas, leading to the kinds of gender differences in the children's own beliefs and task values discussed earlier.

Second, on average, parents provide their daughters and sons with gender-role stereotypic types of toys and activity opportunities, particularly in relation to sport. Not surprisingly, these differential patterns of experiences partially mediate the emergence of gender differences in children's confidence in their own abilities, their interests in participating in different activities, particularly, and their actual emerging competencies Not surprisingly, the extent to which each of these facts holds true is more marked when parents endorse the traditional gender-role stereotypes associated with both ability and interest in these different skills areas.

Conclusion

Research conducted over the past 4 decades by Eccles and colleagues, and by other researchers as well, has provided clear evidence that gender-role related personal and social processes explain, at least in part, the gender differences we see in sport participation. Much less work has been done on exercise. Furthermore, interventions have been created that can help ameliorate these processes, with the result that both girls and women and boys and men are able to make less gender-role stereotypic choices for their own lives.

Jacquelynne S. Eccles

See also Gender; Identity; Parenting; Participation Motives; Self-Determination Theory; Self-Efficacy; Self-Regulation

Further Readings

Eccles, J. S. (1987). Gender roles and women's achievement-related decisions. *Psychology of Women Quarterly, 11,* 135–172.

Eccles, J. S. (1993). School and family effects on the ontogeny of children's interests, self-perceptions, and activity choice. In J. Jacobs (Ed.), *Nebraska Symposium on Motivation, 1992: Developmental perspectives on motivation* (pp. 145–208). Lincoln: University of Nebraska Press.

Eccles, J. S. (2006). Families, schools, and developing achievement-related motivations and engagement. In J. E. Grusec & P. D. Hastings (Eds.), *Handbook of socialization: Theory and research* (pp. 665–691). New York: Guilford Press.

Eccles, J. S., Jacobs, J. E., & Harold, R. D. (1990). Gender-role stereotypes, expectancy effects, and parents' socialization of gender differences. *Journal of Social Issues, 46,* 183–201.

Fredricks, J. A., & Eccles, J. S. (2004). Parental influences on youth involvement in sports. In M. Weiss (Ed.), *Developmental sport and exercise psychology: A lifespan perspective* (pp. 145–164). Morgantown, WV: Fitness Information Technology.

Fredricks, J. A., & Eccles, J. S. (2005). Family socialization, gender, and sport motivation and involvement. *Journal of Sport & Exercise Psychology, 27,* 3–31.

Jacobs, J. E., & Eccles, J. S. (1992). The impact of mothers' gender-role stereotypic beliefs on mothers' and children's ability perceptions. *Journal of Personality and Social Psychology, 63,* 932–944.

Jacobs, J. E., Vernon, M. K., & Eccles, J. S. (2005). Activity choices in middle childhood: The roles of gender, self-beliefs, and parents' influence. In J. L. Mahoney, R. W. Larson, & J. S. Eccles (Eds.), *Organized activities as contexts of development: Extracurricular activities, after-school and community programs* (pp. 235–254). Mahwah, NJ: Erlbaum.

Perkins, D. F., Jacobs, J. E., Barber, B., & Eccles, J. S. (2004). Childhood and adolescent sports participation as predictors of participation in sports and physical fitness activities during adulthood. *Youth and Society, 35,* 495–520.

Rodriguez, D., Wigfield, A., & Eccles, J. S. (2003). Changing competence perceptions, changing values: Implications for youth sport. *Journal of Applied Sport Psychology, 15*(1), 67–81.

EXPERTISE

Expertise refers to the underlying qualities and skills that distinguish highly accomplished people, referred to as experts, from lesser skilled people. Experts are people who are exceptionally skilled in a particular task or domain and their expertise is typically evident across numerous aspects of human performance, including perception, cognition, and motor execution. Interestingly, despite the clarity by which we can identify an expert, definitional inconsistencies of what constitutes an expert are common in the literature. One of the defining features of experts is the amount of practice and effort they have devoted to achieve this status. A number of models detailing the development of expertise have been suggested, creating some confusion for practitioners in the field. Expertise research is conducted in a wide variety of domains, as diverse as sport, medicine, education, the performing arts, and the military.

Why Study Expertise?

There are clear scientific reasons to study expertise. First, discovering the mechanisms underpinning an expert's superior performance in a particular domain, such as sport, provides a broader understanding of the factors that may limit a non-expert's quest to become more skilled. Over time, the collective efforts of expertise researchers have allowed the development of more robust and generalizable theories of expertise and its acquisition (see later section "How Is Expertise Acquired"?). A second key reason to study expertise is to understand what type and volume of practice is critical for the acquisition of skill, and ultimately expertise. Importantly, this information cannot be obtained from the study of non-experts even when trained to perform thousands of practice repetitions in a controlled skill-acquisition experiment.

The scientific study of expertise can assist in providing recommendations to practitioners in the field, such as coaches, teachers, and skill acquisition providers, to assist in the refinement of practice conditions to enhance performance. Similarly, as a higher premium is placed on the identification and subsequent development of talent, testing protocols can be implemented that focus on the domain-specific elements of performance known to be required to achieve expertise.

A Brief History of Sport Expertise Research

While humankind's fascination with expert sport performance can be traced back to at least the time of the first Olympics, quite surprisingly an identifiable program of research investigating sport expertise is only a few decades old. Seminal work investigating chess masters in the mid- to late 1960s and early 1970s proved to be the stimulus for the current interest in sport expertise research. The common experimental paradigm adopted in most studies has involved an expert–novice comparison where a group of experts or highly skilled performers complete a particular task thought to be representative of that completed in the performance setting and their results are compared to those of a lesser skilled group. It is assumed that the performance variables that reliably distinguish the experts from the lesser skilled are elements important to expertise (see later section "Common Features of Expertise").

In 1965, Adriaan De Groot investigated the perceptual attributes of chess players. He found that after providing chess masters with only a brief view of the chess pieces on a chessboard, they were able to reconstruct the locations of those pieces better than lesser skilled players. These early findings were proven to be robust by subsequent researchers and led to William Chase and Herb Simon's 1973 theory of expertise. A key finding central to this theory was that expertise was only evident when the pieces were structurally arranged such that they were in similar positions to those encountered in normal game play. When the same pieces were arranged in completely random configurations, the chess masters lost their reconstruction advantage over lesser skilled players. This finding suggested that expert chess performance was not the result of an enhanced memory capacity but rather of a capacity to overcome the short-term memory limitation of 7 ± 2 pieces (chunks) of information. While the notion of chunking continues to be revised, the superior performance of experts from many domains is grounded in their capability to process larger amounts of task-relevant perceptual information and then use this information to prepare an appropriate movement response.

In addition to the memory-processing explanation of expertise, domain-specific knowledge has also been considered an important underlying mechanism. Declarative knowledge and procedural knowledge have been proposed as the primary cognitive structures underlying skilled performance. *Declarative knowledge* has been defined as the knowledge of factual information, whereas *procedural knowledge* has been defined as the knowledge of how to do things. A declarative knowledge base has been suggested to provide the foundation for the development of the more complex structures present in procedural knowledge. Compared to non-experts, sports experts possess structured knowledge at a more sophisticated level consisting of highly structured offensive and defensive sport concepts, which in turn are thought to facilitate their decision-making processes. However, particularly in sport, the possession of a strong declarative knowledge base does not guarantee equivalent levels of procedural knowledge. For example, players may possess a substantial declarative knowledge about their sport but possess a lower level of procedural knowledge that acts to limit their overall performance capability.

Cognitive approaches to the study of expert performance have been especially influential in the study of experts in sport. However, sport expertise clearly demands not only enhanced cognitive functioning but also well-timed and accurate motor execution. Accounting for the central role of motor skill within sport expertise has been a consistent challenge for researchers, particularly in relation to creating representative tasks that are sufficiently well controlled to permit the underlying components of expertise to be accurately and reliably recorded. However, technological progress in the measurement tools available to researchers has seen a recent shift from laboratory to field-based measurement with a concomitant increase in the use of more representative tasks; this, in turn, has helped build a more complete understanding of sport expertise.

The expert performance approach was first described by Anders Ericsson and Jacqui Smith in 1991. Three stages were proposed within this approach. The first stage involves capturing expert performance or, put alternatively, identifying the domain-specific situations where the expert excels and then developing representative tasks that allow this superior performance to be re-created in experimentally controlled conditions. The second stage aims to assess the underlying mechanisms that account for superior performance on the representative tasks. The identification of processing differences between expert and non-expert performers can be obtained through a variety of experimental techniques, such as gaze tracking, verbal reports, and occlusion techniques. The third and final stage involves examining how the identified expertise was developed through experience and practice, again by using a variety of experimental methods. While the expert performance approach has not been adopted universally, it does provide a logical framework from which to consider some of the common features of expertise that have emerged from research.

Common Features of Expertise

The collective efforts of expertise researchers to understand the nature of the expert advantage have revealed a number of common features of expertise that systematically emerge across sport and other domains. These are summarized below.

Expertise Is Specific

Expertise is not transferable between domains (or across sports) and will only appear when the usual context of the sport task of interest is identical or sufficiently representative of the performance setting. For instance, generalized measures that lack sport specificity, such as a reaction time task where the performer is required to react to a flashing light rather than a sport-specific situation requiring a fast reaction (hitting a baseball), consistently fail to distinguish experts from lesser skilled individuals. Recently, the extent of expertise specificity has been challenged. An intuitive view is that talented performers from one sport have some common skills that transfer across sports or even to other domains. While there is some limited empirical evidence to suggest that some elements (anticipation and decision making) transfer from one related sport to another, much more research is needed before a definitive position can be reached.

Experts Recognize and Recall Patterns From Their Domain of Expertise More Effectively

The chunking capabilities of chess masters described earlier are also consistently found in the team-sport domain with expert players recognizing and recalling structured game patterns more completely than lesser skilled players. It has been suggested this capacity is central to the advanced decision-making skills demanded in time-stressed situations common in such sports as basketball or football. One matter of current debate is whether pattern recall tasks require individuals to use processes they may not otherwise have used, at least explicitly, during a typical game. Accordingly, some researchers have suggested pattern recall is a good example of a task that is not sufficiently representative to elicit true expertise differences in a sport domain despite the demonstration of some expert–novice differences on these types of task.

Experts Possess Knowledge Superior to That of Lesser Skilled Individuals

Not only do experts tend to possess more declarative knowledge or facts about their specific sport, but importantly, experts also appear to know how to navigate an effective course of action in competition (procedural knowledge). Expertise researchers have systematically explored the various connections between different types of knowledge and observable skilled performance to better understand the relative contribution of knowledge to sport expertise. This aspect of sport expertise has been characterized by some innovative research designs where sports experts are compared with expert coaches or spectators who may share similar levels of declarative knowledge but differ in their motor skill proficiency.

Experts Anticipate Their Opponent's Behavior More Effectively Than Non-Experts

In time-stressed tasks, such as returning a tennis serve, an expert player is able to alleviate some of the time stress and in turn allow more definitive response preparation through the reliable anticipation of advance information. The expert performer has been found to pick up two forms of advance information more selectively than lesser skilled performers—situational probability information and opponent movement characteristics. Situational probability information consists of generic information available to a performer before the opponent commences their skill execution. The information typically arises from pre-game knowledge of player strengths, weaknesses, and preferences, as well as court or field position,

and event probability information. The source of the expert performer's attunement to their opponent's movement pattern is argued to stem from a direct link between their perceptual expertise and the pickup of invariant and predictive kinematic information within their opponent's action.

Expert Motor Performance Is More Efficient and Subconsciously Controlled

Expert motor performance has been associated with the ability to produce coordinated movements that are both efficient and effective in terms of meeting the environmental demands of the task or game. The expert's movement coordination superiority over non-experts stems from a range of factors, including the superior recruitment of force, increased fatigue resistance, and the capacity to more effectively control multiple degrees of freedom (limb, joint, and muscle combinations). In contrast to experts, novices tend to approach skills with rigid movements and lock bodily segments at the joints, freezing the degrees of freedom. In a nice illustration of the multidimensional nature of expertise, experts are also able to direct their attention to the external environment to a greater extent than their lesser skilled counterparts as evidenced by their capacity to perform two tasks simultaneously, for example dribbling a basketball while scanning for a passing option). Experts are thought to automate their movement production in that they not have to consciously think about skill execution because of extensive practice relative to lesser skilled individuals. Interestingly, experts can experience skill performance decrements in conditions that force them to process their skills in a more conscious or novice-like manner, leading to what is colloquially referred to as *paralysis by analysis*.

How Is Expertise Acquired?

A long-standing debate within the expertise field concerns determining the most effective pathway to the acquisition of expertise. The most common approach to this question has been to retrospectively examine the practice histories of expert relative to non-expert performers via interviews, training diaries, and questionnaires. Two dominant positions have emerged in regard to the best approach to the development of expertise, that is, a practice-focused approach referred to as the *theory of deliberate practice* and a play-before-specific-practice approach, referred to as the *developmental model of sports participation* (DMSP). In practical terms, these two approaches can also be aligned to the debate on the relative merits of early (deliberate practice) versus late (DMSP) specialization into a sport.

In 1993, Ericsson, Ralf Krampe, and Clemens Tesch-Romer proposed that expertise is primarily a matter of practice rather than reliance on innate talent, albeit acknowledging that height and body size are clearly important to success in many sports. Deliberate practice is considered to have occurred when a well-defined task, set at an appropriate difficulty level for the learner, is completed with access to feedback and opportunities for practice repetition and correction of errors. Such practice requires effort, generates no immediate rewards, is motivated by the goal of improving performance rather than inherent enjoyment, and consequently occurs over an extended period of time (usually in excess of 10 years, referred to as the 10-year rule). Practicing deliberately is argued to incrementally develop the underlying mechanisms that lead to expertise. The key tenets of the deliberate practice framework were originally formulated based on the practice histories of expert-level musicians and research highlighting the plasticity of cognitive skills to the effects of practice. The importance of deliberate practice has been substantiated in some sport settings, albeit with a number of qualifications suggested by those working within the sport domain. For instance, in contrast to the original definition, it has been found that deliberate practice activities can be both highly enjoyable and high in concentration in the sport setting. In addition, squad or team practice, rather than practice alone (or individually with a teacher), has been identified as being most predictive of skill level in team environments.

In contrast to the notions of deliberate practice, others have advocated a more diversified and playful commencement as desirable for the lengthy journey toward expertise. Jean Côté, Joseph Baker, and Bruce Abernethy building on the work of Benjamin Bloom, formulated the DMSP and suggested three chronological stages of sport participation from early childhood to late adolescence. The sampling years (ages 6–13) emphasize fun and excitement through participation in a large number of sport activities. Voluntary participation of the child in activities that are intrinsically motivating, pleasurable, and

provide immediate gratification are key attributes of this stage. These characteristics are typical of pick-up, backyard, or neighborhood-style games that are self-initiated by children with the sole determinant of having fun (commonly referred to as *deliberate play*). In the specializing years (ages 13–15), involvement in other activities gradually decreases and the focus shifts toward only one or two specific sports. Positive experiences with coaches, encouragement from siblings and friends, and the simple enjoyment of the activity influence the child's decision to gravitate toward a specialized sport or sports. Sport-specific skill development is an important feature of the specializing years and marks a transition toward a more deliberate practice approach. The investment years (15 years and older) suggest the intent of an athlete to pursue expertise in a single sport. The sampling and deliberate play activities reported in the previous stages are replaced by large volumes of intense, sport-specific practice (similar to deliberate practice).

While the DMSP has been supported by a number of subsequent investigations in sport, it has also been challenged. In particular, a key issue is whether expertise requires a more focused approach to deliberate play whereby children are encouraged to engage in playful activity primarily related to their preferred sport of interest rather than diversifying or sampling too many sports. It is argued that such an approach may meet the needs of specialization while simultaneously providing sufficient diversification. It has also been suggested that the relative importance of early versus late specialization may be largely sport- and culture-specific.

Conclusion

Research into the development of expertise and expert performance focuses on the identification and understanding of the mechanisms that distinguish experts from lesser skilled performers. Expertise is domain specific and requires the development of representative tasks if it is to be reliably demonstrated and examined in an experimental setting. A number of common features of expertise have been demonstrated in perceptual, cognitive, and motor components of performance. The development of expertise is perhaps the most debated aspect of this research field with two competing approaches being suggested. This debate has important practical implications in regard to whether it is advantageous to specialize early in a sporting task or diversify across a number of sports to reach expert status. There are many fertile areas for future research before a complete understanding of expertise will be gained.

Damian Farrow

See also Anticipation; Automaticity; Chunking/Dechunking; Decision Making; Genetics/Nature–Nurture Determinants; Memory; Pattern Recognition and Recall; Practice; Skill Acquisition; Talent Development

Further Readings

Abernethy, B. (1994). The nature of expertise in sport. In S. Serpa, J. Alves, & V. Pataco (Eds.), *International perspectives on sport and exercise psychology* (pp. 57–68). Morgantown, WV: Fitness Information Technology.

Abernethy, B., Thomas, K. T., & Thomas, J. T. (1993). Strategies for improving understanding of motor expertise (or mistakes we have made and things we have learned!!). In J. L. Starkes & F. Allard (Eds.), *Cognitive issues in motor expertise* (pp. 317–356). Amsterdam: North Holland.

Bloom, B. S. (Ed.). (1985). *Developing talent in young people*. New York: Ballantine.

Côté, J., Baker, J., & Abernethy, B. (2007). Practice and play in the development of sport expertise. In R. C. Eklund & G. Tenenbaum (Eds.), *Handbook of sport psychology* (3rd ed., pp. 184–202). Hoboken, NJ: Wiley.

Ericsson, K. A., Charness, N., Feltovich, P. J., & Hoffman, R. R. (Eds.). (2006). *The Cambridge handbook of expertise and expert performance*. New York: Cambridge University Press.

Ericsson, K. A., Krampe, R. T., & Tesch-Romer, C. (1993). The role of deliberate practice in the acquisition of expert performance. *Psychological Review, 100,* 363–406.

Farrow, D., Baker, J., & MacMahon, C. (Eds.). (2008). *Developing sport expertise: Researchers and coaches put theory into practice*. Oxford, UK: Routledge.

Starkes, J. L., & Ericsson, K. A. (Eds.). (2003). *Expert performance in sports*. Champaign, IL: Human Kinetics.

Williams, A. M., & Ericsson, K. A. (2005). Perceptual-cognitive expertise in sport: Some considerations when applying the expert performance approach. *Human Movement Science, 24,* 283–307.

EXTRAVERSION–INTROVERSION

Extraversion–introversion is a personality factor that refers to the degree to which a person's basic orientation is turned inward (toward oneself) or outward (toward the external world). Introverts are said to be shy and prefer to work alone; they tend to withdraw into themselves, especially when they experience emotional stress and conflict. In contrast, extraverts are said to be sociable and prefer occupations that enable them to work directly with other people; when experiencing stress, they will tend to seek company.

Another related personality factor is *emotional instability–stability* (or neuroticism), which is a continuum of emotionality that varies from moody, anxious, temperamental, and maladjusted persons in the *unstable or neurotic* end, as opposed to *stable* people, who are said to be calm and well adjusted.

These two personality factors are strongly associated with the name of Hans Eysenck. In psychology, the question of which primary source accounts for the apparent variance in human behavior has long been debated. The proponents of the trait approach advocated stable, intraorganismic constructs as the main determinants of behavior. One of the most noted of the trait researchers during the 1960s and the 1970s was Eysenck, who conceived traits as relative. This psychologist used psychiatrists' ratings of patients' characteristics to arrive at two superordinate personality factors ranging on continuums, namely *introversion–extraversion* and *emotional instability–stability* (better known as *neuroticism*); these most significant dimensions emerged from many factor-analytic studies of the intercorrelations between numerous and different traits.

Strictly speaking, these two personality factors only provide phenotypic descriptions; therefore, Eysenck also suggested causal explanations on the biological level. He interpreted the introversion–extraversion dimension as being based on the balance between cortical excitation and inhibition. Excitation is related to the facilitation of perceptual, cognitive, and motor responses in the central nervous system, whereas inhibition is related to the exact opposite effect, namely the suppression of such responses. Emotionality or neuroticism is biophysically explained through the instability of the autonomous neural system; it is assumed that an autonomous response is dependent on a person's constitutional structure, which mediates the strength of his or her responses to incoming stimuli. Thus, it is the autonomous neural system that is most probably the basis of individual differences concerning emotionality.

Trait theorists have typically used objective inventories that involved direct quantification of personality dimensions, without intervening interpretations of participants' responses. Such was the Eysenck Personality Inventory (EPI), which was among the most popular trait inventories taken from general psychology and used during the 1960s and 1970s in early sport personality research. The basic idea here was to try and "match" athletes to sport disciplines; for example, it was argued that an extravert's cortex is less aroused than that of an introvert, and therefore an extravert will need much stronger external stimuli than the introvert, who will in turn suffer from such a strongly stimulating environment; an introvert will clearly prefer a weak environmental stimulation.

According to this line of reasoning, if (a) lower cortical arousal is mostly related to extraversion and higher cortical arousal to introversion, and (b) minor arousal fluctuations are more typical of emotionally stable people and substantial arousal fluctuations are mostly apparent in neurotics, then we could argue that for an elite athlete, although being stable is almost always better than being unstable, the performance quality of introverts versus extraverts will depend on the task (sport discipline) to be performed. Thus, as demonstrated, for example, by J. E. Kane, in a stressful environment when the fulfillment of a complex task is required, as in a basketball game, stable extraverts seem to exhibit motor advantage not only over unstable extraverts, but also over stable introverts (and in particular, of course, over unstable introverts). By contrast, stable introverts will enjoy an advantage in sport disciplines such as marathon running, long-distance swimming, or rifle shooting, which are monotonic and environmentally poorly stimulating.

For the aforementioned reasons, it was particularly the introversion–extraversion dimension that caught the attention of much of the sport-personality research from its earliest days. In general, athletes' personality structures were found to lean toward extraversion, which is not quite surprising given the larger numbers of people actively engaged in extravert sports (team sports such as football or basketball). However, lone athletes like marathon runners were indeed found to be more introverted;

moreover, it was found that top, superior athletes tended to be more introverted in comparison to lower level athletes, even within extravert samples (not to mention introvert ones). Kane contended that superior athletes of all sport disciplines enjoy the advantage of being able to isolate themselves better in order to appropriately concentrate and prepare for task performance, an ability which is clearly related to introverted tendencies.

Despite the fact that Eysenck has been one of the most cited psychologists of his time, and even though his two previously mentioned factors are included among the *Big Five* of personality, it seems that simply knowing someone's personality trait will not really help to predict how that person will perform under specific circumstances. Accordingly, sport-personality research waned toward the 1980s and 1990s, probably because much of this research resulted in what were viewed as statistically significant differences that were often meaningless. However, questions, such as whether extraverts will perform better in team situations and introverts in individual ones, can lead to more accurate predictions of athletes' behavior in comparison to relying only on traits, or alternatively, only on situations.

It may therefore be possible to more usefully apply Eysenck's two factors within an interactionist framework, such as the one suggested by Robin Vealey. Strictly speaking, the basic idea mentioned above, namely that of matching individuals and sports, actually reflects an interactionist perspective. Moreover, transactionist approaches such as Michael Bar-Eli's crisis theory, in which introversion–extraversion and neuroticism were included in a reconceptualization of athletes' prestart states, should be encouraged in order to more fully exploit the potential concealed in these two big personality factors, and further advance our understanding of sport behavior.

Michael Bar-Eli

See also History of Sport Psychology; Models of Emotion–Performance; Personality Tests; Personality Traits and Exercise; Psychological Skills; Psychophysiology

Further Readings

Bar-Eli, M. (1997). Psychological performance crisis in competition, 1984–1996: A review. *European Yearbook of Sport Psychology, 1,* 73–112.

Eysenck, H. J., & Eysenck, M. W. (1985). *Personality and individual differences*. New York: Plenum Press.

Kane, J. E. (1978). Personality research: The current controversy and implications for sports studies. In W. F. Straub (Ed.), *Sport psychology: An analysis of athlete behavior* (pp. 228–240). Ithaca, NY: Mouvement.

McCrae, R. R., & Costa, P. T. (1999). A five-factor theory of personality. In L. A. Pervin (Ed.), *Handbook of personality theory and research* (pp. 139–153). New York: Guilford Press.

Vealey, R. S. (2002). Personality and sport behavior. In T. S. Horn (Ed.), *Advances in sport psychology* (2nd ed., pp. 43–82). Champaign, IL: Human Kinetics.

Eye Movements/Gaze

The eyes perceive spatial information with full acuity when light falls on a small region at the back of the retina called the *fovea*. Because of the small area of the fovea, the area over which we are able to see clearly is only about 2° to 3° of visual angle. Visual angle indicates the size of an image on the retina. It is usually determined by extending lines from the edges of the object as viewed in space through the lens to the retina. One way to estimate the size of this area is to hold your thumb up at arm's length on object in space. The width of your thumb subtends 2° to 3° of visual angle projected into space. Gaze control is the process of directing the eyes to objects or events within a scene in real time and in the service of the ongoing perceptual and cognitive processes. The reason the eyes move is to keep objects of interest projected on the high-acuity fovea. Usually the eyes move before the head, localizing a target first. Head movement follows because of the greater size and inertia of the head compared to the eyes. The movement of the eyes and head to the target is normally smooth, with the processing of visual information occurring within 100 ms of the eyes stabilizing on the new location.

Eye movements were first studied with the head fixed as even the slightest movement of the head could cause large errors in the eye data being collected. Today, with the advent of light mobile eye trackers, it is possible to record accurate eye movements as the participant moves naturally throughout the world, making head movements. Eye-tracking methods permit the measurement of the location of the gaze in space or the eye movements relative to the head. Most eye trackers used in sport are corneal-reflection systems that consist of two video cameras mounted on a headband or glasses. One camera records a video of the eye and the other the scene in front of the performer. The location of the gaze is determined using the center of the pupil and the corneal reflection, which is artificially placed on the eye (using infrared light). Data are collected digitally in *x/y* coordinates, as well as the location of the gaze being shown on the scene video as a cursor or other marker every frame or field of video. The accuracy of most corneal-reflections systems is about 1 degree of visual angle. The most common National Television System Committee (NTSC) data collection is 30 Hz, or 30 frames per second (33.33 ms per frame); or 60 Hz, or 60 fields per second (16.67 per field).

Types of Eye Movements and Gaze

Most eye-tracking systems record fixations, pursuit tracking, and saccadic eye movements. A fixation occurs when the gaze is held on an object or location within 3° of visual angle for 100 ms or longer. The 100 ms threshold is approximately the minimum amount of time the brain needs to recognize or become aware of what is being viewed. Pursuit-tracking eye movements are similar to fixations, except the eyes follow a moving object, such as a ball or a person. The 100-ms threshold still applies for the same reason as it is used for fixations. Saccades occur when the eyes move quickly from one fixated or tracked location to another. Saccades are among the fastest movements that humans can make, exceeding 900 degrees per second. Saccades are ballistic eye movements that bring the point of maximal visual acuity onto the fovea so that an object can be seen with clarity. During saccades, information is suppressed, meaning the information between two fixated locations is not consciously perceived. Instead, the information gained during fixations is maintained in memory thereby ensuring a stable, coherent scene. Saccadic suppression prevents us from seeing a world that is blurry and therefore difficult to comprehend.

The fixated or tracked information falling upon the fovea constitutes focal vision. The focal system is used when fixated or tracked information falls on the fovea and aspects of an object or location are viewed with full acuity or detail.

In contrast, information that falls off the fovea becomes increasingly blurry (of low resolution) and is viewed using ambient or peripheral vision. The ambient or peripheral system is specialized for motion and low light conditions. Both the focal and ambient systems are needed for the visual system to function properly.

Visual Motor Pathways

Visuomotor control is the process whereby visual information is used to direct and control movements. Visual information is registered first on the retina, then passes through the optic nerve, the lateral geniculate nucleus, and the optic or striate radiations to the visual cortex or occipital lobe at the back of the head. Located in the occipital cortex are visual sensors that begin the processing of registering and interpreting what the performer sees, with specific detectors for initial registration (V1), shape (V2), angles (V3), motion (V3a), color (V4), V5 (motion with direction), depth and self-motion (V6), and depth of stereo motion (V7). Once an object, person or location is registered within the visual cortex, visual information moves rapidly forward in the brain, along the dorsal attention network (DAN) and the ventral attention network (VAN). The DAN projects from the occipital lobe to the parietal lobe and forward to the frontal lobe in a journey that goes roughly over the top of the head to the frontal lobe. In contrast, the ventral attention network (VAN) projects forward along the sides of the head through the temporal lobes to the frontal areas. Commands are then sent from the frontal areas to the motor cortex to initiate action. With practice and the development of expertise, it is thought the DAN system sustains attention on critical spatial locations, thereby blocking out competing anxiety-producing stimuli that may intrude from the VAN system while the movement is being performed.

Eye Tracking Methods

Two research methods are widely used in sport, called the *visual-search* and *vision-in-action* paradigms. The visual-search paradigm is the older of the two paradigms, dating back to the beginning of psychology. When the visual-search method is used, eye movements are recorded as the athlete sits or stands and views photographs, videotapes, virtual reality, or computer simulations of events from their sport. Motor responses usually involve a manual key press, step sensor, or pencil-and-paper response. Using this paradigm, it has been established that expert athletes, compared to novices, are superior at recalling and recognizing sport-specific patterns of plays, are faster in detecting specific cues, are more efficient in recognizing objects, and are better at anticipating upcoming events.

The vision-in-action paradigm differs from the visual-search paradigm in recording the athlete's gaze, in situ, under conditions similar to those found in real world play or competition. Elite and non-elite athletes perform well-known tasks, such as golf putting, basketball free throw, and soccer or ice hockey goaltending, in experiments that couple perception and action. Most studies require the athlete to perform the task until an equal number of successful and unsuccessful trials have been completed thus allowing the detection of gaze and perceptual-motor differences during successful and unsuccessful performance. A major finding resulting from this method is the discovery of the *quiet eye,* which is the final fixation or tracking gaze maintained on a specific location prior to a critical movement in the task. Quiet eye onset occurs prior to the movement and quiet eye offset occurs when the gaze deviates off a specific location for more than 100 ms. Numerous quiet eye studies have shown that elite athletes have earlier and longer quiet eye durations than non-elite; a longer duration quiet eye is also a characteristic of more successful performance. Quiet eye training has proven to be effective in improving performance compared to traditional methods in a number of sports and other areas.

A few studies have also tested the same athletes using both the visual search and vision-in-action methods, with different results reported in terms of the gaze and motor performance. When the athletes were tested using the vision-in-action method, they used fewer fixations to fewer locations in the task environment. Their fixations occurred earlier and were longer in duration than when they were tested using the visual-search paradigm and video simulations of the same task. When the vision-in-action paradigm was used, the athletes' anticipatory actions occurred earlier and both their reaction time and movement times were faster than when the visual-search method was used. These results suggest that the demands of real-world performance create a tight coupling between perception and action that can only be detected when the athlete is tested under realistic conditions.

Joan N. Vickers

See also Expertise; Perception; Vision

Further Readings

Aglioti, S., Cesari, P., Romani, M., & Urgesi, C. (2008). Action anticipation and motor resonance in elite basketball players. *Nature Neuroscience, 11*(9), 1109–1116.

Causer, J., Janelle, C. M., Vickers, J. N., & Williams, A. M. (2012). Perceptual expertise: What can be trained? In N. Hodges & A. M. Williams (Eds.), *Skill acquisition in sport: Research, theory and practice* (2nd ed., pp. 306–324). London: Routledge.

Corbetta, M., & Shulman, G. L. (2002). Control of goal-directed and stimulus-driven attention in the brain. *Nature Reviews Neuroscience, 3,* 201–215.

Coren, S., Ward, L. M., & Enns, J. T. (2009). *Sensation and perception* (6th ed.). Hoboken, NJ: Wiley.

Dicks, M., Button, C., & Davids, K. (2010). Examination of gaze behaviors under in situ and video simulation task constraints reveals differences in the information used for perception and action. *Attention, Perception, & Psychophysics, 72,* 706–720.

Hodges, N., & Williams, A. M. (2012). *Skill acquisition in sport: Research, theory and practice* (2nd ed.). London: Routledge.

Müller, S., & Abernethy, B. (2006). Batting with occluded vision: An in situ examination of the information pick-up and interceptive skills of high- and low-skilled cricket batsmen. *Journal of Science Medicine in Sport, 9,* 446–458.

Vickers, J. N. (2007). *Perception, cognition, and decision training: The quiet eye in action.* Champaign, IL: Human Kinetics.

Vickers, J. N. (2009). Advances in coupling perception and action: The quiet eye as a bidirectional link between gaze, attention, and action. *Progress in Brain Research, 174,* 279–288.

Vine, S. J., & Wilson, M. R. (2011). The influence of quiet eye training and pressure on attention and visuo-motor control. *Acta Psychologica, 136*(3), 340–346.

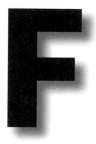

FAIR PLAY

The purpose of fair play is to ensure that every competitor has an equal chance of being successful in any given competition. Fair play is supported by a philosophic belief that every player, team, official, and fan respects and honors (1) the rules of the game (constitutive, regulatory, and sportsmanship), (2) those who play the game (opponents), and (3) those who call the game (officials). This notion of fair play also transcends the actual playing to include all off-field preparation for the game as well as postgame activities for how opponents are treated.

The principle of fair play is ingrained in the Western tradition—fleshed out on the playing fields of English preparatory schools from the late 1700s through the 1800s. In Victorian England specifically, it was argued that young men could learn the important virtues of honesty, fair play, justice, propriety, and decency through the playing of games. Children of the upper classes who attended the elite private schools were taught that sport, played through the virtues of fair play, was a means unto itself. The goal was not about winning but about taking part and being a member of a team. One learned self-control, discipline, and virtue, such as being honest, being fair, and acting properly and decently on the field of play and off the field of play. More importantly, the stated goal was not about victory but about the honorable journey of playing and working together. This was a worthy cause where boys learned to be gentlemen by following rules and being respectful to opponents. This notion of fair play was seen as imperative to the education of gentlemen. Most of the aristocrats from the ages of 13 to 18 attended the elite boarding schools including Eton or Harrow. Students who attended these schools believed deeply in the importance of learning to play fairly, and they noted it as such in their writings. For example, the end of Napoleon's reign occurred following the Battle of Waterloo when the combined armies of Europe under the command of the Duke of Wellington defeated him. Wellington—a graduate of Eton—is often quoted as having said that the Battle of Waterloo was won on the playing fields of Eton. His implication was that the officers at the battle, most of whom had attended Eton, worked together, followed rules, and had a strong sense of fair play and decency, which helped England win the battle.

This concept of learning to be gentlemen through sport was transported to the British colonies that became the United States—and the philosophy was instituted in the elite schools of the time, including Harvard and Yale. This institutional belief in the importance of developing men, and later women, of character blossomed throughout the United States and became part of a mystical belief that sport builds character—the actual virtues of being honest, trustworthy, and fair. This notion continues today in the five U.S. military service academies. The philosophy guiding the programs stems from General Douglas MacArthur, superintendent of the U.S. Military Academy in 1920, who believed that every cadet should play and compete in athletics at their highest level. McArthur said, "On the fields of friendly strife are sown the seeds that on other days and other fields will bear the fruits of victory." This same belief in discipline and athletics sits as the ideal philosophy that sports builds character, and hence a heightened sense of being honest, fair, and respectful, which serves as evidence to include sports and athletics as both curricular and extracurricular activities in U.S. education.

The same fair play philosophy was incorporated by Baron de Coubertin, the founder of the modern Olympic movement, into the overarching purpose of the Olympic Games. Coubertin, classically educated, was highly influenced by Englishman Thomas Arnold (headmaster of Rugby School) that sport was necessary for the balanced education of a person. A balanced education was about developing people of character who knew how to play a game well and fairly. Coubertin spent his life lecturing, writing, and championing the character components of sport. Hence, the Olympic movement worldwide is based in the philosophy of fair play.

The mythical ideal, however, is not always the reality. The institutional and social practices of today support a distorted form of competition—an objectification of the opponents, the game, and the rules in which the one true product valued is the win. One would be hard-pressed to find a fair play standard as noted earlier in most competitive athletic programs in the United States or for that matter in the world today. Instead, sports and athletics are played through a different ethos of competition called *gamesmanship*—getting an advantage using whatever dubious ploys and tactics without getting caught in order to win. Today, it is not the journey that is important, generally, it is the result. "If you ain't cheating, you ain't trying" is a motto today, and often is found pinned to a locker room bulletin board.

In the last year alone, sad unethical practices have occurred at all levels of athletic competition, including youth sport (parents fighting with parents at youth sport events), collegiate sport (famous coaches being fired or censured for not reporting unethical behavior of their players or criminal behavior of their own coaches), professional sport (players placing a bounty on injuring a player), and Olympic sport (athletes being expelled from the games for using illegal performance substances or cheating in relation to the

rules). Few media stories of true fair play exist, and when a story is highlighted that focuses on fair play, it becomes viral through social media because it is so unusual. For example, two softball players carried an injured opposing player around the bases so she could touch the bases and score a run. The opposing player had hit a home run but was injured on rounding first base. She crawled back to first base and asked for a time out. She could not continue, and the rule supposedly stated that she must touch all of the bases. None of her team could aid her to run the bases or take her place. As such, the player would be awarded a one-base hit, and not the home run that she actually earned. Two of her opponents at this point performed an exceedingly unselfish act. They asked if it was legal if they carried her around the bases so she could touch the bases, and thus score the run. It was legal to do so, and so they did. The team of the players who carried the athlete lost the game that day by two runs. They might have won it had they not carried the injured player around the bases.

As noted, fair play does exist, but it can be difficult to find it in the social fabric as defined by the Victorian age. Perhaps a better question is: Can fair play exist and flourish in the highly competitive, gamesmanship world of today? Many observers believe it can, if those individuals who administer and coach athletic programs truly believe in the moral value of fair play. If they do, then missions should be written to support fair play and ethical programs and educational programs should exist for administrators, coaches, athletes, and, in youth sport, parents to support the philosophy of fair play.

In fact, such programs do exist, but they are costly in both resources and time. The World Anti-Doping Agency and U.S. Anti-Doping Agency are presently supporting research to develop fair play intervention programs. Educational programs to recapture the notion of fair play are not a simple process of making rules and expecting people to follow them. Such programs demand reading, writing, and reflection to inspire cognitive change about how we teach, coach, and administer athletic and sport programs. Unless those who are in charge of athletic and sport programs are willing to make the effort, unethical practices are likely to continue while fair play continues to suffer. The problems described here are not unique to the United States. Fair play as a social construct may be expected in sport and competition but is often violated. At the 2012 Olympic Games, two badminton teams from China were disqualified because they violated the Olympic Oath. They conspired to play poorly in early rounds of competition in order to lose. If they lost, they would be placed in a less competitive bracket and would then have a greater chance of making the finals. Officials realized what they were doing, and disqualified the teams from further competition.

Notwithstanding, the belief that sports build character can be found today at all levels of sport, even in the absence of scientific research to support that notion. There may well be reason to suppose that the philosophy of fair play could again become the overarching purpose of sport and athletics—if those who teach, coach, and administer athletics are willing to make it happen.

Sharon Kay Stoll

See also Character Development; Ethics; Moral Development; Moral Reasoning; Moral Values and Attitudes; Sportspersonship

Further Readings

Beller, J., & Stoll, S. K. (1995). Moral reasoning of high school student athletes and general students: An empirical study versus personal testimony. *Pediatric Exercise Science, 7*, 352–363.

Hansen, D., Stoll, S. K., & Beller, J. M. (2004). Four-year longitudinal study of character development in high school sport. *Research Quarterly for Exercise and Sport Supplement,* p. A-32.

Lumpkin, A., Stoll, S. K., & Beller, J. M. (2011). *Practical sport ethics.* Jefferson, NC: McFarland Press.

Shields, D. L. (2009). *What is decompetition and why does it matter?* Retrieved from http://ezinearticles.com/?What-is-Decompetition-and-Why-Does-it-Matter?&id=2285569

Simon, R. L. (2003). *Fair play: The ethics of sport* (2nd ed.). Boulder, CO: Westview Press.

Stoll, S. K. (2011). Athletics: The good it should do. *Journal of College and Character, 12*(4), 1–5.

Stoll, S. K. (2011, September). The problem of ethics and athletics: An illegitimate stepsister. *Journal of College and Character, 12*(3). doi: 10.2202/1940-1639.1817

Stoll, S. K., & Beller, J. M. (2000). Do sports build character? In J. R. Gerdy, *Sports in school: The future of an institution* (pp. 18–30). New York: Teachers College Press.

FATIGUE

Fatigue is an overwhelming sustained feeling of exhaustion and decreased capacity to complete physical and mental work. It is multidimensional with emotional, behavioral, and cognitive components. Feelings of fatigue are associated not only with disease states but also with healthy functioning. Approximately 20% of adults worldwide report current fatigue. When examined in terms of physical activity, feelings of fatigue are related to issues of physical exertion, inadequate rest, and sedentary life style. This entry reviews the evidence regarding the relationship between physical activity and feelings of fatigue and touches on issues of measurement and biological mechanisms.

Conceptualization and Measurement of Fatigue

Italian physiologist Angelo Mosso (1846–1910) began to shift the focus of research from fatigue of the body to fatigue of the mind during the late 19th century. Influenced by the work of Mosso, clinicians began to draw a sharp distinction between objective and subjective fatigue, thus broadening the conceptualization of fatigue. The concept of subjective fatigue raised measurement issues related to the indirect measure of central nervous system activity.

Contemporary theories on physical activity and feelings of fatigue have changed little over the last century and continue to focus on the multidimensional nature of the construct. In addition, the nonspecific, subjective experience of fatigue remains difficult to operationalize through measurement instruments because of the lack of known biological markers. Thus, self-report measures have dominated the clinical and scientific community. These measures range widely in their ability to offer a valid interpretation of fatigue. Despite these limitations, clinicians and researchers recognize exercise as a valuable treatment for fatigue in which the mechanism for the positive effect is likely an interaction among biological, psychological, and psychosocial variables.

Empirical Evidence

Despite the limitations in the measurement of both physical activity and fatigue, the evidence for the effect of physical activity on feelings of fatigue generally is both positive and consistent. Both epidemiological and experimental research in the areas of exercise adoption, exercise cessation, and overtraining support this association.

Population Studies

Epidemiological evidence suggests that people who are physically active in their leisure time have about 40% reduced risk of experiencing fatigue compared with sedentary individuals. There is general agreement among population-based studies of a strong, consistent, temporally appropriate, dose-response relationship between physical activity and feelings of fatigue. Furthermore, feelings of fatigue appear to be alterable in relation to the adoption or cessation of physical activity. The beneficial effects of physical activity appear to be largest for sedentary individuals who initiate and then maintain an exercise program.

Exercise Adoption

Experimental studies examining the effects of exercise training on feelings of fatigue suggest that exercise programs reduce fatigue in previously sedentary individuals. These effects are consistent across both healthy people and patient groups. Physical activity may be especially beneficial in reducing feelings of fatigue in certain patient groups with chronic diseases such as fibromyalgia, cardiovascular disease, and cancer. Exercise may represent a low-cost, efficacious adjunctive therapy that can address other health outcomes beyond fatigue in these patient groups.

Exercise Cessation

Experimental studies examining the effects of temporary exercise cessation by people who regularly exercise suggest that exercisers experience increased feelings of fatigue during periods of exercise withdrawal. These temporary mood disturbances related to fatigue appear to be alleviated with the reintroduction of the exercise regimen.

Overtraining

Overtraining is characterized by an overload in frequency, intensity, or duration of exercise such that an individual's training regime exceeds the recovery capacity. Overtraining can result in decreased performance and symptoms of under recovery or burnout such as fatigue. Increases in training volume during overtraining periods are associated with increased feelings of fatigue, whereas decreases in training volume during tapering periods are associated with decreased feelings of fatigue. Despite increases in negative overall mood in response to overtraining, feelings of fatigue often exhibit the earliest and largest changes in mood state.

Biological Mechanisms

Brain functioning is controlled by genes, but social, developmental, and environmental factors can alter gene expression. These alterations in gene expression can induce changes in brain functioning and behavior. This integrative process supports the conceptualization of fatigue as a multidimensional construct influenced by a variety of biological, psychological, and psychosocial factors. The specific brain mechanisms that generate the feelings of fatigue are unknown, but monoamines, histamine-, acetylcholine-, and gamma-aminobutyric acid (GABA)-mediated neurotransmission have been implicated. There is evidence that physical activity can alter these neurotransmitters and neuromodulators in key brain areas associated with fatigue, such as the dorsolateral prefrontal cortex, striatum, cerebellum, and spinal cord.

Conclusion

Physical activity is a healthful behavior that has promise for combating feelings of fatigue. Historically clinicians have recognized the physiological and psychological aspects of fatigue and have consistently recommended exercise as a treatment. The subjective nature of feelings of fatigue has made conceptualizing and measuring the construct difficult. Despite such limitations, epidemiological and experimental evidence suggests physical activity does reduce feelings of fatigue across both healthy groups and patient populations. However, intensive exercise training can produce feelings of fatigue in the event of overtraining. The biological mechanisms associated with physical activity and fatigue should be considered in relation to the nature of the exercise stimulus.

Timothy W. Puetz

See also Burnout; Mental Health; Neuroscience, Exercise, and Cognitive Function; Overtraining Syndrome; Underrecovery Syndrome

Further Readings

Dittner, A. J., Wessely, S. C., & Brown, R. G. (2004). The assessment of fatigue: A practical guide for clinicians and researchers. *Journal of Psychosomatic Research, 56,* 157–170.

Meeusen, R., Watson, P., Hasegawa, H., Roelands, B., & Piacentini, M. F. (2007). Brain neurotransmitters in fatigue and overtraining. *Applied Physiology, Nutrition, and Metabolism, 32,* 857–864.

Puetz, T. W. (2006). Physical activity and feelings of energy and fatigue: Epidemiological evidence. *Sports Medicine, 36,* 767–780.

Puetz, T. W., O'Connor, P. J., & Dishman, R. K. (2006). Effects of chronic exercise on feelings of energy and fatigue: A quantitative synthesis. *Psychological Bulletin, 132,* 866–876.

St Clair Gibson, A., Baden, D. A., Lambert, M. I., Lambert, E. V., Harley, Y. X., Hampson, D., et al. (2003). The conscious perception of the sensation of fatigue. *Sports Medicine, 33,* 167–176.

FEEDBACK

Feedback, or response-produced feedback, consists of all the information an individual receives as a result of a practice trial of a motor skill, classically divided into two parts—*intrinsic* and *extrinsic*. Intrinsic feedback is all of the information one receives *naturally*, such as vision, audition, and proprioception. Extrinsic feedback is information provided over and above intrinsic feedback, often by a teacher, coach, or experimenter. In the laboratory, tasks or procedures are used such that the learner typically cannot detect how well one has met the task goal, and then extrinsic feedback is manipulated to access its effects on learning. Using this method, *augmented feedback* has been considered a key variable in the learning process, without which learning does not occur at all. It operates to guide the learner to the correct movement pattern. The learner uses this information to correct errors on subsequent trials, until the desired skill level is achieved. Researchers distinguish between two types of augmented feedback: (1) *knowledge of results* (KR), provided after a trial about the movement outcome in relation to its goal, and (2) *knowledge of performance* (KP), provided during or after the movement about the nature of the movement pattern. Even though KR and KP may, on occasion, have somewhat different functions in the learning process, both seem to follow the same principles in the way they affect skill learning. Therefore, here we refer to them both as *feedback*.

Research related to the role of feedback in the learning of motor skills has a relatively long history dating from the early 1900s. The view of the role feedback plays in the learning process has changed throughout this time and continues to change. The following sections describe how our understanding of the functions of feedback has developed from the early views (1900–1970) to the second phase (1980–2000) and current research (2000–present).

Early Views: 1900–1970

Toward the beginning of the previous century, psychologists saw feedback as having primarily a reinforcing role. In particular, Edward Thorndike's law of effect stated that actions tended to be repeated if they had pleasant or rewarding consequences and avoided if they were followed by unpleasant or punishing effects; thereby, it provided an account of feedback's role in learning. Much of this early research was guided by animal (occasionally human) research showing, for example, that feedback delays and feedback frequency had negative and positive effects on animal learning, respectively. Starting in about the 1950s, researchers such as Edward A. and Ina M. Bilodeau focused more on the informational role of feedback. Feedback was considered vital for continued improvement with practice, and learning often did not seem to occur without it. Practice without feedback was thought to allow performance to drift away from the goal movement pattern and to weaken the memory representation of the movement. This view is also reflected in Jack A. Adams's (1971) closed-loop theory and Richard A. Schmidt's (1975) schema theory of motor learning. In both theories, the memory representation of a skill (perceptual trace in Adams' theory; recall and recognition schemata in Schmidt's theory) was thought to develop as a function of practice and feedback. That is, the greater the number of trials with feedback a person had performed, the stronger memory representations were assumed to be, and the better the person's ability both to perform and to detect and correct errors without augmented feedback. According to this view, feedback would be most effective if it was provided frequently and immediately. In the 1980s, these ideas began to be questioned.

Second Phase: 1980–2000

The second major phase of feedback research was initiated and inspired by an influential review of the feedback literature by Alan W. Salmoni, Richard A. Schmidt, and Charles B. Walter in 1984. It became clear that many of the earlier studies had shortcomings, most notably a lack of retention or transfer tests to assess the more permanent, or learning, effects of different feedback manipulations (e.g., temporal delays, frequencies, precision). Inferring learning from the performance of different groups during the practice phase—that is, under the influence of different feedback conditions—became unacceptable. Instead, it was argued, the use of delayed tests under common conditions was crucial to assessing stable learning effects of various experimental variables including augmented feedback. Importantly, Salmoni et al. provided a new conceptual framework for feedback, which was formalized as the *guidance hypothesis*. The term referred to the role of feedback in guiding the performer to the correct movement pattern during the learning process. Aside from this positive function of feedback, several potentially negative effects of frequent feedback were proposed as well. In particular, it was hypothesized that the learner, with very frequent feedback, could become dependent on the augmented feedback, thereby neglecting the processing of intrinsic feedback, which would be necessary for the development of intrinsic error detection and correction mechanisms. Frequent feedback was also assumed to result in excessive variability in performance, as it would prompt learners to constantly correct even small (perhaps acceptable) errors (so-called maladaptive short-term corrections) that perhaps reflected inherent variability in the motor system. The result would be the development of a less stable movement representation. The guidance hypothesis therefore suggested a positive influence of frequent, immediate, or precise feedback during practice while it was present, but it could have a detrimental impact on learning if it were overdone.

Numerous studies examining various feedback manipulations provided support for the guidance idea. These studies typically used feedback manipulations that in some way attempted to reduce the detrimental effects of frequent feedback by encouraging learners to attend to and utilize their intrinsic feedback. For example, reducing the relative frequency of feedback (reduced percentage of trials after which feedback is provided) was found to enhance learning compared with feedback after every trial (100% feedback). Also, summary or average feedback (feedback for individual trials or as an average, respectively, presented only after a set of trials has been completed) have been shown to be more beneficial for learning than feedback after every trial. Furthermore, bandwidth feedback (feedback provided only when errors exceed a certain predetermined bandwidth) appears to reduce movement variability and enhance learning. Finally, delaying feedback, even by a few seconds, and asking learners to estimate their errors prior to receiving feedback have been demonstrated to yield more effective learning outcomes than providing feedback immediately after the completion of the movement, or concurrently with the execution of a movement.

The guidance hypothesis had an important impact on motor learning research. It has contributed to a better understanding of how feedback influences performance and learning. Yet, even though there has been considerable support for the guidance hypothesis, this support comes primarily from studies using relatively simple laboratory tasks or involving situations in which learners were deprived of intrinsic outcome information and therefore had to rely on the augmented feedback provided by the experimenter. In recent years, it has become clear that the guidance view does not provide a comprehensive description of the various functions of feedback in the process of (complex) motor skill learning. One important factor that influences the effectiveness of feedback, and that qualifies the influence of the feedback frequency, is the attentional focus induced by it. Furthermore, there is converging evidence that feedback has not only an informational role, but that its motivational influence on learning is more important than previously thought.

Current Research: 2000–Present

Feedback and Focus of Attention

Studies have consistently shown that feedback or preperformance instructions promoting an external focus of attention—whereby attention is directed to the movement effect on the environment (e.g., the motion of implement, trajectory of a ball)—enhances learning compared with those instructions inducing an internal focus by directing one's attention to one's body movements. That is, a simple change in the wording of feedback can elicit an external or internal focus and produce markedly different learning results. For example, references to the movement of a golf club have been shown to be more effective than those related to the performer's arm movements. External focus advantages for learning have been found for many different types of motor skills, different age groups, and levels of expertise.

Feedback that directs performers' attention to their own body movements causes them to use a more conscious mode of control, which constrains the motor system and interferes with automatic control processes (the *constrained-action hypothesis*). In contrast, by adopting an external focus on the intended movement effect, performers use a more automatic type of control that makes use of unconscious, fast, and reflexive processes. Studies have shown associations of external attentional foci and various measures of automaticity—including reduced attentional demands, reduced pre-movement times (more efficient motor planning), high-frequency (reflexive) movement adjustments, and reduced muscular activity. The result of adopting an external focus is typically enhanced motor performance and learning, as seen in increased movement effectiveness and efficiency.

Not only does feedback promoting an external focus of attention lead to more effective learning than feedback referring to body movements, but the previously found benefits of a reduced relative to a high-feedback frequency have been found to be reversed. That is, despite the informational content being the same, feedback inducing an external focus is most effective when it is provided frequently (e.g., 100%), whereas feedback inducing an internal focus is least effective when it is given frequently. The interaction of feedback frequency and attentional focus, as well as the overall benefits of external relative to internal focus feedback, cannot be explained by extant conceptualizations of feedback (e.g., guidance hypothesis).

One possibility is that at least some of the learning benefits of reduced feedback frequencies found in previous studies were not primarily due to learners' becoming dependent on frequent augmented feedback. Rather, the detrimental effects of frequent feedback may have been because of constant internal focus reminders, with those (negative)

effects being attenuated under reduced feedback conditions. The interactive effects of feedback frequency and attentional focus would be consistent with the concept that experiencing less of a detrimental influence (limited use of an impairing thought such as an internal focus of attention) is good, as more of a good thing (frequent reminders to maintain a beneficial external focus) is good.

It has been suggested that the mere mention of body parts like fingers, arms, or feet—within internal focus feedback or instructions—might provoke a focus on the *self* and ensuing self-regulatory activity. Efforts to manage self-related thoughts and emotions may be so demanding that available attentional capacity is exceeded and performance suffers. In contrast, when feedback promotes an external focus, a focus on the self is reduced. The mechanisms underlying the beneficial effects of feedback inducing an external focus may not be dissimilar to those responsible for the learning advantages seen when feedback is given about successful trials, or when it suggests above-average performance relative to a peer group. These types of feedback are discussed next.

Feedback After Successful Trials

Until recently, most researchers were concerned with the *informational function* of feedback, that is, its role in providing information about an individual's performance relative to the task goal. Similarly, practitioners often see performance feedback from this perspective. For instance, a coach might identify deviations from the optimal technique in an athlete's movement patterns and suggest corrections. While such feedback plays an important role in any learning process, a somewhat underappreciated aspect of feedback has been its influence on the performer's motivational state. Recent findings demonstrate that positive (or negative) feedback affects motor learning via its motivational influence.

Providing learners with feedback after good trials, as opposed to poor trials, has consistently been shown to result in more effective learning. In several studies, feedback about task performance (i.e., accuracy of throwing an object at a target) was provided after each of several blocks of practice trials. However, it was provided on only half of those trials. Unbeknownst to the learners, they were given feedback either about their most effective trials or about their least accurate trials.

Participants receiving feedback after their best trials demonstrated more effective learning on a retention test. Thus, feedback emphasizing successful performance, while ignoring less successful attempts, benefited learning. This effect has been linked to participants' enhanced intrinsic motivation. Learners often appear to have a relatively good feel for how they perform, and instructor feedback indicating errors may not only be superfluous, but it can also irritate learners or heighten concerns about the self that may hamper learning (see below).

Social-Comparative Feedback

Effects of *normative feedback*—which involves norms such as a peer group's actual or false average performance or improvement scores that are provided in addition to the learner's own scores—have been examined in a related line of research. Normative information is a potent basis for evaluating one's own performance. Favorable comparisons with others typically result in perceptions of competence, increased self-efficacy, and motivation, while negative comparisons have the opposite effect. Importantly, normative feedback also has differential effects on motor learning, with learning being enhanced by positive relative to negative or no normative feedback. In other studies, bogus feedback about a peer group's average block-to-block improvement resulted in enhanced learning if it conveyed to the learner that one's own improvement was greater than average, compared to less than average. Thus, favorable social-comparative feedback affects the degree to which task skill is retained.

Positive normative feedback not only leads to improved outcome scores but also produces qualitative differences in participants' control of movements, such as greater automaticity in movement control. It is interesting that positive feedback benefits learning compared with both control conditions without comparison information and negative normative feedback conditions, which have similar effects. This suggests that the latter conditions may trigger thoughts about the self (similar to feedback inducing an internal focus), and ensuing self-regulatory activities in attempts to manage thoughts and affective responses, which hamper learning of the primary task. In contrast, when one is purportedly performing well (above average), such self-related concerns and activities

to suppress them might be unnecessary—with the consequence that learning is enhanced.

For ethical reasons, providing false feedback in practical settings would not seem to be appropriate. However, the findings suggest feedback that implies one is an effective performer, or the provision of positive, competence-affirming feedback is critical for learning. While many practitioners may intuitively provide such feedback, others may be more focused on correcting errors—with unintended consequences for motivation and learning.

Conclusion

The view of how feedback functions in the process of motor skill learning has changed over the past few decades. It is now clear that the role of feedback goes far beyond providing reinforcement or guidance to the goal movement. There is mounting evidence for the motivational role of feedback—which not only has an indirect effect by increasing the amount of practice—but a *direct* impact on motor learning. The learning of motor skills not only involves the fine-tuning of motor programs and movement parameters but requires effective self-regulation of cognitive and affective processes, as well as attentional focus demands. A more integrated perspective on motivational and informational aspects of feedback in motor learning research will benefit future theoretical conceptualizations—and should also yield practical motor skill learning insights, as neutral task information is not easily found in the natural social contexts in which movement skills are learned.

Gabriele Wulf and Richard A. Schmidt

See also Attentional Focus

Further Readings

Lewthwaite, R., & Wulf, G. (2010). Social-comparative feedback affects motor skill learning. *Quarterly Journal of Experimental Psychology, 63*, 738–749.

Salmoni, A. W., Schmidt, R. A., & Walter, C. B. (1984). Knowledge of results and motor learning: A review and critical reappraisal. *Psychological Bulletin, 95*, 355–386.

Schmidt, R. A., & Lee, T. D. (2011). Augmented feedback. In R. A. Schmidt & T. D. Lee (Eds.), *Motor control and learning* (5th ed., pp. 393–427). Champaign, IL: Human Kinetics

Wulf, G., Chiviacowsky, S., Schiller, E., & Gentilini Ávila, L. T. (2010). Frequent external-focus feedback enhances learning. *Frontiers in Psychology, 1,* 190. doi: 10.3389/fpsyg.2010.00190

Wulf, G., & Shea, C. H. (2004). Understanding the role of augmented feedback: The good, the bad, and the ugly. In A. M. Williams & N. J. Hodges (Eds.), *Skill acquisition in sport: Research, theory and practice* (pp. 121–144). London: Routledge.

FEMALE ATHLETE TRIAD

The female athlete triad (triad) refers to the co-occurrence of three interrelated conditions: low energy availability, menstrual dysfunction, and low bone-mineral density. Factors within sport and exercise environments can increase the risk of developing these conditions. Though the prevalence of the full triad is low, many girls and women will experience one or two of the conditions, which can increase their risk of developing the triad. The triad represents a significant health concern, as it can lead to serious and long-lasting health consequences.

Interrelated Conditions

Originally, the triad included disordered eating, amenorrhea, and osteoporosis. However, in 2007, the American College of Sports Medicine revised their position and redefined the triad as low energy availability, menstrual dysfunction, and low bone-mineral density (BMD). *Low energy availability* refers to the amount of energy after exercise or training that is available for physical functioning and may result from excessive exercise, insufficient caloric intake, or other methods of purging, such as laxatives or vomiting. Eating disorders (EDs), including anorexia nervosa (AN), bulimia nervosa (BN), and eating disorders not otherwise specified (EDNOS) may be present and contribute to low energy availability. However, low energy availability can be present without EDs.

Menstrual dysfunction, the second defining condition of the triad, includes primary amenorrhea (delay of menarche), secondary amenorrhea (absence of menstrual cycle, after menarche, for more than three consecutive months) and oligomenorrhea (more than 35 days between menstrual cycles). Abnormal menstrual functioning often results from low energy availability and can contribute to low BMD. *Low BMD* is defined as a BMD of at least one standard unit lower than age-group matched controls, lower than normal levels of estrogen, history of deficient nutrition, and previous bone fractures. Low BMD can result from insufficient accumulation of bone mineral during childhood and adolescence or from bone mineral loss during adulthood.

Prevalence

The prevalence of low energy availability has not been well documented. However, estimates of clinical EDs, which may contribute to low energy availability, range between 0% and 13.4% among college and elite athletes. Prevalence of subclinical levels of disordered eating is much higher, though rates of specific pathogenic weight-control behaviors vary widely. For example, few athletes report using laxatives or diuretics or engaging in self-induced vomiting, but many diet and exercise excessively. Menstrual dysfunction, a product of low energy availability, ranges between 16.6% and 54% among high school athletes and up to 63.9% among college athletes. Low BMD has been found in up to 21.8% of high school athletes and 11% of elite athletes.

Prevalence estimates of the co-occurrence of all three conditions are lacking. Several studies using the original, more narrowly defined, criteria report rates of 1.2% (high school), 2.7% (college) and 4.3% (elite). In a study using the current ACSM guidelines (2007), the triad was found among 15.9% of college runners. When considering the presence of two of the three conditions, prevalence rates can range up to 18% among high school athletes and 26.9% among elite athletes. The presence of any of these conditions may increase the risk of developing the full triad.

Risk Factors

Numerous factors can increase female athletes' risk for developing triad conditions. Distorted attitudes toward food, eating, and body weight and shape are associated with unhealthy eating and weight-control behaviors that can create low energy availability. Athletes in sports that emphasize leanness, low body weight, or appearance, such as distance running, gymnastics, or dance, may be more likely to experience pressures from coaches, teammates, family, and other sport personnel (e.g., judges) about body size or shape. Such stressors may lead athletes to restrict caloric intake and exercise excessively.

Evidence also suggests that sport participation at an elite competitive level increases risk of the triad. Pressure and expectations to consistently perform and achieve at a high level often increase among elite-level athletes. Moreover, there may be serious consequences for poor performance for elite athletes. For example, losing a spot on the national team or losing a sponsorship or endorsement may significantly impact an athlete's livelihood. Thus, athletes competing at elite levels are not only likely to engage in extensive physical training but also may be susceptible to disturbed body image and weight-related pressures, placing them at increased risk for low energy availability.

Health Consequences

All three triad conditions put female athletes at risk for a number of negative health consequences. Disordered eating behaviors, which can contribute to low energy availability, are associated with low self-esteem, anxiety, depression, and a myriad of physical health problems, such as cardiovascular problems, constipation, electrolyte imbalance, muscle cramps, or muscle weakness). Menstrual dysfunction can increase the risk of infertility and result in muscular problems and decreases in BMD. Menstrual irregularities and low BMD increases the risk of stress fractures.

Screening and Prevention

The American College of Sports Medicine recommends screening for the triad during preparticipation and annual health screenings. Additionally, female athletes who present with one triad condition should be screened for the other two. The Female Athlete Triad Pre-Participation Evaluation (Triad PPE), available from the Female Athlete Triad Coalition, can be used to assess eating habits and attitudes, weight and menstrual histories, and history of stress fractures. Potential low BMD can be evaluated via dual-energy X-ray absorptiometry (DXA) when there is a history of low estrogen, disordered eating, or history of stress fractures.

To reduce the risk of the triad, coaches, administrators, and sports medicine professionals can create body-healthy environments by avoiding weigh-ins, weight logs, and weight-related joking, as well as pressures to achieve an unrealistic body size or shape. Moreover, sport governing bodies can promote healthy sport environments by providing triad education and training to officials,

coaches, and athletes. Prevention is important because treatment can be challenging; for example, treatment may not result in restoration of normal levels of BMD and ED recovery rates are low. Education, increased awareness, and early interventions are important steps in triad prevention.

Christy Greenleaf and Trent Petrie

See also Body Dissatisfaction; Body Image; Eating Disorders

Further Readings

Cover, K., Hanna, M., & Barnes, M. R. (2012). A review and proposed treatment approach for the young athlete at high risk for the female athlete triad. *Infant, Child, & Adolescent Nutrition, 4,* 21–27.

Female Athlete Triad Coalition. (2008). *Female Athlete Triad pre-participation evaluation.* Retrieved from http://www.femaleathletetriad.org/~triad/wp-content/uploads/2008/11/ppe_for_website.pdf

George, C. A., Leonard, J. P., & Hutchinson, M. R. (2011). The female athlete triad: A current concepts review. *South African Journal of Sports Medicine, 23,* 50–56.

Nattiv, A., Loucks, A. B., Manore, M. M., Sanborn, C. F., Sundgot-Borgen, J., & Warren, M. P. (2007). American College of Sports Medicine position stand. The female athlete triad. *Medicine and Science in Sports and Exercise, 39*(10), 1867–1882.

FEMINISM

Feminism is a movement to end oppression, especially as it relates to sexism. Feminism can be taken up in many contexts such as sport and exercise, where theorists and practitioners engage with feminist theory, feminist activism, feminist politics, feminist education, feminist class, race, or gender struggle, and global feminism to varying degrees. In this entry, common myths about feminists are explored. This is followed by a discussion of feminist history, theory, and advocacy and some concluding remarks.

Common Myths Surrounding Feminists

Several myths abound related to those who take up feminism and feminist theory. These include (a) feminists are aggressive; (b) feminists hate men; (c) feminists do not wear make-up, are not feminine, are manly, or are ugly; (d) all feminists are lesbian; (e) feminists have no sense of humor; (f) feminists want to take over the world; (g) feminists are obsessed with gender; and (h) we live in a postfeminist age now—we don't need feminism anymore.

In terms of the myth that feminists are aggressive, since the late 1800s, feminists—including some men—have been advocating for equal rights for women in a peaceful and nonviolent way. In fact, the feminist movement is one of the few social movements where there is virtually no documented violence related to protests calling for this type of social change. Regarding the myth that feminists hate men, there are plenty of men who stand side-by-side with women who are involved in feminist movements because they are also disturbed by patriarchy's effect on their lives and on the lives of their mothers, sisters, daughters, wives, female best friends, cousins, and so on. When people say that they think feminists do not wear make-up, are not feminine, are manly or are ugly, what they are referring to is traditional notions of *heterosexual beauty* in a society, which includes (for women) applying foundation, eye shadow, eye liner, mascara, rouge, and other cosmetics, in an effort to fit what is defined as heterosexually *beautiful* or *sexy* for women. Those who do not want to wear make-up are seen as ugly; the next leap that most people make is that because they are not interested in wearing make-up or looking *feminine*, they are not heterosexual. The myth that all feminists are lesbian is related to this leap; however, not all feminists are lesbian just like not all women (regardless of sexual orientation) are political. While it is true that many lesbian and bisexual women were a part of the early feminist movement, it was partially because they themselves had already wrestled with pushing against rigid sexual, gender, class, race, and political categories. There is also the belief that feminists have no sense of humor. This may be because those who advocate feminism do not laugh at jokes made at the expense of women. If they are not laughing when others are, they may be perceived as having no sense of humor; in reality, however, they probably do not find it humorous when women are made fun of. The notion that feminists want to take over the world often comes from the fear (by some) that men will be replaced in positions of power, including in the economic, educational, governmental, and political sectors. While it is true that liberal feminists fight for an equal percentage of men and women in these contexts,

according to recent research, it is also true that successful corporations must have at least one third of their management (e.g., those in power) represented by minority workers, including women. The perception that feminists are obsessed with gender appears related to the fact that feminists are concerned with gender oppression. This is because, in most societies, males are valued over females and masculine interests are privileged over feminine interests. Those who are in the marginalized positions in society are acutely aware of the differences that are highlighted in often taken-for-granted daily encounters. Finally, the myth that we live in a postfeminist age now and we don't need feminism anymore *appears* most prevalent in young women who have grown up in a post–Title IX era. Interestingly, these women are usually college age and may not have experienced sexism in the workplace because they have not yet entered the workforce full time.

Brief History of Feminism, Feminist Theory, and Advocacy

Most researchers agree that there are at least three major waves of feminist movement: (1) from the mid-1800s through 1930; (2) during the 1960s and 1970s; and (3) post-1970s. Feminism actually began as a campaign for women to get the vote. During the first wave in mid-1800s, women advocated for the right to vote first in England, then in France, and then in the United States. In the United States in 1837, Mount Holyoke—the first of the *seven sister colleges*—was founded. This was followed in 1850 by the suffragette movement in the United Kingdom. However, neither England nor the United States was one of the first countries to grant women voting rights; it was New Zealand in 1893, Australia in 1902, the United States in 1920, and the United Kingdom in 1928.

There was a lull in feminist movement in the United States between the first two waves (between 1930 and 1960). This was because men were coming home from World War II in the 1940s and taking back the jobs they once held in factories and other work settings. During the war, these jobs were filled by women participating in the war effort (e.g., working in factories which manufactured parts for the war). However, once the men returned, women were expected to go back into the home, become housewives, and start families.

During the second wave (roughly 1960–1980), the focus was on women taking control of their own bodies, relationships, sexuality, health, and vitality and gaining equality in the workforce. Researchers utilized major feminist theories, including liberal, critical, Marxist, radical, socialist, and ecofeminism, as well as feminist epistemology, empiricism, standpoint theory, and postmodernism. In 1963, Betty Friedan—a wife and mother—wrote a groundbreaking book called *The Feminine Mystique,* which described how "unfulfilled" she was, limited to just those two roles. Friedan and 27 others founded the National Organization for Women (N.O.W.) in 1966. Major theoretical debates were framed around Marxism (e.g., social class issues). In 1970, Shulamith Firestone's *The Dialectic of Sex* was published at the same time that organized marches, demonstrations, bra burnings, and consciousness-raising sessions began. In 1972, Gloria Steinem started *Ms. Magazine.*

Third-wave feminism began post-1980. The focus during this wave was on redefining the feminist movement, especially to include younger women and direct advocacy. While researchers continued to utilize major feminist theories (e.g., liberal, critical, Marxist, radical, socialist, and ecofeminism), many incorporated a hybrid of theorizing that reflected their beliefs about the ways women know what they know (feminist epistemology), how to include women more fully in the scientific process (feminist empiricism), the fact that each woman—particularly those women who have multiple marginal identities—has a unique story to tell (feminist standpoint theory), and a shattering of what was once taken-for-granted notions about *truth* and the structure of gendered *identity* (feminist postmodernism).

Conclusion

Feminism has had at least three distinct waves and has been described as a movement to end sexist oppression. While myths about feminists abound, those who advocate feminism have succeeded in calling attention to gender inequity in the workplace as well as in other contexts such as sport and exercise.

Leslee A. Fisher

Further Readings

Baumgardner, J., & Richards, A. (2000). *Manifesta: Young women, feminism, and the future.* New York: Farrar, Straus & Giroux.

Baumgardner, J., & Richards, A. (2005). *Grassroots: A field guide for feminist activism.* New York: Farrar, Straus & Giroux.

Belenky, M. F., Clinchy, B. M., Goldberger, N. R., & Tarule, J. M. (1997). Introduction: To the other side of silence. In M. F. Belenky (Ed.), *Women's ways of knowing* (pp. 3–20). New York: Basic Books.

Costa, D., & Guthrie, S. (1994). *Women and sport: Interdisciplinary perspectives.* Champaign, IL: Human Kinetics.

hooks, b. (1984). *Feminist theory: From margin to center.* Cambridge, MA: South End Press.

hooks, b. (2000). *Feminism is for everybody: Passionate politics.* Cambridge, MA: South End Press.

Hughes, K. (1998). *Every girl's guide to feminism.* South Melbourne, Australia: Longman.

Krane, V. (2001). We can be athletic and feminine, but do we want to? Challenging hegemonic femininity in women's sport. *Quest, 53,* 115–133.

FLOW

Flow is a special psychological state of total absorption in a task. When in flow, athletes are fully focused on what they are doing, and this heightened attention is associated with a number of positive factors. Accompanying a focused mindset are factors such as knowing exactly what one is going to do and how one is doing, having a sense of oneness with the task being performed, and feeling in control of one's performance. A number of factors have to be in place for flow to occur, and it's not an easy state for most to attain. However, once experienced, individuals are motivated to re-experience flow, because of how intrinsically rewarding an experience it is. Understanding the flow experience is important because it provides a gateway to optimal subjective experience.

Theoretical Background

Mihaly Csikszentmihalyi developed the flow concept in the 1970s, after investigating the experiences of individuals when everything came together during times of involvement with a chosen activity. The types of activities initially investigated by Csikszentmihalyi were diverse, ranging from surgery to dancing to chess and rock climbing. Despite such diversity in setting, there was considerable consistency of responses regarding what was felt during moments that stood out as being special in some way for the individual.

Since his initial investigations where the term *flow* was chosen to denote these special absorbing experiences, Csikszentmihalyi has continued a research program examining this experience. Flow has been examined across diverse settings, from daily living to a state of mind associated with scientific discoveries. There has been remarkable consistency in how flow has been described by individuals across diverse settings. In addition to the enjoyment that flow brings an individual, the experience of flow is associated with many positive psychological characteristics, and is an optimal performance state. Flow has been identified as a key psychological construct in *positive psychology*, a growing field of interest in psychology, particularly with regard to positive subjective experience.

The Experience of Flow

When in flow, one feels strong and positive, not worried about self or failure. Flow can be defined as an experience that stands out as being better than average in some way, where the individual is totally absorbed in what is being done, and where the experience is very rewarding in and of itself. This definition covers several characteristics of flow, and Csikszentmihalyi has detailed the experience of flow into nine dimensions.

The first and perhaps most critical dimension of flow is the concept of challenge–skill balance. Flow is predicted to occur when the individual moves beyond average experience of challenge and skill. The moving beyond average signifies an investment of mental energy into a task. When the perceived challenges are matched by a belief in having the skills to meet the challenge, the stage is set for flow to occur. The perception of challenge, and of skill, is more important than any objective level of challenges or skills in flow state. That is, prediction of the experience of flow is more accurately based on what individuals perceive the levels of challenge and skills are in situations than by reference to the levels of challenges and skills that may actually exist in those situations.

In flow, one is totally involved in the task at hand. Flow can occur at different levels of complexity but, by definition, flow is intrinsically rewarding, regardless of whether it involves a simple task, or a complicated and dangerous gymnastics routine. Csikszentmihalyi categorized the different levels of flow into micro and macro flow experiences.

Micro flow experiences were proposed to fit the patterns of everyday life, whereas macro flow was reserved for experiences associated with higher levels of complexity and demand on the participant. These latter experiences are often associated with peak performance and peak experience.

The Dimensions of Flow

Csikszentmihalyi conceptualized the flow construct in terms of nine dimensions; the first of these dimensions, challenge–skill balance, has already been described. The other dimensions are action–awareness merging, clear goals, unambiguous feedback, concentration on task, sense of control, loss of self-consciousness, time transformation, and autotelic experience. Together, these nine dimensions represent the optimal psychological state of flow; by themselves, they signify conceptual elements of the flow experience.

The action–awareness merging dimension involves a feeling of being at one with the activity being performed. Often used in descriptions by people asked to discuss what it was like being in flow, perceptions of oneness with an activity bring about a sense of peace and harmony to an active engagement with a task. For some performers, feelings of automaticity are described, with well-learned routines enabling them to process subconsciously and pay full attention to their actions.

Clear goals occur in flow, with individuals describing knowing exactly what it is they are supposed to do. Such clarity of purpose occurs on a moment-by-moment basis, keeping a person fully connected to the task and responsive to relevant cues. Closely associated with clear goals is the processing of how performance is progressing in relation to these goals. This is the dimension of unambiguous feedback. When in flow, feedback is easy to receive and interpret. The performer receives clear, unambiguous information that processes effortlessly, keeping performance heading in the right direction.

The next dimension of flow is total concentration on the task at hand. This is one of the clearest indications of being in flow—one is totally focused in the present on the specific task or activity with which one is engaged. Being totally connected to the task in which one is engaged epitomizes the flow state. This connectedness relies on a present-centered focus; flow resides in being in the present moment.

A present-centered focus leads to the next dimension of flow, known as having a sense of control over what one is doing. Being fully connected to the task or activity in which one is engaged allows a person to perceive a sense of control and confidence in what one is doing. This is an empowering feeling, and one that frees a person from a fear of failure that can creep into performance. The absence of thoughts of failure enables an individual to engage in the challenges at hand.

Loss of self-consciousness is another flow dimension, one characterized by a lack of concern about what others may be thinking of them. A lot of the time people live their lives surrounded by evaluations of how they are doing. This sense of evaluation can prevent a full focus on the task at hand. Because flow is defined by being totally focused on the task at hand, it allow for a loss of self-consciousness during engagement in an activity.

A sense of time passing differently defines the dimension of flow known as time transformation. For some, the experience is that time stops. For others, time seems to slow. Or it may be that time seems to pass more quickly than expected. These sensations come about through the intensity of involvement in flow. Because awareness is tightly focused during the intense concentration of flow, people can lose track of time, and afterwards can be surprised by the actual passing of time that has occurred during their task involvement.

Autotelic experience is the final flow dimension, and is the end result of the coming together of the previous eight dimensions. Autotelic experience describes the intrinsically rewarding nature of flow. As described by Csikszentmihalyi, the word is derived from two Greek words that describe doing something for its own sake (*auto,* which means "self" and *telos,* which means "goal"). The idea is that experience of flow is sufficiently enjoyable as to be, in itself, a much sought-after and self-rewarding state. The nine dimensions of flow provide a conceptually coherent framework for understanding optimal experience.

Flow in Sport

Research on sport involvement was a part of Csikszentmihalyi's landmark 1975 book, *Beyond Boredom and Anxiety,* wherein the flow construct was initially conceptualized. Investigation of flow and related concepts (e.g., peak experience, peak performance) in sport started to become evident in the literature the 1980s. In the 1990s, Susan Jackson's systematic qualitative and quantitative efforts to understand the athletic flow experience led to the 1999 publication of the Jackson and Csikszentmihalyi book *Flow in Sports: The Keys to Optimal Experiences and Performances.* Jackson's in-depth qualitative examination of athletes' flow experiences, for example, have demonstrated strong support for Csikszentmihalyi's nine-dimensional model. Across various quantitative studies, positive associations between flow and several important constructs in sport psychology, including task-focused motivation, perceptions of ability, self-determined forms of motivation, hypnotic susceptibility, and use of psychological skills have been reported as well as consistent negative relationships between flow and anxiety. Factors perceived by athletes as influencing flow were identified in Jackson's research that served to provide useful understandings of antecedent and disruptive factors. Examples of factors perceived by athletes to influence whether or not flow occurred during their performance included level of motivation toward the performance, physical preparation and readiness, confidence, and focus. Considerable interest in the flow construct led to development of different ways of empirically studying flow, and this research effort has made flow a more accessible psychological concept for the applied researcher and also to practitioners interested in flow in their performance settings.

Measuring Flow

Interest in the flow concept has led to a range of approaches to tap into this experience. Both qualitative and quantitative approaches have been used to assess flow. In-depth information about the experience of flow has been obtained through interviews. Sampling of experience as it occurs through the use of pagers programmed to sound at random times has been another approach used to assess flow. Self-report questionnaires are part of this approach, known as the experience sampling method. The development of self-report questionnaires that can be administered after performance, as well as more generally, has facilitated assessment of flow along with other psychological constructs, to understand factors associated with the flow experience. The set of Flow Scales developed by Susan Jackson and colleagues provide researchers and practitioners with a range of measurement options for assessing flow. These include scales based on the nine-dimensional flow model, assessed at state and dispositional levels.

Conclusion

Flow is an optimal psychological state that occurs when challenges and skills are balanced and extending an individual. The total focus of flow and the associated positive experiential characteristics of this state provide an opportunity for individuals to move their experience from average to optimal. One outcome of this heightened level of experience is that peak performance is often achieved. However, flow is important not so much for any performance outcomes that may ensue, but primarily for the opportunity it provides to experience full engagement in the present moment.

Susan Jackson and Robert C. Eklund

See also Achievement Goal Theory; Attention–Performance Relationships; Enjoyment; Passion; Self-Determination Theory

Further Readings

Csikszentmihalyi, M. (1975). *Beyond boredom and anxiety.* San Francisco: Jossey-Bass.

Csikszentmihalyi, M. (1990). *Flow: The psychology of optimal experience.* New York: Harper & Row.

Csikszentmihalyi, M. (1997). *Finding flow: The psychology of engagement with everyday life.* New York: HarperCollins.

Jackson, S. A. (1995). Factors influencing the occurrence of flow states in elite athletes. *Journal of Applied Sport Psychology, 7,* 135–163.

Jackson, S. A. (1996). Toward a conceptual understanding of the flow experience in elite athletes. *Research Quarterly for Exercise and Sport, 67,* 76–90.

Jackson, S. A., & Csikszentmihalyi, M. (1999). *Flow in sports: The keys to optimal experiences and performances.* Champaign, IL: Human Kinetics.

Jackson, S. A., & Eklund, R. C. (2002). Assessing flow in physical activity: The FSS-2 and DFS-2. *Journal of Sport & Exercise Psychology, 24,* 133–150.

Jackson, S. A., Eklund, R. C., & Martin, A. J. (2010). *The FLOW manual.* Menlo Park, CA: Mind Garden.

FREEZING

Complex systems in nature are defined as having many individual components that are free to vary and interact with each other, exemplified by a sand pile, a weather system, and social collectives such as animal colonies and sports teams. An athlete can also be studied in this way. In the complexity sciences, the term *degrees of freedom* typically refers to the independent components of a system that can be reorganized in many different ways as surrounding constraints change. When considering the human body as a complex system, an important challenge is to understand how coordination emerges among the large number of motor system degrees of freedom (e.g., the muscles, joints, limb segments). In motor learning, this challenge is known as Nikolai Bernstein's *degrees of freedom problem*: How can humans organize the large number of motor system degrees of freedom to consistently produce functional actions such as catching a ball with one hand? Even a simple movement of reaching and grasping an object with the hand and arm could require a catcher to regulate 7 degrees of freedom (dfs) of the arm, involving flexion–extension, medial–lateral movement, and rotation of joints (3 at the shoulder, 1 at the elbow, and 3 at the wrist). Of course, more degrees of freedom need to be regulated in coordinating more complex actions such as performing a triple somersault in gymnastics.

Bernstein proposed that performers initially cope with the large number of motor system degrees of freedom by rigidly fixing or *freezing* a small number into a basic motor pattern to achieve a task goal. This strategy leads to the characteristic stiffness that many individuals portray early in learning. The freezing of motor system degrees of freedom is a completely understandable coping mechanism when anyone is placed in an unfamiliar performance context and shows how an individual's intentions, perception, and action interact to constrain the movement pattern that emerges. For example, when novices learn to swim their main intention is to remain afloat and maintain stability in the water in order to breathe and not sink. This intention contrasts with those of an Olympic-level swimmer seeking to move rapidly and efficiently through the water to reach a race endpoint in the shortest time possible. An initial coordination mode in the breaststroke corresponds to an iso-contraction of the nonhomologous limbs: the in-phase muscle contraction of arms and legs together. System stability is enhanced by synchronizing the flexion and extension of both arms and legs together, rather like the directional movements of an accordion. The accordion mode of coordination corresponds to a juxtapositioning of two contradictory actions: leg propulsion during arm recovery and arm propulsion during leg recovery. It is not mechanically effective and does not provide high swim speed because each propulsive action is thwarted by a recovery action. However, this freezing coordination strategy is functional for novice swimmers because it is the most stable and easiest to perform early in learning.

As learners become more familiar with a task, their intentions change quickly and they can abandon the coping strategy of freezing degrees of freedom by reorganizing them into specific functional muscle–joint linkages or synergies. Bernstein advocated that these more functional groupings help learners compress the numerous physical components of the movement system to make the relevant dfs for an action become mutually dependent. Synergies between motor system components help make the body more manageable for learners when they discover and assemble strongly coupled limb relations to cope with the huge number of movement system degrees of freedom.

Synergies are functional, being designed for a specific purpose or activity, such as when groups of muscles are temporarily assembled into coherent units to achieve specific task goals, like throwing a ball or performing a triple salchow in ice skating. Good quality perceptual information is necessary in assembling coordinative structures because the details of their specific form or organization are not completely predetermined and emerge under the constraints of each performance situation. Assembling a synergy is a dynamical process dependent on relevant sources of perceptual information related to key properties of the performer (e.g., haptic information from muscles and joints) and the environment (e.g., vision of a target or surface). Synergies emerge from the rigidly fixed configurations that learners use early on to manage the multitude of motor system dfs and become dynamic and flexible as learners use information to tune their functional organization.

Bernstein's ideas were a precursor to recognition of the human body as a complex system and were instrumental for movement scientists seeking to understand how coordination can emerge in human movement systems with their huge number of degrees of freedom, such as muscles, joints, and limb segments. It has been suggested that the degrees-of-freedom problem can be resolved in a human movement system if the human movement system is conceptualized as a complex, dynamical system in which cooperation between subsystem components can lead to a reduction in system dimensionality through the emergence of synergies or more compact movement patterns. Some research on how skilled and unskilled individuals kick a football has supported these ideas. D. I. Anderson and Ben Sidaway's detailed analysis of kicking confirmed the different ways that motor system degrees of freedom are reorganized during learning. They demonstrated that novice kickers did not display the same coordination patterns as skilled individuals. The rigidity of novice movement patterns and the flexible nature of skilled kicking patterns were clearly depicted in their work. Before practice, the joint range of motion (ROM) for knee flexion and extension during kicking by unskilled participants was smaller in magnitude than the values observed in skilled kickers. Smaller ranges of joint ROM tend to signify greater rigidity of movement patterns. After practicing for 10 weeks at 15 minutes per week, the novice group's coordination pattern began to lose its rigidly fixed characteristic and tended to resemble the more flexible pattern of skilled kickers.

Keith Davids

See also Coordination; Motor Commands; Motor Control; Motor Development; Motor Learning; Movement; Task Constraints

Further Readings

Anderson, D. I., & Sidaway, B. (1994). Coordination changes associated with practice of a soccer kick. *Research Quarterly for Exercise and Sport, 65,* 93–99.

Bernstein, N. A. (1967). *The coordination and regulation of movement.* London: Pergamon Press.

Seifert, L., & Davids, K. (2012). Intentions, perceptions and actions constrain functional intra- and inter-individual variability in the acquisition of expertise in individual sports. *The Open Sports Sciences Journal, 5,* 68–75.

FRIENDSHIPS/PEER RELATIONS

Peers have a particularly powerful social influence on youth development, particularly during adolescence. Positive peer interactions can help adolescents acquire a range of skills, attitudes, and behaviors. In sport settings, high levels of peer support and quality friendships have been associated with higher ratings of sport enjoyment, commitment, intrinsic motivation, and perceived competence.

Definitions

Alan L. Smith and Meghan McDonough have generated some important understandings of peer interactions in youth sport contexts. But, as they observed, the term *peer* has rarely been explicitly defined in sport and exercise psychology research. Peer groups are often context specific, which means that individuals can engage with different peer groups in different contexts, such as school, sport teams, or groups people hang out with informally. Peer groups can also change over time as adolescents' interests and habits evolve. This issue makes it difficult to specifically define who are one's peers, but in a general sense, *peers* can be defined as individuals of similar age and with similar interests. For example, in sport teams or schools, teammates or classmates can be considered as peers.

Peer networks reflect the structure of peer connections. For example, individuals on a sport team can identify a network of people they interact with most frequently (e.g., *cliques*). *Peer support* is a concept that stems from the peer network. Support can be viewed in terms of structural, functional, and perceptual dimensions. *Structural* dimensions are represented by the composition of a peer network. *Functional* dimensions refer to specific tangible functions of support provided by others (received support). *Perceptual* dimensions refer to the extent to which individuals feel supported by others (perceived support).

Theoretical Frameworks

The role of peers has been recognized in various theoretical frameworks used in sport and exercise psychology. For example, Susan Harter's *competence motivation theory* considers ways in which social agents influence motivation in achievement domains. Reinforcement, modeling, and approval of mastery attempts can enhance individuals' perceptions of competence and intrinsic motivation to participate in a task. In Albert Bandura's *Social Cognitive Theory*, personal (individual) factors, environmental (social) factors, and behavior are

proposed to influence each other in a reciprocal manner. Peer support is a means by which peers can socially reinforce certain behaviors, such as providing encouragement for individuals to act in certain ways. For example, peers can have a positive influence on children's and adolescents' physical activity behaviors and enjoyment of sport participation.

Kenneth H. Rubin, William Bukowski, and Jeffrey G. Parker put forward a contemporary framework of peer relationships in the developmental psychology literature that has recently been used by sport psychology researchers. Rubin argued that peer experiences are considered across several nested levels of social complexity: individuals, interactions, relationships, and groups. The framework begins with the *individual*. Individuals bring relatively stable social orientations to groups. Individuals involve each other via *interactions* (the simplest level of social complexity), which are short-term social exchanges. Interactions change in response to fluctuating circumstances of the social situation, such as the characteristics and responses of a partner. During interactions youth may cooperate, compete, fight, resolve conflict, or engage in a range of other behaviors.

Interactions are shaped by *relationships* (a higher order level of social complexity). Relationships are influenced by past events and future anticipated events, can take many forms, and have characteristics that are not necessarily found in lower level interactions. But, the nature of a relationship is defined by the characteristics of its members, the types of interactions that take place, and the individual's history of earlier relationships. Friendships are an example of the relationship level, and are discussed with reference to sport psychology research here. Relationships are further embedded in and influenced by *groups*, which are networks of relationships with relatively clearly defined boundaries like a competitive sport team. Peer groups are more than an aggregate of individuals, interactions, and relationships. Rather, groups have norms (e.g., shared cultural conventions), processes (e.g., cohesion) and properties (e.g., hierarchal organization) that are not necessarily found in children's experiences at lower social levels. Groups help define the type and range of relationships that occur within them. Groups therefore influence interactions and relationships and vice versa.

Peer Acceptance

Peer acceptance (or popularity) is based on how a group views the status of an individual. Adolescents with higher levels of athletic ability tend to enjoy more peer acceptance and be more popular in school than adolescents with lower levels of athletic ability. Even within sport teams, the most highly skilled athletes tend to be most accepted and viewed as leaders among their teammates. Additionally, peer comparison and acceptance are important sources of information for judging physical competence. In fact, higher peer acceptance has also been associated with greater physical self-worth, positive affect, and intrinsic motivation for physical activity. Therefore, skilled athletes tend to enjoy high peer acceptance, which is further associated with other positive outcomes.

Friendships

Friendship is a feature of the *relationships* level of peer experiences. There are three fairly distinct aspects of friendships: whether or not a child has friends, who these friends are, and the quality of these friendships. Some of the most influential work on peer friendships in sport was conducted by Maureen R. Weiss, Alan L. Smith, and Marc Theeboomin the United States. Through interviews with 8- to 16-year-olds they identified that the key aspects of *best sport friendships* were companionship and pleasant play, loyalty and intimacy, self-esteem enhancement and supportiveness, things in common, conflict resolution, and conflict. These findings were used by Weiss et al. to develop a questionnaire (the Sport Friendship Quality Scale; SFQS) to assess friendship quality in sport. Research using the SFQS has revealed that adolescent junior tennis players who reported higher quality of sport friendships rated tennis enjoyment and commitment higher than players with lower quality sport friendships.

Peer Conflict

Playing on a team or training with a squad expands adolescents' social networks and requires them to learn to deal with different types of people. Moreover, different types of people may not otherwise be part of the adolescent's social group if it were not for involvement in sport. A recent study of peer relationships among members of early adolescent girls' soccer teams showed that players integrated new members into the team and learned to interact with different types of people, but as the season progressed, they had to manage conflicts that arose. For example, teammates attempted to intervene and mediate conflicts among other teammates, and people learned to accept others' point of view. Over time, a structure of leadership emerged and players learned to work together. Although peer interactions may not always appear to be going smoothly, the ways in which peers learn to deal with each other and manage difficult situations seems to have important implications for their social development, both within sport and beyond.

Constellations of Social Relationships

Peer acceptance, friendship, and conflict are important issues, but artificially separating these issues for the purposes of research may produce only limited understandings of peer experiences. In adolescents' day-to-day lives, they likely experience a complex mixture of peer interactions. Smith has encouraged researchers to consider multiple dimensions of social experiences in youth sport and physical activity settings by highlighting the notion that constellations (or combinations) of social relationships influence adolescents' lives. For example, studies looking at such constellations of social relationships have shown that higher perceptions of adaptive peer group profiles (like high peer acceptance *and* friendship) predicted adaptive motivational responses. Subsequent research has considered an even broader range of social relationships and shown that positive perceptions of issues such as peer friendship quality, peer acceptance, and child–parent relationship were associated with more positive motivational outcomes like enjoyment and perceived competence. Combined, these findings highlight the importance of examining combinations of social relationships in youth sport contexts.

Gender Differences

During the early stages of adolescence, gender differences emerge in peer relations, with females usually assigning higher importance to friendships, intimacy, and emotional support than males. One study conducted in the United States showed that for female high school athletes peer acceptance and friendship quality, along with perceived competence, instrumental, and expressive behaviors, predicted self-ratings of leadership, whereas coach and teammate ratings were primarily related to ability only. For males, the psychosocial variables and ability were related to self, teammates,' and coaches' ratings of leadership. Interestingly, other research has shown girls who play *gender-appropriate* or traditionally feminine sports such as volleyball and gymnastics typically report high social acceptance. Also, physical ability in boys is viewed as a desirable quality associated with popularity and leadership, while in girls it is valued in some groups but not others.

Social Competence and Life Skills

One of the goals of studying peer relationships in sport and physical activity settings is to find ways in which to promote individuals' social competence. Rubin et al. described social competence in peer relationships as adolescents' capacity to engage effectively and successfully with each social level in their framework (interactions, relationships, and groups). Hence, a socially competent adolescent would be able to engage in a peer group structure and effectively participate in group-oriented activities, nurture satisfying relationships based on balanced and reciprocal interactions with others, and fulfill individual goals and needs through these interactions with peers.

Although such dimensions of social competence have yet to be widely explored in youth sport settings, several studies have shown that learning to deal with different types of people and working as a team to achieve common goals are some of the most important life skills people acquire through their involvement in youth sport. In addition, such social life skills seem to readily transfer from sport settings to other areas of adolescents' lives. For example, youth sport participants have reported that learning to interact with people in sport teams has helped them work better in group assignments in academic settings and effectively engage with others in work settings. Hence, the peer relationships and friendships that occur through participation in youth sport have potentially important consequences for youth development.

Nicholas L. Holt

See also Cohesion; Conflict; Fair Play; Group Characteristics; Group Formation; Moral Atmosphere; Moral Behavior; Moral Development; Sportspersonship; Status; Team Attributions; Team Building; Team Communication

Further Readings

Holt, N. L., Black, D. E., Tamminen, K. A., Mandigo, J. L., & Fox, K. R. (2008). Levels of social complexity and dimensions of peer experience in youth sport. *Journal of Sport & Exercise Psychology, 30,* 411–431.

Rubin, K. H., Bukowski, W., & Parker, J. G. (2006). Peer interactions, relationships, and groups. In W. Damon, R. M. Lerner, & N. Eisenberg (Eds.), *Handbook of child psychology: Vol. 3, Social, emotional, and personality development* (6th ed., pp. 571–645). New York: Wiley.

Smith, A. L., & McDonough, M. H. (2008). Peers. In A. L. Smith & S. J. H. Biddle (Eds.), *Youth physical activity and sedentary behavior: Challenges and solutions* (pp. 295–320). Champaign, IL: Human Kinetics.

Weiss, M. R., Smith, A. L., & Theeboom, M. (1996). "That's what friends are for": Children's and teenagers' perceptions of peer relationships in the sport domain. *Journal of Sport & Exercise Psychology, 18,* 347–379.

FUNCTIONAL VARIABILITY

To achieve performance goals in competitive sport there is a need to strike a delicate balance between movement pattern stability and variability because, although athletes need to achieve consistent outcomes, they also need to be able to successfully adapt their movements to changes in the performance environment. To achieve these aims, the theory of ecological dynamics advocates that there is an intertwined relationship between the specific intentions, perceptions, and actions of individual athletes that constrains this relationship between movement pattern stability and variability in each individual performer. This intertwined relation between an individual's intentions, perception, and action processes needs to be carefully understood because of the insights it provides on expert performance in sport.

Traditionally, a high level of expertise in sport has been associated with the capacity to be able to reproduce a specific movement pattern consistently and to reduce attention demands during performance by increasing the automaticity of movement. It was assumed that the central nervous system (CNS) functioned as an executive organizer and prescriber of motor programs and action plans charged with the task of producing stable movement patterns from an individual's effector system. From that viewpoint, expertise in sport was associated with a reduction in deviations in task performance from an ideal standard or movement template which was represented in the CNS. By harnessing integrated feedback systems, athletes were considered to modify the motor program entry parameters until expert behavior was eventually achieved after many hours of practice. Traditionally, therefore, movement variability was considered as noise in performance and learning which should be minimized or eradicated to enable the production of highly functional movement programs (movement variability was considered to be an artifact limiting an individual system's processing of information from input to output).

However, research in ecological dynamics has shown that movement system variability should not necessarily be construed as noise, detrimental to performance. Nor should it always be viewed as error or a deviation from a putative expert model, which should be constantly corrected in learners. Inspired by insights from the Russian physiologist Nicolai Bernstein, movement system variability instead is now considered to exemplify the functional flexibility of a skilled athlete to respond to changes in dynamic performance constraints. For this and other reasons, the concept of functional variability has gained a significant amount of empirical support in the sport psychology field. A key idea is that movement pattern variability can be viewed as a functional property of skilled performers to help them adapt their movement behaviors to changing task constraints (see entry on "Task Constraints"). Traditional research has typically focused on the amount of movement variability exhibited by an athlete during performance, assessed by statistical measures such as the standard deviation or variance around a distribution mean. According to Karl Newell's (1986) *Constraints on the Development of Coordination*, these statistics indicate the amount of noise in a single measurement—that is, the standard deviation only indicates the *magnitude* of variability recorded during task performance (the amplitude, the spatial aspect of the scores in a performance distribution. It provides little information on the

structure of movement variability exhibited by an athlete, which is needed to understand whether it is functional or not. For this reason, Newell and his co-investigators recommended studying the temporal structure of movement pattern variability by analyzing the spectral range of noise, which provides information on the deterministic (preplanned) or stochastic (emergent) nature of movement variability. Also pointed out was that it would be wrong to consider that deterministic processes specify the invariance of a movement pattern and that stochastic processes specify its variance. Given these theoretical advances in understanding movement pattern variability, ecological dynamicists have argued that there is no ideal motor coordination solution (a classical technique) that all athletes should aspire to during learning. Rather, functional patterns of coordination emerge during practice from the interaction of constraints on each individual athlete (task, environmental, and organismic), leading to intra-individual and interindividual movement pattern variability as consistent performance outcomes are achieved.

Recently, the functional role of movement pattern variability has also been supported by research highlighting the property of *neurobiological system degeneracy*, technically defined by Gerald Edelman and Joseph Gally as the capacity of system components that differ in structure to achieve the same function or performance output. This structural property in humans indicates the availability of an abundance of motor system degrees of freedom—that is, the many components of the movement system (alluded to by Bernstein), which can take on different roles when assembling functional actions during sport performance (captured by system degeneracy).

Allied to these ideas on neurobiological degeneracy, research on sport performance has begun to explain why expert performers often display higher levels of intraindividual movement pattern variability than novices in sport, data traditionally viewed as counterintuitive. The movement variability exhibited by skilled individuals can play a functional role. For instance, it highlights an expert athlete's capacity to perform several types of movement or to adopt one of a number of coexisting modes of coordination, that is, exploit system multistability (the many functional states of system organization) and metastability (the capacity to switch between functional states), in order to achieve the same functional performance outcomes. In the past years, empirical research on sport performance has clearly exemplified how intraindividual and interindividual movement variability can play a functional role in the performance of team-based and a range of individual physical activities, such as a cyclical movement task in an aquatic environment (breaststroke swimming) and a continuous discrete task in the wilderness (ice climbing) (see studies by Duarte Araújo, Keith Davids, and Ludovic Seifert and coworkers). These key ideas on functional variability have now been integrated into a motor learning theory by Wolfgang Schöllhorn et al., known as Differential Learning, which advocates adding noise to initial performance conditions to provoke learning by forcing the individual to adapt unexpectedly.

Keith Davids and Ludovic Seifert

See also Adaptation; Coordination; Dynamical Systems; Ecological Theory; Expertise; Freezing; Task Constraints

Further Readings

Bernstein, N. (1967). *The co-ordination and regulation of movements*. New York: Pergamon Press.

Edelman, G.M., & Gally, J. A. (2001). Degeneracy and complexity in biological systems. *Proceedings of the National Academy of Sciences, 98*, 13763–13768.

Newell, K. M. (1986). Constraints on the development of coordination. In M. G. Wade & H. T. A. Whiting (Eds.), *Motor development in children: Aspects of coordination and control* (pp. 341–360). Dordrecht, Netherlands: Martinus Nijhoff.

Schöllhorn, W. I., Beckmann, H., Michelbrink, M., Sechelmann, M., Trockel, M., & Davids, K. (2006). Does noise provide a basis for the unification of motor learning theories? *International Journal of Sport Psychology, 37*, 1–21.

Seifert, L., & Davids, K. (2012, September). Intentions, perceptions and actions constrain functional intra- and inter-individual variability in the acquisition of expertise in individual sports. *The Open Sports Sciences Journal, 5*, 68–75.

Vilar, L., Araújo, D., Davids, K. & Button, C. (2012). The role of ecological dynamics in analysing performance in team sports. *Sports Medicine, 42*, 1–10.

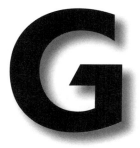

Gaze

See Eye Movements/Gaze

Gender

Gender has a clear and powerful influence in society, and a particularly powerful and persistent influence in sport and exercise. Indeed, the sport world seems to exaggerate and highlight gender. Sport and physical activities remain largely sex segregated and male dominated. Gender is so embedded that trying to be nonsexist and treating everyone the same is difficult. Moreover, trying to treat everyone the same may well do a disservice to participants.

Understanding Gender

Gender refers to psychological, social, and cultural experiences and characteristics associated with being male or female. The terms *sex* and *gender* often are used interchangeably, but they have different meanings. *Sex* refers to biological aspects of being male or female. *Gender*, often mistakenly assumed to be biologically based, is *socially constructed*, which means that characteristics associated with men and women are not innate biological distinctions but develop through social interactions. Moreover, gender is not a dichotomous category. People vary greatly in the extent to which they hold and convey gendered thoughts,

feelings, and behaviors. *Gender expression* refers to the way people convey their gender through mannerisms, behaviors, or expressions.

Gender often is conflated with sex, and considered a naturally determined, unchangeable *gender binary* with two opposing categories. That is, male and masculine (associated with strength, independence, competitiveness, etc.) are the opposite of female and feminine (associated with emotionalism, weakness, nurturance, gracefulness, etc.). When people do not fall neatly into these two categories, sexual orientation is often questioned. That is, a woman whose gender expression reflects masculine characteristics is assumed to be lesbian, and a man whose gender expression reflects feminine characteristics is assumed gay, which further conflates sex, gender, and sexuality. Again, gender is not biological sex, or sexual orientation, but socially constructed roles, behaviors, activities and attributes. Simple, dichotomous gender categories cannot explain gender.

When considering gender, it is important to recognize that gender involves *power relations*. Socially constructed gender roles and expectations lead to inequities and disparities, which reflect power relations. The dominant group has power or *privilege*, and nondominant groups experience *oppression* or discrimination. In gender relations, men have power in society and in sport.

It is also important to note that gender is only one of many sociocultural identities. Everyone possesses many other social identities, such as nationality, class, race and ethnicity, and those multiple identities *intersect*. The mix of multiple, intersecting identities and power relations varies with time and context. Gender affects men as well as women, and gender interacts with other cultural identities. Sport is not only considered male but also considered white, young, middle-class, heterosexual male. A more useful sport and exercise psychology must consider the intersections of gender, race, class, and other power relations.

Gender in Sport and Exercise

Gender is deeply embedded in sport and exercise, not only reflecting the gendered cultural boundaries of society, but also emphasizing physical and biological processes. Sports have separate categories for men and women because of the assumption that men are naturally (biologically) *better* than women, which links to gender disparities and power relations.

Although women's and girls' participation in sport and exercise has exploded in the last generation, the numbers of female and male participants are not equal. More important, gender influences thoughts, feelings, and behaviors within physical activity settings. *Citius, Altius, Fortius*—the Olympic motto—translates as "swifter, higher, stronger," which underscores that sport is competitive and hierarchical (masculine characteristics) as well as physical. Gender disparities reflect power relations. Before 1972 when Title IX was passed, over 90% of U.S. women's athletic teams were coached by women. Today, even though more girls and women participate, less than 50% of their coaches are women.

Sex segregation is not as obvious in exercise, but gender influence is clear. Women and men may exercise in the same fitness center, but the aerobics and yoga classes are predominantly women's spaces, whereas men dominate the free weights area. Public health reports indicate that physical activity is limited by gender, as well as by race, class, and physical attributes. Men engage in more physical activity than women across all age groups and all other categories.

Gender stereotypes are connected to gender disparities. Over 50 years ago, Eleanor Metheny identified gender stereotypes, concluding that it is not socially appropriate for women to engage in contests that involve bodily contact, bodily force, or long distances. Gender stereotypes persist, and media coverage reflects gender bias. Female athletes receive much less coverage, with the emphasis on athletic accomplishments for men, and on femininity and physical attractiveness for women. Men are expected to be bigger, stronger, and faster. Boys who are not athletic often are teased, as with the common insult, "You throw like a girl."

Sport studies scholars have described sport as a powerful force that socializes boys and men into a restricted masculine identity. We expect to see men dominate women, and we are uncomfortable with bigger, stronger women who take active, dominant roles expected of athletes. Gender stereotypes may restrict men in sport even more than women. Men who deviate from the masculine norm within the athletic culture often face ridicule, harassment, or physical violence.

Stereotypes are a concern because people act on them, exaggerating minimal gender differences and restricting opportunities. Both girls and boys can participate in figure skating or ice hockey. Yet children see female figure skaters and male ice hockey players as role models; peers gravitate to sex-segregated activities; and parents, teachers, and coaches support gender-appropriate activities.

The gendered context of sport and exercise has changed, particularly for women and girls, but gender stereotypes and disparities persist. Sport and exercise are clearly linked with masculine values and behaviors. Those gender stereotypes restrict opportunities and behaviors for both men and women, and may encourage unhealthy behaviors, such as overtraining or unhealthy eating behaviors. The limited gender research focuses on women, which highlights neglected issues, but sport and exercise psychology scholars have far to go to understand gender in physical activity settings.

Diane L. Gill

See also Diversity; Feminism; Heterosexism, Homonegativism, and Transprejudice; Sex Differences

Further Readings

Acosta, V. R., & Carpenter, L. J. (2012). *Women in intercollegiate sport: A longitudinal, national study thirty-five year update 1977–2012*. Available from http://www.acostacarpenter.org

Gill, D. L. (2007). Gender and cultural diversity. In G. Tenenbaum & R. C. Eklund (Eds.), *Handbook of sport psychology* (3rd ed., pp. 823–844). Hoboken, NJ: Wiley.

Messner, M. A. (1992). *Power at play: Sports and the problem of masculinity*. Boston: Beacon Press.

GENERALIZED MOTOR PROGRAM

When learning sequential movements, such as those involved in speech production, handwriting, typing, drumming, or sports skills, performers exhibit the ability to modify a learned movement sequence from execution to execution in some ways but not in others. This is thought to occur because a generalized motor program (GMP), which can be used to produce a specific class of movements, has developed and been stored in memory. When the GMP is retrieved, movement parameters must be specified in an effort to scale the program output to meet the specific demands at hand. Because the movement output can be altered by the premovement specification of parameters, the program was termed *generalizable* by Richard "Dick" Schmidt. The notion of a generalizable program is quite different from the more traditional notion of motor program as a prestructured set of central commands that can be used to produce a specific movement.

A generalized motor program is thought to develop over practice and provides the basis for generating movement sequences within a class of movements that share the same invariant features, such as sequence order, relative timing, and relative force. Specific movements are produced by the premovement specification of movement parameters like absolute timing, absolute force, and effectors. For example, when a movement situation requires a learned sequence to be produced either faster or slower than typically practiced, the invariant features remain unchanged, but the absolute timing parameter is changed to accommodate the rate at which the movement is produced. Thus, the relative times used to produce the elements in the sequence remain unchanged, but the absolute time is rescaled to meet the specific demands. Changing the absolute timing parameter results in slower movements that could be considered *stretched out* (in time) copies of faster movements. Likewise, a lower specification of the force parameter would result in a movement sequence generating reduced forces, which could be thought of as a compressed (with respect to force) copy of a more forceful movement.

A common example used to exemplify the notion of a GMP is writing one's signature. Each of us can write our signature under a variety of conditions. According to the GMP perspective, we do this by specifying the movement parameters needed to meet the requirements at hand while maintaining the invariant features of the GMP. For example, if I were asked to write my name (Charles Shea) very quickly on a sheet of paper, the signature maintains the relative timing characteristics invariant to the GMP, but the specification of absolute timing would be reduced. This will result in me taking the same proportion of the total time to write the *Ch*, for example, in my first name when writing quickly as when writing under normal time constraints, but the absolute time used would be reduced. Similarly, if I were asked to write my name in a small box on a sheet of paper or much larger on a white board in the classroom, the invariant features would not change, but the actual timing, actual forces, and even the specific effectors used to produce the movement would change. In the smaller situation, one would use primarily finger movements to produce a signature, while in the larger situation one may use shoulder and arm movements with minimal or no movements of the fingers.

The notion of a GMP has a great deal of intuitive appeal. It seems efficient for each motor program in our movement repertoire to be able to generate a class of movement sequences. This reduces not only the potential storage problems that would result if different programs were needed each time the movement requirements changed but also would reduce potential retrieval problems that would be associated with selecting from among a group of similar motor programs. The notion of a GMP is also consistent with our experience with computer programs and electronic video devices. Indeed, the record player analogy often used to describe the invariant and variant features of the GMP feeds this intuitive appeal. In the record player analogy, a phonograph record is used to illustrate the invariant and variant feature of the GMP. For example, a phonograph record could be played at different speeds (331/3 rpm or 78 rpm), played with different settings on the volume control, or the output directed to different speakers while maintaining the invariant features of the recording. In this analogy, speed is used to indicate absolute time, volume to indicate force, and speakers used to illustrate different effectors.

There is, however, also a good deal of empirical evidence to support the notion of a GMP. Research has demonstrated that learned movement sequences when scaled in time or force exhibit a pervasive tendency toward approximately proportional scaling. Whereas participants are able to rescale learned movement sequences in time and force, variable practice, in which the learner is exposed to various parameter requirements, appears important for the learner to accurately specify the time or force parameter. There is also a good deal of evidence that participants can execute movement sequences using different effectors. As noted earlier, one's signature can be executed with the dominant limb using a variety of difference muscle groups. This literature is, however, a little cloudy especially in terms of transfer to homologous and nonhomologous limbs. That is, when asked to produce a movement sequence with the left hand after learning with the right hand, for example, transfer is not always very effective. Thus, there do seem to be some limits to parameterizing a GMP.

Charles H. Shea

See also Especial Skills; Laws of Movement Learning and Control; Motor Control; Motor Learning

Further Readings

Schmidt, R. A. (1975). A schema theory of discrete motor skill learning. *Psychological Review, 82,* 225–260.

Schmidt, R. A. (1976). Control processes in motor skills. *Exercise and Sport Sciences Reviews, 4,* 229–261.

Shea, C. H., & Wulf, G. (2005). Schema theory: A critical appraisal and reevaluation. *Journal of Motor Behavior, 37,* 85–101.

GENETICS/NATURE–NURTURE DETERMINANTS

Conceptualizations of the factors affecting skill acquisition and the demonstration of expertise generally reflect qualities associated with biological factors such as genes (*nature*) or those related to environmental or experiential factors such as training and coaching (*nurture*).

Historical Background

Although the conceptualization of the nature versus nurture debate can be traced at least to Platonic and Aristotelian discussions of human nature in ancient Greece, more contemporary discussions usually start with Francis Galton's 1874 *English Men of Science: Their Nature and Their Nurture*; Galton may have taken his title from Shakespeare's *The Tempest* (Act 4.1)—"a born devil, on whose nature Nurture can never stick." Galton's approach was very clearly influenced by the work of his cousin, Charles Darwin, and focused on the stable, biological factors that are transferred from one generation to the next (known as *heritability*, the proportion of variance in a population attributed to genetic factors). Alternately, some researchers see human development as starting from a blank slate (tabula rasa) with no innate traits or characteristics, and that all forms of learning and behavior result from interactions with our environment. This extreme nurture viewpoint is demonstrated by behaviorist John B. Watson's famous boast:

> Give me a dozen healthy infants . . . and my own specified world to bring them up in, and I'll guarantee to take any one at random and train him to become any type of specialist I might select— doctor, lawyer, artist . . . regardless of his talents, penchants, tendencies, abilities, vocations and race of his ancestors. (1998, p. 82)

The history of this debate in psychology is marked by radical shifts in opinion, usually driven by social and cultural factors. For example, after World War II, political and intellectual thought changed to reflect the perspective that differences between individuals resulted from opportunities and experience. This perspective was deemed more socially acceptable than ideologies that sought to separate individuals on the basis of biology since this latter approach was so strongly associated with Nazism. A similar social change occurred in 2001, after the publication of the human genome when researchers advanced positions based on the ultimate power of biology for understanding interindividual differences. James Watson, codiscoverer of the structure of DNA and a key developer of the Human Genome Project, said, "We used to think our future was in the stars. Now we know it is in our genes." More recently, we have seen a change in direction, at least in some fields of psychology and education, as researchers focus on the solitary role of deliberate practice (a nurture-related variable) in creating the expert performer. The role of nature and nurture factors in sport and exercise is reviewed as follows.

Nature Determinants

Nature determinants focus on stable biological factors. Each person is the product of a unique sequence of genetic material, half coming from one's mother and the other half from one's father in the form of *chromosomes*. This genetic material (DNA, or deoxyribonucleic acid) is made up of a combination of four chemical bases—adenine, thymine, guanine, and cytosine (abbreviated A, T, G, and C), which group together into base pairs (A with T and G with C) and links of these base pairs form discrete sequences of DNA called *genes*. Each gene corresponds to a specific biological outcome; for example, the COL5A1 gene found in humans on chromosome 9, encodes for a specific collagen protein relevant to flexibility of ligaments and tendons. Within the normal population, there are multiple variants of this gene, which produces the variability seen across a population. This variability results from different *alleles* (a variant in the gene sequence) and is known as a *polymorphism* (the occurrence of many forms of a given gene). Your individual collection of genes (estimated to be between 20,000 and 25,000 genes containing about 3 billion base pairs) is referred to as your *genotype*.

There is strong evidence that genotypic features affect health, fitness, and performance outcomes. For instance, using both heritability statistics and individual genetic markers, data from the HERITAGE Family Study have shown that specific genotypes are better suited for aerobic activities. Since the publication of the human genome in 2001, hundreds of genes and polymorphisms related either directly or indirectly to performance and fitness phenotypes have been identified. Some of these candidates include the COL5A1 gene mentioned earlier as well as genes for the cardiovascular catalyst angiotensin-converting enzyme (ACE), and the skeletal muscle protein alpha-actin type 3 (ACTN3), which have had varying degrees of success explaining interindividual differences in performance. Moreover, despite the considerable attention given to the search for individual genes responsible for athletic achievement, the manifestation of any biological or psychological effect is likely the result of a complex interaction of thousands of genes, and as a result, identification of individual genes that account for meaningful variation in sport- or exercise-related outcomes is extremely difficult.

Nurture Determinants

Few researchers dispute the important role of the environment (nurture) in determining health and fitness related outcomes. In the social and behavioral sciences, few relationships are as robust as the one between practice and achievement. The power law of practice is a mathematical model of this relationship whereby improvements occur quite rapidly at the onset of practice but become more difficult to obtain (requiring greater practice) as the performer becomes more skillful. This law (or derivations of it) has been widely applied and is proposed to describe human learning of perceptual–motor skills ranging from learning to roll cigars and reading text upside down, to scoring a layup in basketball or hitting a bull's-eye in darts.

Studies from the field of human expertise and expert performance have also supported the relationship between training and ultimate achievement. For example, the proposition of deliberate practice, developed by psychologist Anders Ericsson, is based on the notion that proper training (deliberate practice) performed at the appropriate period of biological and cognitive development is a necessity for the acquisition of expertise in any domain, including sports. Ericsson's (1996) extensive work on the acquisition of expert performance has shown that an individual's level of performance in any domain is determined by the amount of time spent performing "a well defined task with an appropriate difficulty level for the particular individual, informative feedback, and opportunities for repetition and correction of errors" (pp. 20–21).

In addition to the primacy of practice or training to explaining human achievement in sport, other environmental factors are important. For example, Joseph Baker and Sean Horton proposed a number of *secondary factors* that facilitate the acquisition of appropriate training and practice, including obvious factors like access to proper coaches and having supportive parents, as well as less obvious factors, such as growing up in talent hotbeds or being born at the right time of year to take advantage of relative age effects.

Interactions of Nature and Nurture

Although discussions in sport and exercise psychology generally focus on nurture-related factors, it is clear that most health, fitness, and performance outcomes result from both nature and nurture. Perhaps the clearest example of nature–nurture interaction (or gene x environment interaction) comes from medicine and relates to the condition phenylketonuria (PKU). This genetic disorder causes brain damage and progressive mental retardation in 100% of individuals with the genetic marker for this condition; however, PKU is highly treatable if individuals eliminate phenylalanine from their diet. In this example, a quality with perfect heritability (PKU) is not expressed because of an environmental manipulation (dietary change). Importantly, the DNA that causes this condition remains unchanged; the individual simply does not express the PKU condition. Although examinations of gene x environment interactions are rarely examined in sport and exercise psychology, it is likely that similar effects occur. For example, the COL5A1 gene, by affecting injury risk, likely constrains the amount and intensity of training individuals in certain sports (e.g., sprinting) can perform throughout their development.

Modern Conceptualizations

Most evolutionary psychologists and geneticists have moved away from the nature–nurture conceptualization on the basis that it is too limited to explain the nuances of the interactions that occur throughout human development. As a result, researchers have developed more comprehensive models of these relationships. For example, *dynamic systems theory* presumes that human behavior is best seen as the interaction of different systems (biologic, social, psychological) with development being emergent, nonlinear and multidetermined. From this theoretical standpoint, genetic diversity is responsible for some variability in the differences between individuals in how they respond to different experiences and beneficial changes like performance adaptations happen when there is a favorable interaction with important environmental constraints. For example, there is growing consensus in the study of human obesity that the contribution of genetic factors is exacerbated in North American environments that are high in caloric availability.

In evolutionary psychology, focus is on the differences between obligate and facultative adaptations. Obligate adaptations occur no matter what environment a person experiences while facultative adaptations are sensitive to environmental variations. The fact that sugar tastes sweet and lemons taste sour (obligate adaptations) does not change if they are experienced in a different environment. Other, more complex qualities reflect facultative adaptations, similar to *if–then* statements. The attachment style one has as an adult

(i.e., how you approach long-term relationships), for example, is affected by the level of trust one had in their caregivers as a child. If a young person often has promises broken by a parent, this may lead to trust issues as an adult. Given that obligate adaptations do not typically vary across development, scientists in this area focus on how different developmental experiences affect the expression of facultative adaptations.

Another important element in this discussion relates to the emerging concept of epigenetics, which shows that changes in gene expression can occur through modifications to the genome that do not involve a change in the underlying DNA sequence. This field of research suggests that experiences provide a stimulus for genes to be turned on or off. For example, a Swedish study showed that a single hard workout resulted in genes involved in energy metabolism being switched on, with harder work resulting in a stronger effect.

Collectively, research on the effects of biology and experience on human behavior and performance indicate that the nature versus nurture dichotomy is ineffective for explaining the dynamics of how these factors interact and the complexity of this process.

Joseph Baker

See also Dynamical Systems; Expertise; Learning; Motor Development; Motor Learning; Practice; Skill Acquisition; Talent Development

Further Readings

Baker, J., & Davids, K. W. (2007). Sound and fury, signifying nothing? Future directions in the nature-nurture debate. *International Journal of Sport Psychology, 38,* 135–143.

Baker, J., & Horton, S. (2004). A review of primary and secondary influences on sport expertise. *High Ability Studies, 15,* 211–228.

Carlsson, S., Andersson, T., Lichtenstein, P., Michaëlsson, K., & Ahlbom, A. (2006). Genetic effects on physical activity: Results from the Swedish twin registry. *Medicine and Science in Sports and Exercise, 38,* 1396–1401.

Davids, K. W., & Baker, J. (2007). Genes, environment and sport performance: Why the nature-nurture dualism is no longer relevant. *Sports Medicine, 37,* 961–980.

Davids, K. W., Button, C., & Bennett, S. J. (2008). *Dynamics of skill acquisition: A constraints-led approach.* Champaign, IL: Human Kinetics.

Ericsson, K. A. (Ed.). (1996). *The road to excellence. The acquisition of expert performance in the arts and sciences, sports and games.* Mahwah, NJ: Erlbaum.

Ericsson, K. A. (2007). Deliberate practice and the modifiability of body and mind: Toward a science of the structure and acquisition of expert and elite performance. *International Journal of Sport Psychology, 38,* 4–34.

Klissouras, V. Geladas, N., & Koskolou, M. (2007). Nature prevails over nurture. *International Journal of Sport Psychology, 38,* 35–67.

Pinker, S. J. (2002). *The blank slate: The modern denial of human nature.* New York: Viking Press.

Watson, J. B. (1998). *Behaviorism.* New Brunswick, NJ: Transaction. (Original work published 1924)

GOAL SETTING

A goal is simply something you are trying to accomplish; it is the object or aim of an action. Although goals can function at an unconscious level, the process of goal setting represents the deliberate establishment and refinement of goals and the evaluation of goal progress. The concept of goals and the practice of goal setting are well known and established within settings where performance enhancement is the objective. It is important to understand goals because they have such a broad function in terms of affecting the thoughts and behaviors of those to whom participation, productivity, and performance are important.

In the broader field of performance psychology where the objective is to enhance productivity in its varying forms, the effectiveness of goal setting as a strategy has consistently been verified across tasks, groups, methods for setting goals, and performance indicators. Although it was assumed that the positive effects of goals would be replicated within sport and exercise settings, research in sport has failed to illustrate unequivocally that goals function as effectively in this domain. The reasons why have been debated widely, with the consensus being that sample and task characteristics were markedly different in sport. Despite this, studies that have described the goal-setting practices in sport performers have confirmed that almost all athletes do set goals and the majority find them to be effective. This entry provides a brief overview of the current state of play with regard to goal setting in sport, and critiques, where appropriate, the transfer of goal-setting concepts to sport and to performers in that domain. The intention is not to present an exhaustive review, but rather to highlight those aspects of goals and goal setting that are most pertinent to the advancement of knowledge in this area from both a theoretical and an applied perspective. The following sections cover definitions and types of goals, proposed mechanisms of effects, parameters of goals, and dispositional and situational antecedents of goals, and the final section addresses future research potential.

Types of Goals

The definition of *goals* as an aim of action serves to portray goals as the drivers (or cognitive regulators) behind goal-directed behavior. Consequently, within the multilayered domain of sport, where the nature and level of engagement varies so much, these underlying drivers of behavior can take many different forms. For example, antecedents of behaviors (goals) might range from winning a gold medal at the next Olympics, through the bending of an injured leg an extra two degrees during a physiotherapy session, to maintaining form through a high knee lift in sprinting.

The sport psychology literature consistently distinguishes between three broad goal types: outcome goals, performance goals, and process goals. *Outcome goals* describe intentions relative to the performance of others involved in the activity. The key delineator of these to other goal types is the notion of social comparison. The objective of winning represents the predominant outcome goal; however, the objective of placing in a race, reaching a final, or simply beating a teammate in an individual race, also represent examples of outcome goals. Unlike outcome goals, *performance goals* are based on *levels* of personal achievement and are entirely self-referenced (subjective). Typical performance goals are to run a race in a certain time, to jump a certain distance, to lift a specific weight, or to do a number of repetitions in a training situation—perhaps within a certain time; they refer to products of performance. These goals are normally based on numeric criteria (e.g., to jump one meter and sixty five centimeters) and refer to a predetermined subjective performance standard. *Process goals* are similarly self-referenced but are distinguished from performance goals because their focus is on the process of performing rather than a product of performance. The variation in process goals is subsequently far broader than that of outcome and performance goals. For example, they might range from the breathing techniques designed to regulate heart rate in a pistol shooter, to imaging in the mind's eye the flight of a golf ball before taking a shot, to focusing on maintaining position while executing a half-court press in basketball. In essence, process goals center on the execution of behaviors regarded as contributing to effective performance.

Relatively few studies have explored the specific effects of using different types of goals. Of those that have, some support, albeit limited, has been found for the use of outcome goals, while moderate to strong support has been provided for the use of performance and process goals. Moreover, it is suggested that combinations of goal types may be more effective than any single type alone. The benefit of performance goals (compared to outcome goals at least) lies in the fact that they are more controllable and flexible than outcome goals; they do not rely on the performance of others to be achieved. However, the achievement of performance goals may still be influenced by external factors, such as environmental conditions, luck, officiating, or even natural fluctuations in personal performance levels. Process goals, conversely, are almost entirely under the control of the individual, and so there is no reason why external factors should disrupt their achievement. Somewhat paradoxically, of those studies which have explored the goal-setting practices of athletes, the majority have found that performers report using outcome and performance goals far more than process goals. This may be a consequence of the less tangible nature of process goals (e.g. regulating breathing or creating a visual image of the trajectory of the ball) and the reassurance that many athletes have in being able to observe or monitor levels of performance directly.

Why Are Goals Effective?

Goal setting is widely regarded as the most popular basic sport psychology technique and is an integral part of any mental training program designed to maximize athletic potential. It is arguably the bedrock of athlete and coach education from a psychological perspective and supports or underpins many other strategies, such as confidence building and enhancing motivation.

In reviewing the literature on goal setting in sport, one is left with two inescapable conclusions: First, goals work; and second, the mechanisms behind their effectiveness are neither well understood nor particularly well documented. The latter has, on occasion, been attributed to early research into goal setting having limited theoretical grounding. Similarly, more recent research has been criticized for not moving beyond confirming performance effects: It has failed to consider factors that might mediate the relationship between goals and actual sport performance. It is to the mechanisms underlying the positive effects of goals that we now turn our attention.

There is an established view that goals facilitate performance through motivational effects. Seminal work into the application of goal setting to sport suggested that goals influence task performance in four main ways; they direct attention to the task, promote increases in effort, encourage persistence in the face of failure, and facilitate the promotion of new task-relevant strategies (In what other way could I achieve this objective?). Anecdotally, this motivational function of goals is supported, yet research in the sport domain is limited. While the motivational effect of goals on performance is largely direct, goals can also exert an indirect effect through changes in confidence. The successful achievement of goals over a period of time is regarded as pivotal in altering individual perceptions of capabilities. As goals are achieved, new goals are identified; as these new goals are achieved in turn, performers develop a stronger and more stable level of confidence. Repeated failure to achieve goals, on the other hand, undermines confidence.

Although it is suggested that the function of different types of goals may vary, there have been few studies exploring the relative effects of different goal types (e.g., performance vs. outcome goals). From the limited work that has been conducted, researchers within sport and exercise psychology have argued that focusing on self-referenced process and performance goals, rather than outcome goals, appears fundamental to the effective use of goals. Somewhat paradoxically, it is also suggested (and strongly supported anecdotally) that outcome goals (e.g., a desire to break into the world's top 10 in a particular sport) appear to facilitate longer term motivation.

Considering the mechanisms of effects, the limited research that has explored the use of process goals suggests that their beneficial effects can be attributed to focusing more on the task, increasing confidence, reducing concerns about evaluation from others, and developing personal interest in learning about the task. However, the narrow scope of this work to date reinforces the importance of research into understanding how goal setting works and ensuring consequently that clear guidelines are provided to promote effective goal setting.

A Framework for Effective Goal Setting

As alluded to in the previous section, early theorizing in relation to goals provided an immediate stimulus for research in sport. This research did not, as one might have expected, attempt to explain how goals functioned to enhance performance, but rather focused on the specific content of the goal and its effects. Consequently, while not necessarily increasing our understanding of how goals work, this research did offer some clarity into the nature of what might be regarded as effective goals. At the very least, this provided practitioners with a useful framework upon which to base future goal-setting interventions. The following paragraphs provide a brief summary and critique of this work as it pertains to educating athletes and coaches on the nature of appropriate goals.

Research on goal content in sport has provided some support for the positive effect of goals and highlighted the importance of a number of qualities of effective goals. These aspects are often referred to as the moderators of the goal setting and performance relationship because they are considered pivotal to describing the qualities of goals that enable them to be effective. The aspects of goals include *goal difficulty, goal specificity, goal proximity,* and *goal collectivity.*

One of the earliest conclusions of research in organizational settings on the relationship between conscious goals and task performance was that individuals striving for goals that were both specific and difficult performed better than those who had goals that were specific and easy, those who had goals that were vague (e.g., "I want to do my best"), and those who had no goals. While there are obvious (and widely debated) contextual differences between business and sport settings, research in sport suggests that moderate levels of goal difficulty were most effective in facilitating performance. Furthermore, responses to extremely difficult goals in sport were very different—instead of withdrawing effort, individuals in sports settings, when faced with relatively difficult goals, modified them

to ensure they remained relevant and achievable. Similarly, in terms of specificity, while specific goals are more effective than no goals or vague goals, those instructed to "do their best" in sport settings do not perform any worse. It is argued that this is because one of the fundamental differences in sport participants is that they actively engage in personal goal setting in response to this type of ambiguous suggestion.

Goal proximity refers to the time aspect of goals, and this can range from immediate intentions to future aspirations. *Long-term goals* have been described as those whose attainment is 6 or more weeks away, whereas goals of shorter duration are termed *short-term goals.* Goal proximity research conducted within sport settings has been rather limited; however, researchers do suggest that combinations of long-term and short-term goals are more effective than using either type alone. Arguably, much of the limited research in this area simply illustrates that having goals is better than not having goals. Nevertheless, in terms of effectiveness, the overriding message is that long-term objectives are most likely to facilitate performance and motivation when short-term goals represent flexible and controllable stepping stones to achieving them. In other words, long-term goals provide direction, while shorter term goals appear to provide opportunities to develop confidence and maintain motivation in pursuit of more distal objectives.

The study of *goal collectivity* concerns itself with the effects of team or group goals on collective performance. Early work on team goals in sport suggested that these goals can facilitate group performance and, in addition, promote team satisfaction, cohesion, and motivation. Specifically, team goals are argued to offer direction for the team and help individual members establish appropriate personal goals to support team objectives. Furthermore, it is logical that team goals should be accompanied by individual goals to ensure task focus and effort levels are maintained by individuals within the team. These individual goals should be based on the individual roles that each player needs to fulfill in order to maximize unit (e.g., a defensive group), and in turn, team effectiveness.

Dispositional and Situational Antecedents of Goals

One important consideration when seeking to more fully understand the nature and function of goals that athletes set is where do the goals come from and what factors lead to individual variations in goal preferences? The concept of the person by situation interaction has been used by many social scientists attempting to explain thoughts and behaviors. Specifically, and of relevance here, it has been applied in the sporting environment to explain variability in goal-setting practices; the personal and situational antecedents of goals are described in the paragraphs that follow.

At a personal level, the goals individuals adopt are argued to give meaning to their behaviors and energize their actions; they reflect the objective of striving and provide a framework through which an individual can interpret performance-related information. According to the predominant goal theory, two categories of achievement goals exist, and these are consistent with personal views of what is required to demonstrate competence in settings where the potential for competition and evaluation occurs. Goals, and the individuals utilizing such goals, concerned with demonstrating capability through personal improvement and learning about a task with reference to personal performance criteria are said to be *task involved*. Conversely, goals that focus on demonstrating competence with respect to others are described as being *ego involved*. The engaged reader may have noted a parallel between what are described here as achievement goals (task- and ego-involved goals) with what were earlier labeled as goal types, such as outcome, performance and process goals. Put simply, ego-involved goals, where the intention is to outperform others, are logically equated to the use of outcome goals. Similarly, task-involved goals are characterized by self-referenced intentions, which might focus on anything ranging from personal performance targets (a performance goal) to successfully executing a skill or action (a process goal).While the goals described reflect moment to moment targets, individuals are also predisposed to pursue goals reflecting their personal theory of what represents achievement. Researchers have labeled these dispositional (or trait-like) tendencies as goal orientations, for example, one predisposed to using ego-involved criteria to judge competence is said to be ego oriented, and those predisposed to using self-referenced criteria are said to be task oriented, and this aspect of achievement goals has stimulated the majority of research in this area.

Broadly speaking, sport-based research in this area has espoused the motivational benefits of a high level of task orientation, and regards high levels of ego orientation as placing the individual motivationally and behaviorally at risk, especially when accompanied by lower levels of perceived competence. One of the key characteristics of task and ego goal orientations is that they are independent. This means that an individual can be high or low in each or both orientations, and thus at a general level make judgments of their competence using a variety of personal and social comparison-based criteria. Although these goal orientations may be regarded as relatively stable, the specific goals used by individuals are dynamic and can change from moment to moment in response to the ongoing stream of information presented within the context of their sport involvement. In other words, specific goals can change during a task or performance.

The preceding paragraph outlines a case for how dispositional preferences affect goal choice. In line with numerous other motivational theories, situational factors also play a role in shaping the goals one adopts. Specifically, in situations where performance is evaluated (achievement settings), the psychological environment (labeled as the *motivational climate*) created by the coach (or those with similar leadership roles), can emphasize or promote, within the individual, a variety of criteria for judging competence; unsurprisingly, these impact individual goal preferences. Based originally on work conducted in education settings, two types of motivation climate have been described and applied to achievement contexts such as sport. A *mastery* climate operates when, for example, individuals perceive that task mastery and self-referenced goals are promoted, effort is rewarded, groupings for training tasks are not based on ability, mistakes are regarded as a natural part of learning, and success is evaluated with regard to personal improvement. Conversely, a *performance* climate exists when, for example, individuals perceive that time constraints limit mastery opportunities, superior performance compared to others in the training group is rewarded, groupings for training are based on ability, mistakes are punished, and success is evaluated with regard to outperforming others. Although motivationally adaptive behaviors are most likely to be associated with a mastery climate, certain individuals, most notably those with high levels of perceived competence, may also flourish in environments that promote social comparison (performance climate).

There is no research examining the direct relationship between motivational climate and goal choice. Nevertheless, one might still predict that the relationship between motivational climate and goal preferences parallels that which has been proposed to exist between achievement goal perspectives and goal types. Athletes exposed to a strong mastery climate are most likely to consider using self-referenced goals focused on personal improvement and learning (performance and process-based goals), whereas athletes in a strong performance climate would more likely lean toward goals based on social comparison (outcome goals). Adopting an alternative perspective, recent research on motivational climate suggests that a mastery climate may actually be promoted by encouraging athletes to adopt self-referenced goals focused on personal improvement and learning or mastery of tasks, that is, performance and process goals, respectively.

Research specifically examining the predictive effects of dispositional and situational antecedents of goal choices has not been forthcoming to date—this is most likely a result of an absence of effective measure of goal choices. Nonetheless, anecdotal evidence and common sense suggest that high levels of task orientation and a mastery motivational climate are likely to promote self-referenced performance and process goals, whereas high levels of ego orientation and an environment emphasizing social comparison are likely to promote outcome goals.

Conclusion

Goal setting is an established technique to increase motivation and enhance confidence. It is used widely across all levels of sport, and goals provide essential direction at both an immediate and long-term level. Goals can take a variety of forms, and they have both personal and situational antecedents. The consensus of research and anecdotal accounts is that an individual's primary focus should be on personal task-focused objectives, rather than social comparison. Nevertheless, factors such as personality, perceived ability, the psychological environment, and support with goals by others significantly influence the motivational and behavioral consequences of goal pursuit. While there is some conjecture regarding the specific nature of effective goals, it is generally accepted that setting and using challenging, specific goals with subgoals formulated to act as stepping stones to longer term objectives seems important. Despite undoubted progress, many questions about goals in sport remain unanswered. More clarity is needed on the functionality of goals and which goal types influence different aspects of personal psychology. Perhaps most importantly, practitioners need to develop methods for process-based goals to be integrated into the day-to-day routines of athletes. Finally, there is a need for much higher quality, theoretically grounded research to provide practitioners with clearer, evidence-based guidance for effective goal setting at an individual and group level.

Kieran Kingston

See also Achievement Goal Theory; Coach–Athlete Relations; Mastery and Control Beliefs; Psychological Skills; Self-Efficacy

Further Readings

Burton, D., & Weiss, C. (2008). The fundamental goal concept: The path to process and performance success. In T. S. Horn (Ed.), *Advances in sport psychology* (pp. 339–375). Champaign, IL: Human Kinetics.

Duda, J. L. (2001). Achievement goal research in sport: Pushing the boundaries and clarifying some misunderstandings. In G. C. Roberts (Ed.), *Advances in motivation in sport and exercise* (pp. 129–182). Champaign, IL: Human Kinetics.

Hall, H. K., & Byrne, A. T. J. (1988). Goal setting in sport: Clarifying recent anomalies. *Journal of Sport & Exercise Psychology, 10,* 184–198.

Kingston, K. M., & Hardy, L. (1997). Effects of different types of goals on processes that support performance. *The Sport Psychologist, 11,* 277–293.

Kingston, K. M., & Wilson, K. (2008). The application of goal setting in sport. In S. D. Mellalieu & S. Hanton (Eds.), *Literature reviews in applied sport psychology* (pp. 75–123). New York: Routledge.

Locke, E. A. (1991). Problems with goal setting research in sport—And their solutions. *Journal of Sport & Exercise Psychology, 8,* 311–316.

Locke, E. A., & Latham, G. P. (1985). The application of goal setting to sports. *Journal of Sports Psychology, 7,* 205–222.

Nicholls, J. G. (1989). *The competitive ethos and democratic education.* Cambridge, MA: Harvard University Press.

Reinboth, M., & Duda, J. L. (2006). Perceived motivational climate, need satisfaction and indices of well-being in team sports: A longitudinal perspective. *Psychology of Sport and Exercise, 7,* 269–286.

Roberts, G. C., & Kristiansen, E. (2012). Goal setting to enhance motivation in sport. In G. C. Roberts & D. Treasure (Eds.), *Advances in motivation in sport and exercise* (3rd ed., pp. 207–227). Champaign, IL: Human Kinetics.

GROUP CHARACTERISTICS

A *group* is defined as a social aggregate of two or more people that involves mutual awareness, interaction, and interdependence of its members. The characteristics of the group shape the beliefs and behaviors of its members. In this entry, two categories of group characteristics are examined, namely (1) characteristics of the group and (2) characteristics of group members.

Characteristics of the Group

Albert V. Carron and Mark Eys examined the many definitions of groups and identified five common characteristics: (1) common fate—sharing a common outcome with other members; (2) mutual benefit—an enjoyable, rewarding experience associated with group membership; (3) social structure—a stable organization of relationships among members; (4) interaction and communication among members; and (5) self-categorization—perceiving oneself as a member of the group. Research in exercise and sport settings was aimed at examining these five characteristics in relation to cognitions and behaviors of its members. A considerable body of research was accumulated about the influence of social structure (e.g., roles and norms of group members) on exercise adherence. In general, the findings support the importance of norms like acceptable forms of behavior and a clear understanding and acceptance of roles to promote exercise behavior. Other research findings pertained to the pattern of communication between coaches and athletes. This research has identified effective verbal and nonverbal communication practices for coaches working with athletes. Research has also begun to focus on self-categorization. Researchers have recently examined how self-categorization influences perceptions, preferences and behaviors in exercise groups.

Kevin S. Spink, Kathleen S. Wilson, and Carly S. Priebe (2010) recently examined all five of the common group characteristics together as a multidimensional construct of *groupness* in relation to adherence in structured exercise settings. Drawing on previous work, Spink et al. viewed groupness as the extent to which the five group characteristics can be perceived by group members. They hypothesized that perceptions of groupness, as captured by the five group characteristics, would be positively associated with individual exercise behavior. Support was found for this hypothesis as enhanced perceptions of groupness were associated with improved frequency and attendance in exercise.

Group Size

In addition to the five common group characteristics conceptualized by Carron and Eys, group size was considered important in this context. Origins of group size research date back to Norman Triplett's first social psychology study in 1898. Triplett examined the influence of others on cycling performance. Since then, research has indicated that as group size increases members report less cohesion, intimacy, satisfaction, and communication, as well as report greater tension, anxiety, competitiveness, being argumentative, feeling more threatened, and displaying more inhibition.

Group Size and Productivity

A topic of considerable interest to researchers has been the relationship between group size and productivity. In 1913, Max Ringelmann investigated the relationship between group size and individual and group performance in a rope-pulling task. Ringelmann's results, coined the *Ringelmann Effect,* revealed that as group size increased, relative productivity of each individual group member decreased. Ivan Steiner later examined the research on group size and productivity and developed a model to illustrate the relationship between the two concepts. Steiner proposed that as the number of members in a group increases, the potential group productivity also increases due to an increase in available resources up a point when the group's productivity plateaus.

Steiner offered two possible explanations for the decrease in individual productivity as group size increases. The first was coordination loss. Steiner proposed that as group size increased, the number of coordination links increased, and it was more difficult to synchronize the efforts of the individuals. The second explanation was the reduction in individual motivation as group size increases. It was hypothesized that as the size of the group grows, personal accountability is reduced, and it is more difficult to motivate individuals. Later work replicating Ringelmann's classic rope-pulling experiment research found support for both explanations.

Based upon the evidence on group size and productivity, it begs the question of what is the ideal group size to maximize productivity? Researchers in many fields continue to struggle with this question. Research in work settings supports smaller groups (three to six members) being more productive than larger groups (more than seven).

Group Size Research in Sport and Exercise Settings

Research on group size in sport and exercise began in the early 1990s in a series of studies conducted by W. Neil Widmeyer, Lawrence R. Brawley, and Albert V. Carron examining group size and cohesion on sport teams. Smaller teams were found to be more optimal for the development of commitment to group goals (task cohesion), while moderate-size groups were best for building strong relationships and friendships among group members (social cohesion). Subsequent work in exercise settings by Carron and Spink found task and social cohesion to be higher in smaller groups. Carron and Spink also found the group-based intervention of team building to offset negative effects of increased group size on cohesion.

Other researchers have examined the influence of group size on affective outcomes in sport and behavioral outcomes, such as attendance and retention in exercise classes. Retention and attendance were greatest in the smallest ($n = 5$–17) and largest ($n = 32$–46) exercise classes, but poorest in the medium classes ($n = 18$–31). Group members' enjoyment, satisfaction, and belief in team's ability tend to progressively decrease with increased group size.

Characteristics of the Group Members

The characteristics of group members individually and collectively (referred to as group composition) have been a topic of considerable interest to researchers and practitioners alike. Group members can differ in age, sex, ethnicity, education, and social status. Further, members can vary in physical size, attitudes, motives, needs, mental and motor abilities, and personality traits. Researchers in social psychology have been interested in understanding how the level of diversity of individual characteristics of group members has implications on group functioning and member cognitions, affect, and behavior. Work in this area has prompted researchers to examine the contextual exercise preferences for adults. In an exercise environment, there is growing support for individuals to prefer to be active with others of similar age and gender. Overweight individuals, in particular, report a greater preference for same-gender exercise classes (versus mixed-gender classes) than normal weight individuals. Research was aimed at examining how intragroup perceptual similarity in surface (age, ethnicity, or physical condition) and deep-level (attitude, beliefs, or values) qualities are related to perceptions of cohesion and exercise adherence within exercise classes. Surface level qualities, notably age, were associated with social cohesion and exercise attendance, while deep level qualities were associated with task cohesion. Collectively, these findings highlight how *similar* we perceive ourselves to be in relation to other group members in terms of various individual characteristics like age can have important implications in terms of our exercise preferences, cognitions, and behavior.

Group Composition

Widmeyer and John W. Loy developed a conceptual framework for group composition suggesting that the properties of sport groups can be considered from three perspectives: (1) amount of group resources, such as skills or personal attributes, present among group members; (2) the variability like homogeneity or heterogeneity in the resources of group members; and (3) compatibility between and among group members.

Strong empirical evidence supports the first perspective as higher individual measures of task ability and motivation have been associated with greater team performance. In regard to Widmeyer and Loy's second perspective, *variability* (e.g., homogeneity vs. heterogeneity in group resources like member attributes) can be considered beneficial or detrimental, or even both depending on the nature of the group and its task. For example, in basketball, effective teams ideally have heterogeneity in playing skills—guards who are gifted at ball handling and forwards who can rebound. Variability in sex, age, and race has also been examined. Among the identified variables, the relationship between race and playing position has been investigated extensively. To date, no conclusive evidence exists to support a relationship between race and playing position.

An area of future consideration in relation to Widmeyer and Loy's first two perspectives is the amount and *variability in team personality composition*. In work groups, researchers have found higher mean levels of extraversion and emotional stability contribute positively to social cohesion.

Researchers have also focused on the variance in team personality composition. This latter approach is based on research suggesting that averaging individual team member personality scores may mask important information, such as the negative effect of a single team member on a group. As such, researchers have used a minimum scores method to examine the personality scores of individual team members. Using this approach, a minimum rather than average score is established for each personality trait for the group. Additional research with work groups revealed minimum levels of conscientiousness and agreeableness to contribute positively to both task cohesion and team performance. Future research in team personality composition in sport and exercise settings is needed.

Widmeyer and Loy's third category is *compatibility in group resources*. Compatibility is described as the ability of an individual to *fit* (e.g., function effectively and in harmony) with other group members. Across social, work, and sport group settings, compatibility contributes to enhanced individual satisfaction and performance. Research on compatibility in sport has predominantly focused on compatibility of coach–athlete relationships (referred to as coach–athlete dyads), member abilities, and group roles. A behavioral approach has frequently been used to examine the compatibility of coach–athlete dyads and teams. This has often involved observations of coach and athlete behaviors. Early work used William Schutz's fundamental interpersonal relations orientation (FIRO) theory to evaluate compatibility of the coach and athlete. Schutz proposed that in interpersonal relationships, individuals need to express three needs—*inclusion, control,* and *affection*. More recent work utilized a novel video observation and analysis approach titled *state space analysis* to examine coach–athlete interactions in youth sport teams over time. The state space approach was adapted from work in psychology examining parent–child relationships.

Collectively, behavioral approaches have attempted to shed light on the compatibility of coach–athlete dyads and group members to achieve effective performance.

Conclusion

Understanding the characteristics of a successful team is a topic of interest shared by researchers and practitioners alike. Further research and the continued integration of theory from other fields, such as organizational psychology or group dynamics, is needed in order to develop a better understanding of the role of group characteristics in sport and exercise settings.

Mark W. Bruner

See also Cohesion; Group Formation; Self-Categorization Theory; Social Identity Theory; Status; Team Building

Further Readings

Beauchamp, M. R., Carron, A. V., McCutcheon, S., & Harper, O. (2007). Older adults' preference for exercising alone versus in groups: Considering contextual congruence. *Annals of Behavioral Medicine, 33,* 200–206.

Beauchamp, M. R., Dunlop, W. L., Downey, S. M., & Estabrooks, P. A. (2012). First impressions count: Perceptions of surface-level and deep-level similarity within postnatal exercise classes and implications for program adherence. *Journal of Health Psychology, 17,* 68–77.

Carron, A. V. (1990). Group size in sport and physical activity: Social psychological and performance consequences. *International Journal of Sport Psychology, 21*(4), 286–304.

Carron, A. V., & Eys, M. A. (2012). *Group dynamics in sport* (4th ed.). Morgantown, WV: Fitness Information Technology.

Carron, A. V., & Spink, K. S. (1995). The group size-cohesion relationship in minimal groups. *Small Group Research, 26,* 86–105.

Dunlop, W. L., & Beauchamp, M. R. (2012). Does similarity make a difference? Predicting cohesion and attendance behaviors within exercise group settings. *Group Dynamics: Theory, Research, and Practice, 15,* 258–266.

Dunlop, W. L., & Beauchamp, M. R. (2012). En-gendering choice: Preferences for exercising in gender-segregated and gender-integrated groups and consideration of overweight status. *International Journal of Behavioral Medicine, 18,* 216–220.

Spink, K. S., Wilson, K. S., & Priebe, C. S. (2010). Groupness and adherence in structured exercise settings. *Group Dynamics: Theory, Research, and Practice, 14*, 163–173.

Steiner, I. D. (1972). *Group processes and productivity.* New York: Academic Press.

van Vianen, A. E. M., & De Dreu, C. K. W. (2001). Personality in teams: Its relationship to social cohesion, task cohesion, and team performance. *European Journal of Work and Organizational Psychology, 10*, 97–120.

Wheelan, S. A. (2009). Group size, group development, and group productivity. *Small Group Research, 40*, 247–262.

GROUP FORMATION

Why do groups form and how do groups develop? In this entry, different perspectives on group development are examined. There are a number of reasons that people join groups. William Schutz theorized humans seek out groups in an effort to fulfill one or more of the following fundamental needs: (1) need for inclusion—desire for affiliation, belonging, and acceptance; (2) need for affection—desire for intimacy; and (3) need for control—desire for power and opportunities to dominate others. Once a group is formed, there are different perspectives on how groups develop.

Group Development Perspectives

Group development involves the evolution of structure, cohesion, and maturity of a group over the course of time. Group dynamics scholars have proposed over a hundred theories to explain group development. Holly Arrow, Marshall S. Poole, Kelly B. Henry, Susan Wheelan, and Richard Moreland reviewed the literature and classified the theories into five general categories: (1) linear (sequential stage) perspective, (2) cyclical (repeating cycles) perspective, (3) robust equilibrium model, (4) punctuated equilibrium model, and (5) adaptive response. The following is an overview of the five perspectives with an emphasis on the linear and cyclical perspectives, which have received the greatest attention in the group dynamics literature.

Linear (Sequential) Perspective

In the mid-1960s, Bruce Tuckman reviewed the literature on group development and proposed that groups progress through four stages of development. The four stages include: *forming, storming, norming,* and *performing.* Tuckman in collaboration with Mary Jensen later added a fifth stage, *adjourning.* In the first stage, forming, group members become familiar with each other and identify the group's task. This stage is similar to an orientation phase as the primary focus of the group members is on inclusion and dependency. Storming is characterized by tension and conflict among members and with the group's leader. Issues of power and authority are focal points as members exert their preferences for the group's approach to a task and question, or even resist, decisions of the leader. During norming, the group members come together to reach a consensus on the group's goals and objectives, and the group's norms, the accepted standards for behavior within the group. The norming stage is also characterized as a period of cooperation, clarification of individual member roles within the group, and development of group cohesion. In performing, the group becomes more stable as group members display a clear understanding and acceptance of their roles. The focus of group members is on the successful achievement of the group's task rather than conflict among members and the leader. Finally, adjourning is highlighted by a termination of roles or duties, reduction of dependency, and breakup of the group. Collectively, this linear perspective has two defining characteristics: (1) the five stages are sequential, and (2) the duration of each stage is variable.

Cyclical (Repeating Cycles) Perspective

One of the defining features of the linear perspective on group development is that groups move through a sequence of stages that begin with formation and end with termination (forming, storming, norming, performing, adjourning). In contrast, the cyclical perspective proposes that group development occurs through a *repeating* cycle of five stages. In the first stage, *discontent,* group members do not yet feel a part of the group or consider the group as part of their identity. An example would be during tryouts for a sport team when new players are vying for a spot on the team. The second stage of *group identification* occurs when individuals display commitment to the group and identify group members from nongroup members. The third stage, *group productivity,* occurs when members strive to contribute toward team goals. The successful attainment of goals often leads to the next stage, *individuation*, in which members seek out recognition for their personal contributions. This may be in the form of an athlete seeking out validation from the coach, fellow teammates, or others for performance. As the group moves through the individuation stage, the group progresses to the final stage, *decay*, where the members become less interested and put less energy toward achieving goals of the group. This often leads the group to cycle back to the first stage of *discontent* beginning the cyclical process again. The group may experience a number of cycles while together.

An analogy to differentiate the cyclical perspective from the linear perspective is a sport team progressing through various segments over the course of a season (preseason, regular season, playoffs). For example, during the preseason, a basketball team may display signs of *decay*, the final stage of the cyclical perspective, for example, lack of interest toward the team's goals, and cycle back to the initial stage of *discontent*. However, the start of the regular season may reinvigorate the group and push the group to the stage of *group identification* as members have renewed interest and seek out their roles for the team to be successful. Conversely, a linear perspective would not describe the team as cycling back to early stages in group development during the preseason. Rather, a linear perspective would view the team as progressing sequentially over the season (forming and storming during the preseason, norming and performing during the regular season).

Additional Perspectives on Group Development

Three alternative group development perspectives identified by Arrow and colleagues include the robust equilibrium model, punctuated equilibrium model, and adaptive response. The robust equilibrium perspective is characterized by group development (e.g., delineation of norms and roles) during the early time periods of the group's formation. Then the structure of the group becomes relatively stable over time. The punctuated equilibrium model is a variation of the robust equilibrium perspective where group development is perceived to consist of stable periods that are interrupted by sudden bouts of instability. During bouts of instability, the group is restructured and may involve a turnover in group members or reassignment of roles within the group. The final perspective, adaptive response, rejects the notion that all groups move through a similar progression of stages. The adaptive response perspective proposes that groups develop in their own unique manner based upon the stressors and challenges each group needs to overcome. As such, each group's pattern of development is idiosyncratic and a response to environmental constraints and opportunities.

Integrated Model of Group Development

Susan Wheelan examined the group development literature and developed an Integrated Model of Group Development that built upon Tuckman's linear model of group development and the early work of Wilfred Bion. Similar to Tuckman's model, there is a linear progression of stages. Conversely, Wheelan's perspective emphasized that groups achieve maturity as the group members work together rather than simply going through stages of activity. Group development in early stages in the model is associated with dependency, counterdependency, and trust while the later, more mature stages are where productivity is a focus.

To reflect the characteristics of each stage in the Integrated Model of Group Development, Wheelan relabeled the stages beginning with the first stage—*dependency and inclusion*. Similar to Tuckman's model, the stage is characterized by the member's concerns for inclusion and dependency on the group's leader for direction. Within the second stage, *counterdependency and fight*, there is conflict among the group members about the group's goals and procedures. If the group can work through the conflict with open communication, the group can foster commitment and trust, and progress to the third stage, *trust and structure*. The structural component of the third stage reflects the negotiation of roles and conformity to norms (acceptable procedures) within the group. This stage also highlights the establishment of positive work relationships. The final or *work* stage is a period of enhanced productivity and effectiveness, whereby previous deleterious issues within the group have been resolved and the focus of group members' energy is on the tasks and achievement of group goals. An emphasis of Wheelan's model is the link between the productivity of the group and the different stages, whereby lower productivity is evident during Stage 1 and higher productivity is evident during Stage 4.

Group Development Assessment

Several attempts have been undertaken to assess group development. Susan Wheelan and Anthony Verdi developed the Group Development Observation System (GDOS). This approach involves transcribing, coding, and analyzing the patterns of communication of group members based upon seven group-development categories (dependency, counterdependency, fight, flight, pairing, counterpairing, and work). GDOS has been used to examine the patterns of communication between sexes, whereby researchers have compared same-sex (homogeneous) and mixed-sex (heterogeneous) groups during progressive phases of group life. In this work, no significant differences were found to exist between same-sex groups. However, mixed-sex groups differed from same-sex groups but this was attributed to a larger group size rather than sex composition. In sum, sex composition does not appear to influence group developmental patterns.

Susan Wheelan and Judith Hochberger used the integrated model of group development to create the Group Development Questionnaire (GDQ). The GDQ includes four scales that correspond to the four stages of Wheelan's integrated model. The items in each scale are designed to assess the characteristic behaviors of groups in each stage (e.g., Stage 1 scale assesses dependency and inclusion). Calculating group mean scores for the four scales can be used to determine each group's stage of development, productivity, and effectiveness. Higher group mean scores on the higher stages are indicative of greater productivity and group effectiveness.

Wheelan has conducted group development research with the GDQ in a number of settings, such as work and schools. One study in elementary schools found greater staff group development (e.g., when teachers displayed more trust and cooperation) to be positively associated with student learning and performance. More recently, Wheelan used the measure to examine the relationship between group size, development, and productivity in over 300 work groups. Results revealed that group size is an important factor in group development and productivity. Smaller groups of three to eight members were found to be significantly more productive and more developmentally advanced and with higher mean scores in more mature stages on GDQ than larger groups of nine or more members. Groups consisting of three to four members were found to be most productive and developmentally advanced.

Empirical Evidence in Sport and Exercise

Although there has been an abundance of work on group development in organizational and work settings, research on group formation and development in sport and exercise is relatively limited in scope. The vast majority of research in this area has focused on the relationship between managerial and team member turnover and team effectiveness. In general, longitudinal examinations of team success after a managerial change in a number of professional and intercollegiate sports, such as baseball, basketball, and hockey, have revealed higher managerial turnover to be associated with lower team effectiveness (e.g., poorer win–loss, league standing) or only short-term improvement in team performance, that is, no long-term effects beyond the season.

Similar to managerial turnover, research on the relationship between athlete turnover and team effectiveness has revealed that higher athlete turnover is associated with lower team effectiveness (e.g., poorer win–loss, league standing) in a number of professional sports (baseball, basketball, football). Nevertheless, contradictory evidence also exists, with one review of professional ice-hockey teams, from 1950 to 1966, revealing that both coach and athlete turnover were unrelated to team performance. Indeed, some coaches and researchers have suggested that turnover is not always problematic as too little turnover can lead to complacency and diminished motivation among team members. The ideal time and level of player turnover with regard to team success has been a related area of study and found to vary by sport and position. Given that player turnover can happen for a variety of reasons—injury, retirement, trade—and can potentially impact the group's development and team effectiveness, it is likely to be a topic of future research interest.

Conclusion

Social scientists have highlighted the importance of groups for individuals. While group development has been a topic of considerable interest in organizational settings, this topic has received much less attention in sport and exercise settings. A fruitful line of research would involve examining the influence of group development on group effectiveness, such as team morale and performance, and on individual members' satisfaction or adherence. in exercise and sport settings.

Mark W. Bruner

See also Cohesion; Group Characteristics; Norms; Roles; Team Building

Further Readings

Arrow, H., Poole, M. S, Henry, K. B., Wheelan, S., & Moreland, R. (2004). Time, change, and development: The temporal perspective on groups. *Small Group Research, 35,* 73–105.

Carron, A. V., & Eys, M. A. (2012). *Group dynamics in sport* (4th ed.). Morgantown, WV: Fitness Information Technology.

Forsyth, D. R. (2010). *Group dynamics* (5th ed.). Belmont, CA: Wadsworth, Cengage Learning.

McTeer, W., White, P. G., & Persad, S. (1995). Manager/ coach mid-season replacement and team performance in professional team sport. *Journal of Sport Behavior, 18,* 58–68.

Tuckman, B. W., & Jensen, M. A. C. (1977). Stages in small group development revisited. *Group and Organizational Studies, 2,* 419–427.

Verdi, A. F., & Wheelan, S. A. (1992). Developmental patterns in same-sex and mixed-sex groups. *Small Group Research, 23*(3), 356–378.

Wheelan, S. A. (2009). Group size, group development, and group productivity. *Small Group Research, 40*(2), 247–262.

Wheelan, S. A., & Hochberger, J. M. (1996). Validation studies of the group development questionnaire. *Small Group Research, 27,* 143–170.

Wheelan, S. A., & Kesselring, J. (2005). Link between faculty group development and elementary student performance on standardized tests. *The Journal of Education Research, 98*(6), 323–330.

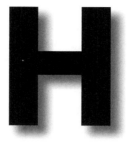

Habit

Repetition can make a simple behavior very powerful. Improving your physical health by exercising, increasing body strength by working out, or building up your potting skills in playing snooker can only be achieved by frequently executing these behaviors. However, people often struggle to maintain such regimes; sport schools typically see a decline in attendance a few weeks after the season start, and many training programs fail due to a lack of perseverance. Turning a beneficial behavior or practice into a habit is therefore the key to success. Unhealthy or ineffective habits may form barriers for change and may prevent establishing positive outcomes or improvements.

In the psychological literature, *habit* has always been defined in terms of frequency of behavior, which was inherited from the behaviorist school. However, there are problems with this definition. The first problem is that it is unclear how frequently behavior must be executed in order to qualify as a habit; does a habit exist after 2, 4, or 20 repetitions? Secondly, frequent behavior is not necessarily a habit. An athlete may regularly attempt to break the world record in sprinting, but few would consider this as a habit. We therefore need a better definition.

Such a definition of habit rests on three pillars. The first pillar obviously is *repetition*. Habits are formed by repeating behavior with satisfactory outcomes and without repetition there is no habit. However, repetition is a necessary but not a sufficient condition for behavior to qualify as

habit, hence a second pillar, which is *automaticity*. Habits are typically executed with relatively little mental effort, awareness, and conscious intent. These qualities make habits being experienced as *easy* or *fluent*; there is not much thought involved or needed to carry them out. While habits are forms of automatic behavior, they are functional and goal directed; we develop habits that serve us in one way or another, no matter whether these goals are constructive or unconstructive. If a habit has been developed, the recognition or activation of a goal may thus automatically elicit the accompanying habit. This relates to the third pillar of habit, which is *context stability*. This pillar is not so much a feature of the habit itself, but rather of the conditions and environments where habits occur. Habits are often elicited by specific cues, such as a particular time, location, physiological state, or the presence of an object or person. Habits thrive in stable conditions, where the same cue elicits the habitual response time and again. For instance, a person may have developed the habit of running twice a week after work and before having dinner. Such a habit may flourish if this person has a stable pattern of returning from work and having dinner at the same time and location but would be difficult to maintain in the face of irregular work times or if this person would travel a lot.

Some Caveats

Measurement. If we accept that behavioral frequency is an inadequate definition of habit, the traditional way of using behavioral frequency as a measure of habit should be replaced by one that is commensurate to the new definition. The Self-Report Habit Index has been developed for that purpose. It is a 12-item scale, which assesses habit as a psychological construct. It incorporates the various facets of habit, such as the experience of repetition and the lack of awareness and conscious intent.

Locus of control. The fact that habits are dependent on and elicited by cues in the environment where the behavior takes place points to a shift in locus of control when behavior becomes habitual. Whereas new or deliberate behaviors are controlled by conscious intentions and *willpower*, which is very much in line with prevalent socio-cognitive models such as the theory of planned behavior, habits are to a much larger degree controlled by the external environment. Habits are thus less likely to change through motivation and attitude change. Although motivation and attitude change may certainly help make changes, managing the environments in which behavior occurs may be paramount to success if strong habits are involved. This implies identifying and changing or removing the cues that trigger old habits and engineering the environment for new habits to establish and flourish. Habits may thus be planned in a particular environment and may be promoted by, for instance, the use of implementation intentions.

Where is the habit? One may wonder whether habits really exist in the domain of sport and exercise. After all, many who practice sport and exercise do that intentionally and mindfully. These activities are characterized by repetition, but seemingly not so much by automaticity. It is therefore important to analyze precisely where exactly habits may reside. Take for instance exercising. While exercising may be executed intentionally and mindfully, it is often the *decision* to exercise where the problems lie. If we would deliberate every time whether or not to exercise, we would be vulnerable to our well-developed skills to rationalize and find excuses to stay home. On the other hand, if we make the decision to go exercising a habit and build this into our daily or weekly routines, we would not need to deliberate whether or not to exercise, but rather which route to take or which clothes to wear. In other words, while the activity itself may be executed in a mindful, and hopefully joyful fashion, the decision to exercise is the critical habit.

Opportunities to break and create habits. As breaking old habits often requires rearrangements of the environment where habits reside, we may look for opportunities to break habits that sometimes naturally arise. This happens particularly when people undergo life course changes, such as moving to a new house, starting a family, changing a job, or starting retirement. These events provide short windows of opportunity where old habits are temporarily broken, and individuals may be looking for new ways to arrange their lives. In those situations, people may consider making changes that they have contemplated all along. These may also provide opportunities where behavior change interventions may be more effective and thus provide more value for money.

Mental habits. We have not only habits of doing but also of thinking. Mental habits are repetitive patterns of thought, which may possess the crucial features of behavioral habits such as described by the three pillars. Mental habits may involve negative thoughts, which then may get in the way of good performances and may affect outcomes such as one's self-esteem or mental health. Mental habits may also involve positive thoughts, which may then play constructive roles in keeping up one's motivation and believing in oneself.

Bas Verplanken

See also Automaticity; Decision Making; Goal Setting; Interventions for Exercise and Physical Activity; Leadership in Sport: Social Cognitive Approaches; Learning; Mental Health; Mindfulness; Positive Thinking; Thought Stopping

Further Readings

Orbell, S., & Verplanken, B. (2010). The automatic component of habit in health behavior: Habit as cue-contingent automaticity. *Health Psychology, 29,* 374–383.

Verplanken, B. (2006). Beyond frequency: Habit as mental construct. *British Journal of Social Psychology, 45,* 639–656.

Verplanken, B., & Orbell, S. (2003). Reflections on past behavior: A self-report index of habit strength. *Journal of Applied Social Psychology, 33,* 1313–1330.

Wood, W., & Neal, D. T. (2007). A new look at habits and the habit-goal interface. *Psychological Review, 114,* 843–863.

HEALTH ACTION PROCESS APPROACH

Theories of health behavior change are needed to explain, predict, and improve self-regulation of physical activity. Such theories are being divided into continuum models and stage models. In continuum models, people are positioned along a range that reflects the likelihood of action. Influential predictor variables are identified and combined within one prediction equation. The goal of an intervention is to move the person along this route toward action. Health promotion, then, focuses on increasing all model-inherent variables in all persons, without matching treatments to particular audiences. The *theory of planned behavior* (TPB), developed by Icek Ajzen, is one such *continuum model.*

In contrast, according to *stage models,* health behavior change consists of an ordered set of categories (or stages) into which people are classified. These categories reflect cognitive or behavioral characteristics, such as the intention to perform a behavior. The main purpose of applying stage models lies in the identification of relatively homogeneous target groups for interventions and the design of stage-matched treatments. The most popular stage theory of health behavior change is the *transtheoretical model* (TTM), developed by James Prochaska, that proposes five stages of change.

Both continuum models and stage models have their advantages and disadvantages. Continuum models have been found useful for explanation and prediction, whereas stage models are often preferred to guide interventions. For health promotion, the continuum models are often too general because all variables involved in such a model need to be addressed in interventions, without considering the special needs of particular subgroups of participants. However, it is possible to integrate both approaches when researchers use a continuum model as a theoretical template and,

when it comes to interventions, subdivide the audience into stage groups to allow for stage-matched treatments. The *health action process approach* (HAPA), developed by Ralf Schwarzer, is such a *hybrid model* with a continuum layer as well as a stage layer.

Mediating Mechanisms

The traditional continuum models have been criticized mainly because of the so-called intention–behavior gap (referring to the frequent failure of intention to predict behavior). HAPA explicitly includes postintentional factors to overcome this gap. It suggests a distinction between (1) preintentional motivation processes that lead to a behavioral intention, and (2) postintentional volition processes that lead to the actual health behavior. Within the two phases, different patterns of social cognitive predictors may emerge (see Figure 1). In the initial motivation phase, a person develops an intention to act. In this phase, *risk perception* is seen as a distal antecedent (e.g., "I am at risk for cardiovascular disease"). Risk perception in itself is insufficient to enable a person to form an intention. Rather, it may set the stage for a contemplation process and further elaboration of thoughts about consequences and competencies. Similarly, *positive outcome expectancies* (e.g., "If I exercise five times per week, I will reduce my cardiovascular risk") are chiefly seen as being important in the motivation phase, when a person balances the pros and cons of certain behavioral outcomes. Further, one needs to believe in one's capability to perform a desired action, *perceived self-efficacy* (e.g., "I am capable of adhering to my exercise schedule in spite of the temptation to watch TV"). Perceived self-efficacy operates in concert with positive outcome expectancies, both of which contribute to forming an intention. Both beliefs are needed for forming intentions to adopt difficult behaviors such as regular physical exercise.

After forming an intention, the volitional phase is entered. When a person is inclined to adopt a particular health behavior, the *good intention* has to be transformed into detailed instructions on how to perform the desired action. Once an action has been initiated, it has to be maintained. This is not achieved through a single act of will but involves self-regulatory skills and strategies. Thus, the postintentional phase is further broken down

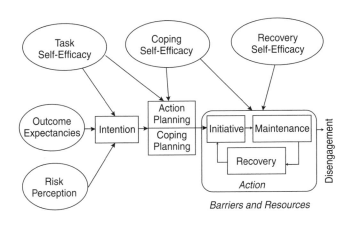

Figure 1   Health Action Process Approach

Source: Copyright © 1992 by Ralf Schwarzer. Used by permission.

into more proximal factors, such as *planning, coping self-efficacy,* and *recovery self-efficacy.* Additional volitional constructs that have been included in HAPA research are *action control* and *social support.*

Including planning and self-efficacy as volitional mediators renders the HAPA into an implicit stage model because it implies the existence of at least a motivational and a volitional phase. The purpose of such a model is twofold: It allows a better prediction of behavior, and it reflects the assumed causal mechanism of behavior change. Research that is based on this continuum layer of the model employs path-analytic methods.

Preintenders, Intenders, Actors

When it comes to the design of interventions, one can consider turning the implicit stage model into an explicit one. This is done by identifying individuals who are located either in the motivational stage or in the volitional stage. Then, each group receives a specific treatment that is tailored to this group. Moreover, it is useful and theoretically meaningful to subdivide the volitional group further into persons who perform and those who only intend to perform. In the postintentional–preactional stage, individuals are labeled *intenders,* and in the actional stage *actors.* Thus, a pragmatic subdivision within the health behavior change process yields three groups: preintenders, intenders, and actors.

The term *stage* in this context was chosen to allude to the stage theories, but not in the strict

definition that includes irreversibility and invariance. The terms *phase* or *mindset* may be equally suitable for this distinction. The basic idea is that individuals pass through different phases on their way to behavior change. Thus, interventions may be most efficient when tailored to these particular mindsets.

For example, preintenders are supposed to benefit from confrontation with outcome expectancies and some level of risk communication. They need to learn that the new behavior like becoming physically active has positive outcomes, such as well-being, weight loss, and fun, as opposed to the negative outcomes that accompany the current (sedentary) behavior, such as developing an illness or being overweight. They also need to develop an optimistic belief that they are capable of performing the critical behavior.

In contrast, *intenders* should not benefit much from health messages in the form of outcome expectancies because, after setting a goal, they have already moved beyond this mindset. Rather, they should benefit from planning to translate their intentions into action.

Finally, *actors* should be prepared for particular high-risk situations in which lapses are imminent. Interventions help them if they desire to change their routines by adopting or altering a behavior, for example.

Five Principles

The HAPA is designed as an open architecture that is based on principles rather than on specific testable assumptions. Developed in 1988, it was an attempt to integrate the model of action phases by Heinz Heckhausen and Peter Gollwitzer, with social cognitive theory developed by Albert Bandura, based on five principles.

Principle 1: Motivation and volition. The health behavior change process is divided into two phases. There is a switch of mindsets when people move from deliberation to action. First comes the motivation phase in which people develop their intentions. Afterwards, they enter the volition phase.

Principle 2: Two volitional phases. In the volition phase, there are two groups of people: those who did not yet translate their intentions into action, and those who did. Thus, there are inactive as well as active persons in this phase. In other words, in the volitional phase one finds intenders as well as actors who are characterized by different psychological states. In addition to health behavior change as a continuous process, one can also create three categories of people with different mindsets, depending on their current location within the course of behavior change: preintenders, intenders, and actors.

Principle 3: Postintentional planning. Intenders who are in the volitional preactional stage are motivated to change, but they do not act because they might lack the right skills to translate their intention into action. Planning is a key strategy at this point. It serves as an operative mediator between intentions and behavior.

Principle 4: Two kinds of mental simulation. Planning can be divided into action planning and coping planning. Action planning pertains to the when, where, and how of intended action. Coping planning includes the anticipation of barriers and the design of alternative actions that help to attain one's goal in spite of impediments.

Principle 5: Phase-specific self-efficacy. Perceived self-efficacy is required throughout the entire process. However, the nature of self-efficacy differs from phase to phase. This is because there are different challenges as people progress from one phase to the next one. Goal setting, planning, initiative, action, and maintenance all pose challenges that are not of the same nature. Therefore, we distinguish between preactional self-efficacy, coping self-efficacy, and recovery self-efficacy. Sometimes the terms *task self-efficacy* instead of preaction self-efficacy, and *maintenance self-efficacy* instead of coping and recovery self-efficacy are preferred.

Assessment of Constructs

Risk Perception. Risk perception can be measured by items such as "How high do you rate the likelihood that you will ever get one of the following diseases: (a) cardiovascular disease (e.g., heart attack, stroke), (b) diseases of the musculoskeletal system (e.g., osteoarthritis, herniated vertebral disk)?" Any other health risk can be added, if relevant to the research context.

Outcome Expectancies. Positive outcome expectancies (pros) and negative outcome expectancies (cons) can be assessed, for example, with the stem "If I engage in physical activity at least three times per week for 20 minutes . . ." followed by pros such as "then I feel better afterwards," or "then I meet friendly people," and followed by cons such as "then every time would cost me a lot of money," or "then I would be financially depleted."

Self-efficacy. Perceived motivational and volitional self-efficacy can be composed of items such as the following. Motivational self-efficacy (task self-efficacy) refers to the goal-setting phase and can be measured with the stem "I am certain . . ." followed by items like "that I can be physically active on a regular basis, even if I have to mobilize myself," or "that I can be physically active on a regular basis, even if it is difficult." Volitional self-efficacy refers to the goal-pursuit phase. It can be subdivided into coping self-efficacy and recovery self-efficacy. Coping self-efficacy has been measured with the stem "I am capable of strenuous physical exercise on a regular basis . . ." followed by barriers like "even if it takes some time until it becomes routine," or "even if I need several attempts until I will be successful." Items on recovery self-efficacy can be worded "I am confident that I can resume a physically active lifestyle, even if I have relapsed several times," "I am confident that I am able to resume my regular exercises after failures to pull myself together," or "I am confident that I can resume my physical activity, even when feeling weak after an illness."

Intention. Intention to perform a behavior is assessed in correspondence to the behavior itself: for example, "I intend to perform the following activities at least 3 days per week for 20 minutes: strenuous (heart beats rapidly, sweating) physical activities," "moderate (not exhausting, light perspiration) physical activities," and "mild (minimal effort, no perspiration) physical activity." Answers can range, for example, from not at all true (1) to absolutely true (6). Alternatively, intention can be assessed in terms of frequency and duration of more specific behaviors: (a) physiotherapeutic exercises (e.g., back training), (b) fitness activities (e.g., using an exercise bike), (c) resistance training (training muscle strength, e.g., on machines), and (d) physical activity while commuting (e.g., going by bicycle or walking for longer distances).

Planning. Action Planning can be assessed with items addressing the when, where, and how of the activity: for example, "I have already planned . . ." (1) "which physical activity I will perform (e.g., walking)," (2) "where I will be physically active (e.g., in the park)," (3) "on which days of the week I will be physically active," and (4) "for how long I will be physically active." Coping planning, on the other hand, can be measured with the item stem "I have made a detailed plan regarding . . ." and the items (1) "what to do if something interferes with my plans," (2) "how to cope with possible setbacks," (3) "what to do in difficult situations in order to act according to my intentions," (4) "which good opportunities for action to take," and (5) "when I have to pay extra attention to prevent lapses." Another option is to ask participants to actually generate their plans, which, however, confounds measurement and treatment.

Action Control. While planning is a prospective strategy, that is, behavioral plans are made before the situation is encountered, action control is a concurrent self-regulatory strategy, where the ongoing behavior is continuously evaluated with regard to a behavioral standard. Action control can be assessed with a six-item scale comprising three facets of the action control process: *self-monitoring* ("I consistently monitored myself whether I exercised frequently enough," or "I consistently monitored myself when, where, and how long I exercise"), *awareness of standards* ("I have always been aware of my prescribed training program," or "I often had my exercise intention on my mind"), and *self-regulatory effort* ("I really tried hard to exercise regularly," or "I took care to practice as much as I intended to").

Staging. When using the continuum model for the prediction of behavior, these variables are being specified as predictors and mediators in a path model (see Figure 1). When employing the stage variant to conduct an intervention study, an assessment of stages is necessary. Stage theories employ algorithms for the staging procedure which can be regarded as a *fast and frugal tree* with satisfactory validity. For a three-stage procedure, one needs two steps. First, behavior is assessed on the basis of a context-specific dichotomous criterion (yes = already active, no = not yet sufficiently active). Those who meet the preselected criterion are defined as *actors*. Those who don't are subject to

the second step by asking them whether they intend to become active or not. If they do intend, they are defined as *intenders*; if they don't, they are *nonintenders* (or *preintenders*). Such straightforward diagnostic procedures may be too simple to account for response bias and temporal fluctuation. However, when subdividing large samples to assign stage-matched treatments, such a pragmatic procedure results in more homogeneous subgroups that allow for more effective interventions.

Conclusion

In sum, the HAPA has two layers: a continuum layer and a phase (or stage) layer. Depending on the research question, one might choose one or the other. HAPA is designed as a sequence of two continuous self-regulatory processes, a goal-setting phase (motivation) and a goal-pursuit phase (volition). The second phase is subdivided into a preaction phase and an action phase. One can superimpose these three phases on the continuum model as a second layer and regard phase as a moderator.

This two-layer architecture allows switching between the continuum model and the stage model, depending on the given research question. The stage layer is useful for designing stage-matched interventions. For preintenders, one needs risk and resource communication, for example by addressing the pros and cons of a critical behavior. For intenders, planning treatments are helpful to support those who lack the necessary skills to translate their intentions into behavior. And for actors, one needs to stabilize their newly adopted health behaviors by relapse prevention strategies.

The HAPA allows both the researcher and the practitioner to make a number of choices. Although it was initially inspired by distinguishing between a motivational and a volitional stage, and later expanded to the distinction between preintenders, intenders, and actors, one need not necessarily group individuals according to such stages. If the purpose is to predict behavior change, one would specify a mediator model that includes postintentional constructs (such as planning and volitional self-efficacy) as proximal predictors of performance.

For stage-tailored interventions, however, usually three stage groups would be established. This does not exclude the possibility of generating more than three stages. For example, for some research questions, one might subdivide the preintenders into precontemplators and contemplators, according to the TTM. Or one might opt for a distinction between preintenders, who are (a) unaware of an issue, (b) aware but unengaged, or (c) still deciding. Thus, HAPA is not a puristic stage model, but a principle-based framework that allows for a variety of approaches. Evidence from intervention studies shows good results, in particular for patients with various chronic illnesses and disabilities. Planning interventions and action control programs proved especially successful.

Ralf Schwarzer

See also Adherence; Control Theory; Interventions for Exercise and Physical Activity; Self-Regulation; Social Cognitive Theory; Theory of Planned Behavior; Transtheoretical Model

Further Readings

Fleig, L., Lippke, S., Pomp, S., & Schwarzer, R. (2011). Exercise maintenance after rehabilitation: How experience can make a difference. *Psychology of Sport and Exercise, 12,* 293–299. doi: 10.1016/j.psychsport .2011.01.003

Gellert, P., Ziegelmann, J. P., & Schwarzer, R. (2012). Affective and health-related outcome expectancies for physical activity in older adults. *Psychology & Health, 27,* 816–828. doi: 10.1080/08870446.2011 .607236

Heckhausen, H., & Gollwitzer, P. M. (1987). Thought contents and cognitive functioning in motivational versus volitional states of mind. *Motivation and Emotion, 11,* 101–120.

Lippke, S., Ziegelmann, J. P., Schwarzer, R., & Velicer, W. F. (2009). Validity of stage assessment in the adoption and maintenance of physical activity and fruit and vegetable consumption. *Health Psychology, 28,* 183–193. doi: 10.1037/a0012983

Luszczynska, A., Schwarzer, R., Lippke, S., & Mazurkiewicz, M. (2011). Self-efficacy as a moderator of the planning-behaviour relationship in interventions designed to promote physical activity. *Psychology & Health, 26,* 151–166. doi: 10.1080/08870446.2011.531571

Parschau, L., Richert, J., Koring, M., Ernsting, A., Lippke, S., & Schwarzer, R. (2012). Changes in social-cognitive variables are associated with stage transitions in physical activity. *Health Education Research, 27,* 129–140. doi: 10.1093/her/cyr085

Prochaska, J. O., & DiClemente, C. C. (1983). Stages and processes of self-change of smoking: Toward an integrative model of change. *Journal of Consulting and Clinical Psychology, 51,* 390–395.

Scholz, U., Nagy, G., Schüz, B., & Ziegelmann, J. P. (2008). The role of motivational and volitional factors for self-regulated running training: Associations on the between- and within-person level. *British Journal of Social Psychology, 47,* 421–439.

Schwarzer, R. (1992). Self-efficacy in the adoption and maintenance of health behaviors: Theoretical approaches and a new model. In R. Schwarzer (Ed.), *Self-efficacy: Thought control of action* (pp. 217–243). Washington, DC: Hemisphere.

Schwarzer, R. (2008). Modeling health behavior change: How to predict and modify the adoption and maintenance of health behaviors. *Applied Psychology, 57,* 1–29.

Sniehotta, F. F., Schwarzer, R., Scholz, U., & Schüz, B. (2005). Action planning and coping planning for long-term lifestyle change: Theory and assessment. *European Journal of Social Psychology, 35,* 565–576.

Wiedemann, A. U., Lippke, S., Reuter, T., Ziegelmann, J. P., & Schüz, B. (2011). The more the better? The number of plans predicts health behaviour. *Applied Psychology: Health & Well-Being, 3,* 87–106. doi: 10.1111/j.1758-0854.2010.01042.x

HEALTH BELIEF MODEL

The health belief model, grounded in John Atkinson's expectancy–value theory of achievement motivation, proposes that people are rational decision makers who, during decision making, take into consideration advantages and disadvantages associated with physical activity. The theory also posits that motivation is unidimensional and that the construct of intentions, which represents motivation, is one of the most immediate determinants of physical activity. Therefore, the health belief model is a *motivational theory* that explains intention formation. It does not explain the processes by which people carry out their previously formed intentions.

The health belief model proposes that an individual's readiness (intention) to engage in physical activities is a function of the perceived vulnerability to a health condition and the probable severity of that condition. Consistent with the expectancy–value model, the model posits that readiness is determined by a person's beliefs about the benefits to be gained by a particular behavior such as exercise weighted by one's perceived barriers associated with physical activity. Finally, the model predicts that readiness to action may not result in physical activity unless some instigating event occurred to set the action process in motion. Irwin M. Rosenstock termed such instigating events as *cues to action*.

Overall, the health belief model predicts that strong intentions emerge when individuals feel vulnerable to an illness, the illness is perceived to be severe, and individuals believe that physical activity will reduce the health threat associated with the illness. For example, individuals may feel susceptible to cardiovascular disease because they have a poor diet and had been told by their physician that they have hypertension. They may also believe that regular exercise may reduce the threat of cardiovascular disease. According to the model, these perceptions are likely to motivate the individual to participate in physical activity.

Thus far research has shown that perceived severity and beliefs about the benefits of physical activity exert strong influences on readiness to engage in that behavior, while perceived severity and barriers have lesser impact. In addition, evidence suggests that the direct effects of perceived vulnerability, severity, susceptibility, benefits, and barriers on physical activity are small and are mediated by readiness. Further, there is evidence to suggest that the health belief model does not sufficiently capture all of the psychological determinants of physical activity and that the model may benefit from considering effects of other constructs such as self-efficacy on intentions and behavior.

One limitation of the health belief model is that it does not define perceived vulnerability clearly, nor does it specify how different variables combine in influencing readiness and physical activity. For example, it is unclear what type of vulnerability to disease should be measured. Shall we measure vulnerability to cardiovascular disease or vulnerability to back pain? In addition, vulnerability to cardiovascular disease may not predict the physical activity behavior of young individuals, given that getting a heart attack is a remote prospect for youth. Moreover, the model does not explicitly state whether perceived vulnerability would facilitate exercise or healthy dieting given that both behaviors would be effective in ameliorating cardiovascular disease risk. Hence, the model does not address behavioral choice. As a result, empirical evidence related to health belief model varies greatly across studies because different studies have used different operational definitions for psychological constructs or populations.

An important function of research is to provide information about the content of interventions. Generally speaking, the greater the relative importance of a factor in predicting physical activity intentions, the more likely it is that changing that factor will influence intentions and ultimately physical activity behavior. Given that studies adopting the health belief model have shown that appraisals related to perceived vulnerability and perceived severity, and appraisals related to benefits and barriers influence intentions to exercise, it can be suggested that attempts to change exercise behavior should try manipulate threat appraisals alongside perceived benefits and barriers. An important question, therefore, is how health appraisals can be influenced.

Threat appraisals can be manipulated through fear-arousing communications that highlight (a) the painful and debilitating effects of an illness (perceived severity) and (b) that people who do not exercise regularly are vulnerable to heart disease (perceived vulnerability). Physical activity benefits can be manipulated by exposing people to information that explains the effectiveness of exercise in preventing disease. The negative impact of perceived barriers on exercise can be circumvented by asking people to engage in types of physical activities that are relatively easy to perform or by prompting people to invent coping strategies that help them cope with barriers.

One caveat of interventions based on the health belief model is that although they may be successful in strengthening intentions, they may not always bring substantial changes in exercise behavior. Therefore, it cannot be expected verbatim that application of this model will produce strong effects on exercise behavior. Instead, the effectiveness of the health belief model in changing exercise behavior may be enhanced through the implementation of volitional techniques that can help people translate intentions into actions. Another limitation of the health belief model is that the threatening messages can sometimes undermine rather than enhance intentions. Generally speaking, people have a desire to protect or enhance sense of self. As a consequence, they may not easily accept and endorse health-threatening messages. Therefore, fear-arousing communications should be designed and applied with caution. Health messages should not be too threatening because otherwise interventions will elicit a maladaptive coping response. For example, telling individuals that exercise reduces the risk of cardiovascular disease may be more easily accepted than telling individuals that they will have a heart attack if they do not exercise on a regular basis. It is therefore always desirable to pilot intervention strategies in a small group of people before conducting large-scale interventions.

Nikos L. D. Chatzisarantis, Svetlana Kamarova, Masato Kawabata, and Martin S. Hagger

See also Health Action Process Approach; Social Cognitive Theory; Theory of Planned Behavior; Transtheoretical Model

Further Readings

Abraham, C., Clift, S., & Grabowski, P. (1999). Cognitive predictors of adherence to malaria prophylaxis regimens on return from a malarious region: A prospective study. *Social Science and Medicine, 48,* 1641–1654.

Ajzen, I. (1991). The theory of planned behavior. *Organizational Behavior and Human Decision Processes, 50,* 179–211.

Becker, M. (1974). The health belief model and sick role behavior. *Health Education Monographs, 2,* 409–419.

Courneya, K. S., & McAuley, E. (1995). Cognitive mediators of the social influence-exercise adherence relationship: A test of the theory of planned behavior. *Journal of Behavioural Medicine, 18,* 499–515.

Gollwitzer, P. M. (1990). Action phases and mind-sets. In E. T. Higgins & R. M. Sorrentino (Eds.), *Handbook of motivation and cognition: Foundations of social behavior* (Vol. 2, pp. 53–92). New York: Guilford Press.

Harrison, J. A., Mullen, P. D., & Green, L. W. (1992). A meta-analysis of studies of the health belief model with adults. *Health Education Research, 7,* 107–116.

Milne, S. E., Orbell, S., & Sheeran, P. (2002). Combining motivational and volitional interventions to promote exercise participation: Protection motivation theory and implementation intentions. *British Journal of Health Psychology, 7,* 163–184.

Norman, P., Conner, M., & Bell, R. (1999). The theory of planned behavior and smoking cessation. *Health Psychology, 18,* 89–94.

Quine, L., Rutter, D. R., & Arnold, L. (1998). Predicting and understanding safety helmet use among schoolboy cyclists: A comparison of the theory of planned behaviour and the health belief model. *Psychology & Health, 13,* 251–269.

Rosenstock, I. M. (1974). Historical origins of the health belief model. *Health Education Monographs, 2,* 328–335.

Smith, B. N., & Stasson, M. F. (2000). A comparison of health behavior constructs: Social psychological predictors of AIDS-preventive behavioral intentions. *Journal of Applied Social Psychology, 30,* 443–462.

HEALTH PROMOTION

Health promotion has been defined in a number of different ways and used in reference to a constellation of behaviors, such as eating, exercise, and stress management. For the purposes of this entry, we consider *health promotion* to be defined as strategies that (1) facilitate awareness of the benefits of, and opportunities for, physical activity; (2) enhance exercise motivation and skills; and (3) intervene to make environments supportive for active living. Within this definition is the explicit acknowledgment that both individual- and environmental-level factors are related to health promotion. In this entry, we focus on health promotion strategies to increase exercise or physical activity that focus on individuals, groups, and specific settings.

Individual-Level Interventions

Strategies that are based on underlying theories appear to be more effective than strategies that are not. Social cognitive theories that include outcome expectations, control beliefs, and social influences are the typical underlying theories for individual-level physical activity promotion interventions. Using these models, participants develop goals and plans to achieve these goals. This personal action planning is essential to many of the individual-level interventions.

Personal Action Planning

Personal action planning can be useful in health promotion interventions targeting physical activity. Action plans allow the participants to focus on personally relevant motives as to why they should increase physical activity. For example, one person may list that engaging in an exercise routine will maintain or improve health while another may list the desire to stay young with one's children. These personally relevant motives are directly related to the outcome expectations a person may have relative to a given behavior. Personal action plans also allow for the behavior changes to be goal directed, meaning a person may cite specific and measurable goals and activities to increase their physical activity. To overcome barriers that may decrease a person's self-efficacy, or the belief in ability or competence to perform a certain action, a person may brainstorm ways to overcome obstacles that may impede personal goals. For example, if one cites not enjoying exercise because it is boring, that person may want to try different activities at the local YMCA until finding something stimulating. A personal action plan process works well to assist participants in resolving these issues. It is also a key tool in a goal setting and feedback loop that can be initiated between a participant and a health professional.

There are a number of effective individual-level interventions that vary in the way they are delivered. It is clear that one-on-one counseling can be an effective method to increase physical activity and that the more frequent and longer duration of the intervention, the more likely it is to lead to behavior changes. One-on-one counseling has been done successfully using face-to-face methods, telephone methods—both live and automated—and, more recently through computer interactive sessions and mobile phones.

The ALIVE! study provides a good example of an individual-level intervention that includes action planning. The study used a computerized program to motivate participants to increase their physical activity as well as a number of other behaviors. The intervention included assessing participants' health behaviors and then encouraging them to set a goal in the area of greatest behavioral need (the behavior that they were currently not doing). Over the next three months, the program facilitated a series of small goals to provide participants with an opportunity to be successful before progressing to more challenging goals. During the program, participants received feedback on their accomplishments. The results of ALIVE! showed that people who participated in the intervention increased their physical activity more than those in a control group.

Group-Based Interventions

Group-based interventions are those that use a group-dynamics approach to promote physical activity. It is important to distinguish between individual-level interventions that are delivered to an aggregate of people—like a group-education class—and a group-based intervention that includes strategies that consider the positive and negative forces that reside within groups and target those forces to enact behavior change.

For group-based interventions, one of the driving concepts is that group cohesion is key in the process of behavior change and that three general areas of influence can be used to facilitate group cohesion. First, the group environment, which includes the sense of distinctiveness participants hold within the group and the size of the group, is thought to influence group cohesion and adherence. It appears as though the ideal exercise class size is 5 to 17 members, and the most common method used to generate a sense of distinctiveness is to create a group name. Some use games to create member proximity to remove barriers that are typical when people exercise together. Second, the structure of a group, including norms, roles, and even location of members within group meetings, facilitate group cohesion. Group norms are often developed through the public sharing of individual behavior and goals. Roles can be developed formally to aid in participants feeling a stronger responsibility toward the group (e.g., attendance tracker, warm-up leader) and participants can be encouraged to exercise in the same space at each group meeting to give a sense of belonging and fit within the group. Third, specific group processes that included communication, cooperation, and competition in the pursuit of a common group goal can enhance group cohesion. The common goal can be an aggregate of the individual goals of people within the group so that they feel accountable to the group. A group goal is critical and perhaps the most important aspect of group dynamics strategies to promote physical activity.

When a physical activity promotion strategy includes components that focus on group environment, structure, and process, it will typically lead to large changes in behavior. In fact, when compared to individual interventions (with or without social support) group-based interventions lead to significantly larger changes. Interestingly, unlike individual-level interventions, group-based interventions seem to be effective regardless of the intensity and duration of the intervention program. Early research that focused on group-based approaches typically used interventions that included three to five sessions per week over a 3- to

6-month period. These interventions were successful in improving adherence, outcome expectations, and control beliefs as well as increasing exercise participation. These types of interventions also demonstrated improved maintenance of exercise after the sessions were completed.

At the other end of the spectrum, studies like Move More tested the degree to which group-based interventions could increase and maintain physical activity with just two, 2-hour sessions spaced a month apart with the focus of the second session on increasing exercise once the program was completed. Move More targeted insufficiently active adult patients, and the participants were randomly assigned to either a group-based intervention, which used group dynamic strategies, or an enhanced-standard care group, which used social cognitive theory and a self-directed approach (action planning workbook, information on resources in the community, a follow-up telephone call). The results showed that although both interventions succeeded in increasing physical activity over the first 3 months, the participants in the group-dynamics approach were able to sustain and further increase their physical activity 6 months after the intervention ended while those in the enhanced-standard care group did not.

Site-Specific Interventions

The next sections discuss health promotion efforts across a number of different sites. In each case, individual-level strategies, group-based strategies, or both could be applied. As you will note in the examples below, site-specific interventions also regularly use social (e.g., policy changes) and physical (e.g., development of walking paths) environmental strategies to support physical activity.

School-Based Interventions

Children spend much of their time in school, and school provides a great place to offer health promotion activities. As children get older, their time doing physical activity significantly declines. In the Healthy Youth Places Project, an intervention rooted in social cognitive theory, researchers wanted to increase the availability and acceptability of physical activity for middle-school students. The underlying proposition of the Healthy Youth Places Project was that engaging student, staff, and faculty leaders within the intervention would enhance the likelihood that intervention strategies

would be effective. Change teams made up of these key stakeholders received training on effective strategies to promote physical activity and implemented a number of different environmental strategies to improve student perceptions of connection, autonomy, skill building and healthy norms related to physical activity. The results of the Healthy Youth Places project demonstrated that students in the schools with change teams increased their physical activity over 3 years significantly more than those students in the control group.

Worksite Interventions

Like schools for children, worksites are the location that adults spend most of their waking hours. Worksite wellness has a long history because of the role of health in worker productivity and satisfaction. Worksites also provide a wide variety of avenues for intervention strategies (e.g., interpersonal relationships, group settings, organizational structure and policy). The Active for Life work-based physical activity intervention provides a good example of a typical approach for this setting. The intervention included changes to the physical environment in the form of posters and onsite health fairs and individually targeted materials in the form of regular newsletters, goal setting, self-monitoring, and incentives. It also included a group-based approach that was facilitated by site captains and included interoffice friendly competitions. The program reached about a third of the employees and lasted for 10 weeks. By the end of the intervention, the proportion of employees who were meeting the recommended guidelines for physical activity increased from 34% to 48%. However, 6 months following the intervention most of the employees had returned to a less active level. This lack of maintenance of physical activity change is common across health promotion strategies and provides an area in need of considerable research focus.

Health Care–Based Interventions

Medical clinics have the potential for broad reach into the U.S. population. Furthermore, clinicians are considered credible and objective sources of health information for patients. A number of researchers have attempted to take advantage of the credibility of physicians to promote physical activity. Unfortunately, it appears as though a simple prescription for physical activity is insufficient to initiate physical activity change. Some researchers have attempted to increase the amount of time that physicians spend counseling patients on physical activity and have also used techniques such as motivational interviewing. While there has been some success with these approaches in efficacy trials, there is limited evidence that physicians have the time necessary to even insert a 2- to 3-minute counseling session for each patient that presents with a low level of physical activity. Where the most promise appears to be in regard to clinic-based physical activity promotion is at the intersection of health information technology and community resources. With the growing prevalence of the electronic health record and the push to include exercise as a vital sign, clinics have moved to the forefront as a location to identify people who could benefit from more physical activity. Still other researchers have shown that when physicians refer patients to a proactive community physical activity organization like the YMCA, the results are typically quite good in terms of increased physical activity.

Faith-Based Interventions

The rationale for intervening in faith-based institutions is not very different than some of the other place-based or settings-based interventions mentioned above. A large proportion of the American population attends a weekly faith-based service, and these services provide a great opportunity to promote physical activity. Just as with worksites, there are a number of different levels of potential intervention in a faith-based organization—sermons, socials, and service opportunities. Guide to Health provides a strong example of an effective intervention that was evaluated across 14 churches in southwest Virginia. The intervention prompted congregates to create weekly step-count goals, and when step counts were met, the future goals changed by an additional 500 steps. If a congregant failed to meet a weekly goal, helpful self-regulation strategies were used to help that person meet personal goals. The intervention was successful in initiating physical activity among congregation members.

Paul A. Estabrooks and Erin M. Smith

See also Ecological Theory; Group Characteristics; Group Formation; Social Cognitive Theory; Team Building

Further Readings

Dzewaltowski, D. A., Estabrooks, P. A., Welk, G., Hill, J., Milliken, G., Karteroliotis, K., et al. (2009). Healthy youth places: A randomized controlled trial to determine the effectiveness of facilitating adult and youth leaders to promote physical activity and fruit and vegetable consumption in middle schools. *Health Education & Behavior, 36*(3), 583–600.

Estabrooks, P. A., & Glasgow, R. E. (2006). Translating effective clinic-based physical activity interventions into practice. *American Journal of Preventive Medicine, 31*(Suppl. 4), S45–S56.

Green, B. B., Cheadle, A., Pellegrini, A. S., & Harris, J. R. (2007). Active for life: A work-based physical activity program. *Preventing Chronic Disease, 4*(3), A63.

O'Donnell, M. P. (2009). Definition of health promotion 2.0: Embracing passion, enhancing motivation, recognizing dynamic balance, and creating opportunities. *American Journal of Health Promotion, 24*(1), iv.

Winett, R. A., Anderson, E. S., Wojcik, J. R., Winett, S. G., & Bowden, T. (2007). Guide to health: Nutrition and physical activity outcomes of a group-randomized trial of an Internet-based intervention in churches. *Annals of Behavioral Medicine, 33*(3), 251–261.

Hedonic Theory

Hedonic theory, or theory of psychological hedonism, is the idea that human behavior is motivated by the pursuit of pleasure and the avoidance of *pain* (or, more accurately, displeasure). Its origins can be traced to the beginnings of Western philosophy. Although its prominence within psychology waned during the 20th century, updated versions of hedonic theory have emerged in behavioral economics and neurology. As researchers in exercise psychology have begun searching for postcognitivist explanations for variations in exercise behavior, hedonic theory has attracted attention as a perspective of considerable potential value.

History

Early expressions of hedonism can be found in Aristippus (435–366 BCE) and Epicurus (341–270 BCE), both of whom considered pleasure as the ultimate good. Aristippus emphasized physical pleasures, whereas the Epicureans promoted a holistic view of pleasure that included serenity, a sense of belonging, and overall well-being. Holistic views of pleasure were also promoted by Plato (428–348 BCE), who believed in the balance of the rational, emotional, and appetitive parts of the soul, and Aristotle (384–322 BCE), who coined the term *eudaimonia* to signify the pleasure derived from a virtuous and fulfilling life.

Hedonism reemerged during the Renaissance, with thinkers struggling to align hedonistic ideas with the stern doctrine of the Church. Erasmus (1466–1536) and Thomas More (1478–1535) argued that the pursuit of pleasure is consistent with religion. René Descartes (1596–1650) accepted that passions, including pleasures, influence human behavior but maintained that the mind must control these passions in its pursuit of higher ideals.

In Britain, hedonism was at the core of debates on the appropriate goal of societies and political systems. Thomas Hobbes (1588–1679) and David Hume (1711–1776) accepted that humans are motivated to pursue pleasure and avoid pain. Hume further claimed that reason, which previous thinkers from Plato to Descartes considered capable of keeping passions under control, is powerless. French philosophers La Mettrie (1709–1751) and Helvétius (1715–1771) also endorsed hedonism, arguing that pursuing pleasure and avoiding pain are and should be the primary human motives.

Hedonistic ideas gained wide exposure in utilitarianism, a movement pioneered by Jeremy Bentham (1748–1832) and continued by James Mill (1773–1836) and his son John Stuart Mill (1806–1873). Utilitarianism was an ethical philosophy, according to which the goal should be the maximization of *utility*. In Bentham's hedonic calculus, the utility (usefulness) of each action is computed as the algebraic sum of the pleasure to be obtained minus the pain to be caused. The *fundamental axiom* of utilitarianism was that "the greatest happiness of the greatest number . . . is the measure of right and wrong." In the opening lines of his book *Introduction to the Principles of Morals and Legislation*, Bentham famously wrote that "nature has placed mankind under the governance of two sovereign masters, pain and pleasure; it is for them alone to point out what we ought to do, as well as to determine what we shall do."

The utilitarian pursuit of pleasure was criticized for encouraging unprincipled self-interest and a disregard for costs to others. Critics argued that this emphasis on pleasure abolished any distinction between humans and animals, characterizing hedonism a doctrine "worthy only of swine." This attack prompted John Stuart Mill to revise Bentham's earlier undifferentiated view of pleasure by distinguishing between *lower* and *higher* forms (e.g., education, art), the latter being of higher utility.

The ideas of the utilitarians greatly influenced the psychologists of the 19th and early 20th century. Herbert Spencer (1820–1903) emphasized the evolutionary advantage of hedonism, insisting that the only type of behavior that is conducive to life is the behavior that ensures a surplus of pleasure over pain. This evolutionary advantage was also highlighted by Alexander Bain (1818–1903), William James (1842–1910), and William McDougall (1871–1938). Their opinions diverged on the question of whether the pursuit of pleasure and the avoidance of pain are the only (the ultimate) human motives, with Bain supporting and James and McDougall rejecting this notion. The writings of Bentham also influenced Sigmund Freud's (1856–1939) *pleasure principle*.

Fragments of hedonic theory can even be found during behaviorism and cognitivism, periods during which psychology largely ignored subjective states, such as pleasure, focusing instead on overt behavior and cognitive appraisals, respectively. According to Edward L. Thorndike's (1874–1949) law of effect, when a behavior is paired with pleasure, it becomes more likely to be repeated, whereas, if it is paired with displeasure, it becomes more likely to be avoided. Similarly, for Albert Bandura (1925–), pleasant and unpleasant emotional states can have an influence on behavior, albeit not directly but rather by influencing self-efficacy.

Contemporary Iterations

References to hedonic theory in contemporary psychology are rare because, in the prevailing view, behavior and decision making are driven by the rational cognitive analysis of information. Among the exceptions have been emotion theorist Silvan Tomkins (1911–1991) and his students, who have considered affects, including pleasure and displeasure, as the prime human motives. Revivals of psychological hedonism have come mainly from disciplines outside of psychology proper. In behavioral economics, Nobel laureate Daniel Kahneman proposed that, because human rationality and cognitive ability are limited compared to the complexity of the problems that humans face, decision making is aided by *heuristics,* including the *affect heuristic,* that is, people do what makes them feel better and avoid what makes them feel worse.

In neurology, Antonio Damasio, working with patients with focal brain lesions, showed that when areas involved in affective processing are damaged, one may be able to list the pros and cons of various behavioral options but has difficulty making decisions. According to Damasio, different behavioral options are associated with pleasant or unpleasant configurations of bodily state, called *somatic markers,* which influence the decision-making process.

Application in Exercise Psychology

Prompted by the limited variance in exercise behavior explained by cognitive variables, researchers have begun exploring the potential of hedonic theory. Data show that exercise enjoyment (which partly reflects pleasure from exercise), affective associations (pairing the idea of exercise with positive or negative descriptors), and ratings of pleasure–displeasure obtained during exercise are significant correlates and predictors of exercise behavior.

Panteleimon Ekkekakis

See also Affect; Affective Responses to Exercise; Enjoyment, as Mediator of Exercise Behavior Change; Pleasure

Further Readings

Damasio, A. R. (1994). *Descartes' error: Emotion, reason, and the human brain.* New York: Putnam.

Ekkekakis, P., & Dafermos, M. (2012). Exercise is a many-splendored thing but for some it does not feel so splendid: Staging a resurgence of hedonistic ideas in the quest to understand exercise behavior. In E. O. Acevedo (Ed.), *The Oxford handbook of exercise psychology* (pp. 295–333). New York: Oxford University Press.

Kahneman, D. (1999). Objective happiness. In D. Kahneman, E. Diener, & N. Schwarz (Eds.), *Well-being: The foundations of hedonic psychology* (pp. 3–25). New York: Russell Sage Foundation.

Mees, U., & Schmitt, A. (2008). Goals of action and emotional reasons for action: A modern version of the theory of ultimate psychological hedonism. *Journal for the Theory of Social Behaviour, 38,* 157–178.

Slovic, P., Finucane, M. L., Peters, E., & MacGregor, D. G. (2002). The affect heuristic. In T. Gilovich, D. W. Griffin, & D. Kahneman (Eds.), *Heuristics and biases: The psychology of intuitive judgment* (pp. 397–420). New York: Cambridge University Press.

HETEROSEXISM, HOMONEGATIVISM, AND TRANSPREJUDICE

Heterosexism, homonegativism, and transprejudice are prejudices aimed at lesbian, gay, bisexual, or transgender (LGBT) people. These beliefs and actions are common in sport and negatively impact all participants, regardless of their sexual orientation or gender identity. This entry discusses common types of prejudices faced by LGBT sport participants, defines related terminology, and notes the effects of biased sport climates.

Heterosexism is a belief system in which it is assumed or expected that all people are heterosexual. In a heterosexist environment, heterosexuality is viewed as the natural or normal sexual orientation. This belief creates the assumption that people are inherently *straight* (heterosexual), and that those individuals who do not meet this expectation are deviant. As a result, nonheterosexuality is considered strange or abnormal. Heterosexism forms a climate where heterosexuality is privileged or rewarded with high social status and respect not readily granted to nonheterosexuals.

In sport, heterosexism is common. The prevailing silence about the existence of LGBT athletes or coaches renders them invisible. For example, heterosexual privilege is provided when locker rooms are divided by sex. This separation is based on the assumption that through creating all-male and all-female spaces, all sexual innuendos, harassment, or relationships among teammates will be prevented since everyone is expected to be heterosexual. That people in sport tend to only imagine and recognize male athletes as having girlfriends or wives and female athletes solely in relationships with males shows how extensive heterosexism is. Nonheterosexuals participating in heterosexist sport climates may feel excluded from or invisible to their teammates, coaches, or other sport personnel. Heterosexism provides the foundation for climates perceived as unwelcoming for LGBT sport participants.

Homonegativism refers to purposeful negative stereotypes, prejudice, and discrimination toward nonheterosexuals, whereas *homophobia* is an irrational fear of LGBT people. Unlike homophobia, the term *homonegativism* signifies that the bias against nonheterosexuals often is rooted in personal belief systems and maintains social and political functions. Therefore, the term *homonegativism* more accurately addresses the social issues embedded in the discrimination that takes place in sport and connects it to other "isms" in sport (e.g., sexism, racism). Examples of homonegativism in sport include name calling, stereotyping athletes, physical violence, bullying, and benching or cutting LGBT athletes from teams. Additionally, coaches may be fired or overlooked for jobs if they are perceived as LGBT.

Often such negative treatment is based on stereotypes equating masculinity in females with being lesbian and femininity in males with being gay. The application of these stereotypes has serious implications, including causing some people to avoid or quit sport. LGBT athletes and coaches in heterosexist or homonegative sport settings often experience high levels of stress and monitor themselves to conceal their sexual identity. Other consequences of homonegativism in sport include a decline in self-confidence, increased anxiety, difficulty focusing, dejection, and decreased athletic performance.

Heterosexism and homonegativism can only continue to function as long as the gender binary exists in sport. This binary acknowledges only two categories: *male/masculine* and *female/feminine*. These categories are considered distinct and opposite of one another. This sorting system appears throughout sport. For example, youth sport leagues are divided by gender and some sport uniforms and rules change based on the gender of the participant. Boys are often demeaned through phrases like "You throw like a girl," which further suggests that boys should throw differently (and better) than girls. Through sport, boys and girls learn how to speak and behave appropriately in relation to their gender. Those who do not conform to these heterosexist rules may encounter homonegative treatment.

One's gender identity refers to the internal sense of one being a girl or boy, woman or man. For many individuals, gender identity aligns with their outward appearance. However, some people have an identity that is outside of the female–male binary. For transgender individuals, gender identity is not consistent with their biological sex (anatomy), is fluid (changeable), or is perceived as something other than male or female. Intersex individuals are born with anatomical, hormonal, or genetic characteristics of both female and male bodies. Transsexual people intend to undergo or have completed hormone therapy or sex reassignment surgery so gender identity and sex are compatible. They go through a transition period in which they begin hormone therapy to make physical changes to their body while they live full-time consistent with their gender identity. During this time, their physical body is not consistent with binary gender conforming bodies. After surgery, and with sustained hormone therapy, transsexual athletes can compete in the gender category consistent with their reassigned sex. All of these *trans* people challenge the gender binary because, instead of following the belief that one is born into a prestructured gender classification system, these individuals move across the boundaries. Yet, there is no place for trans people in a heterosexist sport environment and they often face transprejudice (bias based on gender identity, also called *transphobia*). Most sport policies do not include trans and transitioning individuals.

Though the negative effects of heterosexism, homonegativism, and transprejudice persist, they do not describe all sport settings. Some organizations are working to create more inclusive sport climates that do not privilege one particular sexual orientation or gender identity. Many coaches also are working diligently to provide inclusive environments that allow all of their athletes to be successful in and out of the playing arena. More LGBT sportspeople are coming out, or letting others know of their nonconforming sexual orientation or gender identity than in previous decades. That more people are feeling comfortable to do so suggests that, at least in some contexts, the climate of sport is becoming more open and welcoming to diverse people.

Vikki Krane and Mallory Mann

See also Cultural Competence; Diversity; Gender; Multiculturalism

Further Readings

Canadian Association for the Advancement of Women and Sport and Physical Activity. *Seeing the invisible, speaking the unspoken: Addressing homophobia in sport.* Retrieved from http://www.caaws-homophobiainsport.ca/e/index.cfm

Gay, Lesbian, & Straight Education Network. (2012). *Changing the game: The GLSEN sports project.* Available from http://sports.glsen.org

Griffin, P., & Carroll, H. J. (2010). *On the team: Equal opportunity for transgender student athletes.* Retrieved from http://www.nclrights.org/site/DocServer/TransgenderStudentAthleteReport.pdf?docID=7901

HIERARCHICAL SELF

Researchers and practitioners have long believed that how people feel about and describe themselves can strongly influence motivated behavior in sport and exercise. Two key constructs studied in the sport and exercise psychology literature are self-esteem and self-concept. Since many people have argued that judgments about the self will influence the selection and maintenance of physical activity behavior, it is critical to distinguish between self-concept and self-esteem. *Self-esteem* or self-worth refers to how a person feels about oneself. It is a self-evaluation that provides a sense of how an individual assesses worth. *Self-concept* refers to self-perceptions of personal attributes such as skills, abilities, and physical characteristics.

Historically, researchers studied both self-esteem and self-concept from a very broad global perspective. Modern work, however, recognizes that self-esteem, and especially self-concept, is best viewed from a multidimensional and hierarchical perspective. Starting with the work of Richard J. Shavelson and colleagues in the 1970s, self-concept has been conceptualized as a multifaceted hierarchy consisting of the global self at the top, with specific domains (e.g. academic, social, and physical) and subdomains nested underneath. For example, one important domain of global self is the physical self, which can be further divided into several subdomains, such as flexibility, endurance or conditioning, sport skills, strength, and appearance. Each subdomain can be further differentiated into more discrete components. For example, physical flexibility can be further separated into facets such as leg flexibility, back flexibility, hip flexibility, and shoulder flexibility. Typically, subdomains of physical self-concept have moderate to strong interrelationships. Aspects of the physical self, especially body appearance, demonstrate moderate correlations with perceptions of global self across the life span.

Although there is strong support for the multidimensional view of self-concept, support for the hierarchical perspective is less compelling. Work by Herb Marsh and others has found that relationships among some specific domains or subdomains are low or non-existent. Furthermore, global self-concept also has low correlations with specific self-concept domains or subdomains. A hierarchical model also implies either a top-down or bottom-up direction of causal flow. The bottom-up approach proposes that situation-specific and task-oriented experiences influence perceptions in specific subdomains, which in turn will influence domain specific self-concept and overall global self-concept. Researchers conducting interventions using this model would target a specific facet of physical self (e.g. leg strength) and would expect changes in the facet to effect perceptions of a specific physical subdomain (e.g. physical strength). Changes in the specific physical subdomain would then result in expected changes to global physical self, which would effect change in global self-concept.

The top-down model hypothesizes that changes in global self-esteem will influence lower order domains (e.g. physical self), which will impact specific subdomains and in turn would influence specific physical activity behaviors. Therefore, top-down interventions target global self-esteem as it is assumed that individuals with higher self-esteem would be more confident to engage in physical activity behaviors regardless of experience and perceived competence in that domain. A top-down model implies that changes in global self-concept (or self-esteem) should cause changes in lower order domains and influence subsequent situation specific experiences. Unfortunately, longitudinal and experimental research has found little evidence of either top-down or bottom-up causal flow between the domain level and global level.

Measurement of Hierarchical Self

Investigating the causal relationship between self-esteem, self-concept, and physical activity behaviors has been greatly enhanced by multidimensional models and subsequent measurement instruments. Many instruments have been developed, evaluated, and modified for various populations and age groups. Within sport and exercise research, there are a few instruments that have consistently demonstrated strong measurement properties. Susan Harter and colleagues developed the Self-Perceptions Profiles for various age groups. These instruments were based on hierarchical models with global self-esteem and various domains (e.g., social, athletic, appearance) depending on the age group. Separate work by Kenneth Fox and Herb Marsh sought to capture the physical self in more detail. Kenneth R. Fox and Charles B. Corbin developed the Physical Self-Perception Profile, which consists of four subdomains of physical self-concept and one global domain of physical self-worth. The subdomains include sport competence, attractive body, physical strength, and physical conditioning. Marsh and colleagues developed the Physical Self-Description Questionnaire, which specifies physical self-concept as nine unique physical self-dimensions (strength, body fat, activity, endurance or fitness, sports competence, coordination, health, appearance, and flexibility) nested under general physical self-concept and global self-esteem. Marsh and colleagues also developed the Elite Athlete Self-Description Questionnaire to assess physical self-concept in elite athletes using six different dimensions. Elite athlete self-concept dimensions include skill, body, aerobic fitness, anaerobic fitness, mental competence, and overall performance.

Self-Esteem, Self-Concept, and Physical Activity Behavior

Researchers in sport and exercise psychology recognize the importance of self-esteem and self-concept as not only significant mental health outcomes, but also as potential determinants of physical activity behavior. There is solid evidence, in both youth and adults, that physical activity behavior is correlated with aspects of physical self-concept and sometimes with global self-concept and self-esteem. For example, many researchers have found that conditioning and endurance self-perceptions predict objective physical fitness and physical activity levels. Similarly, self-perceptions of body fat or physical appearance self-concept predict objective measures of body mass index or body composition. Physical self-concept measures are far superior compared to global self-concept or self-esteem measures in predicting physical activity behaviors. However, self-perceptions of body appearance and body fat are often unrelated to physical activity behaviors.

Many physical activity intervention studies in children, youth, and adult populations have primarily focused on global self-esteem or self-concept and physical activity. In studies with children and youth, the majority of these studies have found a modest short-term significant intervention effect. However, many of these studies have been criticized for being poor quality. In adults, John Spence, Kerry McGannon, and Pauline Poon conducted a meta-analysis of over 100 exercise intervention studies and reported that exercise intervention seemed to have a small but significant effect on either global self-concept or self-esteem. Overall, researchers suggest that physical activity interventions can produce small changes in global self. However, there is little consistent evidence about the characteristics of the physical activity intervention (intensity, duration, types) required to produce changes.

Physical activity intervention research targeting changes in the various levels of the hierarchical self is more limited. In one review of intervention studies in various populations, Kenneth Fox concluded that physical activity conferred significant improvements in some components of the physical self. Typically, the intervention effect was stronger for physical self-perceptions compared to global measures. More recent work in adults suggested that interventions have a stronger impact on physical self-concept compared to global self.

Based on a mix of findings, researchers seem to suggest that physical activity can cause changes in both global and physical self. Intervention studies often indicate a bottom up model in that physical activity will cause a change in self-concept or self-esteem. However, recent work by Herbert W. Marsh and Rhonda G. Craven and Marsh and other colleagues strongly suggests there is a reciprocal relationship between achievement behaviors and domain level self-concept. Using longitudinal designs and complex modeling, they found that self-concept and physical activity are both a cause and effect for each other. The reciprocal model suggests that previous physical activity behavior would influence physical self-concept, which would in turn impact physical activity behavior even after controlling for previous physical activity behavior. This reciprocal effect was found in several studies using various physical activity contexts, such as elite swimming, physical education, and extracurricular activities. The work of Marsh and colleagues in various populations and achievement domains indicates that the reciprocal effect occurs primarily at the domain level. The use of the reciprocal model has implications for research and applied practice. For instance, it implies that interventions should be targeted at both the self-concept level and at specific physical skills or perceptions related to the targeted domain. Also, the level at which self-concept is measured needs to be considered, as reciprocal effects are stronger when the domain in self-concept is congruent with the achievement domain.

Gender and Cultural Differences

Researchers have consistently found that males have more positive global and physical self-perceptions than females in both youth and adults, although there are large variations within each gender. This parallels the findings in the physical activity literature. However, there is no consistent evidence of the relationship between self-concept and physical activity behaviors being different across genders. Some researchers have argued that gender stereotypes, cultural beliefs, and the dominance of traditional boys' sports in school systems and community organizations results in sports being more highly valued for males and thus more prominent in the development of their self-concept and self-esteem. There is, however, no reliable evidence that physical activity interventions are more effective in enhancing self-perceptions for either females or males.

Understanding cultural differences in the global and physical self-concept is challenging. Most studies comparing samples from various countries show similar results in terms of physical self-concepts being meaningfully related to physical activity behaviors and there is strong evidence that males have more positive self-perceptions across groups. However, most studies compared nationality (e.g., Turkey vs. United Kingdom) rather than assessing cultural values, such as filial piety, familism, collectivism, fatalism, and machismo. Overall, there are few quality longitudinal or intervention studies in this area to make any definitive statements.

Conclusion

Self-esteem and self-concept are best understood from a multidimensional perspective. Physical self-concept is an important dimension in understanding motivated behavior in sport and exercise

settings. Males tend to have more positive perceptions of physical self as well as higher levels of physical activity behaviors. Physical activity interventions have a stronger impact on enhancing the physical self-concept compared to the global self. There is growing evidence, however, that there is a reciprocal effect between physical self-concept and physical activity behavior over time. Cultural differences are not well-understood.

Peter R. E. Crocker and Carolyn McEwen

See also Body Self-Esteem; Self-Appraisal/Assessment/ Perception; Self-Awareness

Further Readings

Crocker, P. R. E., Kowalski, K., & Hadd, V. (2008). The role of self and identity in physical (in)activity. In A. Smith & S. J. Biddle (Eds.), *Youth physical activity and inactivity: Challenges and solutions* (pp. 215–237). Champaign, IL: Human Kinetics.

Fox, K. R. (Ed.). (1997). *The physical self: From motivation to well-being.* Champaign, IL: Human Kinetics.

Fox, K. R. (2000). The effects of exercise on self-perceptions and self-esteem. In S. J. H. Biddle, K. R. Fox, & S. H. Boutcher (Eds.), *Physical activity and psychological well-being* (pp. 88–117). London: Routledge.

Marsh, H. W., & Craven, R. G. (2006). Reciprocal effects of self-concept and performance from a multidimensional perspective: Beyond seductive pleasure and unidimensional perspectives. *Perspectives on Psychological Science, 1,* 133–162.

Spence, J. C., McGannon, K. R., & Poon, P. (2005). The effects of exercise on global self-esteem: A quantitative review. *Journal of Sport & Exercise Psychology, 27,* 311–334.

History of Exercise Psychology

The history of exercise psychology is closely intertwined with the history of sport psychology. Although discussed in separate entries in this encyclopedia, the history of sport and exercise psychology can be considered as one history, with some differing paths and forks, but continual connections. That history has roots going back into classical times, as reflected in the classical ideal of *mens sana in corpore sano* (a sound mind in a healthy body), highlighting the mind-body connection, which is the essence of sport and exercise psychology. Hippocrates, widely acknowledged as the father of Western medicine, clearly connected mind and body in citing the role of exercise in health. As Janet Buckworth, Rod Dishman, Patrick O'Connor, and Phillip Tomporowski note in their 2013 exercise psychology text, the major religions emphasized healthy lifestyles in the early writings. In the Hebrew Bible, one can find, "She girdeth her loins with strength and strengthened her arms," and 12th-century Jewish philosopher Maimonides cautioned that anyone who leads a sedentary life and does not exercise will have painful days.

We can find research on physical activity and health in the early physical education and psychology work, but as an identifiable academic area, sport and exercise psychology is relatively young, emerging as a subdiscipline within physical education in the 1960s. Sport psychology emerged in the 1970s, and exercise psychology began to develop in the 1980s. Still, from the classical times, through the early roots around 100 years ago, through the development over the last 50 years, to today's expansive academic discipline, sport psychology and exercise psychology have always been connected. This entry focuses on the history of the *exercise* psychology side of the disciplinary area that might better be termed *psychology of physical activity*.

W. Jack Rejeski and Lawrence R. Brawley were first to formally define and delimit exercise psychology in 1988 as "the application of the educational, scientific, and professional contributions of psychology to the promotion, explanation, maintenance, and enhancement of behaviors related to physical work capacity." A few years later, Rejeski and A. Thompson suggested a slightly broader scope by substituting *physical fitness* for physical work capacity. Today, most scholars who might adopt the exercise psychology label would take an even broader approach and substitute *health-related physical activity*. As the following historical review suggests, health-related physical activity could well describe the emphasis in the early roots stage of sport and exercise psychology 100 years ago. As the discipline developed, sport psychology narrowed to focus on competitive sport performance, and subsequently, exercise psychology split off to connect with exercise science and focus on physical fitness. It should be noted that the sport psychology–exercise psychology separation is a North American development. International sport psychology has maintained the sport psychology title but gradually incorporated more exercise and fitness topics since the 1980s. With more recent rapid growth and expansion of research and practice, the sport psychology–exercise psychology categorization does not capture the rich diversity of topics, populations, outcomes, contexts, perspectives, and approaches within the psychology of physical activity today.

Early Roots: Late 1800s to Early 20th Century

Psychology and kinesiology (then physical education) both began to organize as academic disciplines over 100 years ago, and that early work includes evidence of the psychology of physical activity. Scholars who have described the history of sport and exercise psychology have noted the words of G. Stanley Hall, founding president of the American Psychological Association, who clearly connected physical activity with psychology in his 1908 statement in the *Proceedings of the National Education Association* that physical education makes "the intellect, feelings and will more vigorous, sane, supple and resourceful" (p. 1015). Similarly in 1899, William James wrote about the importance of the "well-trained and vigorous body" for a "well-trained and vigorous mind" and explicitly highlighted the importance for men and women alike. Hall's and James's statements portend some current exercise psychology topics, such as the role of exercise in mental health, and influence of exercise on cognitive performance.

Many sport and exercise psychology texts cite Norman Triplett's 1898 study of social influence and performance as a widely recognized early contribution. Triplett observed that cyclists seemed motivated to perform better with social influence (pacing machine, competition), and devised an experiment to test his ideas. Other early scholars from both psychology and physical education espoused psychological benefits of physical education and conducted isolated studies, including George W. Fitz of Harvard, who conducted experiments on the speed and accuracy of motor responses in the late 1800s.

Sport and Exercise Psychology: 1920s–1940s

The pioneering sport psychology work of the 1920s to the 1940s is discussed in more detail in the entry

"History of Sport Psychology." Coleman Griffith was a prolific researcher who established a lab at the University of Illinois and published widely. Although Griffith's applied work with athletes is most often cited, he actually was more concerned with developing the research and knowledge base. In his 1930 article, "A Lab for Research on Athletics," he noted the abundance of anecdotal reports and explicitly called for a more scientific and experimental approach to psychological issues such as skill acquisition and the effects of emotions on performance. Griffith clearly connected sport and exercise. He closed the 1930 article with a list of 25 specific topics that might be investigated in his lab. Notably, that list included several topics that we might now call *exercise psychology*, although Griffith clearly did not make that distinction. The first topic listed was the relation between physical exercise and learning, and the list included effect of exercise on length of life and resistance to disease, the nature of sleep among athletes, photographic analysis of muscle coordination during fear, sex differences in motor skill tests, and effects of nicotine and other toxins on learning—to name just a few. Not only did Griffith merge topics that many today separate into sport and exercise, he included motor skills, coordination, and development and covered a range of topics that fit into the psychology of physical activity.

Around the same time that Griffith was working in the United States, Robert Werner Schulte in Germany and Avksenty Cezarevich Puni in Russia were developing sport psychology labs and active research programs. Although both clearly identified their pioneering work as sport psychology, like Griffith, their research often included topics such as exercise and memory that could be considered exercise psychology.

C. H. McCloy, one of the early scholars bringing research and a scientific perspective to physical education during Griffith's time, explicitly called for an end to debates on *of* the physical versus *through* the physical, which reflect the old mind–body dualism. According to McCloy, mind and body cannot be separated. As McCloy understood, mind and body are connected, *of* and *through* the physical are connected, and sport and exercise are connected. The dualism of sport psychology versus exercise psychology is artificial and inaccurate. The full range of physical activities and related issues, including positive health, youth development, life skills, quality of life, and lifestyle physical activity, belong in psychology of physical activity. In his own pioneering research, McCloy investigated character building through physical education as well as his many studies of motor skills and development, topics that fall within a psychology of physical activity.

From Griffith's and McCloy's time through the late 1960s when an identifiable specialization emerged, sustained programs were non-existent. After World War II, several scholars developed research programs in motor behavior that incorporated sport and exercise psychology topics, but research was sporadic.

Emergence of Sport and Exercise Psychology as an Academic Discipline: 1950s–1970s

Despite the innovative work during the first half of the 20th century, sport and exercise psychology did not emerge as an identifiable field until the late 1960s, when several individuals, typically in physical education departments, developed research programs, graduate courses, and eventually, specialized organizations and publications. Notably, these emerging programs and scholars were housed in physical education (now kinesiology).

The International Society of Sport Psychology (ISSP) formed and held the first International Congress of Sport Psychology in Rome in 1965. The ISSP, and international sport psychology, was more closely connected to applied psychology and performance enhancement than in North America, but exercise psychology can be found even in the early development stages. For example, the proceedings of the second ISSP congress in 1968 include several papers on *emotional health*, and another large section of papers on *the child and physical activity*. Specific papers included "Physical Activity Attitudes of Middle-Aged Males" by Dorothy V. Harris, and "Drug Therapy and Physical Performance in Emotionally Disturbed Children" by William P. Morgan, as well as several papers on motor behavior that do not clearly fall into sport or exercise psychology but fit within psychology of physical activity. The inclusion of exercise and physical activity, as well as motor behavior, is not unusual, and around the world, sport psychology is typically understood as including all forms of sport, exercise, and physical activity.

As international sport psychology was organizing, North American scholars also began to organize, and the North American Society for the Psychology of Sport and Physical Activity (NASPSPA) was officially incorporated in 1967. The organization of NASPSPA reflected the overlapping of sport and exercise psychology and motor behavior in the 1960s and 1970s, with subareas of motor learning, motor development, and social psychology of physical activity (now the sport and exercise psychology area).

As graduate programs and organizations developed, research expanded and sport and exercise psychologists developed specialized publications. The *International Journal of Sport Psychology* began publishing in 1970. The *Journal of Sport Psychology* (JSP) appeared in 1979 (*Journal of Sport & Exercise Psychology,* since 1988) and was immediately recognized, as it is today, as the leading publication outlet for sport and exercise psychology research.

Development of Sport Psychology and Exercise Psychology: 1980s–2000

From the 1970s through the 1990s, sport and exercise psychology gradually became the largest and most diverse of the three areas within NASPSPA. Rainer Martens's 1975 text, *Social Psychology and Physical Activity,* reflects the content and orientation of those early years. Major psychological theories framed the content; most supporting research was from psychology; and the sport psychology work cited seldom involved *sport* (or exercise), but more often involved laboratory experiments with motor tasks. Martens also clearly described physical activity as an inclusive term, not limited to competitive sport, but encompassing varied forms of movement in a wide range of settings.

Separation of Sport Psychology and Exercise Psychology

Sport and exercise psychology from 1975 to 2000 was characterized by *narrowing* and *separating.* As noted, in North America the field began as social psychology and physical activity. Soon, the academic focus shifted, and in the 1970s and 1980s, the field became more sport specific. Sport psychology (exercise was not part of the label or the scope) began to narrow its focus and shifted away from social influence toward psychology of the individual. Before 1980, application largely meant physical education; but with the 1980s, it came to imply psychological skills training with elite competitive athletes. Following a NASPSPA vote to include only research presentations at the conference, a group split off to form a new organization focused on *applied sport psychology.* October 1985 marked the beginning of the Association for the Advancement of Applied Sport Psychology, shortened to the Association for Applied Sport Psychology (AASP) in 2006. As summarized in the first issue of the *AAASP Newsletter* in 1986, "AAASP provides a forum for individuals interested in research, theory development, and application of psychological principles in sport and exercise." From the beginning, however, AASP meetings and publications have been dominated by the focus on competitive sport with little attention to exercise or physical activity. Meanwhile, NASPSPA maintained its research focus, including research on exercise and physical activity.

International sport psychology, reflected in ISSP and the European Federation of Sport Psychology (FEPSAC) which was formed in 1969, began with an emphasis on sport and competitive athletes, and thus did not experience such a dramatic narrowing and separation. Instead, international sport psychology maintained its emphasis on sport and continued to develop applied programs for athletes, often within psychology.

Emergence of Exercise Psychology

Just as some scholars chose to split off to focus on applied sport psychology, others (a smaller number) shifted to align more closely with exercise science and focus on psychology of exercise and fitness. Several exercise psychology sources refer to the fitness craze of the 1970s and 1980s as a key factor in the growing interest in exercise psychology. Activities such as aerobics, jogging, and weight training gained more popularity, and the fitness industry grew to meet that interest. NASPSPA and the *JSP* concentrated on strong research and maintained connections with exercise and motor behavior. In 1988, *JSP* added exercise to the title, becoming the *Journal of Sport & Exercise Psychology,* and more explicitly sought research on health-oriented exercise as well as sport.

The American Psychological Association (APA) organized an interest group, and in 1986, Division 47—on Exercise and Sport Psychology—became a formal division of APA. Although many in APA were interested in applying psychology in competitive sport, it is notable that the group highlighted *exercise* in the division name. William P. Morgan, a key leader in the emerging exercise psychology research was the first president of Division 47.

Morgan, who spent most of his career at Wisconsin, might well be considered the father of exercise psychology. Certainly Morgan and his many students, particularly Rod Dishman, conducted much of the early research in the 1980s and 1990s and set the standard for continuing exercise psychology research. Like Morgan, most exercise psychology researchers were aligned with kinesiology programs, often collaborated with exercise physiology researchers, and adopted similar research approaches. For example, studies might investigate the influence of type, duration, and intensity of exercise on psychological outcomes such as mood state. On the other side of the exercise–psychology relationship, the role of psychological factors in exercise adherence was an early exercise psychology topic. That early research was connected with the medical model that dominated exercise science at the time. As exercise psychology research expanded, scholars brought in more psychological theories and turned to the *biopsychosocial* model that dominates health behavior research. However, the social aspect was largely ignored at that time, and remains understudied today.

Psychology of Physical Activity in the 21st Century

The psychology of physical activity continued to expand rapidly though the 1990s and into the 21st century, and in many ways became more diverse, for example, including exercisers as well as athletes and a larger settings and psychological perspectives. However, rather than encompassing diverse participants, settings, and issues, sport and exercise psychology researchers, organizations, and programs split into separate, and often intentionally separated, subareas with little connection to each other. Moreover, the separate factions tended to be elite with little connection to the traditional physical education base or wider physical activity contexts. The sport psychology faction focused on elite athletes. Meanwhile, the exercise psychology faction moved to exercise physiology labs with a focus on young, fit exercisers.

The editor who initiated the name change to *Journal of Sport & Exercise Psychology,* Diane

Gill, also coauthor of this entry, fully supports the exercise psychology movement but firmly believes the sport psychology–exercise psychology split is artificial and destructive. *Psychology of physical activity* is more encompassing and more appropriate for this area. Stuart Biddle and Reinhard Fuchs clearly took a psychology of physical activity approach despite the title of their 2009 chapter, "Exercise Psychology: A View From Europe." After describing the expansion from sport to sport and exercise psychology in the 1980s, and citing the early definition of *exercise psychology* as referring to "behaviors related to physical work capacity," they clearly defined the scope and major issues in the field as psychology of physical activity. They referred to physical activity throughout their excellent article, and the few times they cited exercise psychology, the term was in quotes.

Again, the separation of sport and exercise is not so dramatic at the international level. Rather than develop a separate exercise psychology, international sport psychology has gradually incorporated more research and issues related to exercise and physical activity, particularly in the 21st century. Notably, ISSP, the first and still dominant international organization, changed its official journal to the *International Journal of Sport and Exercise Psychology* in 2002 explicitly recognizing the expansion of sport psychology into the psychology of exercise and physical activity and health issues. As Gershon Tenenbaum and Dieter Hackfort (2003) noted in their opening editorial statement,

> The *IJSEP* encourages researchers and practitioners from all the sub-disciplines of sport and exercise psychology to share their contributions and views through this outlet. It is through integration of the specific knowledge gained by scholars in different fields, and through sharing of different views that our domain will benefit. (p. 8)

Similarly, the European FEPSAC and newer (1989) Asian South Pacific Association of Sport Psychology have maintained the sport psychology title but increasingly incorporated exercise, physical activity, health research, and programs.

Today, the psychology of physical activity has matured and moved in many directions. Despite the multiple facets and factions in the 21st century, there are promising directions and many connections. During the 1980s and 1990s, attention shifted to competitive *sport* and applied work with athletes. Attention has now shifted back to *exercise,* meeting the public concern for health and fitness with increased research and applied emphasis on physical activity and health promotion. Both sport psychology and exercise psychology have moved toward a broader psychology of physical activity. *Sport psychologists* investigate mental health and eating behaviors of participants, stress and injury, and adherence to rehabilitation exercise as well as sport performance. *Exercise psychologists* have expanded beyond fitness training to consider the relationship of physical activity to quality of life among older adults and clinical populations and the role of reducing sedentary behavior in health. Some researchers focus on exercise parameters and adopt methodologies of exercise science. Others adopt public health models and approaches with a wide range of target populations to investigate lifestyle physical activity and psychological outcomes ranging from cognitive performance to quality of life. In many ways, we have returned to the mind–body connection, albeit with a wider range of measures, models, and methods. Traces of our roots and development are evident, but today's psychology of physical activity is multifaceted and diverse in research and practice and truly global.

Conclusion

The history of exercise psychology is inextricably intertwined with the history of sport psychology and best understood within a broader psychology of physical activity perspective. Although relatively young as an identifiable area, we can trace our roots back over 100 years with early connections between psychology and physical education. Sport and exercise psychology emerged in the late 1960's and expanded rapidly during the 1970s, creating a knowledge base and specialized publications. During the 1980s, with sport psychology narrowly focusing on applied research and competitive sport, some scholars turned attention to the relationship between exercise and psychological factors. Exercise psychology has continued to grow and expand into new populations and contexts, and today is more appropriately considered as the psychology of physical activity. Today's global psychology of physical activity is multifaceted and diverse in research and practice, while continuing to address mind–body connections and the role of physical activity in health and well-being.

Diane L. Gill and Erin J. Reifsteck

See also Adherence; Affective Responses to Exercise; History of Sport Psychology

Further Readings

Biddle, S. J. H., & Fuchs, R. (2009). Exercise psychology: A view from Europe. *Psychology of Sport and Exercise, 10,* 410–419.

Buckworth, J., Dishman, R. K., O'Connor, P. J., & Tomporowski, P. D. (2013). *Exercise psychology* (2nd ed.). Champaign, IL: Human Kinetics.

Gauvin, L., & Spence, J. C. (1995). Psychological research on exercise and fitness: Current issues and future challenges. *The Sport Psychologist, 9,* 434–448.

Gill, D. L. (2009). Social psychology and physical activity: Back to the future. *Research Quarterly for Exercise and Sport, 80,* 685–695.

Tenenbaum, G., & Hackfort, D. (2003). A new journal for the international perspective on sport and exercise psychology. *International Journal of Sport and Exercise Psychology, 1,* 7–8.

Weiss, M. R., & Gill, D. L. (2005). What goes around comes around: Re-emerging themes in sport and exercise psychology. *Research Quarterly for Exercise and Sport, 76*(Suppl. 2), S71–S87.

HISTORY OF SPORT PSYCHOLOGY

In many ways, the history of sport psychology mirrors the history of other longstanding disciplines, including psychology, physical education, and other kinesiology-related disciplines, and has been influenced by larger sociocultural trends for decades, for example, the growth of the Olympic movement, professionalization of sport, and women's liberation. Progressing through a number of eras, sport psychology has grown into a dynamic and continually advancing field. Although there are many detailed written histories of sport psychology, the purpose here is to provide a brief overview. Specifically, this entry begins with a summary of major time periods and key contributors and concludes with general remarks on sport psychology and its development. Importantly, most historical accounts of the field are described from a North American or European white male perspective. However, recent efforts have aimed to recognize and share a more holistic history inclusive of diverse individuals all over the world. Attempts are thus made here to present these global contributions. Finally, the history of sport psychology cannot truly be divorced from the history of exercise psychology. However, to highlight the historical accounts that uniquely shape these disciplines today, the history of exercise psychology is described in a separate entry of this encyclopedia.

Eras in the History of Sport Psychology

The history of sport psychology has often been organized into six key eras or time periods that mark the field's development. These eras serve as rough guidelines for retrospectively examining events that have shaped sport psychology today. The eras include (1) the prehistory of the field from antiquity to the early 1900s, (2) the development of sport psychology as a specialty in the 1920s and 1930s of the 20th century, (3) preparation for the discipline between the 1940s and 1960s, (4) the establishment of the academic discipline in the late 1960s and 1970s, (5) the science and practice of sport psychology between the late 1970s and 1990s, and (6) contemporary sport psychology over the last decade.

Era 1: Pre-History (Antiquity–Early 1900s)

While most accounts of the history of sport psychology start in the late 1800s, interest in the area can be traced back to ancient times. For example, with the start of the Olympic Games around 776 BCE, the ancient Greeks embraced the mind–body connection and discussed both physical and mental preparation of athletes. In fact, the ancient Greeks are said to be among the first to systematically explore athletic performance with much of the work paralleling modern-day study in the areas of sports medicine and sport psychology. For instance, comparisons have been made between the Greek tetrad system used to prepare athletes for competition (preparation, concentration, moderation, and relaxation) and the contemporary concept of periodization where training occurs in phases.

Fast forwarding to the Victorian era of the late 1800s in the United States and Great Britain, athletes, educators, journalists, and others demonstrated interest in the many topics studied in sport psychology today, such as the psychological characteristics of high-level athletes as well as cultural issues in the sporting world. By 1894, French physician Philippe Tissie and American psychologist Edward Scripture had published some of the first studies in the field. While Tissie studied psychological changes in endurance cyclists, Scripture examined reaction time in fencers and runners. Notably,

Scripture's work reflected efforts to establish a *new psychology* that focused on data collection and experimentation versus subjective opinion as well as an emphasis on applying scientific findings to the real world (e.g., enhancing athletic performance). Although less recognized, Harvard professor G. W. Fitz was also examining reaction time in athletes around the same time. In 1898, American psychologist Norman Triplett conducted the first known experiment to blend the principles of sport and social psychology. Examining the influence of others on cycling performance, Triplett's study contributed to the development of social facilitation theory often studied in contemporary sport and exercise settings. Researchers continued to explore these and related topics throughout the early 1900s; American psychologists Karl Lashley and John B. Watson conducted a series of studies on skill acquisition in archery.

Perhaps the person who demonstrated the most consistent interest in sport psychology during this era was the French founder of the modern Olympic movement, Pierre de Coubertin. A prolific writer, Coubertin wrote numerous articles relevant to topics studied in sport psychology today, such as the reason children participate in athletics, the importance of self-regulation, and the role of psychological factors in performance improvement. He was also the catalyst in organizing several Olympic Congresses, two of which focused on the psychological aspects of sport. Interested in the blend between body, character, and mind, Coubertin's efforts garnered publicity around the critical role of psychology in sporting activity and continued to influence the field's development well into the 1940s.

The contributions of this era involved several noteworthy psychologists, physical educators, and physicians whose work demonstrated interest in what is now referred to as the field of sport psychology. However, while the work of these scholars dabbled in the world of sports, none of these individuals were considered sport psychology specialists who made consistent contributions. Few concerted efforts were made to systematically study the area until the 1920s.

Era 2: The Development of Sport Psychology as a Specialty (1920s–1930s)

In the 1920s and 30s, professionals continued to show interest in the psychological aspects of sport through periodic writing, research, and exploration. For example, baseball great Babe Ruth was brought to Columbia University in 1921 and psychologically tested to determine the reasons for his exceptional hitting skills. In 1926, American psychologist Walter Miles, his student B. C. Graves, and legendary football coach Pop Warner conducted an interesting study on the influence of signal calling on charging times among the offensive line players.

However, it is also in this era that individuals from around the world began to specialize in the area by developing more systematic lines of research, presentations, and publications that marked a more sustained interest in the psychological aspects of sport. In Charlottenburg, Germany, Robert Werner Schulte started one of the first sport psychology laboratories in 1920 at the Deutsche Hochshule für Leibesübungen where he wrote a book titled *Body and Mind in Sport* and continued his work until his untimely death in 1933. In Russia, notable scholars Piotr Antonovich Roudik and Avksenty Cezarevich Puni began work at the Physical Institutes of Culture in Moscow and Leningrad, respectively. Roudik conducted studies on perception, memory, attention, and imagination while Puni examined psychological preparation and the effects of competition on athletes.

Around the same time, Coleman Griffith was directing the Research in Athletics Laboratory at the University of Illinois. Griffith, who is recognized as the father of North American sport psychology, published approximately 25 studies on topics ranging from motor learning to personality and character. He also published two classic books, *Psychology of Coaching* (1926) and *Psychology of Athletics* (1928), and outlined the key functions of the *sport psychologist*. Griffith's laboratory closed during the Great Depression of the 1930s, but in 1938, he was hired by the Chicago Cubs to assist in improving the team's athletic performance. Unfortunately, Griffith's applied work is said to have been far from successful because of resistance from players and coaches.

The 1920s and 1930s were characterized by not only scholars who dabbled in sport psychology work, but also those across the globe who set up sport psychology laboratories and devoted significant portions of their career to studying the area. Interestingly, with the exception of some Russian scholars whose work continued through the 1960s, the research findings of these early pioneers

had little direct influence on the scientific advancement of the field. Griffith, for example, was ahead of his time but worked in isolation with few students to immediately build upon his work. Still, the emergence of sport psychology as a discipline was ready to begin.

Era 3: Preparation for the Discipline (1940s–1960s)

Scholars who trained future generations of students and professionals set the stage for the development of sport psychology as an academic discipline. As previously mentioned, Puni's work in Russia continued well into the 1960s and 70s and is still recognized today. The same is true in North America where Franklin Henry of the University of California at Berkeley established a psychology of physical activity program and trained physical educators. Upon earning their graduate degrees, these students initiated systematic lines of research across the country. While much of Henry's work focused on what would now be considered motor learning and control, some of his students examined social psychology topics such as athlete personality and the arousal–performance relationship. This era of sport psychology research was also likely influenced by sociocultural events, such as increasing emphasis on performance at the Olympic Games, the Cold War, and the space race, which spurred considerable interest in the development of science in many fields.

On the applied front, the work of David Tracy is noteworthy as he consulted with semipro baseball players as well as the St. Louis Browns' major league team. Tracy helped athletes improve their performance by teaching relaxation skills, using confidence building techniques, autosuggestion, and hypnosis. His work is crucial to this era in that it garnered a great deal of publicity for the practice of sport psychology. It was reported that the Browns' front office believed that if other industries used psychologists, then it would be logical for professional baseball to do so as well. This may have helped initiate a shift in the attitudes of sportspersons and administrators toward the usefulness of sport psychology practitioners.

In addition to Tracy, the work of female pioneer Dorothy Hazeltine Yates is also noteworthy. Best known for her consulting with university boxers, Yates emphasized the use of positive affirmations and relaxation to enhance performance. She also taught a psychology course for athletes and aviators. Embracing the science–practitioner model, she went on to conduct an assessment of her interventions with boxers. A reflection of her work reveals that Yates made important contributions in an otherwise male-dominated field.

Era 4: Establishment of Academic Sport Psychology (Late 1960s–1970s)

The latter part of the 1960s was marked by a major occasion. The First World Congress of Sport Psychology was held in Rome, Italy, in 1965. While few delegates were considered *sport psychologists* given that the field was only emerging as a discipline, this event marked the beginning of worldwide interest and institutionalization of the field. It was here that the International Society of Sport Psychology (ISSP) was born. With Ferruccio Antonelli of Italy as its first president, the inaugural issue of the *International Journal of Sport Psychology* arrived just five years later in 1970. Serving as a model, ISSP inspired the development of several other professional organizations of sport psychology across the globe, including the North American Society for the Psychology of Sport and Physical Activity in 1966, the British Society of Sports Psychology in 1967, the French Society of Sport Psychology in 1967, the Canadian Society for Psychomotor Learning and Sport Psychology in 1969, and the German Association of Sport Psychology in 1969. Born out of disagreements within ISSP, the European Federation of Sport Psychology (FEPSAC) was founded in 1969 with female pioneer Ema Geron of Bulgaria as its first president. Both ISSP and FEPSAC remain prominent influences on the field today.

In the late 1960s and 70s, physical education as an academic discipline was firmly taking hold in the United States. Professors were asked to begin research programs in all the sport sciences, curriculums were revised to include more academic sport science coursework, and graduate programs were developed. Sport psychology, now considered distinct from motor learning and control, was a part of this change. Increased activity on the applied side of the field was also occurring during this era, albeit not without controversy. In 1966, clinical psychologists Tom Tutko and Bruce Ogilvie wrote a controversial book, *Problem Athletes and How to Handle Them,* and developed the Athletic Motivation Inventory, a personality assessment that was said to predict athletic success. The book was controversial because it suggested that athletes

were problematic and needed to be controlled, while some scholars felt that their personality test was based on questionable science. Despite the controversy, Ogilvie was active in working with elite athletes and teams and was seen as a role model for many young professionals with an interest in applied work. In fact, he has been called the father of applied sport psychology in North America.

Era 5: Bridging Science and Practice in Sport Psychology (Late 1970s–1990s)

As the name of the era implies, it was between the late 1970s and 1990s that sport psychology came of age as both a science and an area of professional practice. This era was characterized by increasing interest in the field with scientists devoting their entire careers to the field, and a growing number of practitioners working directly with athletes and coaches. For example, the U.S. Olympic Committee developed a sport psychology advisory board, hired its first resident sport psychologist, and sent its first sport psychologist to the Olympic Games. New academic journals, including the *Journal of Sport Psychology* (1979; known as the *Journal of Sport & Exercise Psychology* since 1988), *The Sport Psychologist* (1986), the *Journal of Applied Sport Psychology* (1989), and the *Korean Journal of Sport Psychology* (1989), were published. The development of organizations to meet the needs of a growing field continued. For example, the Japanese Society of Sport Psychology was developed in 1973 followed by the Korean Society of Sport Psychology in the 1980s. Following the dissolution of other related organizations, the British Association of Sport and Exercise Sciences was developed in 1984 with *The Sport and Exercise Scientist* becoming its official publication. The Association for Applied Sport Psychology (formerly the Association for the Advancement of Applied Sport Psychology) was established in 1986, established its Certified Consultant designation in 1991, and continues to be the largest applied sport psychology organization in the world. In 1986, the American Psychological Association formed a new division, Division 47, devoted specifically to exercise and sport psychology. Born out of the First National Congress of Sport Psychology in Barcelona, the Spanish Federation of Sport Psychology was founded in 1987. Shortly thereafter, the Australian Psychological Association was developed with sport and exercise psychology as a specialization in 1988, followed by the creation of the Asian South Pacific Association of Sport Psychology in 1989.

Finally, women of this era were afforded more opportunities and entered the field in greater numbers thanks to the concerted efforts of several female pioneers, including Ema Geron, Dorothy Yates, Dorothy Harris, Jean Williams, Carole Oglesby, Tara Scanlan, Maureen Weiss, and Diane Gill, to name just a few. Recently, determined efforts have been made to write these female pioneers into the history of the field and recognize their many contributions.

Era 6: Contemporary Sport and Exercise Psychology (2000–Present)

Contemporary sport psychology is a firmly established discipline. The popularity of the field was evidenced by over 700 delegates from 70 countries attending the 2009 World Congress of Sport Psychology held in Morocco. A large number of universities now offer specializations at the graduate level with hundreds of research studies being conducted every year. Reflecting a shift in the field's focus toward the inclusion of both sport and exercise contexts, the *International Journal of Sport Psychology* changed its name to the *International Journal of Sport and Exercise Psychology* (IJSEP) in 2002. The British Psychological Society also developed a sport and exercise psychology division in 2004. Greater attention is being paid to the practice of sport psychology with the development of an applied journal, *The Journal of Sport Psychology in Action*, published by the Association for Applied Sport Psychology in 2010. As sport psychology becomes increasingly popular through media outlets and social networking, Olympic and professional athletes continue to work with sport psychology specialists, as do a number of developing and recreational athletes.

With the growth of both the science and practice of sport psychology, a number of major changes are occurring in the field today. For example, fueled by rising obesity rates and a decrease in physical activity in many Western countries, there has been an explosion of interest in health and exercise-related research in the last decade. Exercise motivation and adherence, the role of physical activity in mental health, and the psychology of athletic injuries have all been topics of considerable interest (see also the entry "History of Exercise Psychology"). Life skill development,

cultural issues, and diversity in the sport context have also become popular areas of inquiry. In addition to the topics studied, the methods employed are also expanding. An increase in qualitative research methods in particular is evidenced by the development of new journals solely devoted to this type of research like *Qualitative Research in Sport, Exercise, and Health*.

At the same time sport psychology has seen tremendous growth and advancement, several important challenges face the field. For example, although they are more widely accepted, qualitative research methods have been criticized for their subjective nature and have led to some debate over the best way of gaining knowledge. Economic support for higher education in many Western societies has declined and caused sport psychology laboratories to become more conscious of the need to secure external funding (e.g., grants, fellowships) to support their research efforts. Tension between researchers and practitioners of sport psychology continues, which has led various professional organizations to purposefully attempt to bridge the gap. Other concerns include the job outlook for many being trained in the field. While sport psychology has certainly grown, academic positions are somewhat limited, and few practitioners will land full-time positions working with athletes and teams. Finally, perhaps the greatest challenge is defining the educational training necessary to become a practitioner in sport psychology. Disagreement over the role of kinesiology versus counseling-based training has led to heated debates among professionals. Increasing attention paid to certifications, licensures, and ethical standards are intended to safeguard against those who may unethically practice sport psychology without the appropriate competencies. Addressing these challenges and embracing the aforementioned successes of the field will fuel the growth of sport psychology in the future.

Conclusion

While sport psychology emerged out of other disciplines, the field certainly has a longer and deeper history than has often been described. Recent efforts have unveiled the contributions of individuals who demonstrated interest in the psychological aspects of sport long before Coleman Griffith and brought to light a history characterized by diverse and global influences not previously recognized. Sport psychology is a worldwide phenomenon with strong research and practice components that parallels the growth of other established disciplines, including psychology and physical education.

Daniel Gould and Dana K. Voelker

See also History of Exercise Psychology

Further Readings

Green, C. D., & Benjamin, L. T. (2009). *Psychology gets in the game: Sport, mind, and behavior, 1880–1960.* Lincoln: University of Nebraska Press.

Kornspan, A. S. (2012). History of sport and performance psychology. In S. M. Murphy (Ed.), *The Oxford handbook of sport and performance psychology* (pp. 3–23). New York: Oxford University Press.

Krane, V., & Whaley, D. E. (2010). Quiet competence: Writing women into the history of U.S. sport and exercise psychology. *The Sport Psychologist, 18,* 349–372.

Ryba, T. V., Schinke, R. J., & Tenenbaum, G. (2010). *The cultural turn in sport psychology.* Morgantown, WV: Fitness Information Technology.

Vealey, R. S. (2006). Smocks and jocks outside the box: The paradigmatic evolution of sport and exercise psychology. *Quest, 58,* 128–159.

Weinberg, R. S., & Gould, D. (2011). *Foundations of sport and exercise psychology.* Champaign, IL: Human Kinetics.

HOME ADVANTAGE

The association of being at home with feelings of increased physical comfort, safety, and psychological well-being are reflected in a wealth of popular expressions and sayings, such as *Home free; Home is where the heart is; East–west, home is best; Home sweet home; There's no place like home.* Thus, it is hardly surprising that the term *home advantage* has been adopted in sport to represent two related phenomena—both of which are founded on the belief that a team's own park, stadia, or venue is, indeed, a good place in which to compete.

One phenomenon pertains to (for lack of a better term) *competition location.* In most professional sports in North America, for example, teams play a full schedule of regular season games to determine final league standings. Those teams ranking higher in the final standings are awarded one extra competition in their home venue in every 3-, 5-, or 7-game playoff series. That extra opportunity to compete at home is referred to as a *home advantage* (e.g., "New York will have the home advantage in its playoff series against Boston"). If the team happens to lose one of its extra competitions at home, it is said to have lost its home advantage. Although competition location can represent a home advantage, it does not always turn out to provide that advantage. For example, in the first round of the National Hockey League (NHL) playoffs in 2010, home teams won 22 games and lost 27 games; in 2011, they won 23 games and lost 26 games. So, certainly from the perspective of competition location, home teams in those 2 years were not able to capitalize on their home advantage.

A second phenomenon, flowing directly from the first, pertains to *probability for a successful outcome.* In almost every instance where large sets of data have been examined—for team and individual sports, for female and male competitors, for international competitions between nations, for athletes and teams from across the age and experience spectrum—the home competitors have had a superior winning percentage that is beyond chance (discussion of these findings in the section that follows).

During the 2011–2012 NHL season, ice-hockey fans closely followed the Detroit Red Wings as they obtained an exceptional 75.6% success rate at home. In their 41 home games, they won an NHL-high of 31, including a league-record 23 straight. This success rate is atypical, of course, but does serve to illustrate an exceptional instance of home advantage.

In this entry, discussion of the home advantage phenomenon is limited to results pertaining to an increased probability for a successful outcome. To this end, discussion is focused on the extent of the home advantage in team and individual sports over a variety of contexts and the explanations that have been advanced by fans, the media, athletes, and sport scientists to help explain its causes. Also, the implications of competing at home for the psychological states and behaviors of athletes and coaches are examined.

The Extent of the Home Advantage

In almost every sport examined, teams have better results when they compete at home. In professional sport, for example, over a recent 5-year period, the winning percentage was 53.7% in baseball, 61.0% in English football (soccer), 54.6% in ice hockey, 58.2% in American football, and 61.0% in basketball.

In most sports examined, athletes competing individually also have superior results when they compete in their home territory. For example, in World Cup Alpine Skiing, skiers competing in their home country on average improved 16% from where they were seeded going into the race to where they actually finished. Interestingly, professional golf and tennis are the only two individual sports where a home advantage has not been found.

In terms of international competitions, there also seems to be evidence of a home advantage for host countries in both the Summer and Winter Olympic Games, as well as the Fédération Internationale de Football Association (International Federation of Association Football; FIFA) World Cup. In the case of the Winter Olympics, for example, host countries showed an average improvement of about four medals over the previous Olympiad. The only host country in the history of the Winter Olympics that failed to improve was Italy (in Torino in 2006); it won 11 medals compared to 13 in Salt Lake City in 2002.

In the case of the Summer Olympics, host nations show an average improvement of approximately five medals over their previous Olympiad. This respectable improvement, however, is dwarfed by China's performance in the 2008 Summer Olympics held in Beijing; China improved its medal count by 37 (for a total of 100 medals) from Athens in 2004.

The FIFA World Cup has also yielded results that seem to show that host nations benefit from competing at home. The first World Cup took place in Uruguay in 1930 and there have been 19 competitions every 4 years since; the most recent World Cup was in 2010 in South Africa. There were no tournaments in 1942 and 1946. The host nation has reached the semi-finals in 12 of 19 tournaments, the finals in 8 of 19 tournaments, and has won 6 out of 19 times. (Given that FIFA is now making an effort to provide a host opportunity to countries and regions that based on their world rankings have minimal chance of winning a medal [e.g., United States, 1994; South Africa, 2010], the overall results are impressive from a home advantage perspective.) The six host countries that have won the FIFA World Cup include Uruguay (1930), Italy (1934), England (1966), West Germany (1974), Argentina (1978), and France (1998). The runners-up include Brazil (1950) and Sweden (1958). Finally, Chile (1962), Italy (1990), and Germany (2006) all finished third when they hosted.

Causes of Home Advantage: Popular Beliefs

The benefits that accrue to host teams have given rise to considerable discussion, speculation, and inquiries among fans, athletes, media, and coaches about *why*. What are the principal factors that underlie the home advantage? As might be expected, there is some overlap among the groups in the explanations advanced.

For example, crowd support was the first choice of fans in one survey and one of the top three choices advanced in another conducted with intercollegiate athletes. Two other choices (endorsed by athletes) were familiarity with the home court and the elimination of the need to travel. The belief that greater familiarity with the nuances of the home venue provides home competitors with the major source of their advantage also was the top reason advanced by coaches.

After working for years as a sabermetrician in major league baseball (*sabermetrics* is the specialized study of baseball through objective statistics), Craig Wright, with the assistance of Tom House, a major league pitching coach, offered his appraisal. Wright and House estimated that 5% of the home advantage is due to a psychological lift from the crowd, 5% results from the advantage of batting last, 10% is due to familiarity with the stadium, 10% is due to the ability of the home team to select and use personnel best suited to its home stadium, 30% is due to a regime regularity, and 40% is due to an umpire bias that favors the home team.

Causes of Home Advantage: Empirical Analyses

Figure 1 is a framework Albert Carron, Todd M. Loughead, and Steven R. Bray offered to systematically examine the home advantage. As a starting point, they proposed that the location of the competition (home vs. away) differentially influences four main factors—the degree of crowd support (and through crowd support, possible favorable officiating decisions), the need to travel, learned familiarity with the venue, and some rule advantages (e.g., batting last in baseball).

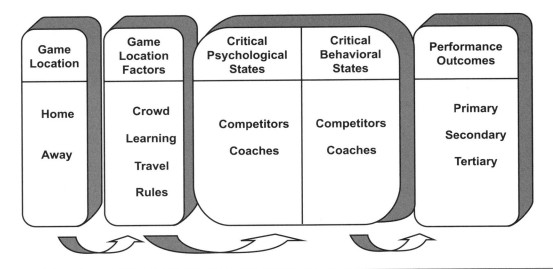

Figure I   Conceptual Framework of the Home Advantage

Source: Adapted from Carron, A. V., Loughead, T. M., & Bray, S. R. (2005). The home advantage in sport competitions: Courneya and Carron's (1992) conceptual framework a decade later. *Journal of Sports Sciences, 23,* 396.

Note: The term *officials* was originally presented in the Carron and Courneya (1992) model. Upon revision of the model in 2005, the terms was removed from the boxes because, unlike coaches and athletes, officials do not have a home or away status.

Game Location Factors

As is the case with many areas of scientific inquiry, results from studies examining the nuances of each of the game location factors have been consistent in some cases but have shown mixed results in the case of other factors. For example, studies that have examined the influence of the rules factor have been consistent; the home team does not have an advantage from the rules.

Insofar as crowd support is concerned, the results have been mixed. At the risk of oversimplification, the following generalizations seem reasonable:

- Absolute crowd size is generally unrelated to the home advantage.
- Crowd density is consistently positively related to the home advantage.
- The nature of crowd behavior (i.e., booing versus cheering the home team) has no consistent influence on the home advantage.
- Laboratory studies have shown that the home crowd has an influence on officiating decisions (i.e., home teams receive more favorable calls). However, field studies and archival research have not supported these results. In well controlled studies, there is no evidence that crowd support produces more favorable officiating for the home team.

The need for a visiting team to travel to compete has also received a great deal of research attention. Again, the results are mixed. At the risk of oversimplification, the following generalizations seem reasonable:

- Distance traveled (e.g., a 120-mile trip to compete versus a 100-mile trip to compete) does not influence the visiting team's disadvantage (and, of course, the home team's advantage).
- The duration of the road trip does not influence the visiting team's disadvantage in professional basketball and baseball. In professional ice hockey, visiting teams are less successful in the initial games of a road trip.
- Travel across time zones can be a source of disadvantage for visiting teams. The adage "traveling west is best" does seem to have some validity. Professional teams traveling from western to eastern regions of North America are at a greater disadvantage than teams traveling from the east westward.

The final game location factor in the framework illustrated in Figure 1 is the home team's learned familiarity with its own venue. There are a number of elements that fall under this category; these can be categorized as either *stable* or *unstable.* The latter are elements in the home team's environment that can be manipulated to one's own advantage. For example, anecdotal accounts in the media have reported a professional baseball team competing at home providing excess water to the base paths to reduce the speed advantage possessed by the visiting team. Another reported a visiting professional basketball coach's concern that the home team might overly inflate the balls to facilitate a higher dribble that would favors the preferences of its point guard.

Stable elements are idiosyncratic aspects of the home team's venue. The Green Monster in Boston's Fenway Park would be one example. Presumably Boston outfielders, as a result of their greater opportunities to practice and play in that environment, would be more familiar with caroms. As another example, professional ice-hockey teams competing on an ice surface at home that is smaller or larger than the league average could benefit from increased familiarity.

The following generalizations about the role that familiarity might play in the home advantage seem reasonable:

- Professional soccer teams with a playing surface larger or smaller than the league average have a greater home advantage.
- Professional baseball teams with artificial turf have a greater home advantage than those teams without artificial turf.
- Professional baseball, basketball, and ice-hockey teams moving to a new facility (thereby temporarily losing their superior knowledge of their own venue) experience a reduction in their home advantage. This result is moderated by team quality. Teams with a superior home advantage prior to relocation (a home advantage greater than 50%) experience a temporary significant reduction. Conversely, teams with an inferior home advantage prior to relocation (a home advantage less than 50%) have a temporary significant improvement in their home advantage.

As Figure 1 illustrates, the game location factors are thought to contribute to different critical psychological states for the home versus visiting athletes and coaches.

Critical Psychological and Physiological States

There is relatively consistent evidence that supports the conclusion that coach and athlete psychological states are superior when playing at home. The generalizations that seem reasonable are as follows:

- Both athletes and coaches have greater personal confidence and confidence in their team prior to competitions at their home venue.
- Athlete emotions and mood states are superior at home. For example, cognitive and somatic anxiety, depression, tension, anger, and confusion are lower prior to a home competition.
- Athletes feel more vulnerable at competitions held away from home because they know they will have to deal with the taunting of away fans (commonly seen in basketball).

Critical Behavioral States

As Figure 1 illustrates, competing at home versus away is also thought to have a differential influence on the behaviors of home versus visiting athletes and coaches. A sense of *territoriality*, which refers to an animal's occupation and defense of a geographical area where it feeds, nests, and mates, has been used to explain the home advantage. Athletes do have higher levels of testosterone prior to home competitions. They are thought to compete more aggressively, expend more effort, and persist longer.

The studies that have been carried out comparing athlete and coach behaviors at home versus away contribute to the following generalizations:

- From a strategy and tactics point of view, coaches adopt more defensive tactics for away games and more aggressive strategies for home games.
- Home versus away teams do not differ in defensive behaviors, such as errors, shots blocked in basketball, or double plays in baseball, but home teams do exhibit more aggressive offensive behaviors like shots taken in ice hockey and basketball.
- Home and visiting teams do not differ in number of aggressive penalties, such as penalties that have intent to injure, as their critical component.

Studies have found trends that away teams seem to be penalized more often and home teams get away with more. In addition, star players seem to get away with more at home.

Conclusion

The aspect of group territoriality known as the *home advantage* has undoubtedly been one of the most examined phenomena in the sport context by coaches, athletes, researchers, administrators, and consultants alike. Generally speaking, the home advantage seems to share some consistency in prevalence across all sport types. Although it would be fair to say that while the home advantage is enjoyed throughout all sport, it is not necessarily enjoyed by all teams within those sports. Certain factors like team quality do moderate the effects of the home advantage. Additionally, it is likely fair to assume that questions going forward surrounding the home advantage would not be to determine *whether* such a phenomenon exists; as outlined in this entry, the pervasive evidence demonstrating a superior winning percentage for the home team goes beyond chance. The fact that the home advantage has also been well documented over the last 100 years should calm any uncertainties. Future directions on investigating the home advantage should maintain a primary focus on why this phenomenon continues.

The conceptual framework presented in this entry is intended as a useful guide to further investigation. No claim is made, however, that it encapsulates everything and all factors pertaining to the home advantage. What it does provide is a simple depiction of what is presumably a dynamic construct (in that it fluctuates) depending on a wide variety of variables and factors specific for each sport and each team.

Albert V. Carron and Kyle F. Paradis

See also Aggression; Competition; Group Characteristics

Further Readings

Balmer, N. J., Nevill, A. M., & Williams, A. M. (2001). Home advantage in the Winter Olympics (1908–1998). *Journal of Sports Sciences, 19,* 129–139.

Balmer, N. J., Nevill, A. M., & Williams, A. M. (2003). Modelling home advantage in the Summer Olympic Games. *Journal of Sports Sciences, 21,* 469–478.

Carron, A. V., & Eys, M. A. (2012). *Group dynamics in sport* (4th ed.). Morgantown, WV: Fitness Information Technology.

Carron, A. V., Loughead, T. M., & Bray, S. R. (2005). The home advantage in sport competitions: The Courneya & Carron conceptual framework a decade later. *Journal of Sport Sciences, 23,* 395–407.

Courneya, K. S., & Carron, A. V. (1992). The home advantage in sport competitions: A literature review. *Journal of Sport & Exercise Psychology, 14,* 13–27.

Pollard, R., & Pollard, G. (2005). Long-term trends in home advantage in professional team sports in North America and England (1876–2003). *Journal of Sport Sciences, 23,* 337–350.

HUMAN FACTORS

Human factors (HF) is a multidisciplinary area that aims to understand and support the interactions between a human user and other elements of a sociotechnical system. Because human factors research addresses psychological, social, biological, and other task-related parameters of interactions between humans or between a human and a technical system in the context of work and industrial production, such disciplines as psychology, robotics, industrial design, engineering, anthropometry, biology, and graphic design are incorporated. Sport psychology can contribute to the field as well because of its knowledge concerning performance acquisition and the development of psychological skills like routines, inner speech, or the regulation of stress; all are useful in designing an optimal work environment. The term *ergonomics* is often used interchangeably with human factors.

The goal of HF research is to develop human-oriented technology that adapts to the physical and psychological needs of the human operator. Because humans must interact with technical and production-oriented systems, the research and applied discipline *human factors science* (HFS) exists to optimize and maintain the health and well-being of humans in particular tasks and work environment constellations. Another related goal is to develop and maintain productivity in a particular interaction between the system and the human. Therefore, experts and practitioners in *human factors engineering* (HFE) work to design an optimal fit between the technical production system and the human action system. Dimensions of such an optimal fit between human and technical systems are, for instance, task- and person-related equipment (e.g., body-oriented shape and flexibility of equipment), the presentation and change of information in accordance with human perceptual systems, and a working structure that considers the biological needs of humans.

From a person-related view, *human factors* are cognitive, motivational, perceptual, physical, or biomechanical properties of individuals and their behavior that may influence the interaction between the human and the technological system. Many approaches in HF research, therefore, explicitly address the structure and cognitive basis of human action and human motion as a main factor in the production process. For instance, research concerning attention in technological systems is based on a close interaction between psychologists and engineers. Psychologists use their knowledge about attention, perception, information processing, and memory to inform engineers, who design products based on these principles, for instance, to improve aviation safety or for constructing new cars.

There are many links between human factors science and sport psychology. For example, performance plays a central role in both areas. Therefore, both disciplines have some potential links to *action theory*. The action theory approach has a number of historical roots; one of which is a book on planning and the structure of behavior, which was written by American psychologists George A. Miller, Eugene Galanter, and Karl H. Pribram in 1960. This book broke away from behaviorist concepts and formulated preliminary ideas about the functional construction of action. Further roots can be found in Russian and German psychology. Thus far, the action theory approach has been formulated most elaborately for human factors by American researchers such as Donald A. Norman and German scientists like Winfried Hacker. Action theory addresses, for instance, the finding that the various elements of a behavior that can be observed externally are based on a deep hierarchical structure and are carried out in order to attain a specific action goal. Hence, activities in production processes or sport environments are always performed relative to a goal and are directed toward this goal. This gives all of the psychological processes and structures (emotions, representations, etc.) within a human–machine interaction or a particular sport setting an action-regulating function. Based on such a common background, it is possible for sport

psychology to inform human factors researchers about well-investigated elements of action and performance and vice versa. While human factors research topics like perception, cognition, attention, and motivation in human–machine interaction are well investigated, important topics often investigated in sport psychology like emotion are mostly ignored. In 2011, David W. Eccles, Paul Ward, Christopher Janelle, and other researchers addressed this discrepancy. They argued that the development of emotional self-regulatory skills in human operators could support system performance, explain risk-taking behavior in human–machine interaction, and may also influence motor planning and motor control in the context of technical systems.

In recent years, the expanding field of cognitive robotics has offered new opportunities to study the construction and functionality of human factors like cognitive representations, attention, and communication with technical platforms, and in doing so has changed some perspectives in human factors research. The long-term goal of newly developed human factors disciplines like *cognitive interaction technology* is to develop robots with unprecedented sensorimotor, emotional, and cognitive intelligence to assist human activities in the industrial production process. Interestingly, current robot technology has matured to the point of being able to approximate a reasonable spectrum of specialized perceptual, cognitive, and motor capabilities, allowing researchers to explore the bigger picture that is the architecture for the integration of these functions into robot action control. This provides the opportunity to fit existing human models of perception, representation, motor control, and decision making together with architectures generated for robot actions. Cognitive interaction technology research labs have produced impressive humanoid robots, robot musicians, dancing robots, robot arms, and brain–machine interfaces, among others, to study the organization and functioning of human action and human–machine interaction in more detail. Based on such platforms, HF researchers are not only addressing the attention of a human user as the guiding factor of human–machine interaction, but furthermore, they wish to create a shared action and a shared attention between humans and robots. This research aims to systematically investigate the principles needed to build artificial cognitive systems based on the human archetype that can interact with a human in an intuitive way, including the acquisition of new skills by learning.

Thomas Schack

See also Attentional Focus; Biofeedback, Neurofeedback; Task Constraints

Further Readings

Eccles, D. W., Ward, P., Woodman, T., Janelle, C. M., Le Scanff, C., Ehrlinger, J., et al. (2011). Where's the emotion? How sport psychology can inform research on emotion in human factors. *Human Factors, 53,* 180–202.

Norman, D. A. (1981). Organization of action slips. *Psychological Review, 88,* 1–15.

Schack, T., & Ritter, H. (2009). The cognitive nature of action—Functional links between cognitive psychology, movement science, and robotics. *Progress in Brain Research, 174,* 231–250. doi: 10.1016/S0079-6123(09)01319-3

HUMOR

In the year 2000, psychologists Martin Seligman and Mihaly Csikszentmihalyi were authors of an influential article proposing a new focus in the field of psychology: the positive psychology movement. Since that time, researchers have begun to explore the positive aspects or strengths of life such as satisfaction, optimism, happiness, and other positive emotions. Included in this repertoire of constructive attributes is the sense of humor. Humor can simply be described as the quality of being funny, laughable, amusing, or comic. However, how humor is utilized, that is sense of humor, is of main interest in exercise and sport psychology because of humor's ability to serve as a powerful, robust coping mechanism, cohesion enhancer, and communication technique. Humor has also shown to have positive benefits in many other domains, such as therapy, marriage, job satisfaction, education, leadership, and health. People who use humor are usually better able to successfully build relationships and tend to be more popular.

Over the years, several theories of humor have been proposed. Four of these theories are briefly mentioned here. The release theory proposed by Sigmund Freud stated that humor is used as a coping mechanism to release sexual or aggressive tensions. Many of the other humor theories attempt to explain why humor is found in various circumstances. The incongruity theory states that humor is found in situations where a particular action or outcome is expected, yet an unexpected action or outcome occurs. In other words, the element of surprise plays a role in humorous events. The superiority theory of humor states that persons feel *sudden glory* over another when the other person is the target of a joke. Finally, the benign violation theory states that humor is found when norms or expected behaviors are violated (similar to incongruity theory) without any serious or threatening consequences.

There are numerous forms or types of humor—sarcastic, self-deprecating, hyperbolic, parodic, ironic, and situational—to name just a few. Each may have various effects on the sender and receiver. In other words, although many believe humor has several positive mental and physical benefits, when used differently humor may serve to increase stress, humiliate, or decrease motivation. Used in a positive manner, however, humor may be an effective cognitive strategy (particularly in dealing with stressful situations) and help people to reassess life situations by allowing them to see the problem more realistically—providing psychological distance from the situation. Also, humor may be categorized as reactive or productive. Reactive humor is the ability to accurately appreciate and respond to humorous events (i.e., understand, laugh). Productive humor represents the capacity to devise, create, or use humor in situations not initially seen as humorous.

The sense of humor may be considered to have trait and state components. Measurement instruments have been developed to measure these various aspects of humor, such as the Humor Perceptiveness Test, Coping Humor Scale, Humor Styles Questionnaire, Multidimensional Sense of Humor Scale, Sense of Humor Questionnaire 6, Sense of Humor Scale, and Situational Humor Response Questionnaire. These scales measure facets of the sense of humor: the ability to appreciate various types of humor, humor creativity, use of humor to cope, styles of humor, and the relationship of humor to certain personality characteristics.

As early as the 1960s, studies were conducted on the effects of humor on teaching. Humor has been found to assist in information recall and is valued by both the teachers and students. Teachers who use appropriate humor usually receive higher teaching evaluations, are seen as more approachable, and are better able to establish rapport with students. Interestingly, although coaching is seen by many as similar to teaching, very few studies have been conducted on the use of humor by coaches. Also, there are very few studies of the use of humor in sport and exercise in general. The few studies found in coaching indicated head coaches who use appropriate humor were more liked by their players—particularly by female athletes. Also, coaches who use humor were found to be perceived as having higher abilities and evaluated more positively.

Future investigations of the effectiveness of humor as a coping mechanism in sport and exercise may provide valuable insight to this often discussed, yet not fully understood behavioral characteristic. How humor may be used by leaders and participants to assist in adhering to exercise programs would significantly impact the fitness and medical industries. Discussions of the use of humor by teammates and coaches to enhance team relationships, cohesion, enjoyment, or satisfaction, as well as for coping with sport circumstances, would be valuable additions to the literature.

Kevin L. Burke

See also Adherence; Coach–Athlete Relations; Coaching Efficacy; Cohesion; Coping; Enjoyment; Friendships/ Peer Relations; Optimism

Further Readings

Burke, K. L., Peterson, D., & Nix, C. L. (1995). The effects of the coaches' use of humor on female volleyball players' evaluation of their coaches. *Journal of Sport Behavior, 18,* 83–90.

Grisaffe, C., Blom, L. C., & Burke, K. L. (2003). The effects of head and assistant coaches' use of humor on collegiate soccer players' evaluation of their coaches. *Journal of Sport Behavior, 26,* 103–108.

Hurley, M. H., Dennett, D. C., & Adams, R. B. (2011). *Inside jokes: Using humor to reverse-engineer the mind.* Cambridge: MIT Press.

Ruch, W. (Ed.). (1998). *The sense of humor: Explorations of a personality characteristic.* New York: Mouton de Gruyter.

Seligman, M., & Csikszentmihalyi, M. (2000). Positive psychology. *American Psychologist, 55,* 5–14.

HYPNOSIS

The term *hypnosis* is often shrouded in misconception, myth, and apprehension because most views about hypnosis are influenced by entertainment stage shows. These shows often highlight participants' engaging in strange and often embarrassing behaviors. However, hypnosis is consistently reported to be an effective and reliable technique in many domains (including medicine, dentistry, and psychology) for the treatment of a number of physical and psychological issues, including pain management and addictive behaviors. Hypnosis is a cognitive behavioral process using the influence of suggestion to bring about changes in thoughts, perceptions, feelings, memory, and behavior. Successful hypnosis is associated with situations in which (hypnotic) suggestions are more readily accepted and acted upon by the participants. Indeed, hypnosis is a psychological technique available to athletes and exercisers to facilitate the mindset for peak performance and regular exercise. The nature of hypnosis, hypnotic procedures, theories of hypnosis, and the applications of hypnosis to sport and exercise are outlined in the following sections.

Nature of Hypnosis

Hypnosis is a process that involves an interaction between the hypnotherapist and participant and typically combines the procedures of visualization, relaxation, and the presentation of hypnotic suggestions. Hypnosis is usually characterized by extreme relaxation, intense concentration, and an increased responsiveness to hypnotic suggestion. Suggestion is an important facet of hypnosis and refers to the issuing of verbal statements—that is, words and metaphors of how a person would like to think, feel, or behave—by the hypnotherapist to a participant. Suggestions are provided during hypnosis to alter perceptions, thoughts, feelings, sensations, and behavior. Further, post-hypnotic suggestions may be presented to participants during hypnosis that are intended to trigger responses affecting behavior during a normal waking state. For example, post-hypnotic suggestions may be presented to help a soccer player feel more calm, composed, and confident during training and competition situations.

Fundamental to hypnosis is determining the degree to which individuals are susceptible to hypnosis. Therefore, many measures of hypnotic capacity and susceptibility have been developed and evidence demonstrates that from 10% to 15% of all individuals are highly responsive, 10% to 15% are almost completely unresponsive, and the remaining majority of individuals are able to respond to some but not all hypnotic procedures.

Hypnotic suggestions are considered effective when they are presented to participants when they are in or entering a trance. Participants in a trance may look as though they are asleep, but a hypnotic trance is different from sleep. Indeed a person in a trance is aware of their environment, is relaxed, will respond to suggestions, and can usually remember later what transpired in the trance. Trance allows access, via suggestions, to the unconscious mind that holds memories and feelings that are below the level of conscious awareness but exert an influence on behavior, thoughts, and emotions. The properties of trance typically include intense relaxation, time distortion, and an increased tolerance of discomfort and pain.

Hypnotic Procedures

Hypnosis usually includes four phases. Phase 1 is based around preparing the participant for hypnosis by educating them about hypnotic procedures. In Phase 2, a process of induction and deepening occurs that typically involves relaxation procedures to enhance participants' susceptibility to hypnotic suggestions. Phase 3 is where the therapy or change will happen. When a participant reaches a deep level of hypnosis, suggestions and also posthypnotic suggestions are presented about the way the participant thinks and behaves when alert. Phase 4 of hypnosis is about bringing the participant out of hypnosis and alerting them to the surroundings. In addition, participants may then use self-hypnosis to further increase the acceptance and the effects of suggestions. To illustrate, athletes can use self-hypnosis procedures as part of a preperformance routine, further enabling them to acquire an optimal performance state.

Theories of Hypnosis

Generally, theories of hypnosis fall into one of two camps: state and nonstate. A *state* perspective presents the effects of hypnosis as a result of trance states, altered or divided consciousness, or dissociation. For example, a trance state is posited to be responsible for increasing a participant's acceptance of hypnotic suggestions. In contrast, a *nonstate* perspective views the effects of hypnosis as a consequence of positive attitudes, motivations, and expectations held by both the hypnotherapist and participant. To illustrate, a hypnotherapist may create expectancy in participants that hypnosis will be effective for them and that they will have certain experiences and responses.

Applications of Hypnosis

The amount and breadth of sport and exercise psychology literature demonstrating the efficacy of hypnosis is currently somewhat scant. However, the research to date has revealed positive effects for hypnosis in increasing optimal performance states like flow and peak performance, augmenting the use of mental imagery, reducing precompetition anxiety, influencing perceptions of effort and physiological responses at rest and during treadmill running exercise, and enhancing athletes' self-confidence. For example, in a recent study using a controlled group design, data revealed the immediate and long-term effects of hypnosis interventions on soccer players' self-confidence and shooting performance. Future researchers should consider evaluating the efficacy of hypnosis on other important psychological factors necessary for optimal sport performance (e.g., concentration, anxiety, and motivation) using controlled group designs.

In sum, hypnosis is a potentially viable and effective strategy available to coaches, athletes, and exercisers for bringing about meaningful psychological and performance gains. To illustrate, during preparation for an important competition, hypnosis could be used to increase relaxation and concentration, therefore reducing muscle tension and distraction. Further, the presentation of positive suggestions prior to and during competition about the feelings and emotions that relate to performing successfully may increase the likelihood of an athlete's experiencing increased motivation and feelings of confidence as well as reducing anxiety.

Jamie Barker

See also Imagery; Interventions for Exercise and Physical Activity; Mindfulness; Psychological Skills; Relaxation; Self-Regulation

Further Readings

Barker, J. B., Jones, M. V., & Greenlees, I. (2010). Assessing the immediate and maintained effects of hypnosis on self-efficacy and soccer wall-volley performance. *Journal of Sport & Exercise Psychology, 32,* 243–252.

Heap, M., & Aravind, K. A. K. (2002). *Hartland's medical and dental hypnosis* (4th ed.). London: Churchill Livingstone.

Lynn, S. J., Rhue, J. W., & Kirsch, I. (Eds.). (2010). *Handbook of clinical hypnosis* (2nd ed., pp. 641–666). Washington, DC: American Psychological Association.

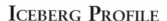

ICEBERG PROFILE

The *iceberg profile* in sport is a visual representation of desirable emotional health status, characterized by low raw scores on the *tension, depression, anger, fatigue,* and *confusion* scales and above norms (the "water line") on *vigor* as assessed by the Profile of Mood States (POMS). The iceberg profile as a metaphoric image has been employed for better understanding of emotion–performance relationships and well-being in competitive and high-level athletes. This entry examines the utility of the iceberg profile in description of interaction effects of multiple negative and positive mood states affecting preparation and athletic performance.

Iceberg Profile as a Metaphor

An iceberg (*ice mountain,* from Middle Dutch *ijsberg*; Norwegian *isberg*) is a large mass of ice floating in the sea. The iceberg image is often used metaphorically to represent the notion that only a very small amount (the tip) of information about a situation is available or visible whereas the real bulk of data is either unavailable or otherwise hidden. The principle gets its name from the fact that only about one tenth of an iceberg's mass can be seen above the water's surface, while about nine tenths of it is submerged and invisible. Another interesting feature of the iceberg profile, which should be emphasized, is its ability to identify the interactive effects of the components of different phenomena. That is why the

iceberg profile as an image, principle, or a model is popular in various contexts. The *iceberg diagram* has also been helpful to identify some of the crucial aspects and influences in management and organizational settings. The iceberg graphically demonstrates the idea of having both visible and invisible structures interact. It is also helpful for understanding of global issues and is often used in systems thinking. In this case, at the tip above the water are events happening in the world; below the waterline there are often patterns or the recurrence of events. Patterns are important to identify because they indicate that an event is not an isolated incident. Like the different levels of an iceberg, deep beneath the patterns are the underlying structures or root causes that create or drive those patterns.

Profile of Mood States-Based Iceberg Profile in Sport

William Morgan introduced the term *iceberg profile,* as a metaphor, in sport in the late 1970s; it was based on his systematic research and monitoring of overtraining and staleness in competitive and elite athletes across different sports. In his assessments, Morgan used the 65-item POMS and noticed that elite athletes and active individuals in general tend to score below the population average on the tension, depression, anger, fatigue, and confusion scales. Moreover, these individuals usually scored about one standard deviation above the population average on *vigor.* This profile has been called the iceberg profile because the resulting configuration resembled an iceberg. All five negative mood states fell below the population average (*T*-score of 50), and one positive mood state was one standard deviation above the population mean (see Figure 1). (It has been observed that it was good luck that the developers of the POMS placed the vigor subscale *fortuitously* in the middle, or there would be no iceberg profile at all!)

The POMS yields five negative mood states measures, one positive mood state, and a global measure of mood. A *global score* is computed by adding five negative mood states (tension, depression, anger, fatigue, and confusion) and subtracting the one positive mood state (vigor). Since this computational procedure sometimes yields negative values a constant of 100 is added (*Ten + Dep + Ang + Fat + Con + 100 – Vig*). These values are employed as a baseline for individual athletes (and in groups) to estimate the dynamics of staleness during the season. If the athlete suffers from chronic fatigue and is unable complete a workout session, his POMS profile can become *inverted*. The inverse iceberg profile is characterized by a lower level of vigor and higher levels of tension, depression, anger, fatigue, and confusion than the average individual. This type of mood profile is associated with a poor state of physical and mental functioning.

The POMS has several response sets depending on the focus in the assessment of mood states. These sets include *statelike* (*right now, today,* or *prior to your last competition*) and *traitlike* (*generally, usually, typically* during a week or a month) *foci*. For instance, if the athlete is asked to respond to the question "How have you been feeling *during the past week, including today?*" rather than "How have you been feeling *today?*" then both statelike and traitlike aspects of emotional state are assessed.

Iceberg Profile and Mental Health Model

The POMS-based iceberg profile represents visually the *interaction of multiple* mood *states*, and it is grounded in Morgan's mental health model (MHM). Briefly described, the MHM assumes that performance is inversely correlated with psychopathology. Thus, positive mental health is associated with high performance levels whereas mood disturbances are predicted to result in performance decrements. The basic premise of the model is that positive aspects of mental health should be associated with broadly defined success in sport.

There are several concerns with the application of POMS-based iceberg profiles for testing the

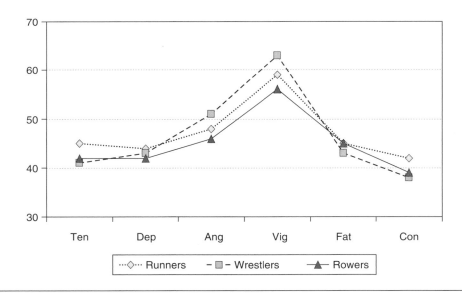

Figure 1   Profile of Mood States Iceberg Profiles in High-Level Runners, Wrestlers, and Rowers

Source: Adapted with permission from Morgan, W. P. (1985). Selected psychological factors limiting performance: A mental health model. In D. H. Clarke & H. M. Eckert (Eds.), *Limits of human performance* (pp. 70–80). Champaign, IL: Human Kinetics.

Note: Ten = tension. *Dep* = depression. *Ang* = anger. *Vig* = vigor. *Fat* = fatigue. *Con* = confusion.

validity of the MHM in prediction of athletic performance, especially at the individual level. First, POMS emotion descriptors are predominantly negative (five negative versus one positive mood state). Second, the researcher-generated mood descriptors are "fixed" and thus do not capture the idiosyncratic nature of athletes' individual emotional experiences. Third, POMS-based iceberg profiles as measures of mood states are not related directly to preperformance and midperformance situations. Neither are they focused on optimal and dysfunctional impact of mood states on performance. Fourth, population average (norms) rather than individually optimal and dysfunctional profiles serve as criteria to evaluate postperformance emotion impact. Finally, there is a need to examine the effectiveness of deliberately created iceberg profile based on other than POMS assessment measures—for instance, idiosyncratic emotion-centered and action-centered profiles.

Extension of Iceberg Profile Applications

The utility of POMS-based iceberg profiles can be enhanced by adding context-specific and relevant response sets. These response sets include *recalled* iceberg profiles of past emotional experiences ("How did you feel prior to your season best competition?"); *anticipatory* profiles ("How do you think you will feel prior to the upcoming competition?"); *performance related* (pre-, mid-, post-event) profiles; *interpersonal* profiles ("How do you feel while interacting with your coach or a teammate?"), and *intragroup* profiles ("How do you feel in this team and in your previous team?").

Iceberg profile applications can also be extended by the assessment of emotions other than POMS mood states. For instance, does the iceberg principle work for other multiple emotion measures, such as CSAI-2 (with self-confidence, cognitive and somatic anxiety) or the individualized *emotion-centered profiling*? Some of these concerns were addressed empirically in the individual zone of optimal functioning (IZOF) model that predicts high probability of individually successful performance if the intensity of athlete's optimal pleasant (P+) and optimal unpleasant (N+) emotions interacts with low intensity of dysfunctional unpleasant (N−) and dysfunctional pleasant (P−) emotions. Figure 2 depicts two individualized iceberg profiles based on the assessment of personally

relevant and performance-related idiosyncratic emotions. These iceberg profiles were constructed by deliberately placing optimal positively toned and negatively toned emotions in the middle and dysfunctional emotions (negative and positive) by their sides (N− > N+ and P+ > P−).

Individualized emotion-centered profiling captures the fact that one athlete may perform quite well when angry or anxious whereas another athlete with the same mood may perform poorly. That is why it is crucial to use task and personally relevant items (idiosyncratic emotion descriptors). In both cases, the predominance of functionally optimal positively toned and negatively toned emotions (P+N+) over the dysfunctional negatively toned and positively toned emotions (N−P−) serves as a predictor of high probability of individually successful performance (well-functioning). On the other hand, predominance of positives (well-being P+P−) over the negatives (ill-being N+N−) characterizes the athlete's situational mental health status. A distinction between well-being (vs. ill-being) and well-functioning (vs. ill-functioning) is made by identifying both positive and negative emotions that have optimal and dysfunctional impact on mental health and athletic performance.

Variability of optimal intensity zones for each emotion descriptor and their interaction are identified during the repeated (recalled and current) assessments of emotion profiles prior to several successful performances in a single athlete. Prior to unsuccessful performance, the profiles are "flat" or positively skewed or negatively skewed. Consistent results suggest that there are two success-related and two failure-related iceberg profiles based on measures of multiple positively toned and negatively toned emotions. These four profiles are the summary of intraindividual emotion dynamics contrasting individually successful and unsuccessful performances (Figure 3).

Enhancing the Utility of Individualized Emotion Profiling

There are several ways to enhance the utility of the iceberg profile and its applications.

1. "Ideal" emotion iceberg profiles should be identified by multiple intraindividual profiling of five to seven personally successful (self-referenced) performances.

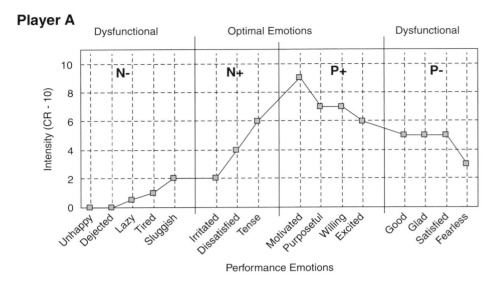

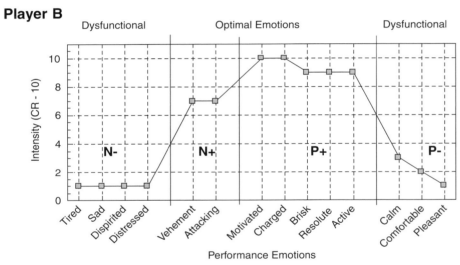

Figure 2   Individualized Pre-Game Zone of Optimal Functioning Emotion Profile of Soccer Players A and B

Source: Adapted from Hanin, Y. L. (2000). Soccer and emotions: Enhancing or impairing performance? In J. Bangsbo (Ed.), *Soccer and science—In an interdisciplinary perspective* (pp. 69–89). Munskgaard, Copenhagen, Denmark: Institute of Exercise and Sport Sciences, Copenhagen University.

2. Emotion descriptors should be idiosyncratic and self-generated by the athlete rather than fixed researcher-generated markers

3. To create iceberg profile, these multiple success-related factors should be placed in the middle; poor performance factors are located by the sides.

4. The main focus in research and applications should be on distinguishing intraindividually between the profiles related to success and poor performance.

5. Action-centered profiling is also recommended in considering successful and unsuccessful performances processes.

Conclusion

The findings suggest that iceberg profile predicting successful performance is possible to create by using idiosyncratic athlete-generated and aggregated researcher-generated emotion descriptors. Successful performances are predicted by two predominant types of profiles (P+) or (P+N+) that are similar for most athletes even if they have different emotion markers. On the other hand, inverse ("flat," "cavity-shape," N-skewed, or P-skewed) iceberg profiles predict high probability of individually poor performances. A future challenge in sport psychology (SP) is the development of

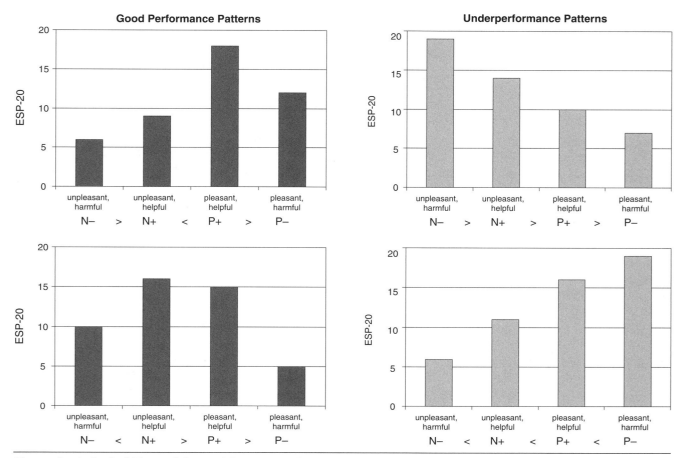

Figure 3   Individual Zone of Optimal Functioning Emotion Profiles Before Successful ("Iceberg") and Poor (N-Skewed or P-Skewed) Performances

Source: Adapted from Hanin, Y. L. (2011, July 9). *Emotions in sport: Current issues and perspectives.* Paper presented at the invited symposium "Emotions in Sport," 16th ECSS Congress Liverpool, UK.

individualized emotion scales capable of capturing interactive effects of emotions on athletic performance. Iceberg profile provides a partial solution to this challenging task.

Yuri L. Hanin

See also Affect; Basic Emotions in Sport; Emotional Responses; Individual Response Stereotype; Mental Health; Overtraining Syndrome; Psychological Well-Being; Stress Management

Further Readings

Hanin, J., & Hanina, M. (with commentators). (2009). Optimization of performance intop-level athletes: An action-focused coping. *International Journal of Sport Sciences & Coaching, 4*(1), 47–91.

Hanin, Y. L. (Ed.). (2000). *Emotions in sport.* Champaign, IL: Human Kinetics.

McNair, D. M., Lorr, M., & Droppleman, L. F. (1971). *Profile of mood state manual.* San Diego, CA: Educational and Industrial Testing Service.

Morgan, W. P. (1985). Selected psychological factors limiting performance: A mental health model. In D. H. Clarke & H. M. Eckert (Eds.), *Limits of human performance* (pp. 70–80). Champaign, IL: Human Kinetics.

Morgan, W. P., Brown, D. R., Raglin, J. S., O'Connor, P. J., & Elickson, K. A. (1987). Psychological monitoring of overtraining and staleness. *British Journal of Medicine, 21*(3), 107–114.

Morgan, W. P., & Pollock, M. L. (1977). Psychological characterization of the elite distance runner. In P. Milvy (Ed.), *Annals of the New York Academy of Science, 301,* 382–403.

Raglin, J. S. (2001). Psychological factors in sport performance. The mental health model revisited. *Sports Medicine, 31*(12), 875–890.

Terry, P. (1995). The efficacy of mood state profiling with elite performers: A review and synthesis. *The Sport Psychologist, 9,* 309–324.

IDENTITY

Exercise identity is a construct that captures the extent to which one sees exercise as a part of one's self-concept, or who one is. This self-perception has been related to exercise behavior and may be of interest to researchers and practitioners who are invested in understanding and promoting exercise adherence. Adhering to recommended levels of exercise has been reliably linked to the procurement of health benefits, yet the majority of the population remain insufficiently active to benefit from exercise. Consequently, researchers and practitioners alike pursue a variety of solutions to the widespread and complex problem of exercise nonadherence. As one avenue to address this problem, researchers have begun to investigate how self-perceptions, or how one views oneself, influence exercise behavior. This approach to understanding exercise behavior is consistent with the position advocated by social psychological theorists that self-views have implications for the motivation and execution of goal-directed behavior. One self-perception that has received increased research attention relative to exercise adherence is *identity.*

Identity and Identity Theory

Identity is a construct appreciated and studied in a wide range of contexts. For example, the term *identity* has been applied relative to, among other categories, cultures, nations, groups, and individuals. When applied with the goal of understanding how identity influences the self-regulation or management of goal-directed behavior, the conceptualization of identities as provided by Peter J. Burke is useful. Burke, an influential proponent of identity theory, views identities as role meanings, or what it means for an individual to hold a particular role in society. Socialization is thought to result in shared conceptualizations among individuals about what it means to hold a particular role in society that, in turn, prescribes acceptable behavior for a given role. Given shared social knowledge, most people are able to describe what it means to hold particular roles in society, such as exerciser (e.g., an exerciser is someone who engages in regular exercise). Identification involves classifying oneself as holding that societal role and internalizing the meanings associated with that role (e.g., I am an exerciser, and exercisers engage in regular exercise. Engaging in regular exercise is a part of who I am).

Burke has suggested that identities function as self-regulating control systems that encourage identity-consistent behavior. Because the meanings associated with an identity are incorporated into one's sense of self, identities serve as a personally relevant standard for behavior; individuals are motivated to maintain consistency between their identity (e.g., I am an exerciser. Exercisers engage in regular exercise) and their behavior (e.g., I will engage in regular exercise). According to identity theory, when an individual perceives that his or her behavior is at odds with his or her identity, he or she should experience negative affect (e.g., dissatisfaction, guilt) that, in turn, motivates the individual to verify the identity through his or her behavior. As an example, an individual who perceives herself as an exerciser (and therefore someone who exercises regularly) who also perceives that her exercise identity has not been verified through her behavior (she has not exercised for over a week) should experience negative affect and resume exercise as a means of verifying the identity. When no discrepancy between identity and behavior is detected, identity verification should be in place and no adjustment in behavior is necessary. While an identity is theorized to serve as a self-regulatory control system for all individuals who identify with a behavior variations in identity strength or salience are thought to influence the effectiveness of the self-regulatory control system; identity theorists posit that individuals are more likely to behave consistent with an identity when it is strongly endorsed.

Exercise Identity and Exercise Behavior

Researchers and practitioners interested in understanding and promoting exercise adherence recognize the behavioral self-regulatory implications of the identity construct. Consequently, the relationship between exercise identity (or related variations of the construct such as physical activity [PA] identity) and exercise behavior has been examined. It has been well established that exercise identity is positively associated with a variety of exercise-related outcomes. For example, strength of exercise identity has been associated with how many minutes and how frequently people exercise in a week, how hard people exercise (perceived exertion) and physiological outcomes of exercise including measures of cardiorespiratory fitness (e.g., VO_2 max), and anthropometric variables (e.g., percentage of body fat). While most of the research on exercise identity has been done on university and community samples, support for the ameliorative effect of identity on exercise behavior extends to older adults.

In addition to being associated with exercise behavior, exercise identity has also been associated with variables known to influence the self-regulation of exercise. For example, when compared to individuals with lower scores on exercise identity, individuals with higher scores also report holding their intentions for future exercise more strongly and exhibit higher scores of self-regulatory efficacy—or one's confidence in one's a ability to manage (e.g., schedule, plan) exercise behavior. Further, when studied over time, exercise identity appears to serve as a mechanism through which exercise identity exerts its influence on exercise adherence. Specifically, having a strong exercise identity predicts self-regulatory efficacy for exercise that, in turn, predicts frequency of exercise behavior. Planning of exercise also appears to explain in part the relationship between exercise identity and exercise behavior; PA identity has been found to predict planning of exercise that then predicts individual perceptions of progress toward PA goals.

Researchers from the self-determination theory (SDT) literature also suggests that exercise identity may be related to variables that are known to be important in the self-regulation of exercise. SDT, a psychological theory conceptualized by Deci and Ryan, suggests that when individuals engage in a behavior for self-determined reasons, such as enjoyment or because doing so is in line with one's personal goals (as opposed to external reasons such as external pressure or pursuit of reward), positive behavioral outcomes such as adherence result. Stronger endorsement of exercise identity positively relates to engaging in exercise for self-determined reasons. According to SDT, exercise identity may encourage exercise adherence through its association with adaptive motives for exercise.

Further support for the idea that exercise identity promotes the successful self-regulation of exercise comes from research examining how individuals respond when their exercise identity is challenged. Individuals who report high and those who report moderate levels of exercise identity who are asked to imagine that they have been much less active than usual both respond in a manner that suggests they would self-regulate to bring their exercise back in line with their identity. For example, individuals report that they would experience negative affect such as disappointment and guilt, would intend to increase their exercise, and would employ self-regulatory strategies to help get their exercise back on track if they found themselves in a situation where they had been much less active than usual. However, individuals who report higher levels of exercise identity have reported a *stronger* self-regulatory response to the scenario than individuals who report moderate levels. These findings hold regardless of whether the individual perceives the cause of the identity-inconsistent behavior to be within (e.g., poor time management) or outside (e.g., exercise facility unavailable) his or her personal control. Individuals react similarly to *real-life* perceptions that their recent exercise has not been consistent with their exercise identities. For example, strength of exercise identity moderates affective reactions to one's perceptions that recent behavior is at odds with one's exercise identity; negative affect increases as perceptions of identity-behavior inconsistency increases but this relationship is stronger for individuals with stronger exercise identity scores. It also appears that participants who identify as exercisers exhibit a self-regulatory response to identity-challenging feedback when feedback about exercise identity comes from *others* (e.g., others in a situation perceive that the participant is not an exerciser). Finally, among members of running groups, strength of exercise identity (specifically, runner identity) appears to promote adaptive responses to the possibility of the running group disbanding. For example, strength of runner identity has been associated with self-efficacy for running and less difficulty running in the face of group disbandment. Taken together, these findings are in accordance with identity theory; exercise identity appears to act as a self-regulatory control system that helps people adhere to identity-congruent behavior even in the face of challenges and the effectiveness of this system may be influenced by strength of exercise identity.

Based on what is known about exercise identity to date, exercise identity can be considered a reliable correlate and predictor of exercise adherence. Further, exercise identity is associated with a variety of variables that are recognized for their ameliorative influence on exercise adherence. In the case of some of these adherence-related variables (e.g., self-efficacy, planning), exercise identity may exert its influence on exercise adherence through these variables. Together these findings support identity theory propositions regarding the role of exercise identity in promoting the successful self-regulation of exercise.

Practical Implications

Given that exercise identity has been established as a reliable correlate and predictor of exercise regulation and adherence, a logical and practical question to ask is how can we promote the strengthening or formation of exercise identities as a means for fostering exercise adherence? A first concern for the enterprise of building and strengthening identities is whether or not this construct is amenable to change. Proponents of identity theory such as Burke describe identities as being relatively stable and, by their very nature, resistant to change. Indeed, previous research has demonstrated that once established, people work hard to protect and confirm their exercise identities. Efforts at changing identities may be best targeted at situations where identity change is most probable such as when individuals are embarking on an exercise program and a few studies have demonstrated exercise identity change in these settings. These preliminary findings suggest that change in exercise identity is a possibility.

As reviewed previously, many correlates of exercise identity have been identified (e.g., self-efficacy, intentions). Deborah Kendzierski and her colleagues offered a formal model, the PA self-definition model, aimed at outlining factors associated with PA self-definition, a construct conceptually similar to exercise identity. This model demonstrates that when studied cross-sectionally, perceived commitment and ability relative to exercise directly relate to PA self-definition while enjoyment of exercise, perceived wanting, and trying to exercise are indirect determinants. This model makes a contribution by imposing some order on some of the many correlates of exercise identity and suggesting how they may work together in association with this construct. Further, this model holds potential as a basis for

intervention efforts aimed at increasing exercise identity.

Importantly, researchers are also beginning to determine which variables are associated with *change* in exercise identity. Preliminary efforts to this end employ both quantitative and qualitative research and suggest a number of variables are associated with change in exercise identity. These variables include perceptions of changes in skill mastery, physical changes in the body, progress toward exercise goals, perceived achievement, control, and belonging. Thus, research is starting to point to factors that may be important in strengthening or building exercise identities. Future intervention efforts that target these variables to bring about change in identity will help determine the best path to identity change. Exercise identity appears to be an important construct related to exercise adherence and further research exploring the role of this construct in the promotion of exercise, including intervention efforts, is likely and warranted.

Shaelyn M. Strachan

See also Self-Appraisal/Assessment/Perception; Self-Categorization Theory; Self-Construal; Self-Discrepancy; Self-Regulation; Self-Schema

Further Readings

Burke, P. J., & Stets, J. E. (2009). *Identity theory.* New York: Oxford University Press.

Cardinal, B. J., & Cardinal, M. K. (1997). Changes in exercise behavior and exercise identity associated with a 14-week aerobic exercise class. *Journal of Sport Behavior, 20,* 377–386.

Carraro, N., & Gaudreau, P. (2010). The role of implementation planning in increasing physical activity identification. *American Journal of Health Behavior, 34,* 298–308.

Hardcastle, S., & Taylor, A. H. (2005). Finding an exercise identity in an older body: "It's redefining yourself and working out who you are." *Psychology of Sport and Exercise, 6,* 173–188. doi: 10.1016/j.psychsport.2003.12.002

Kendzierski, D., & Morganstein, M. S. (2009). Test, revision, and cross-validation of the physical activity self-definition model. *Journal of Sport & Exercise Psychology, 31,* 484–504.

Strachan, S. M., & Brawley, L. R. (2008). Reactions to a perceived challenge to identity: A focus on exercise and healthy eating. *Journal of Health Psychology, 13,* 575–588. doi: 10.1177/1359105308090930

Strachan, S. M., Brawley, L. R., Spink, K. S., & Jung, M. E. (2009). Strength of exercise identity and identity-exercise consistency: Affective and social cognitive relationships. *Journal of Health Psychology, 14,* 1196–1206. doi: 10.1177/1359105309346340

IMAGERY

Imagery involves internally experiencing a situation that mimics a real experience without experiencing the real thing. As a conscious process that is deliberately employed by an athlete or exerciser to serve a specific function, it is distinctly different from daydreaming or just thinking about something. The terms *mental rehearsal* and *visualization* are sometimes used to refer to imagery, but this can be misleading for two reasons. First, although imagery is a popular type of mental rehearsal, this term encompasses a variety of mental techniques athletes and exercisers employ such as observation and self-talk. Therefore, imagery and mental rehearsal are not synonymous, but imagery use does fall within the category of mental rehearsal. Second, the term *visualization* implies that imagery only contains a visual component. However, it is well known that mentally simulating an experience can involve multiple sensory modalities. As well as being able to see the scenario, imagery allows an individual to feel associated movements and bodily sensations, and experience the sounds, smells, and even tastes related to the actual situation. Consequently, imagery is the most appropriate term to describe this cognitive process.

Imagery is deliberately employed by athletes and exercisers to achieve a range of affective, cognitive, and behavioral outcomes. When used effectively, this technique results in better performance, both directly and indirectly via improvements to, among other things, motivation, confidence, and attentional focus. Moreover, the frequency of imagery use is a marker of success in sport as well as level of engagement in physical activity. It is well established that athletes competing at a higher level and more active exercisers report greater use of imagery. Consequently, imagery has emerged as a popular topic within sport and exercise psychology and is extensively researched. This entry summarizes key research findings including (a) the main imagery modalities and perspectives characterizing athletes' and exercisers' imagery use,

(b) the functions and outcomes this imagery use can serve, and (c) how imagery can be used most effectively.

Imagery Modalities and Perspectives

Although imagery can be experienced through different sensory modalities, within movement domains such as sport and exercise, the two most commonly used are visual and kinesthetic. The visual modality refers to what the individual sees in the image and is therefore commonly referred to as the mind's eye. Visual imagery can be performed from either a first-person perspective or a third-person perspective. In a first-person perspective, also referred to as an *internal visual imagery perspective,* the individual views the scenario through their own eyes as if they were performing the movement. An athlete who is imaging herself kicking a ball from this perspective may see the ball down on the ground, her feet running toward the ball, her foot making contact with the ball, and the ball rising up in front of her. In a third-person perspective, also referred to as an *external visual imagery perspective,* the individual views the movement as if they were adopting someone else's point of view to see the scenario. This can be done from different viewpoints or angles, with the most common being in front, behind, the side, and above. Returning to the ball-kicking example, if the athlete was to view herself from a third-person perspective, she may see her entire body performing the kicking movement.

Kinesthetic imagery refers to how it feels when experiencing the situation. Most commonly this internal sensation refers to the muscles associated with performing a movement. A runner may image how his legs feel while performing the running action. However, kinesthetic imagery can also encompass other bodily feelings including body limb positioning, tactile information (e.g., the feet make contact with the ground), physiological responses (e.g., an increase in heart rate, pain, fatigue), and emotions (e.g., excitement, anxiety).

Historically, there has been some confusion related to the concept of imagery perspective and the terminology used. Initially, the first-person–internal visual imagery and third-person–external visual imagery perspectives were known simply as internal imagery and external imagery. However, these terms and how they were defined conveyed the impression that kinesthetic sensations could only be experienced using internal imagery. By confounding perspective with modality, this led to the assumption that *internal imagery* was the more effective way to image by providing the individual with a realistic and complete sensory experience (i.e., a movement could be both seen and felt). It has now been established that kinesthetic imagery can also accompany visual imagery performed in the third person. Furthermore, adopting the position of an observer appears to be particularly beneficial when imaging tasks with a focus on form or body positioning. This allows the individual to see information that otherwise would not be available from the first person perspective. If a figure skater is trying to improve her performance of a spiral, imaging the scenario from a third-person perspective is likely to help her better see the arch in her back, the height of her leg, and whether her toes are pointed. Alternatively, a first-person perspective is considered more beneficial when perception and timing are important to the skill being performed. A canoeist might view his slalom run from a first-person perspective to determine how to time the turns needed through different gates on the course. In other words, the benefits of imaging from a particular visual perspective will depend partly on the demands of the task being imaged and/or reasons for imaging.

Individual preferences also appear to matter, with some favoring a first-person perspective while others prefer a third-person perspective. It is likely that adopting the preferred visual perspective will make it easier to generate more vivid and controllable images, which in turn, would result in greater benefits from imaging. Individuals able to easily switch between perspectives would be able to maximize the benefits of imagery by appropriately matching the visual perspective to the task being imaged. Moreover, while the visual and kinesthetic senses can be used in isolation, combining these will create more effective images. During such multisensory imagery, individuals can experience both modalities simultaneously or switch their attention between what they are experiencing visually and kinesthetically to focus on a different modality at a particular time.

Imagery Use and Outcomes

Due to imagery's flexible nature, it is used at different times and in various locations. The most frequent occurrences for athletes are just prior to competing or during training, but they will use imagery throughout the season including during the off-season. Exercisers similarly report using imagery during an exercise session but will commonly use it beforehand. Both types of individuals will typically image within the sport and exercise environment where the benefits of this technique are maximized; for example, it would be more effective for a swimmer to mentally rehearse her race start by adopting the appropriate position on the starting block at the swimming pool, compared with sitting on a chair at home. However, athletes and exercisers should still be encouraged to use imagery in other locations, particularly when injured, ill, or traveling. Indeed, imagery is reportedly used at home, work, and school and in rehabilitation sessions.

Similarly to when and where imagery is used, what is imaged may vary greatly between individuals. Common images range from skills and strategies to those involving thoughts and emotions as well as one's own appearance and health. This content can be very specific and short in duration (e.g., imaging the action of throwing a ball) or be more complex and/or longer by combining different types of content (e.g., imaging an entire gymnastics floor routine with the appropriate attentional focus and emotions associated with best performances). Alongside the duration and complexity of the image, this content can take on different characteristics including the sensory modality, visual perspective, viewing angle, agency (e.g., imaging oneself vs. imaging other individuals), and timing (e.g., slow motion vs. real time). For example, a basketball player might image his teammates and therefore hear them calling for the ball during the scenario.

When deliberately employed, the imagery content is usually intended to serve a particular function or functions. These are most typically categorized as being either cognitive or motivational that, in turn, are classified at specific or general levels resulting in five main functions: (1) cognitive specific, (2) cognitive general, (3) motivational specific, (4) motivational general-arousal, and (5) motivational general-mastery (see Table 1 for definitions and examples).

Although imagery is most frequently used for motivational rather than cognitive functions, individuals typically use imagery for all five functions. Furthermore, reasons for imaging are not only

Table I   Cognitive and Motivational Imagery Functions

Imagery Function	Description	Athlete Example	Exercise Example
Cognitive Specific	To learn, improve, or maintain performance of specific skills	Improving performance of a tennis serve	Maintaining performance of a dumbbell curl
Cognitive General	To learn, improve, or maintain performance of strategies, game plans, or routines	Learning a new offensive play	Improving a strategy for a 5K run
Motivational Specific	To achieve specific process, performance, and outcome goals	Winning a race	Performing a set of 10 leg extensions
Motivational General-Arousal	To regulate emotions, mood, and arousal and anxiety	Reducing precompetition anxiety	Psyching up for a training session
Motivational General-Mastery	To modify cognitions	Improving confidence	Enhancing motivation to train

Source: Jennifer Cumming.

limited to these functions. Additional functions include those associated with injury rehabilitation (e.g., facilitate healing and pain management) and artistic endeavors (e.g., to choreograph a routine and understand how to interpret movements to music). The different imagery functions are intended to achieve various cognitive, affective, and behavioral outcomes. An exerciser might use imagery to improve his weight lifting technique and enhance his confidence to lift a particular weight for a number of reps. What is imaged to improve this technique and/or raise confidence will depend on both the individual and the situation. It is most common for individuals to closely match the content of their imagery to the function (e.g., image the skill for the purpose of improving that skill), but this is not always the case (e.g., image the skill for the purpose of reducing anxiety). Furthermore, imagery content can mean different things to different individuals. An image of winning a competition might be used by one athlete to motivate herself to train hard, but the same image might be used by another to maintain focus. The same imagery content can also be used in different situations to achieve varying functions. For example, a gymnast might image herself performing a routine correctly at practice to help improve her performance but image the same scenario immediately prior to competition to improve her confidence.

Effective Imagery

When imagery is combined with physical practice it can lead to greater improvements in the performance of a skill compared with just physical practice. Additionally, imagery can maintain performance levels in the absence of physical practice such as when injured or unable to train. The most contemporary explanation behind imagery's effectiveness is based on the partial overlap of certain neural networks involved with the planning and execution of motor movements during both imagery and execution of a particular skill. More simply put, some areas of the brain that are active when a skill is imaged are also active when the skill is physically performed. Researchers have described this partial overlap as a functional equivalence existing between the two activities. These similarities have also led to the suggestion that imagery might serve to prime performance of a skill by enabling neural networks to activate more accurately or more readily during actual performance.

Other theoretical explanations to imagery's benefits also exist, including the psychoneuromuscular theory, the symbolic learning theory, the bioinformational theory of emotional imagery, the triple code theory, dual coding theory, the action-language imagination (ALI) model, and the arousal or attentional set theory. Each theory has helped shape our understanding of imagery in different ways, but with the exception of the bioinformational theory, few of these have received empirical support.

Beyond merely improving the physical performance of skills and strategies, imagery also allows someone to rehearse and experience a scenario before it happens for real. This can help an individual mentally prepare for what they are likely to experience in the actual situation. Imagery can therefore allow the individual to anticipate what to expect. For example, a long jumper preparing for his first national championship might try to create a realistic preview of demands unique to this event by including in his imagery the presence of a loud crowd and distractions. By rehearsing how he will perform optimally in this situation, the athlete will likely feel prepared and more confident in his ability to cope when he actually experiences the situation for real.

A factor strongly influencing the effectiveness of imagery in serving its intended function is the individual's ability to image. Although everybody has the capacity to image to some extent, this ability will vary between individuals. For example, elite athletes tend to display a better imagery ability compared with lower level athletes. These differences can be reflected in a number of ways reflective of the imagery process, including how clear and vivid the image is, how realistic it is, and how well it can be modified and maintained once generated. Consequently there are a number of different methods used to assess imagery ability such as self-report questionnaires, computer tasks, and even brain imaging techniques. It is important to include some measure of imagery ability when conducting interventions because research demonstrates that individuals with higher levels of imagery ability experience greater benefits from imagery use compared with their lower-level counterparts who can experience few or sometimes no benefits. Moreover, although termed *ability,* an individual's capacity to create and control vivid and realistic images can be improved or enhanced with invested time and effort, similar to physical skills. It is

therefore thought that while some individuals may inherently find it easier to image compared with others, imagery can be honed with practice.

Making Imagery Effective

When imagery for skill learning and development is used to best effect, it will closely reflect the actual situation where the skill will take place. There are a variety of methods and techniques that can be used to improve imagery ability and maximize imagery's effectiveness. These methods can involve certain triggers or cues such as physical performance, sport or exercise equipment, observations and demonstrations, and imagery scripts to help prompt or guide the imagery scenario.

Physical performance can be done prior to imaging to remind an individual what it looks and feels like to perform a particular movement or action. This can help make the imagery more realistic. A soccer player might physically perform a penalty shot, then use this experience to help her image herself taking a penalty in the shoot-out of a championship tournament. As well, adopting physical characteristics associated with a scenario, actually incorporating certain pieces of equipment can facilitate more effective imagery. A javelin thrower who images himself throwing a personal best while holding a javelin and standing in the stance he would adopt before his run-up would likely prompt certain feelings and sensations associated with the situation thus creating a more vivid and realistic image.

Similarly to physical practice, observation clips and demonstrations can act as a template for the image and provide the individual with specific information or details about what the imaged movement or situation should look like. Unlike physical practice, however, this can be done for movements the athlete is not yet capable of performing. A novice golfer learning to perform a tee shot may use a coach's demonstration, either performed live or played back on video, to remind him of the positioning of his grip or head during the swing and follow-through. Additionally, these prompts may also help the imager work out some of the feelings associated with the image. The novice golfer may watch the smooth swing action of a demonstration to work out the feelings he or she should experience during the swing phase of the image. A few studies also suggest that observations can also be used when trying to image certain situations. Showing a video of a group of athletes performing a ski run on a particular course may help athletes image themselves performing on the same course.

Imagery scripts are used by athletes and exercisers to help them keep more focused on the scenario they are imaging. These scripts usually provide details of what and how the individual should image and guides them through the experience. Although typically audio recorded, some individuals may prefer to have a written script. Regardless of the format, scripts provide a clear beginning, middle, and end to the scene and prompt the individual to focus on specific modalities (e.g., by referring to your heart beating faster or hearing your teammates call to you). This can be particularly helpful for individuals who find it difficult to control or focus their imagery appropriately.

Finally, personalizing the imagery can make it more emotively meaningful to the athlete or exerciser. Including the relevant emotions in an image allows the individual to be able to draw from memories of their own real experiences more readily. In turn, these memories help make the imagery more vivid, detailed, and realistic. If an athlete or exerciser is unable to relate to the scenario, they are much less likely to be able to image the scenario clearly, making it unlikely to be effective.

Jennifer Cumming and Sarah E. Williams

See also Mental Rehearsal; Mirror Neurons; Modeling; Multimodal Mental Training; Simulation Training

Further Readings

Cumming, J., & Williams, S. E. (2012). The role of imagery in performance. In S. Murphy (Ed.), *Handbook of sport and performance psychology* (pp. 213–232). New York: Oxford University Press.

Hall, C. (2001). Imagery in sport and exercise. In R. N. Singer, H. Hausenblas, & C. M. Janelle (Eds.), *Handbook of sport psychology* (2nd ed., pp. 529–549). New York: Wiley.

Hall, C., Mack, D., Paivio, A., & Hausenblas, H. (1998). Imagery use by athletes: Development of the sport imagery questionnaire. *International Journal of Sport Psychology, 29,* 73–89.

Holmes, P. S., & Collins, D. J. (2001). The PETTLEP approach to motor imagery: A functional equivalence model for sport psychologists. *Journal of Applied Sport Psychology, 13,* 60–83.

Martin, K. A., Moritz, S. E., & Hall, C. (1999). Imagery use in sport: A literature review and applied model. *The Sport Psychologist, 13,* 245–268.

Implicit/Self-Theories of Ability

Implicit or self-theories of ability refer to individuals' views on the stability and changeability of personal attributes. Two lay theories are argued to exist: an entity theory, whereby individuals consider qualities and attributes of the self or others to be fixed and traitlike, and an incremental theory, whereby qualities and attributes are thought to be dynamic and changeable, and which can be developed. People can thus be described as entity or incremental theorists in relation to their beliefs about specific human qualities. In this entry, the pioneering work of Carol Dweck in the domain of intelligence is discussed. This body of work essentially examines how the two sets of beliefs lead to the adoption of different goals, which in turn, result in different outcomes in educational settings. This section will be followed by a presentation of key issues and empirical findings in sport and school physical education, demonstrating the theoretical and practical relevance of this area of research in sport and exercise psychology.

Research in the Education Domain: Beliefs About Intelligence

Interested in why children of similar ability respond to challenging tasks and achievement setbacks in a very different manner, Carol Dweck proposed that a mastery response (characterized by responding to challenge and setbacks with increased effort and determination to succeed) is underpinned by the pursuit of learning goals, which themselves are undergirded by the belief that intelligence can be improved. In contrast, the helpless response (characterized by responding to challenge and setbacks with negative affect and withdrawal from the task at hand) is underpinned by the pursuit of performance goals, which themselves are undergirded by the belief that one's level of intelligence is fixed. Learning goals refer to striving to develop competence in a self-referenced fashion whereas performance goals refer to striving to prove one's competence to others. Thus, beliefs and goals combine to create a meaning system or personal framework in achievement settings such as education. Adopting an incremental view of intelligence sets in motion an adaptive (mastery) response in which children, *irrespective* of actual ability, try hard, value the giving of effort, and are more likely to achieve their potential. On the other hand, adopting an entity view of intelligence sets in motion an adaptive response *only* when children are confident in their ability. When doubts about competence exist, a maladaptive (helpless) response is predicted, as children are unlikely to believe in their ability to demonstrate normative competence, and thus reveal to others their lack of (fixed) intelligence. It is thought that individuals do not possess a generalized cognitive style; instead, domain-specific frameworks exist within the person. This idea has led researchers to consider incremental and entity perspectives in the physical domain and, in particular, the notion of implicit beliefs about athletic ability.

Research in the Physical Domain: Beliefs About Athletic Ability

Initial research in the area of implicit beliefs in the physical domain has centered on youth sport and school PE. Essentially, researchers were interested in whether the two theories could be identified with reference to *athletic ability*. Thus, the concept of intelligence was substituted with physical competence in sport and PE activities. In order to discover whether processes of goal adoption and resultant outcomes were evident in the manner found in the classroom setting, it was necessary to devise a reliable measure of self-theories of athletic ability. Early efforts in this regard identified three components underpinning both incremental and entity theories. In relation to the incremental view, children and adolescents responded to items tapping learning, improvement, and specific aspects of athletic ability; in relation to the entity view, participants responded to items assessing gift, stable, and general aspects of athletic ability. Subsequent research resulted in the subscales of general and specific components of ability being dropped. The Conception of the Nature of Athletic Ability Questionnaire–Version 2 (CNAAQ-2) conceptualizes and measures the two theories as higher-order constructs underpinned by notions that ability in PE and sport can be learned and improved upon through hard work (incremental),

and by notions that ability is a genetic gift and immutable (entity). Work in the physical domain implicitly adopts the perspective that individuals' self-systems are domain-specific and not uniform across broad life domains (e.g., relationships, morality, stereotyping).

Correlational Research

Findings from correlational research with young people in sport and PE have generally supported the theoretical and empirical work of Dweck and colleagues in education. First, psychometric work with the CNAAQ-2 has supported the existence of the two implicit theories. Second, these theories have been linked with achievement goals and important outcomes. More specifically, an entity belief has been shown to positively predict amotivation in PE and sport (a maladaptive form of motivation characterized by a lack of purposeful intent and behavior—e.g., "I don't know why I'm doing this"). In contrast, an incremental belief has been shown to positively predict enjoyment. In both cases, these effects were partially mediated by performance and learning goals respectively. Work has also provided evidence of reliable links with affective responses, self-handicapping, and self-regulated learning in PE classes. For example, among Norwegian PE students, an entity conception of ability has been associated with increased anxiety and reduced satisfaction, regardless of perceived competence. In the same study, an incremental conception of ability predicted increased feelings of satisfaction among students.

Qualitative Research

In addition to correlational research with the CNAAQ-2, investigators in this area have undertaken qualitative forms of inquiry both to substantiate prior findings in regard to links with goals and outcomes but importantly to identify the socialization factors responsible for the development of theories within individuals. One study with low handicap golfers revealed the role of the coach in facilitating the view of golf ability as acquirable, the importance of high-profile role models such as Tiger Woods, learning about the game, and player's own practice and development. Peers were viewed as potentially endorsing either belief. Exposure to talented and dedicated golfers helped to formulate the view that natural talent could be built upon. Unexpected development in golf ability, as well as the notion that players with little all-round sporting ability could improve their golf, also underpinned the theme of developing natural attributes. Moreover, this study explored the idea of a ceiling effect (an upper limit at which the individual believes further improvement is not possible) and the potential specificity of golf beliefs (e.g., some aspects or components of the game may be seen as more fixed than others).

A second interview-based investigation has examined elite (Olympic standard) track and field athletes, specifically with respect to sprinters and throwers. As with golfers, the socialization of athletes' beliefs is complex, illustrating the value of conducting both quantitative and qualitative methods of inquiry in this area. In accordance with previous findings, athletes endorsed the importance of key social agents including family members and coaches in shaping beliefs. Interestingly, these studies have also identified psychological attributes, such as confidence and motivation, as components of achievement that are subject to entity and incremental perspectives.

One area of interest in sport, as in education, is how individuals respond to setbacks and the role played by implicit theories of ability in formulating a response. Setbacks have been found to revolve around injury, poor performance, and relationships. An incremental theory may help to buffer against setbacks and lead to a more optimistic view of the future—that is, that injury can be overcome, that performance can improved upon, that relationship issues can be resolved. However, more research is necessary to validate these notions.

Longitudinal Research: Are Young People's Implicit Theories Stable?

There has been some interest in whether and how implicit theories of athletic ability change as children transfer to secondary school. This work, although limited, has shown that both beliefs decline across the transition. Similar work has found evidence for a decline in athletic ability beliefs among older secondary school students. More longitudinal work is required—both to illuminate the direction and extent of changes in implicit beliefs that occur and to link these changes with important outcomes (e.g., goals, behavior) along with the factors that might explain instability in beliefs. One promising line of inquiry is to examine possible change in motivational climate

(the extent to which environmental cues in school PE classes or sports teams endorse either learning or performance goals) as a predictor of instability in incremental and entity theories.

Experimental Research: Can Ability Beliefs in Sport and Exercise Be Changed?

From an applied perspective, it is vitally important to investigate whether implicit theories themselves can be changed—that is, whether an incremental belief can be fostered in individuals. Studies have shown that school and college students' beliefs about athletic ability can be altered, at least temporarily. In experimental studies, beliefs are typically manipulated through participants reading a passage that espouses either an entity or incremental view of the ability concerned, such as golf putting ability or another novel exercise task. After conducting a manipulation check, links with cognitive, affective, and behavioral outcomes are examined. For example, attributions to ability following failure have been found to be higher among school students exposed to an entity theory manipulation than students exposed to the incremental condition. Researchers need to investigate alternative means of manipulating beliefs using video and Internet sources, as well as conduct longer-term interventions with PE classes, sports teams, and exercise groups. Research with adults in this regard is sorely lacking. Changing adults' perspectives on ability may prove more challenging compared with young people.

Conclusion

This entry has sought to discuss the concept of implicit or self-theories of ability in the physical domain. Building on original research in the education domain, it has been shown that incremental and entity perspectives of athletic ability can be identified and have important links with achievement-relevant outcomes. In addition, work in physical settings using multiple methods has sought to identify the antecedents of the beliefs, the role played by beliefs in dealing with setbacks or adversity, temporal characteristics of beliefs among young people, and the susceptibility of beliefs to experimental manipulation. More work in this area is warranted, not least because of the applied implications for coaches, exercise instructors, teachers, and, indeed, parents. Evidence to date suggests that identifying key socialization influences, and in particular, finding ways to foster and cement incremental views of ability, could have positive consequences for motivation and behavior in the physical domain.

Christopher M. Spray

See also Achievement Goal Theory; Attribution Theory; Personality and Psychological Characteristics of Athletes; Social Cognitive Theory; Youth Sport, Participation Trends in

Further Readings

Biddle, S. J. H., Wang, C. K. J., Chatzisarantis, N. L. D., & Spray, C. M. (2003). Motivation for physical activity in young people: Entity and incremental beliefs about athletic ability. *Journal of Sports Sciences, 21,* 973–989.

Dweck, C. S. (1999). *Self theories: Their role in motivation, personality, and development.* Philadelphia: Psychology Press.

Dweck, C. S., & Leggett, E. L. (1988). A social-cognitive approach to motivation and personality. *Psychological Review, 95,* 256–273.

Kasimatis, M., Miller, M., & Marcussen, L. (1996). The effects of implicit theories on exercise motivation. *Journal of Research in Personality, 30,* 510–516.

Slater, M. J., Spray, C. M., & Smith, B. M. (2012). "You're only as good as your weakest link": Implicit theories of golf ability. *Psychology of Sport and Exercise, 13,* 280–290.

Spray, C. M., Wang, C. K. J., Biddle, S. J. H., Chatzisarantis, N. L. D., & Warburton, V. E. (2006). An experimental test of self-theories of ability in youth sport. *Psychology of Sport and Exercise, 7,* 255–267.

Impression Management

See Self-Presentation

Individual Response Stereotype

Research and application in sport and exercise psychology (SEP) has relied heavily on psychophysiological applications. Heart rate (HR), blood pressure (BP), skin conductance (SC), and measurement of brain activity through sophisticated techniques such as positron-emission tomography (PET), electroencephalography (EEG) and magnetoencephalography (MEG), and functional magnetic resonance imaging (fMRI) are only a few of the many psychophysiological measures that have been successfully used to better understand psychological phenomena and clarify mechanisms in exercise and sport settings. For instance, studies examining the relationship between arousal and performance in sport have relied heavily on HR in order to classify individual performance at various levels of physiological activation or arousal. This area of research has led to the idea that individuals perform best when they are at an optimal level of arousal, not too over- and not too under-aroused. Physiological measures have also been employed in exercise psychology to better understand the effects of exercise on a wide variety of psychological and mental health outcomes including mood, anxiety, depression, cognitive function, and stress reactivity. In all of these studies, subtle changes in sensitive physiological measures are used to infer changes in readiness to perform or psychological state. These subtle physiological responses are believed to be a function of the demands of a situation or particular stimuli, an individual's predisposition to respond in a specific fashion, and the interaction between the two. Individual response stereotypy (IRS), or the tendency of individuals to evidence particular physiological response patterns from one condition or situation to another, is an important consideration in all studies or applications incorporating psychophysiological measures. The construct of IRS, also referred to as autonomic response patterning, has led to a growing recognition that the psychological and health significance of certain psychophysiological states are better reflected by the overall pattern of activity across multiple measures of physiological state, rather than from an acute response or sensitive change across only one or a select group of response domains, such as fluctuations in HR or SC. Complex patterns of physiological responses, which are determined by multiple factors, are thus best studied by incorporating multiple measures of physiological responding.

According to IRS, some individuals will respond to certain situations or conditions (e.g., anticipation of an upcoming event, performance of a difficult cognitive task, drawing of blood from the finger, rest) with the greatest degree of activity in the same physiological measure, regardless of the situation or stressor. This is particularly relevant for studies or applications that rely only on a few or unitary situations and response measures. As an example, in the area of stress reactivity, researchers have been interested in determining whether exercise or fitness are associated with blunted or altered cardiovascular responses to stress. When assessing BP responses to stress following acute aerobic exercise, it is important to determine not only baseline BP values (in order to assess change in stress-related BP following exercise) but also any individual difference variables that might influence BP responding. Individuals with borderline hypertension or essential hypertension tend to respond to stressful situations with greater increases in BP, particularly when compared to normotensive individuals. Assessing hypertension status would therefore be important. It is also important to note that individuals differ widely in both resting (tonic) and task-related (phasic) physiological responses. Understanding the factors that predispose some individuals to respond in unique ways helps inform the design of research studies as well as understand for whom and under what situations one person may perform optimally or realize the greatest benefits from exercise. This individual, unique pattern of responding has led to IRS being conceptualized as a physiological trait, or an enduring disposition of the body to show specific elicited physiological states or responses.

Although not all studies are in agreement, the notion of IRS points to several important implications. First, it is important to realize that individuals do not vary haphazardly in their physiological reactivity in a given response measure, nor do they vary haphazardly in their pattern of reactivity. Rather, some individuals may respond with maximal physiological activation in the same response measure or to a particular stimulus while another may be considered a low responder or nonresponder. Also, a strong tendency exists for a unique pattern of physiological response to be reproduced from situation to situation. This is so even though the physiological and psychological demands of the different situations may be unrelated. Second, IRS has resulted in a better understanding of the specific situational factors, familiarity with the situation, and range of behavioral choices that contribute to the expression of physiological responses. These factors can be used to strengthen future experimental designs and justify caution in oversimplifying physiological measures. Future studies should aim to elucidate the specific determinants of these unique patterns of response and consider IRS and situational

demands simultaneously. The problem of IRS does not currently appear to be a serious concern as long as careful consideration is given to the number and selection of physiological responses to be measured in psychophysiological studies. Also, a focus on IRS highlights the importance of studying *individual differences* in SEP research.

Brandon L. Alderman

See also Autonomic Nervous System; Biofeedback, Neurofeedback; Cardiac Function; Emotional Reactivity; Neuroscience, Exercise, and Cognitive Function; Psychophysiology; Stress Reactivity

Further Readings

Davis, R. C. (1957). Response patterns. *Transactions of the New York Academy of Sciences, 19,* 731–739.

Lacey, J. I. (1956). The evaluation of autonomic responses: Towards a general solution. *Annals of the New York Academy of Sciences, 67,* 125–163.

Stern, R. M., Ray, W. J., & Quigley, K. S. (2001). *Psychophysiological recording* (2nd ed.). New York: Oxford University Press.

INFORMATION PROCESSING

During the early part of the 20th century, psychology was dominated by the school of thought known as *behaviorism,* which emphasized that psychological processes could only be examined at the level of observable behaviors. This approach assumed that all behaviors could be understood in terms of simple stimulus–response (S–R) relationships and that references to mental processes were neither useful nor valid. To this extent, the behaviorists viewed all mental processes as a *black box* whose internal workings are not directly observable, and are inconsequential to understanding how behaviors are governed by environmental stimuli.

Driven in part by the inability to explain more complex behaviors, the field of psychology underwent a major paradigm shift in the 1950s, which later became known as the *cognitive revolution.* The internal processes of the black box once ignored by the behaviorists now became the primary interest in the emerging field of cognitive psychology. Consequently, understanding what occurs *inside* the "box" (the human mind) was viewed as essential for explaining complex human behaviors. Coinciding with this new direction, researchers began to observe similarities between human cognition and the early computers of the time. Both humans and computers could be viewed as general symbol manipulators, which can "take in" information, perform mental operations on the data, and finally output the information via behaviors and actions (e.g., images on a monitor). As a result, references to computers became a central metaphor for exploring human cognition, as it could provide direction and useful analogies for how humans process information mentally.

Humans as Information Processors

Based on this perspective, humans are fundamentally considered to be processors of information, with cognition understood as a sequence of computational processes. That is, information in the environment, such as words on a page, are taken in; stored in various memory systems; and processed via mental operations that encode, transform, and give meaning to the information through comparison with previously stored information (i.e., memory). Central to this approach is the suggestion that all information is encoded as internal symbolic representations of the external reality. These mental representations are constructed for all knowledge, information, ideas, and memories and are the subject of mental operations.

Systematic attempts have been made to study the capabilities and limitations of human information processing. Just as computers have certain limitations regarding speed of processing and how much information can be processed at any one time, similar limitations have been investigated with regards to human information processing. Given that mental operations occur within a black box, and thus are not directly observable, researchers have adapted and created a number of experimental methods from which overt behaviors are used to infer knowledge about the underlying cognitive processes. Chief among these approaches has been the use of *chronometric methods,* which emphasize the use of reaction times (RTs) to infer the temporal properties of mental operations. The Dutch physiologist F. C. Donders was the first to use such RT tests to determine the time needed for certain mental operations. Specifically, Donders argued that the duration of mental operations could be determined by subtracting the RTs of various types of tests

(e.g., simple RT, choice RT, go or no go RT) that have different cognitive processing requirements.

Three Stages of Information Processing

Every conscious action by humans, including those of athletes during action execution, is believed to be a consequence of response selection from long-term memory (LTM). LTM consists of a hierarchical structure neural network, which stores information after interacting with the environment. By definition, response selection indicates adaptive behavior based upon the capacity to solve problems. This "behavioral effectiveness" is directed by cognitive processes and mental operation. The effectiveness of these processes consists of the richness and variety of perceptions processed at a given time—that is, the system capacity to encode (store and represent) and access (retrieve) information relevant to the task being performed. From an information-processing perspective, motor behaviors consist of encoding relevant environmental cues through the utilization of attentional strategies, processing the information through an ongoing interaction between working memory and LTM, making an action-related decision, and executing the action while leaving room for refinements and modifications. Under pressure, changes in each of these components are seen. These changes are sequential in nature (i.e., they begin with the perceptual components, continue with the cognitive components, and end with the motor system).

Based on Donder's *subtractive method,* a number of different processing stages are conceived to exist between the presentation of a stimulus and the initiation of a response (see Schmidt & Lee, 2011). Specifically, at least three information-processing activities must occur during RT. First, the presentation of a stimulus must be detected and identified—the *stimulus-identification stage.* Next, the proper response to the stimulus must be chosen—the *response-selection stage.* Finally, the selected response must be prepared by the motor system and initiated—the *response-programming stage.* In the past 50 years, a number of studies have been conducted to determine the processing limitations of each of these stages as well as the factors that influence processing performance.

The *stimulus-identification stage* consists of the mental operations concerning the sensing and encoding of environmental information. As a stimulus contacts the body's sensory systems, it is taken in and encoded such that the neurological impulses activate the appropriate mental representation and knowledge associated with the information. A number of stimuli-related characteristics have been found to impact the speed at which the system is able to detect and encode relevant environmental stimuli. The *clarity* of the stimulus (i.e., how distinct and clear the stimulus appears) has been found to significantly impact the speed at which processing occurs during this stage. Specifically, RTs have been found to be slower when the stimulus is less defined compared to when the stimulus is presented with increased clarity (e.g., blurry vs. sharp picture). Similarly, the *intensity* at which the stimulus is presented impacts the speed of identification, with more intense stimuli resulting in faster RTs. Likewise, the modality of stimulus presentation has been found to influence the speed at which a stimulus is detected, as tactile and auditory stimuli have been found to result in faster RTs compared to visually presented stimuli. Once the stimulus is detected, it must also be correctly identified. In real life, the stimuli are often complex, and decisions must be made regarding a complex set of features. The ability to *recognize patterns* or features within the information set is important. Research indicates that task familiarity significantly influences the ability to quickly identify relevant features and patterns within the environment.

Following the detection and identification of the stimulus, a decision must be made regarding how to respond (i.e., what action to take). This stage is referred to as the *response-selection stage*. As with the previous stage, research has identified a number of different factors that influence the speed and selection of responses during this stage of processing. Not surprisingly, the time it takes for a person to decide upon a response has been shown to be influenced by the number of possible response choices they have. As the number of *S–R alternatives* increases, associated increases in choice RTs are observed. The mathematical relationship between RT and the number of response alternatives is given by Hick's law, which states that choice RT is linearly related to the Log_2 of the number (N) of S–R alternatives. Additionally, the *compatibility*, or the degree of fit, between the stimulus and response has been shown to influence RTs. For example, when the presentation of a stimulus and the required motor response are

spatially congruent (e.g., left stimulus and left response), RTs are quicker compared to when the stimulus and response are spatially incongruent (e.g., left stimulus and right response).

The final processing stage concerns the programming and initiation of the selected response, known as the *response-programming stage*. During this stage, the selected response must be compiled and transformed into overt muscular activity. F. M. Henry and D. E. Rogers demonstrated that the *complexity* of the movement required during the response is a critical factor in the latency of RTs during this stage. Specifically, responses that require more complex movements show larger latencies before the initiation of the response. This increased latency in responding is suggested to result from the additional time needed to prepare and program the upcoming motor action. A number of key factors relating to movement complexity have been identified which significantly influence this stage of processing. First, as the number of movement parts increases, corresponding increases in RT latencies are observed. For instance, responding to a stimulus with a simple finger movement is initiated faster compared to a response in which the whole arm must be utilized. Additionally, the accuracy requirements of the movement affect RT. As the precision demands of the movement response increase, increases in RT and movement time (MT) latency are likewise observed. Finally, responses with longer movement durations display increased RT and MT to initiate the motor response.

Conclusion

With the emergence of cognitive psychology, the view that humans are processors of information became the dominant framework from which to consider mental operations. In this regard, mental operations are viewed to consist of a series of information processing steps that begin with the taking in of information from the environment, processing that information, and then outputting the information via movement responses. Based on this framework, significant advancements have been made in the areas of intelligence, attention, decision making (DM), linguistics, and memory. Although more recent theoretical perspectives, such as ecological psychology and dynamical systems, provide alternative accounts of cognitive functions, the theoretical roots of information processing remain a strong influence in modern psychology.

William Land and Gershon Tenenbaum

See also Decision Making; Knowledge Structure; Memory; Motor Commands; Motor Control; Motor Development; Motor Learning

Further Readings

Donders, F. C. (1969). On the speed of mental processes. In W. G. Koster (Ed. & Trans.), *Attention and performance II*. Amsterdam: North-Holland. (Original work published 1868)

Henry, F. M., & Rogers, D. E. (1960). Increased response latency for complicated movements and a "memory drum" theory of neuromotor reaction. *Research Quarterly, 31*, 448–458.

Schmidt, R. A., & Lee, T. D. (2011). *Motor control and learning: A behavioral emphasis* (5th ed.). Champaign, IL: Human Kinetics.

Tenenbaum, G. (2003). Expert athletes: An integrated approach to decision making. In J. L. Starkes & K. A. Ericsson (Eds.), *Expert performance in sports* (pp. 191–218). Champaign, IL: Human Kinetics.

Tenenbaum, G., Hatfield, B., Eklund, R. C., Land, W., Camielo, L., Razon S., et al. (2009). Conceptual framework for studying emotions-cognitions-performance linkage under conditions which vary in perceived pressure. In M. Raab, J. G. Johnson, & H. Heekeren (Eds.), *Progress in brain research: Mind and motion—The bidirectional link between thought and action* (pp. 159–178). Oxford, UK: Elsevier.

Injury, Psychological Susceptibility to

Sport and recreational-related injuries have become a significant public health concern for physically active persons. For example, in 2006 the Centers for Disease Control and Prevention estimated that participation in high school sports will result in approximately 1.4 million injuries reported to medical staff at a rate of 2.4 injuries per 1,000 athlete exposures (i.e., practices or competitions). As sport and other physical activities continue to be promoted as part of maintaining and restoring health, there will continue to be an increase in sport-related injuries. These trends have resulted in multifactorial perspectives of injury prediction and prevention. Advances in safety of equipment, improvement to the physical environment, and new policies to protect sport participants have been implemented. Of relevance to this resource, but not likely as well known, are those approaches that involve the monitoring and modifying of psychological factors associated with sport injury.

Psychological Stress and Sports-Related Injury

In the 1960s, Thomas Holmes and colleagues suggested that changes in social stress, as measured by assessing accumulated stressful life events, were a precursor to changes in overall health. Essentially, life events often evoked changes in psychological status that required increased efforts to cope. This response to stress, or stress reactivity, was the mechanism underpinning the relationship between stress and health, whereby as stress demands and coping efforts increased, health would be compromised (e.g., onset of illness, progression of disease). In the 1970s, Holmes and later S. T. Bramwell and colleagues were the first to explore this notion in sport. They surveyed American football players and found greater levels of stress were associated with increased likelihood of athletic injury. This prompted further exploration of the relationship between stress and sport injury, yet much of what followed failed to replicate Holmes and Bramwell's findings. The literature lacked a unifying framework until 1988, when Mark B. Andersen and Jean M. Williams's model of stress and athletic injury filled an important gap and provided direction for future efforts.

Model of Stress and Injury

The stress-injury model posits that three categories of psychological risk factors (i.e., personality, history of stress, and coping resources) influence athletes' response to stressful athletic situations that, in turn, influences the likelihood of athletic injury through various stress-response mechanisms (see Figure 1). In addition to proposing psychological risk factors, their model offered specific avenues for psychological interventions and skills training to buffer adverse stress-related consequences for athletes' health and to minimize, or ideally prevent, athletic injury.

Stress Response Mechanisms

Cognitive Appraisal

Central to the stress and injury model is one's cognitive appraisal. Based upon the pioneering

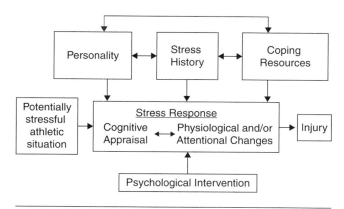

Figure 1 Stress and Injury Model

Source: Williams, J. M., & Andersen, M. B. (1998). Psychosocial antecedents of sport injury: Review and critique of the stress and injury model. *Journal of Applied Sport Psychology, 10*(1), 5–25. Adapted and reprinted with permission.

work of Richard Lazarus and Susan Folkman, the cognitive appraisal involves a balance (or imbalance) between two perceptions. The primary appraisal reflects perceived demands or threat of the stressor whereas the secondary appraisal reflects perceived personal and situational resources to cope with those demands and/or threat. When coping resources are perceived to be adequate to manage threat or demands, stress reactivity is minimal. In contrast, an imbalance occurs where one's perception of stress demands exceeds available coping resources, at which point stress reactivity is heightened.

Physiological Considerations

Very little attention has been given to physiological considerations. Within the model, stress responses that were initially described involved increase in muscle tension, which was thought to potentially impair motor control and slow reaction time (RT) that, in turn, may heighten injury vulnerability when engaged in sport competition and/or training. Over time, three additional pathways emerged associating psychological stress to physiological response. Perturbations in visual attention involving peripheral narrowing of visual field were described among highly stressed athletes and were hypothesized to heighten risk for injury (i.e., being blindsided). The other pathways linking stress to injury involved excess autonomic activity (e.g., increases in stress hormones) that were posited to increase injury risk by impairing immune

function and other cellular processes necessary for muscle repair following strenuous exercise training, or by altering sleep and associated secretion of growth factors also required for muscle anabolism. To date, excess elevation in psychological stress-related autonomic activity remains as the leading mechanism associated with athletic injury, but the specific causal pathway(s) remains unknown.

Attentional Considerations

In contrast to physiological factors, research studies have explored stress-related implications on attentional performance. Measures of visual and attentional indices have included peripheral narrowing and increased distractibility. In 1999, Mark Andersen and Jean Williams first demonstrated that peripheral narrowing mediated the relationship between injury outcomes and high stress in college athletes, and this was later replicated among high school athletes in 2005 by Traci Rogers and Dan Landers. While stress-related effects upon attentional and visual performance have been examined, there are other avenues (e.g., working memory capacity) that may be very relevant yet remain unexplored in the psychological injury vulnerability literature.

Psychological Factors That Influence Stress Response

Athletes who have a history of stress, a personality that amplifies perceptions of stress demands and/or reactivity to stress, and few available or effective coping resources are more likely to have cognitive appraisals of athletic situations that heighten their stress-reactivity. For those athletes, the consequences of heightened stress reactivity experienced within a sporting environment increase their risk of injury.

Personality

Research examining personality has measured patterns of behavior likely to exaggerate perceptions of stress demands and/or responses. In the original 1988 model, six likely personality variables were proposed and those included hardiness, locus of control, sense of coherence, competitive trait anxiety (TA), and achievement motivation. After nearly a decade of research, only four of those had received any attention and other characteristics had emerged that seemed appropriate that were not originally included (e.g., dispositional optimism). Today, well over 20 different personality factors have been explored as potentially associated with injury vulnerability. While evidence for an injury-prone athlete personality type has not emerged from any of this literature, very few personality variables have been examined in more than one study. Those exceptions that have been explored across multiple studies are anxiety, locus of control, mood states, and anger. Anxiety is the most frequently measured, and while operational definitions vary considerably across studies, those studies examining competitive TA have consistently demonstrated significant associations with injury. In contrast, the research on locus of control, mood states, and anger remains inconclusive.

Associated with personality, other characteristics and sport-related patterns of behavior involving behavioral genetics may also influence the athletes' psychological stress and injury vulnerability. Genome-wide association studies (GWAS) have found particular single nucleotide polymorphisms (SNPs) associated with sport-related ligament injuries. GWAS has not been applied to the study of possible mechanisms linking personality or psychological stress factors to athletic injury. However, behavioral genetic findings associated with mood regulation and conscientiousness identified in the general population may have relevance to athletes' emotional response to injury and behavioral adherence to recovery protocols. As an emerging area of inquiry, further research is necessary.

History of Stress

Stress history was the initial and continues to be the most commonly examined psychological risk factor associated with injury. Athletes' history of stress has been examined through measuring three different variables: major life events, daily hassles or minor life events, and prior injury history. Early studies by Holmes and Richard S. Rahe and colleagues measured accumulated life events (or total life stress) irrespective of the specific nature or impact of those events. Over the years, a focus has shifted away from measuring only accumulative life events and toward measures that examine the impact and valence of stressful events, as well as both life and sport-related stressful events typical of athletic populations. The evidence supporting a relationship between life events' stress and athletic injury is by far the clearest and most consistent.

In contrast to these findings, research examining minor life events or daily hassles has been less clear. By definition, daily hassles occur frequently and therefore contribute to sustained stress activation. Unfortunately, daily hassles have not always been measured in a manner that captures its reoccurring nature; when it has, it has been significantly associated with injury. The third variable, prior injury history, influences athletes' stress reactivity in a few important ways. Athletes who have been injured previously may be physically and/or psychologically vulnerable to re-injury due to returning to sport prematurely either because physical and/or psychological recovery was not yet complete. For example, athletes may be physically recovered but may still have considerable self-doubt and anxiety. Either independently or conjointly, cognitive and physiological symptoms of anxiety further heighten stress reactivity and may have a more pronounced impact upon cognitive, attentional, and/or physiological functioning. In recent reviews of the literature done by Jean Williams as well as our own recent work, approximately 80% to 90% of studies have documented significant relationships between stress history and sport injury. Collectively, the evidence supports the centrality of athletes' stress reactivity in determining stress-related vulnerability to sport injury.

Coping Resources

Compared to stress history and personality, less attention has been given to coping resources in the injury vulnerability literature. Coping resources involve both internal or personal factors as well as external or environmental factors, which collectively reflect the strengths and vulnerabilities in managing demands of stress. Internal coping resources examined have involved measuring athletes' general coping behaviors or self-care (quality of nutritional intake, sleep, etc.) and psychological or sport coping skills (regulation of one's thoughts, energy, attention, emotion, etc.). Researchers have not always been able to demonstrate a significant relationship between internal or personal coping resources and sport injury. When significant links have been reported, they have almost always reflected a protective effect—greater coping was directly or indirectly associated with lower injury risk.

External coping resources have primarily been evaluating the quality, quantity, and/or effectiveness of athletes' social support networks. In contrast to personal coping resources, results from studies examining social support are quite contradictory. Some studies have reported stress-buffering effects of social support while others have demonstrated increased stress-reactivity and injury risk with greater social support. These contradictory findings are perhaps suggestive of different stress-injury mechanisms across different sports.

Psychological Interventions for Health Promotion in Sport

The most exciting avenue of research is the efficacy of psychological interventions to prevent athletic injury. Intervention studies, based on Donald Meichenbaum's cognitive behavioral stress management (CBSM), involve the provision of education and skills training to athletes aimed to foster adaptive cognitions (e.g., thought stopping, restructuring) and/or manage physiological and attentional functioning (e.g., relaxation, mental rehearsal). To date, intervention studies have yielded medium to very large effects (e.g., 0.67–0.99), and the quality of this research has occurred at the highest level for therapeutic interventions (i.e., a randomized clinical trial). Findings provide strong support for psychological services for athletes to mitigate negative health-related consequences of sport participation (e.g., reduced injury or illness, time loss due to injury).

Renee N. Appaneal, Frank M. Perna,
and Leilani Madrigal

See also Autonomic Nervous System; Biopsychosocial Model of Injury; Stress Management; Stress Reactivity

Further Readings

Appaneal, R. N., & Habif, S. (in press). Psychological antecedents to sport injury. In J. Waumsely, N. Walker, & M. Arvinen-Barrow (Eds.), *The psychology of sport injury rehabilitation* (pp. 6–22). Oxford, UK: Routledge.

Johnson, U. (2007). Psychosocial antecedents of sport injury, prevention and intervention: An overview of theoretical approaches and empirical findings. *International Journal of Sport and Exercise Psychology, 5,* 352–369.

Perna, F. M., & McDowell, S. L. (1995). Role of psychological stress in cortisol recovery from exhaustive exercise among elite athletes. *International Journal of Behavioral Medicine, 2,* 13–26.

Petrie, T. A., & Perna, F. M. (2004). Psychology of injury: Theory, research, and practice. In T. Morris & J. J. Summers (Eds.), *Sport psychology: Theory, application, and issues* (2nd ed., pp. 547–551). Hoboken, NJ: Wiley.

Wade, C. H., Wilfond, B. S., & McBride, C. M. (2010). Effects of genetic risk information on children's psychosocial wellbeing: A systematic review of the literature. *Genetic Medicine, 12,* 317–326.

Wiese-Bjornstal, D. M. (2010). Psychology and socioculture affect injury risk, response, and recovery in high-intensity athletes: A consensus statement. *Scandinavian Journal of Medicine & Science in Sports, 20,* 103–111.

Williams, J. M., & Andersen, M. B. (2007). Psychosocial antecedents of sport injury and interventions for risk reduction. In G. Tenenbaum & R. C. Eklund (Eds.), *Handbook of sport psychology* (3rd ed., pp. 379–403). Hoboken, NJ: Wiley.

INJURY, RETURN TO COMPETITION FOLLOWING

Evidence suggests the challenges of injury recovery may not cease at the completion of athletes' physical rehabilitation. Over the past decade, researchers have uncovered a range of psychosocial issues, challenges, and demands associated with the return to competition following injury. In this entry, athlete experiences returning to competition, the motivational issues surrounding return, and options for evaluating athletes' mental readiness to resume competitive activities are examined. Throughout this entry, the phrase *return to competition* refers to injured athletes' transition from injury rehabilitation to sport-specific training and competition.

Athlete Experiences of the Return

In an attempt to examine athlete experiences in returning to competition following injury, researchers have solicited the perspectives of athletes, coaches, and sport medicine practitioners. Issues of competence, autonomy, and relational concerns prominently appear throughout published literature. Competence refers to a sense of being capable or proficient in one's pursuits. Competence concerns comprise the most commonly reported sources of athlete apprehension during the return to competition transition.

Competence issues are salient in athlete expressions of anxiousness over re-injury, concerns about the impact of injury on skill execution or loss of overall physical fitness. Athletes also typically report uncertainties about performing at pre-injury levels. Concerns over re-injury and competing at pre-injury levels are not surprising, given elite athletes' interest in athletic attainment and the inability to pursue goals over a potentially prolonged absence during injury recovery.

Research has also highlighted the salience of autonomy issues among returning athletes. Autonomy pertains to an individual's sense of choice or control over one's actions and behaviors. During the return to competition transition, athletes may experience varying degrees of choice and control over the timing and circumstances of their return. Whereas some athletes may be free to return at a time and manner of their own choosing, evidence suggests that many athletes face external pressures to return from coaches, teammates, or even sport medicine practitioners. Such pressures appear to be largely a function of the temporal proximity of upcoming competitions and the importance of the athlete in attaining desired team outcomes. Further complicating the situation are the internal pressures athletes place upon themselves to return to competition. Internal pressures may stem from intraindividual concerns regarding an inability to perform sport skills, self-generated worry that one is losing considerable fitness, or self-induced distress over "falling behind" fellow competitors during one's sport absence. Unfortunately, indicators of functional capacity (e.g., proprioception, joint range of motion) or consideration of the athlete's long-term health and well-being can sometimes be a secondary concern.

Finally, relational issues pertaining to the lost sense of connection to others and one's sport have been reported in the psychology of sport injury literature. Athlete perceptions of inadequate social support have also been highlighted. In particular, feelings of detachment and isolation, occurring during rehabilitation, may persist until such time as athletes are able to fully resume competitive play and contribute to valued team outcomes. Inadequate levels of social support may also contribute to relational concerns. For example, athletes report some coaches to be distant and insensitive to injury, uninterested in providing desired rehabilitation guidance, or as lacking a belief in their ability to return. Such distancing

by a coach may contribute to the perception that one is not a valued member of the team and that only those who are competing are deserving or worthy of the coach's attention. Confronted with this reality, it is not surprising that athletes all too commonly feel a sense of estrangement from their sport.

A lack of social support may also come in the form of insufficient information about recovery progressions and the requirements for attaining return to competition readiness. Specifically, some athletes have reported a lack of guidance and information from coaches and physiotherapists regarding adequate rehabilitative training to facilitate re-entry to the competitive arena. Such instances are unfortunate, given substantial evidence supporting the benefit of social support for injured athletes. Social support from coaches, family members, and athletic trainers may be essential in enabling the athlete to overcome the demands and uncertainties inherent in the return to competition.

Given the apparent relevance of competence, autonomy, and relational issues, Leslie Podlog and colleagues examined the impact of rehabilitation environments that satisfy athletes' need to feel competent, volitional, and connected to relevant others. Findings reveal that support for athletes in these three areas promotes enhanced well-being and effective return-to-competition outcomes. In particular, athletes who experienced a sense of competence and autonomy during rehabilitation had more positive emotions, which likely fostered a "renewed perspective on sport" following the return to competition (e.g., greater sport appreciation, heightened motivation for success, enhanced mental toughness). Moreover, those who felt a sense of connection to relevant others indicated less negative affect and greater self-esteem—both of which decreased the likelihood of athletes' experiencing "return concerns" (e.g., increased competitive anxiety, re-injury concerns). These findings highlight that the satisfaction of injured athletes' needs may facilitate perceptions of well-being and positive return to competition outcomes. Given these findings, it seems reasonable to suggest that interventions targeting competence, autonomy, and relatedness needs may help mitigate the challenges inherent in the return to competition. Further applied research aimed at minimizing athletes' return to competition concerns is needed, however, to explore the merits of this contention.

Motivational Issues

Motivational researchers Edward Deci and Richard Ryan suggest that the reasons why people engage in a behavior (i.e., their motives for action or involvement) may have important implications for the sustainment of such behaviors and the extent to which individuals experience optimal functioning or well-being. A wealth of evidence across various life domains including education, work, and relationships supports this line of reasoning. Operating from a similar assumption, Leslie Podlog and Robert Eklund recently examined the implications of athlete motives to return to competition on perceptions of post-injury performance. In an investigation with high-level athletes from Canada, Australia, and England, the researchers found that intrinsic motives to return to competition such as a love of the game or the excitement of participation were positively associated with a "renewed perspective on sport." On the other hand, athletes who were extrinsically motivated—that is, those who returned to competition because they wanted to attain external rewards or to avoid punishments, such as exclusion from participation—experienced greater "return concerns." Return concerns included, but were not limited to, diminished confidence, unsatisfying performances, and heightened competitive anxiety. Similarly, in an experimental investigation with professional Australian football league players, Podlog and Eklund found that greater intrinsic (versus extrinsic) motivations resulted in more positive thoughts and emotions regarding a return to competition. Interestingly, athletes who returned for intrinsic reasons such as a love of the game reported diminished perceptions of threat, unfairness, and potential damage to one's ego than their extrinsic counterparts. These findings suggest that the motivations underlining athletes' return to competition may have important consequences for the quality and nature of their return. In particular, the aforementioned studies by Podlog and Eklund indicate that intrinsic reasons for returning to competition may be associated with positive perceptions of a return to competition and enhanced post-injury performances.

Assessing Psychological Readiness to Return to Competition

Taking into account the abundant challenges and motivational demands placed upon returning athletes, the need for psychological evaluation is critically important. Several options presently exist for assessing athletes' psychological status upon return to competition. One option is D. W. Creighton and colleagues' three-step return to competition decision-making model. In Step 1 of the model, the health status of the athlete is assessed through the evaluation of medical factors (e.g., medical history of the patient, lab tests such as X-rays or MRIs, severity of the injury, functional ability, psychological state). Step 2 involves consideration of the risks associated with participation by assessing variables such as the type of sport played (e.g., collision, noncontact), the position played (e.g., goalie, forward), the competitive level (e.g., recreational, professional), the ability to protect (e.g., bracing, taping, padding), and the limb dominance of the patient. Step 3 in the decision-making process includes consideration of nonmedical factors that can influence return to competition decisions. Relevant considerations here include the timing in the season (e.g., playoffs), pressure from the athlete or others (e.g., coach, athlete's family), ability to mask the injury (e.g., pain medications), conflict of interest (e.g., potential financial gain or loss to the patient or clinician), and fear of litigation (e.g., if participation is restricted or permitted). The model provides a framework outlining the complex interaction of factors ultimately contributing to return-to-competition decisions. Utilizing the three-step process can help guide clinician decisions regarding athletes' return to competition.

In an effort to assess athletes' psychological state mentioned in stage 1 of Creighton and colleagues' model, researchers and practitioners are encouraged to use Douglas Glazer's Injury–Psychological Readiness to Return to Sport scale. The inventory is a valid and reliable scale consisting of six questions designed to assess athlete confidence regarding various aspects of their return to competition. For example, athletes are asked to rate their overall confidence to return to competition, their confidence to play without pain, and their confidence to give 100% effort. Given its concise nature, the readiness to return questionnaire can be easily administered by sport psychologists and health practitioners in the rehabilitation setting.

Another possibility in assessing psychological readiness to return to competition is Natalie Walker and colleagues' Re-Injury Anxiety Inventory. The questionnaire contains 28 statements aimed at uncovering the extent to which athletes experience uncertainty regarding re-injury. Fifteen of the questions pertain to re-injury anxieties during rehabilitation. These 15 questions require athletes to reflect upon the extent to which they are worried or feel nervous about becoming re-injured during rehabilitation. Another 13 questions assess re-injury worries upon return to competition. These 13 questions ask athletes to indicate how "worried" or "nervous" they are about becoming re-injured during re-entry into competition. Walker and her collaborators made efforts to distinguish fear (a flight-or-fight response to danger) from anxiety (uncertainty, worry, or concern) indicating the latter is a more accurate description of the athlete's state of mind.

Both the readiness to return and re-injury anxiety questionnaires may facilitate assessment of athletes' psychological state as they approach a return to competition. Low scores on either scale may alert health practitioners to the fact that athletes may not be psychologically prepared to resume competitive activities. Initial evidence suggests that athletes who experience heightened re-injury anxiety may have an elevated risk for poorer return-to-competition outcomes such as heightened competitive anxiety and diminished confidence in performing sport skills. It is also possible that re-injury anxieties or a lack of confidence in return-to-competition abilities increase athletes' actual risk of re-injury. This suggestion, however, requires further research.

Conclusion

Returning to competition following injury may entail a range of psychosocial challenges and demands. Issues pertaining to athletes' sense of proficiency, perceptions of autonomy, and feelings of connection to relevant others appear to predominate during the re-entry period. Evidence also reveals that athlete motivations to return to competition following injury may have important consequences for post-injury performances. Given the plethora of demands and motivational challenges associated with a return to competition, ensuring a holistic assessment of athletes' physical and psychological readiness is imperative. Creighton and colleagues' three-step decision making model can be a useful tool in determining an athlete's ability to safely and successfully compete after injury. Finally, two questionnaires, the Injury–Psychological Readiness to Return to

Sport scale and the Re-Injury Anxiety Inventory, show promise in facilitating evaluation of athletes' mental preparedness to return to competition.

Leslie Podlog and Robert C. Eklund

See also Injury, Psychological Susceptibility to; Intrinsic/Extrinsic Motivation, Hierarchical Model of; Psychological Well-Being; Self-Determination Theory; Self-Doubt; Self-Efficacy

Further Readings

Bianco, T., & Eklund, R. C. (2001). Conceptual considerations for social support research in sport and exercise settings: The instance of sport injury. *Journal of Sport & Exercise Psychology, 2,* 85–107.

Creighton, D. W., Shrier, I., Shultz, R., Meeuwisse, W. H., & Matheson, G. O. (2010). Return-to-play in sport: A decision-based model. *Clinical Journal of Sport Medicine, 20,* 379–385.

Podlog, L., & Eklund, R. C. (2005). Return to sport following serious injury: A retrospective examination of motivation and outcomes. *Journal of Sport Rehabilitation, 14,* 20–34.

Podlog, L., & Eklund, R.C. (2007). The psychosocial aspects of a return to sport following serious injury: A review of the literature. *Psychology of Sport and Exercise, 8,* 535–566.

Podlog, L., & Eklund, R. C. (2010). Returning to competition following a serious injury: The role of self-determination. *Journal of Sports Sciences, 28,* 819–831.

Roderick, M. (2004). English professional soccer players and the uncertainties of injury. In K. Young (Ed.), *Sporting bodies, damaged selves: Sociological studies of sports-related injury.* Oxford, UK: Elsevier.

INTERDEPENDENCE THEORY AND THE COACH–ATHLETE RELATIONSHIP

In sport, and sport coaching more specifically, the connection between coach and athlete is instrumental for optimal functioning, be it physical, psychological, mental, or social. In fact, there is strong evidence to suggest that success in sport is the product of the combined interrelating between the coach and the athlete. Athletes are unlikely to produce top-level performances without the direction and encouragement of their coaches, and coaches are unlikely to be successful without their athletes' hard work, commitment, and enthusiasm. Thus, coaches and athletes who are locked into a relationship that is harmonious and stable are also more likely to achieve sport success (e.g., skill development, tactical awareness, trophies, medals) and make the journey to success more pleasurable, satisfying, and personally fulfilling.

Interdependence Theory

Interdependence theory (IT) is an important framework for understanding the processes of personal and social relationships including a central relationship in sport—namely, the coach–athlete relationship. It focuses on how those in relationships, such as coaches and athletes, cause one another to experience positive versus negative outcomes. Positive outcomes are reflected in the *rewards* the relationship and its members experience such as happiness, gratification, and pleasure while negative outcomes are reflected in the *costs* the relationship and its members experience, such as anxiety, conflict, and antagonism. *Interdependence* is a fundamental element because it can affect how, for example, a coach and an athlete influence one another's outcomes through the processes of exchanging, communicating, and interacting. Moreover, these processes allow relationship members to understand themselves and one another.

Interdependence in the Coach–Athlete Relationship

The notion of interdependence in the coach–athlete relationship was recently captured by the constructs of *closeness, commitment, complementarity,* and *co-orientation,* known in the literature as the 3 + 1 Cs model. Closeness represents coaches' and athletes' affective bond and is reflected in such relational properties as mutual trust, respect, appreciation, interpersonal liking, as well as emotionally caring and supporting one another. Commitment represents coaches' and athletes' thoughts of maintaining an athletic partnership that is close over a long period of time (e.g., the emphasis is on staying near to each other physically or symbolically; to want to coach the athlete or be coached by the coach now and in the future). Complementarity represents coaches and athletes' behavioral exchanges that are (a) affiliative and corresponding, such as members being friendly, responsive, and comfortable in each

other's presence, and (b) organized and reciprocal, such as members assuming their specific and respective roles in a suitably and effective manner (e.g., coach instructs and athlete executes). Finally, co-orientation reflects the degree to which athletes and coaches are perceptually similar (i.e., have a similar understanding as this may relate to the relationship and its outcomes). The 3 + 1 Cs model provides a conceptual and operational model to study the degree to which relationship members are interdependent.

Interdependence Structures

According to IT, the *interdependence structure* in dyadic relationships such as the coach–athlete relationship can be defined by examining the main effects and interaction of each relationship member's behaviors, including (a) actor control (e.g., a main effect of athlete's actions on athlete's outcomes), (b) partner control (e.g., a main effect of coach's actions on athlete's outcomes), and (c) joint control (e.g., an interaction of coach's and athlete's outcomes). Interdependence structure is composed of four properties known as degree of dependence, mutuality of dependence, basis of dependence, and correspondence of interests.

Degree of dependence reflects the extent to which an athlete depends on his or her coach and, thus, the degree to which an athlete's outcomes depend on his or her coach's actions. Dependence is a psychological significant relational characteristic that can exert positive and negative effects on the coach and the athlete as well as their relationship. Research has shown that, for example, coaches' and athletes' dependence on each other in terms of the 3 + 1 Cs can promote open channels of communication and self-disclosure, skill and performance development, physical self-concept, motivation, passion, team cohesion, collective efficacy (CE), and well-being, to name a few. However, coach–athlete dependence can also have negative consequences. For example, low levels of dependence in terms of the 3 + 1 Cs have been found to be detrimental to athletes' morale, performance, satisfaction of basic psychological needs, and well-being. In this case, athletes and coaches would appear to be uncomfortably dependent on one another and more often than not they perceive one-sided dependence (caused by situational factors such as power struggles and/or individual difference factors such as personality, age, maturity).

Mutuality of dependence describes the extent to which a coach and an athlete are mutually rather than separately dependent on one another for generating enjoyable or fulfilling outcomes. Healthy, harmonious, and stable coach–athlete relationships as characterized by the 3 + 1 Cs are expected to involve a considerable degree of mutual dependence (e.g., we support each other) rather than one-sided dependence (e.g., I support him, but he doesn't support me). Mutually dependent relationships and interactions tend to yield rewards. There is evidence in the literature that when coaches and athletes are mutually dependent (both relationship members experience and perceive mutually high levels of 3 + 1 Cs), personal and interpersonal rewards are yielded. However, when coaches and athletes have been found to be nonmutually dependent, upset and discomfort were more readily experienced. In one study, it was found that athletes feel less dependent and satisfied with the relationship (while coaches may continue to feel highly dependent and satisfied), when they perceive that their coaches' resources (e.g., experience, skills, knowledge) are depleting or their self-interests lie elsewhere (e.g., more emphasis is given to other athletes in the team or squad).

Basis of dependence describes the way in which coaches and athletes influence one another's outcomes or whether dependence results from, for example, one's member control (e.g., coach). There are many empirical and anecdotal examples that highlight coaches' power to have control over their athletes, but there are also examples whereby both coaches and athletes have joint control over each other's outcomes. Coordinated forms of interaction whereby, for example, the coach orchestrates the proceedings of training, instructs, and supplies advice while the athlete receives the instructions and advice positively and responsively are indicators of relationship members' comfort with the basis of dependence. If discomfort was experienced due to a member being unwilling to interact in a coordinated fashion (instead interacted in a one-sided or competitive fashion) the likely result would be poor individual and relationship outcomes. Finally, *correspondence of interests* describes the extent to which an athlete's and a coach's actions yield rewards for both members in a corresponding fashion. While interaction is relatively easy when both a coach and an athlete's interests correspond (e.g., we want to win an Olympic title; we want to maintain an effective and successful partnership), interaction is relatively tricky when their interests conflict (e.g., Coach wants me to go to a summer camp but I don't; athlete never talks, opens up, shares news). Correspondence of interests may range from perfectly correspondent to perfectly noncorrespondent and may be reflected by the degree to which coaches and athletes perceive high or low and corresponding or noncorresponding levels of the 3 + 1 Cs. An open channel of communication has been viewed as a major factor that leads to correspondence of interests and has been found to be a major contributor to enhancing interdependent coach–athlete relationships.

Comparison Level and Comparison Level for Alternatives

IT posits that relationship members' evaluations of their relationships are influenced by two standards: *comparison level* (CL) and *comparison level for alternatives* (CL-alt). CL is a criterion against which coaches and athletes evaluate how satisfactory the relationship is whereas CL-alt is a criterion coaches and athletes are likely to use to decide whether to stay in or leave the relationship. Within IT, satisfaction with a relationship per se is a function of comparing the rewards and costs of that relationship with some type of internal standard (CL). In contrast, deciding whether to stay in a relationship is a function of comparing the rewards and costs of that relationship with the rewards and costs of other relationships that are available (CL-alt). For example, someone may remain in a dissatisfying relationship (below his or her CL) because the satisfaction available in other relationships (CL-alt) is less. Alternatively, someone may leave a satisfying relationship (above his or her CL) because the satisfaction available in other relationships (CL-alt) is greater. Research that focuses on the links between interdependence and satisfaction has found that a coach's and an athlete's interdependence as measured by the 3 + 1 Cs are positively related to satisfaction with training, instruction, and performance accomplishments, as well as satisfaction with personal treatment and athletic relationship. Moreover, it has been found that interdependence (as defined by the 3 + 1 Cs) and satisfaction with training, instruction, and personal treatment were weaker for lower-level (i.e., club) competitors than for higher-level competitors (i.e., regional, national, and international). Finally, associations between interdependence and satisfaction were stronger for longer relationships and same-gender dyads (all male and all female coach–athlete dyads) than mixed-gender dyads (female coach–male athlete and male coach–female athlete). Collectively the findings of these studies underline that coaches and athletes depend on each other for obtaining valued outcomes; this is reflected in their evaluations of developing a positive relationship and in their beliefs that the other relationship member meets important outcomes.

Conclusion

From an IT point of view, coaches and athletes are likely to be both attracted to a relationship and satisfied with it as the rewards associated with the relationship increase and costs decrease. The research evidence to date suggests that more interdependent relationships (defined by the 3 + 1 C) may be more satisfying because they fulfill basic human needs, heighten positive affect, and enhance self. The application of IT can provide a framework to understand and explain important research questions that relate to complex processes within the phenomenon of the coach–athlete relationship.

Sophia Jowett

See also Attachment Theory and Coaching; Coach–Athlete Relations; Commitment; Conflict; Passion; Relational Efficacy Beliefs in Coach–Athlete Relations; Self-Determination Theory; Team Communication

Further Readings

Jowett, S. (2003). When the honeymoon is over: A case study of a coach–athlete relationship in crisis. *The Sport Psychologist, 17*, 444–460.

Jowett, S. (2008). Outgrowing the familial coach–athlete relationship. *International Journal of Sport Psychology, 39*, 20–40.

Jowett, S., & Cockerill, I. M. (2003). Olympic medalists' perspective of the athlete–coach relationship. *Psychology of Sport and Exercise, 4*, 313–331.

Jowett, S., & Nezlek, J. (2012). Relationship interdependence and satisfaction with important outcomes in coach–athlete dyads. *Journal of Social and Personal Relationships, 29*, 287–301.

Kelley, H. H., & Thibaut, J. W. (1978). *Interpersonal relations: A theory of interdependence.* Toronto: Wiley.

Rusbult, C. E., Kumashiro, M., Coolsen, M. K., & Kirchner, J. L. (2004). Interdependence, closeness, and relationships. In D. J. Mashek & A. Aron (Eds.), *Handbook of closeness and intimacy* (pp. 137–162). Mahwah, NJ: Lawrence Erlbaum.

Rusbult, C. E., & Van Lange, P. A. M. (2003). Interdependence, interaction and relationships. *Annual Review of Psychology, 54*, 351–375.

Thibaut, J. W., & Kelley, H. H (2007). *The social psychology of groups* (4th ed.). New York: Wiley.

INTERFERENCE

The need for consistency in training, motor learning, technical preparation, and competition is well understood by coaches, athletes, and applied sport psychology (SP) consultants. A number of factors, however, can interfere with athletes' ability to perform or learn at an appropriate level during training, technical preparation, and competition. The term *interference* addresses the decrease in performance due to conflicts between different cognitive modules or motor structures within the human action system in a specific environmental constellation.

Interference in Cognitive Learning and Verbal Memory

In the psychological realm, interference is mostly discussed in the context of memory and learning. Interference is addressed as a memory problem that occurs when a learning process is impaired because of an existing, stabilized memory structure or when the activation of consolidated memory representations is affected because of newly learned material. Interference in learning with verbal material has been observed and studied for more than 100 years. Notably, the studies of the German psychologist Georg Elias Müller opened up new perspectives on the topic of memory consolidation. While the studies of Hermann Ebbinghaus (1885) hypothesized forgetting as a function of time, Müller and his student Alfred Pilzecker provided evidence for interference-based memory loss and an interference-based decrease of learning. The term *retroactive interference* was coined by Müller and describes the phenomenon seen in memory in which newly learned material affects the recall performance of previously learned information. In the opposite direction, *proactive interference* specifies the phenomena that—depending on the task—previously learned information potentially impairs the learning of new information. Proactive interference is commonly explained as competition between two learning processes that are based on the same cognitive resources. From this point of view, in the case of retroactive interference, the learning of new material influences the consolidation of previously learned material in memory. During proactive interference, consolidated memory information is challenged by new information and inhibits the consolidation of new information in memory. Subsequent studies have found that similarity between the information already stored in memory and the new material affects the learning process and causes interference.

Interference in Motor Learning and Motor Memory

In motor control research, interference is mostly discussed in the context of motor learning. The learning of new skills is based on previously learned sensory-motor patterns that are stored in memory. In general, there are two possible types of interactions between previously learned skills and recently acquired skills: (1) a positive and supportive interaction called *transference* or (2) a negative interaction called *motor interference*. Transference was originally addressed by researchers like Nikolai A. Bernstein and is explained as the facilitation of learning as a result of similarity between the required motor pattern and the existing stored pattern, while conversely, motor interference is mostly hypothesized as a negative overlap (i.e., dissimilarity) between the coordination patterns of previously learned motor actions and the structure of a recently acquired skill. From this point of view, learning to crawl could generally facilitate skills like canoeing because of similarities in motor structures (transference), while techniques in sports like tennis and badminton at the same time seem to be related at a surface level but suffer from interference because of significant differences between the relevant sensory-motor structures at a functional level.

Charles H. Shea and other researchers addressed the topic of *contextual interference* and compared performance during practice of a motor task under randomized and blocked conditions. They found that practicing the task in a blocked order, repetitively and under stable conditions (low contextual interference), resulted in better performance than did practicing the task under randomized conditions (high contextual interference). Interestingly, however, when the performance between random and blocked practice was compared, these and other studies revealed that the random practice group showed superior performance to the blocked practice group. It has been hypothesized that in the short term, reduced interference supports the learning process of simple motor skills, but in the long term, randomized practice supports the establishment of more stable representations in motor memory and leads to better performance compared to the more artificial (low contextual interference) conditions.

Interference Between Motor Control and Verbal Memory

Until now, the phenomenon of interference has been mostly investigated in the area of verbal memory research, isolated from motor learning and vice versa. Interference in the context of motor learning has often been discussed as it relates to memory resources, but it remains unclear whether or not motor planning and verbal working memory share common cognitive resources. In our daily life, verbal memorization and motor action are often performed together—for instance, remembering a list of consumables in a shop while walking along the shop floor and searching for the next product.

In the research area concerning the learning and storage of lists in working memory, the *serial position effect* is a stable finding. This effect is observed when subjects memorize and recall a sequence of items. Subjects are best able to memorize the items presented at the beginning of the list (primacy effect) and the end of the list (recency effect). This recall paradigm has often been used to learn about interference in verbal memory. Combining a motor task and a verbal memory task could lead to two kinds of interference: *cognitive interference* or *motor interference*. In the case of cognitive interference, the memorization of verbal lists would decrease the motor performance; conversely, the opposite would be true in the motor interference scenario. In a variety of tasks such as replanning of motor actions and sequential motor planning in unimanual and bimanual coordination, researchers like Matthias Weigelt, Mark G. Fischman, and Marnie A. Spiegel have investigated in recent years the interference between motor planning and recall performance. In multiple experiments, they found evidence for the so-called *motor interference hypothesis*—that is, that motor planning reduces memory performance of verbal items because of the challenge between these two entities.

Thomas Schack

See also Attentional Association and Dissociation; Automaticity; Memory

Further Readings

Logan, S. W., & Fischman, M. G. (2011). The relationship between end-state comfort effects and memory performance in serial and free recall. *Acta Psychologica, 137,* 292–299.

Shea, J. B., & Morgan, R. L. (1979). Contextual interference effects on the acquisition, retention, and transfer of a motor skill. *Journal of Experimental Psychology: Human Learning & Memory, 5,* 179–187.

Spiegel, M. A., Koester, D., Weigelt, M., & Schack, T. (2012). The costs of changing an intended action: Movement planning, but not execution, interferes with verbal working memory. *Neuroscience Letters, 509,* 82–86.

INTERVENTIONS FOR EXERCISE AND PHYSICAL ACTIVITY

Interventions in the field of exercise or physical activity (PA) psychology focus on issues related to health rather than on issues related to performance in sport. Exercise, by definition, suggests a form of PA that is often structured and undertaken with the aim of improving fitness. However, health benefits can be obtained from more incidental modes of PA that are not primarily done for fitness benefit such as gardening, dog walking, or bicycling to work. Such activity may have different determinants than those that could be defined as exercise and so, to encompass both, the term *PA–exercise psychology* is used in this entry. PA–exercise psychologists employ a wide range of skills, some of which overlap with the skills used by sport performance psychologists, to assist individuals and groups achieve sufficient PA to gain health benefits. PA–exercise psychologists also engage in research to further understand what constitutes effective interventions that may influence population health. When psychologists intervene with individuals, groups,

or communities, they use approaches that have a strong evidence base for successfully increasing PA levels. This health-related aspect of sport and exercise psychology (SEP) is growing in importance because of the global public health risk posed by lack of sufficient PA. This entry summarizes the importance of PA for health, discusses the need to decrease sedentary time, introduces the global call to action in the Toronto Charter for Physical Activity, describes a series of interventions that have global support and represent good investments for countries seeking to increase population levels of PA, and finally makes a recommendation that all interventions should be properly evaluated.

The Importance of Physical Activity for Health

Physical inactivity is the fourth leading cause of mortality from chronic diseases such as heart disease, stroke, diabetes, and cancers, and inactivity contributes to the rising obesity levels noted around the world. For children, the recommended minimum amount of activity shown to be beneficial is 300 minutes of moderate intensity activity over the course of a week, and for adults, the recommended minimum is 150 minutes of moderate intensity activity over the course of a week. Public health physical inactivity is a serious challenge: Inactivity is a risky health behavior and, because the majority of Western populations do not achieve the minimum amount of activity for health, it is also a very prevalent risk. There is also a considerable challenge in increasing the levels of PA within a country's population. Psychologists are part of a team of professionals contributing to determining how best to increase population levels of activity.

The New Issue of Sedentary Behavior

A new aspect of this health-related field is the developing understanding that lengthy periods of sedentary time, such as those experienced in many desk jobs or through TV viewing, may be detrimental to health even if the person achieves the currently recommended minimum amount of activity for health. There is therefore also a need for interventions to focus on how people might decrease the number of minutes they spend in sedentary activities. Exercise and PA psychology has a clear role to play in the design, implementation, and evaluation of interventions that promote PA behavior or decrease sedentary time.

The Toronto Charter for Physical Activity

The Toronto Charter for Physical Activity, which was launched in May 2010 by the Global Advocacy Council for Physical Activity (GAPA), is an important milestone in the history of PA and public health. The aim of the charter is to create sustainable opportunities for physically active lifestyles for everyone. Within the Toronto Charter there are nine guiding principles listed for a population-based approach to PA. Psychologists should use the charter to guide their role in developing interventions to increase PA and decrease sedentary time. The charter's principles identify the importance of evidence-based approaches—of embracing equity by reducing social and health inequalities or removing disparities in access to PA. Importantly, the principles acknowledge the need to move beyond the individual to include environmental and social determinants of physical inactivity. Other principles identify sustainability, a life-course approach to promoting activity, and the need to garner political support and resource commitment at the highest level.

What Kinds of Interventions Are Appropriate?

One common framework for understanding the various levels at which intervention aimed at improving health may take place is known as the socioecological model. This model suggests that there are multiple influences on PA and sedentary behavior, such as individual psychology, social circumstances, the surrounding physical environment, and wider sociopolitical influences such as culture and policies. This suggests that interventions aimed at increasing individuals' activity levels must take into account these wider influences, and psychologists need to work in partnership with other agencies to advocate for environments that encourage activity, such as the creation of foot paths and bicycle lanes. In addition, exercise psychologists must also work at the policy level and advocate for the creation of local and national policies that lay out strategic objectives for raising the level of PA. However, the issue of which interventions to use for greatest effect is not easy to resolve because the evidence base is relatively young, and one cannot say with certainty which approaches are best. Agencies such as the Centers for Disease Control and Prevention in the United States and the National Institute for Health and Care Excellence (NICE) in the United Kingdom

issue guidance from time to time, which is based on thorough and critical reviews of the available evidence, and these resources are useful starting points for psychologists wishing to understand the current evidence. For example, NICE issued a set of guidelines on the best approaches to changing the environment to promote PA.

Which Interventions to Use?

GAPA and leading academics and practitioners from around the world have reviewed evidence for interventions that were effective in increasing PA levels. This review led to the production of a companion document to the Toronto charter, titled "Seven Investments That Work" (www.globalpa .org.uk/investments). These seven approaches are as follows:

1. *Whole-of-school programs*. In these programs, schoolchildren of all ages are encouraged to be active in a variety of ways such as on the journey to and from school, during school break times, and after school and via quality physical education (PE) programs.

2. *Transport policies and systems*. By intervening at the level of transport systems, people might be encouraged to use public transport, which is almost always a more active journey than a car, or they might be encouraged to actively commute from place to place by foot or by bicycle. Transport policies that prioritize walking and cycling and provide safe infrastructure, such as well-lit pavements and off-road cycle paths, could have a substantial impact on population levels of PA. Scandinavian countries provide good examples of this approach.

3. *Urban design regulations and infrastructure*. Towns and cities that provide for equitable and safe access to recreational PA, such as playgrounds and sports facilities, with opportunities for all ages to participate, support lifelong involvement in PA.

4. *Primary care programs*. Every patient in a health service scheme, who is visiting a doctor or nurse for whatever reason, should be asked about his or her current level of activity and given encouragement and opportunities to increase activity to benefit health.

5. *Public education*. Many people simply do not know the risks of inactivity nor the amount of

activity needed to gain health benefits. Public education is therefore needed and might include mass media to raise awareness and change social norms around PA to help create a culture in which being physically active is normal behavior.

6. *Community-wide programs.* Offering opportunities to be active in one's local community and mobilizing community engagement and resources is seen as an effective route in helping people be more active.

7. *Sports systems and programs that promote "sport for all."* When sport is taught within schools and communities, coaches should employ a "sport for all" ethos that encourages participation across the life span in preference to an ethos that only promotes elite-level sport.

How Should Physical Activity–Exercise Psychologists Design and Evaluate Interventions?

When PA–exercise psychologists intervene, perhaps in one of the seven areas listed previously, to promote PA or reduce sedentary behavior, they should base their work on a recognized theory of behavior change and use the principles of that theory to develop appropriate materials. They must also consider a framework to guide the evaluation of their intervention. At a minimum, all interventions must measure PA behavior, ideally with an objective monitor such as a pedometer or accelerometer, to determine if improvements have occurred.

Nanette Mutrie

See also Adherence; Affective Responses to Exercise; Energy, Effects of Exercise on; Intrinsic/Extrinsic Motivation, Hierarchical Model of; Obesity; Quality of Life; Sedentary Behavior; Stress Management

Further Readings

Biddle, S. J. H., & Mutrie, N. (2008). *Psychology of physical activity: Determinants, well-being, and interventions* (2nd ed.). London: Routledge.

Craig, P., Dieppe, P., MacIntyre, S., Mitchie, S., Nazareth, I., & Petticrew, M. (2008). Developing and evaluating complex interventions: The new Medical Research Council guidance. *British Medical Journal, 337,* 979–983.

Katzmarzyk, P., Church, T., Craig, C., & Bouchard, C. (2009). Sitting time and mortality from all causes,

cardiovascular disease, and cancer. *Medicine & Science in Sports & Exercise, 41*(5), 998–1005.

Sallis, J., & Owen, N. (2002). Ecological models of health behavior. In K. Glanz, F. Lewis, & B. Rimer (Eds.), *Health behavior and health education: Theory, research, and practice* (3rd ed., pp. 462–484). San Francisco: Jossey-Bass.

Intrinsic/Extrinsic Motivation, Hierarchical Model of

The hierarchical model of intrinsic and extrinsic motivation (HMIEM) is a comprehensive theory that seeks to describe human motivation and its determinants and outcomes from a multilevel perspective. Its major premise is that in order to more completely understand the motivation of sport participants (e.g., athletes, coaches, referees, fans), one needs to consider their motivation in various contexts and at various levels of generality. In line with self-determination theory (SDT), the HMIEM posits the existence of three types of motivational constructs: intrinsic motivation (behaving out of pleasure and free choice), extrinsic motivation (behaving to obtain rewards or avoid punishments), and amotivation (the relative absence of motivation). These motivational constructs are organized both vertically and horizontally within the HMIEM. This structural arrangement serves to integrate knowledge on the personality (vertical axis) and social psychological (horizontal axis) determinants of motivation.

First, the vertical organization of elements in the HMIEM specifies that the three types of motivation (intrinsic, extrinsic, and amotivation) exist at three different levels of generality: global, contextual, and situational. The most stable level is situated on top (the global level) and the most ephemeral (the situational level) at the bottom. The global level corresponds to a person's usual way of functioning at the personality level (e.g., Susan is typically intrinsically motivated). The next level is the contextual level. It corresponds to one's usual motivation in a particular context such as sports, education, leisure, or interpersonal relationships. This type of motivational orientation is moderately stable and can vary from one context to another. For instance, Susan may be intrinsically motivated to play sports but extrinsically motivated to go to school. Finally, the situational level is the most specific and refers to one's motivational state in the present moment, the here and now. For instance, you may observe that Susan is intrinsically motivated to play tennis right now.

Top-Down and Bottom-Up Effects

Importantly, the HMIEM postulates that relationships exist between the levels of the hierarchy such that the type of motivation one has at a given level influences his or her motivation at the other levels. The relationships between motivation at the different levels of the hierarchy take place through the *top-down* and *bottom-up effects*. Top-down effects refer to the influence of higher levels in the hierarchy upon lower levels. Specifically, global motivation influences both contextual motivation and situational motivation whereas contextual motivation influences only situational motivation. Each level has the strongest influence on the level immediately below (i.e., the proximity principle). In other words, global motivation will have a stronger influence on contextual motivation than on situational motivation. For example, if Susan has a high global intrinsic motivation, all else being equal, she is also likely to have a high level of intrinsic motivation at the contextual level (next level below) such as in sports. Research supports this top-down hypothesis showing that the more athletes have a high level of contextual intrinsic motivation for sports the more they have a high level of situational intrinsic motivation during a game. Similar findings have been obtained in physical education (PE) settings.

Second, bottom-up effects represent the influence of lower levels in the hierarchy upon higher levels. This effect explains how repeated motivational changes at a given level instigate changes in motivation at the next higher level. For example, if Susan repeatedly experiences increases in intrinsic motivation (e.g., during many tournaments), she may become more prone to adopt an intrinsically motivated orientation in the context of sports. In turn, this increase in intrinsic motivation at the contextual level in sports may also lead to increases in intrinsic motivation at the personality level (i.e., the global level). The proximity principle applies here as well. Thus, situational motivation will have a stronger effect on contextual motivation than it will on global motivation. Longitudinal research provides support for these hypotheses.

Social Psychological Processes

The HMIEM also describes a horizontal organization of elements that describe the nature of the social psychological processes through which changes in motivation take place and lead to outcomes. The same sequence takes place at all three levels of the hierarchy: "Social Factors→Psychological Needs→Motivation→Outcomes." At the beginning of the sequence, it is postulated that motivation is determined first and foremost by social factors. For instance, global social factors are so pervasive that they are present in most areas of a person's life. One example is parenting, which represents a rather continuous influence on children because it spans many life contexts and situations. The way parents raise their children determines, in part, whether the children will adopt an intrinsic or extrinsic way of interacting with the environment (i.e., a global motivation). Second, contextual social factors are recurrent factors but only in a specific context such as in basketball (i.e., a basketball coach) or in school (i.e., a teacher). Third, situational social factors are present at a single point in time. For example, winning a basketball game on a Sunday afternoon may have an impact on one's situational motivation to join another scrimmage match when the opportunity comes up. Importantly, global social factors determine global motivation, contextual factors determine contextual motivation, and situational factors determine situational motivation.

Next, the HMIEM postulates that the influence of social factors on motivation occurs through basic psychological need satisfaction. Need satisfaction acts as a mediator between social factors and motivation at every level of generality in the model. The more an individual's psychological needs are met in general, in a given context or in a specific situation, the more he or she will engage in activities in an intrinsic way at the global, contextual, or situational level. For example, the more athletes perceive their coach as supporting their needs for autonomy, competence, and relatedness, the more they will develop an intrinsic motivation for sports. Much empirical support exists for the role of need satisfaction as mediators of the effects of social factors (e.g., the coach's behavior) on athletes' motivation. Of additional importance is that motivation in different contexts can interact in different ways. For instance, motivation in a given context (e.g., education) may add to, or even conflict with, motivation in another context (e.g., sport). In other words, there might be compensation or additive effects among different contexts. Research in sport and education empirically supports the presence of such effects.

Finally, the social psychological process ends with the effects of motivation on outcomes of three types: affective, cognitive, and behavioral. Such effects take place at every level of the hierarchy and are specific to the level of generality. In other words, global motivation produces global outcomes, contextual motivation produces contextual outcomes, and situational motivation produces situational outcomes. For example, Susan may generally experience positive emotions, enhanced concentration, and better performance when playing sports because she has an intrinsic motivation in this context. However, she may experience less desirable consequences such as negative emotions, decreased concentration, and poorer performance in another context (e.g., at school) because she is more extrinsically motivated in this context. At all levels of generality, intrinsic motivation leads to the most positive outcomes whereas extrinsic motivation produces the least positive consequences. Once again, research supports these postulates.

In sum, the HMIEM offers a comprehensive explanation of athletes', coaches', referees', and fans' motivation from multilevel, personality, and social psychological perspective.

Daniel R. Lalande and Robert J. Vallerand

See also Passion; Self-Determination Theory

Further Readings

Blanchard, C. M., Mask, L., Vallerand, R. J., de la Sablonnière, R., & Provencher, P. (2007). Reciprocal relationships between contextual and situational motivation in a sport setting. *Psychology of Sport and Exercise, 8,* 854–873.

Ntoumanis, N., & Blaymires, G. (2003). Contextual and situational motivation in education: A test of the specificity hypothesis. *European Physical Education Review, 9,* 5–21.

Vallerand, R. J. (1997). Toward a hierarchical model of intrinsic and extrinsic motivation. *Advances in Experimental Social Psychology, 29,* 271–360.

Vallerand, R. J. (2001). A hierarchical model of intrinsic and extrinsic motivation in sport and exercise. In G. Roberts (Ed.), *Advances in motivation in sport and exercise* (pp. 263–319). Champaign, IL: Human Kinetics.

Vallerand, R. J. (2007). A hierarchical model of intrinsic and extrinsic motivation for sport and physical activity. In M. Hagger & N. Chatzisarantis (Eds.), *Intrinsic motivation and self-determination in exercise and sport* (pp. 255–363). Champaign, IL: Human Kinetics.

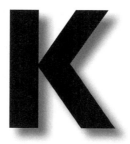

KNOWLEDGE STRUCTURE

Knowledge about tasks and the environment is organized hierarchically in the human cognitive system, involving the diverse long-term memory (LTM) systems and working memory. Knowledge structures underlying task performance are fundamental elements of action control in sports. Experts' skills are often based on the efficient access to relevant task knowledge as well as on enhanced physical abilities. In the history of research in general psychology, motor control, and sport psychology (SP), knowledge structures have been addressed in different ways, focusing on their significance for task performance from different perspectives.

Structured Motor Programs, Schemata, and Events

In the field of motor control, Richard A. Schmidt's generalized motor program (GMP) theory has been one of the most prevalent theories used to explain how we control coordinated movements and how we therefore develop structured plans and knowledge. GMP theory is based on feedback-based models, such as James A. Adams's closed-loop theory of motor learning, and adopts the concept of schema, making it more adaptable and thereby a more realistic explanation of motor learning, especially as it occurs in sporting contexts. Schmidt describes GMPs as templates that serve as abstract plans for basic movements. GMPs can be adapted to individual situations by modifying variant and invariant parameters. Parameters such as absolute timing, absolute force, and building blocks (individual muscle actions) within the GMP can vary (variant parameters). In contrast, the sequence, relative timing, and relative force of these building blocks are thought to remain invariant.

Schmidt uses the term *schemata* (recall schema, recognition schema) to explain how movements can be learned on the basis of GMPs. Support for a structured organization comes from research investigating the underlying neuronal structures of movement. According to these studies, the basic definition describes organization principles in action and perception that are based on neuronal structures but include functional levels of behavior and cognition up to and including language. According to Michael A. Arbib's theory, motor schemata and perceptual schemata interact in complex ways but are coordinated by control programs that generate and control action performance on a higher level.

More recently, event segmentation theory, developed by Jeffrey M. Zacks, has provided an interesting approach to studying structure and modularity in perception and knowledge memory, showing that the way in which a person spontaneously segments an observed action determines the understanding and later memorizing of this action. This approach can be well applied to sporting contexts. When watching a basketball match, we spontaneously segment the observed stream of movements performed by the different athletes into meaningful actions. Our understanding of the scenario is based on the way we store an event in memory and segment what we see, the number of segmentation points, the choice of cues, and so on. Naturally, the quality of our understanding is strongly influenced by our own experience and our structured knowledge about the type of action.

Declarative and Procedural Knowledge Structures

A very interesting and often-cited distinction of knowledge quality and structure has been provided in the adaptive components of thought (ACT) theory by John Anderson, a psychologist at Carnegie Mellon University. ACT and later versions such as ACT-R have been inspired by the idea of Allen Newell to develop a cognitive architecture of knowledge. Such a cognitive architecture is computationally implemented in a technical system and is able to simulate a wide range of tasks. ACT is based on production systems. As do other psychological theories, it differentiates between declarative knowledge and procedural knowledge. Knowledge about facts (e.g., a BMW is a German car) has been called *declarative knowledge*. The relevant knowledge elements are facts and events. This knowledge has been characterized as explicit knowledge and as *knowing that*. *Procedural knowledge* about, for instance, bicycle riding is implicit knowledge about how to perform a task. It has been therefore characterized as *knowing how*. Both declarative and procedural knowledge are stored in LTM and are related to each other especially in the learning process. Neurophysiological research has shown that their storage and retrieval are based on different brain structures.

Anderson has described the development of knowledge structures within three phases of motor skill learning. The first phase is characterized as a cognitive phase. In this phase, the learning agents are developing a declarative encoding of the motor skill. They store a lot of facts and explicit elements of the learning process in memory. The second phase is an associative phase. In this phase, single elements of procedural and declarative knowledge become more strongly interconnected, and motor production rules are created. In this phase, it is possible to perform some motor acts step by step and to develop a declarative frame for motor activities. The last phase is the autonomous phase. In this phase, the motor procedures become faster and more and more automated.

Based on perspectives coming mostly from the ACT theory, a number of researchers have addressed the question of how declarative knowledge is structured and networked in sport actions. The major issue of relevance in the SP domain is whether we can confirm that improved performance is accompanied by a higher degree of order formation in the sense of knowledge structuring and hierarchies. Research has therefore been undertaken to confirm expertise-dependent differences in the classification and representation of context-specific problem states in, for instance, springboard divers, judokas, triathletes, and weight lifters. Research on springboard diving has revealed that the nodes of the representation structures in experts possess far more features than those of novices. This result replicates findings in the problem-solving domain. Likewise, expert springboard divers show a greater number of connections between nodes, just as do experts in problem solving. An interesting study about the development of declarative knowledge structures and performance in sports was conducted by Karen E. French and Jerry R. Thomas. They assessed various components of basketball performance (e.g., control of the basketball and cognitive decisions, dribbling and shooting skills) along with declarative knowledge in children ages 8 to 12. Declarative knowledge was measured via a paper-and-pencil test. Results confirmed relationships between knowledge and the decision component of performance, suggesting that knowledge plays an important role in skilled sport performance.

Studies using categorization tasks have shown that experts classify problems according to underlying functional principles, whereas novices operate more strongly with superficial features. Furthermore, questionnaire methods and interviews have revealed the structure and organization of movement knowledge in sports.

Mental Knowledge Representation and Hierarchies in Memory

The idea that actions are mentally represented in functional terms as a combination of action execution and the intended or observed effects is well established in cognitive psychology and has received growing acceptance in the fields of motor control and SP. Perceptual-cognitive approaches, such as the ideomotor approach to action control, propose that motor actions are formed by mental knowledge representations of target objects, movement characteristics, movement goals, and the anticipation of potential disturbances. David A. Rosenbaum and coworkers demonstrated that movements can be understood as a serial and functional order of goal-related body postures, or goal postures, and their transitional states. The link between movements and perceptual effects is bidirectional and based on information that is typically stored in a hierarchical fashion in LTM. Complex movements can be conceptualized as a network of sensorimotor information. The better the order formation in memory, the more easily information can be accessed and retrieved. This leads to increased motor execution performance, which reduces the amount of attention and concentration required for successful performance. The nodes within this knowledge network contain functional subunits or building blocks that relate to motor actions and associated perceptual (including related semantic) content. These building blocks can be understood as representational units in memory that are functionally connected to perceptual events or as functional units for the control of actions, linking goals to perceptual effects of movements.

Research in complex actions in sports, dance, rehabilitation, and manual action has demonstrated that basic action concepts (BACs) are fundamental building blocks at the cognitive level of representation. BACs are based on the chunking of body postures related to common functions in the realization of action goals and are conceptualized as representational units in LTM that are functionally connected to perceptual events. From this point of view, action control is organized as perceptible event through a structures representation of anticipated characteristic (e.g., sensory) effects, with the corresponding motor activity automatically and flexibly tuned to serve these effects.

The integration of representation units, like for instance BACs, into structures of representation has been studied with a wide range of methods. Based on a new experimental approach, Thomas Schack and Franz Mechsner studied the tennis serve to investigate the nature and role of LTM in skilled athletic performance. In high-level experts, these representational frameworks were organized in a distinctive hierarchical treelike structure, were remarkably similar between individuals, and were well matched with the functional and biomechanical demands of the task. In comparison, action representations in low-level players and nonplayers were organized less hierarchically, were more variable between persons, and were less well matched with functional and biomechanical demands.

The results of different studies in golf, soccer, windsurfing, volleyball, gymnastics, and dancing have shown that the mental representation structures in place relate clearly to performance. As different studies have shown, these representations are also position- and thereby task-dependent. These representation structures are the outcome of an increasing and effort-reducing formation of order in LTM. This order formation reveals a clear relation to the structure of the movement. With increasing expertise, the representation of the movement corresponds more and more exactly to its topological (spatiotemporal) structure. At this level, the representation has nothing to do with a muscle-oriented effector code. Evidently, the representation structures are formed through the sensory movement effects of distinctive node points (body postures) of the movement. Therefore, the representation structure itself possesses spatiotemporal properties, corresponding with the structure of the movement. Accordingly, movement control becomes possible by representing the anticipated intermediate effects of the movement and comparing them with incoming effects. Importantly, this also means that no special translation mechanism is required between perception, representation, and movement.

Results from another line of experimental research have showed that not only the structure formation of mental representations in LTM but also chunk formation in working memory is built up on BACs and relates systematically to movement structures. These studies have revealed a plausible relation between chunking and priming processes in working memory and the structure of human movements, suggesting a movement-based chunking. Such findings provide experimental evidence that structures in movement and memory mutually overlap.

These results and perspectives are of central meaning for the understanding of cognitive learning and coaching processes. A disadvantage of traditional procedures in mental training (imagery) is that they try to optimize the performance through repeated imagination of the movement without taking the athlete's mental knowledge representation into account (i.e., they are representation-blind). Problems arise if the movement's cognitive reference structure has structural gaps or errors, as these will tend to be stabilized rather than overcome by repeated practice. The alternative approach is to measure the mental representation of the movement before mental training and then integrate these results into the training. This mental training based on mental representations has now been applied successfully for several years in professional sports such as golf, volleyball, gymnastics, and windsurfing and recently in the rehabilitation of hand functions in patients after stroke.

Thomas Schack and Bettina Bläsing

See also Chunking/Dechunking; Expertise; Information Processing; Memory; Pattern Recognition and Recall

Further Readings

Adams, J. A. (1971). A closed-loop theory of motor learning. *Journal of Motor Behavior, 3,* 111–150.

Anderson, J. R. (1976). *Language, memory, and thought.* Mahwah, NJ: Lawrence Erlbaum.

Arbib, M., Conklin, E., & Hill, J. (1987). *From schema theory to language.* New York: Oxford University Press.

French, K. E., & Thomas, J. R. (1987). The relation of knowledge development to children's basketball performance. *Journal of Sport Psychology, 9,* 15–32.

Koch, I., Keller, P., & Prinz, W. (2004). The ideomotor approach to action control: Implications for skilled performance. *International Journal of Sport and Exercise, 2,* 362–375.

Rosenbaum, D. A., Meulenbroek, R. G., Vaughan, J., & Jansen, C. (2001). Posture-based motion planning: Applications to grasping. *Psychological Review, 108,* 709–734.

Schack, T., & Hackfort, D. (2007). An action theory approach to applied sport psychology. In G. Tenenbaum & R. C. Eklund (Eds.), *Handbook of sport psychology* (3rd ed., pp. 332–351). Hoboken, NJ: Wiley.

Schack, T., & Mechsner, F. (2006). Representation of motor skills in human long-term-memory. *Neuroscience Letters, 391,* 77–81.

Schmidt, R. A. (1975). A schema theory of discrete motor skill learning. *Psychological Review, 82,* 225–260.

Zacks, J. M., Kumar, S., Abrams, R. A., & Mehta, R. (2009). Using movement and intentions to understand human activity. *Cognition, 112,* 201–216.

KÖHLER EFFECT

See Social Processing Effects

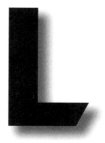

LAWS OF MOVEMENT LEARNING AND CONTROL

Various laws of movement learning and control have been proposed on the basis of research. In this entry, the focus is on three of the most firmly established of these laws: the law of practice, Fitts's law, and Hick's law. These laws are of interest to sport and exercise psychologists because they specify relatively simple relationships between different variables related to movement learning and control. The defining feature of these laws is that the relationships they specify apply to many different populations (e.g., males and females, the young and the elderly) and types of movement in sport and exercise. The laws are useful because they afford the identification of practice-related conditions that promote movement learning and predictions about how individuals will perform in various situations requiring movement. As such, the laws provide a basis for the design of practice and training curricula, schedules, and environments and also for the design of equipment for sport and exercise. The laws are described here, in turn.

The Law of Practice

The *law of practice* states that more practice of a motor task will lead to more learning of that task. This definition is usually accompanied by a second statement: Changes in motor task performance that follow practice are generally large and rapid at first and become gradually smaller with continued practice. As an example, consider a scenario in which 30 novice gymnasts are each provided with 10 practice sessions, in which the gymnast attempts to stand one-footed on the beam, with the other leg bent at the knee, without wobbling or falling off the beam. Each practice session is separated by a 3 days' rest, lasts 2 hours, and begins with one test of how long, in seconds, the gymnast can do the task before they experience an obvious wobble or a fall. Consider then that the average of the 30 gymnasts' test scores is calculated for each of the 10 days' tests and the average values are plotted on a graph against the practice sessions undertaken. The law of practice predicts that the graph would look something like the (hypothetical) example graph shown in Figure 1. Note from the graph that, consistent with the law of practice, the increase in time spent balanced one-footed on the beam is greatest early in practice, between Practice Sessions 1 and 2, and becomes smaller with more practice; the smallest increase occurs between Practice Sessions 9 and 10. One interpretation of this effect is that the rate of improvement at any point in practice is determined by how much learning remains. Early in the practice of a given task, much remains to be learned and thus the rate of learning is very rapid. After extensive practice, there is not much left to be learned, so learning is much slower. At this late stage of learning, it can take months or even years of practice before any noticeable gain in performance is attained. As with all of the laws described here, the law of practice applies to many different populations and types of

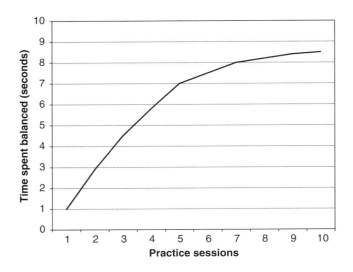

Figure 1   A Hypothetical Example Demonstrating the Relationship Between Task Performance (Time Spent Balanced One-Footed on a Gymnastics Beam) and Amount of Practice as Predicted by the Law of Practice

Source: David W. Eccles.

movement task, from turns in skiing to throws in discus.

It is important to define practice in relation to the law of practice. Practice activities can differ widely, and these differences are not always appreciated, leading some individuals to engage in what they consider to be practice activities only to be disappointed when little or no learning follows. While the exact qualities of practice activities affording optimal learning in sport and exercise are in contention, Anders Ericsson and his colleagues have proposed the term *deliberate practice* to capture some of the qualities that appear associated with learning. Deliberate practice is structured, purposeful practice relevant to improving performance. It requires concentration and/ or effort and is often undertaken alone to allow the learner to concentrate; these characteristics make the *process* of engaging in deliberate practice inherently unenjoyable, even if the *result* of deliberate practice is enjoyable, such as the acquisition of a new skill. Deliberate practice activities are often focused on improving weaker components of current performance—for example, a backhand volley in tennis. Coaches are often employed to identify these components and prescribe specific deliberate practice activities to improve them— for example, drills to practice backhand volleys at various distances from the net. These components

are often practiced in isolation from other components of the sport, which affords an increase in the rate of attempts to practice the component; a tennis player might devote an entire practice session to practicing her backhand volley.

Thus, the deliberate practice of a task contrasts with mere engagement in, and experience of, a task. A common example of this difference concerns golf. A golfer seeking to improve his game adds a nine-hole round with friends to his weekly golf schedule, which he considers extra practice but no improvement in his game results. On closer inspection, however, the holes are played in a relaxed way and the "practice" session lacks the qualities of deliberate practice. Thus, this golfer's addition of nine holes to his weekly golf schedule affords him the opportunity to obtain more experience of the game but does not involve its deliberate practice. Hence, there is no improvement in the golfer's game.

Fitts's Law

Fitts's law describes in more formal terms what is known in everyday terms as the speed-accuracy trade-off; that is, it describes the relationship between the speed of a movement and its accuracy. In the 1950s, researcher Paul Fitts created an experiment in which two targets were laid upon a table-type surface in front of a participant; one target was positioned slightly to the left of the participant and the other slightly to the right. The participant's task was simply to tap anywhere on the surface of the left target and then the right target using a stylus, which was a penlike rod, held in one hand, and then repeat this (i.e., left target, right target, left target) as fast as possible for a specific time such as 30 seconds. The task was like hitting one drum with a drumstick, and then another drum (with the same drumstick in the same hand), then the first drum, and so on, as fast as possible. In the experiment, the width of the two targets could be varied; for example, they each might be small, at 2 cm in width, or large, at 10 cm in width. Also, the distance between the targets could be varied; for example, they might be closely spaced, with 10 cm between them, or farther apart, with 20 cm between them. The task was scored as the number of taps the participant could make in the time allowed. Accuracy was stressed by asking the participant to make sure that no more than 5% of the taps fell outside of a target. Fitts calculated the average time taken between two consecutive taps by dividing the time over which the participant was requested to tap (e.g., 30 seconds) by the number of taps made: If 30 taps were made in 30 seconds, the average time between 2 consecutive taps was 1 second. In other words, it took the participant a second on average to tap one target and then move his or her hand to the other target and tap that target. Fitts called this variable *movement time* (MT).

Fitts explored what happened to MT when the width of each target and the distance between the targets was varied. When targets at a fixed distance apart (e.g., 10 cm) each had their width reduced (e.g., from 4 cm to 2 cm), MT increased; participants appeared to need to move slower to be more accurate in the spatial positioning of their taps. Also, when targets of a fixed width (e.g., 4 cm) were moved farther apart (e.g., from 10 cm to 20 cm), MT slowed. Participants appeared to need to take longer to move their hand over the extra distance if they were to maintain the spatial accuracy of their tapping. While these findings were interesting, Fitts's really important finding was that MT increased by a constant amount whenever the distance between the targets was doubled or the size of each target was halved. Furthermore, this finding was basically the same for all the participants tested. This meant that Fitts was able to predict, with reasonable accuracy, the MT of participants he had not yet tested, based simply on the width of the targets and their distance apart. Of course, not every task involving movement is like Fitts's tapping task, but since his research, studies involving different populations and different types of movement task have yielded findings consistent with his own. These consistent findings have led to Fitts's early observations being considered a law of motor control.

One explanation for Fitts's law, in simple terms, is as follows. An increase in the speed with which a given limb (e.g., an arm) is moved requires an increase in the impulse applied by the muscles to that limb; note that an impulse is the amount of force applied multiplied by the time for which that force is applied. A characteristic of the human movement system is that there is a slight and unavoidable difference between the impulse an individual intends to apply to a limb to make it move and the impulse that the individual actually applies to the limb. This difference can be considered error. Research has indicated that the larger the impulse applied, the greater the error. Now let us put these separate statements together: When humans attempt to move a limb faster, they must apply a larger impulse to the limb: The larger the impulse applied to the limb, the larger the error in the impulse applied; the larger the error in the impulse applied, the greater the inaccuracy in the spatial positioning of the limb.

While tasks involving simple movements like Fitts's tapping task offer the researcher a chance to study motor control under controlled laboratory conditions, these movements might seem at first glance to be of limited relevance to sport and exercise. However, simple movements form the basis for the more complicated movements made in sport and exercise and, as such, Fitts's law is reflected in sport- and exercise-related movements. For example, pole-vaulters take a long time to learn to place the pole tip into the box (i.e., the hole in the ground) correctly at speed; until then, they use a shorter approach, which affords a relatively slow approach run, to achieve an accurate tip placement. In addition, rock climbers who attempt to reach up very quickly to grab the next hold, because they feel their other points of contact with the rock are tenuous, are less likely to accurately place their fingers on the desired hold.

Hick's Law

Hick's law describes the relationship between the time taken to prepare a movement response and the number of possible movement response alternatives. In more everyday terms, the law states that individuals are slower to react when required if it is not clear *before* they are required to react exactly *how* they should react—that is, if it is not clear what kind of movement response is required. An example of Hick's law can be seen in football. Consider a down in which the defense is unclear about what type of offensive play the opponent is likely to run: When the ball is snapped, the defense will be relatively slow to react with an appropriate response. In contrast, if the defense knows exactly what offensive play the opponent is going to run, the defense will be relatively fast to react with an appropriate response when the ball is snapped.

In the 1950s, researchers William Edmund Hick and Ray Hyman studied reaction time (RT) using what has become known as a "choice reaction time" task. In one type of this task, the participant is seated, with one hand laying palm-down on a "response panel," and each of the four fingers of the hand resting on a separate button mounted in the panel. In front of the participant, four lights are presented in a row (i.e., horizontally) at head height. Each light is considered a *stimulus*, to which the participant must respond as fast as possible with a movement. Specifically, when a light is lit, the participant must press the button, from the four available, that corresponds to the lit light. Thus, if the leftmost light is lit, she must press the leftmost button with her index finger (if she is right-handed), whereas if the rightmost light is lit, she must press the rightmost button with her little finger, and so on. Usually, participants are unable to predict exactly which light will be lit or when it will be lit and thus are unable to initiate a response in advance of a light being lit. RT is measured as the time taken from a light being lit to the beginning of the participant's finger movement on the button.

In the choice RT task presented previously, there were four "stimulus–response" (S–R) choices or alternatives; that is, the participant could be presented with one of four stimuli, and each of these stimuli required a unique response. For example, when the second-to-left light was lit, a press of the second-to-left button was required by the middle finger. Hick and Hyman studied the relationship between RT and the number of S–R alternatives by presenting various numbers of lights associated with an equal number of buttons to be pressed. One study condition presented to the participant might feature two S–R alternatives, involving two lights and two buttons, whereas the next study condition presented might involve four S–R alternatives, as in the previous example. The researchers found that RT slowed as the number of S–R alternatives increased. In other words, when it was less clear how they would be required to respond, participants were slower to react.

However, Hick and Hyman's findings extended beyond identifying that RT slowed under these circumstances. What these researchers discovered was that RT slowed by a constant amount, which was approximately 150 milliseconds on average for the type of choice RT task described here, every time the number of S–R alternatives was doubled. Of course, RT was also quickened by this amount every time the number of S–R alternatives was halved. Thus, when a "one light and one button condition" was changed to a "two lights and two

buttons" condition, RT slowed by 150 milliseconds on average, and when an "eight lights and eight buttons" condition was changed to a "two lights and two buttons" condition, RT quickened by 300 milliseconds on average.

Researchers have found that Hick and Hyman's findings apply to different populations and different types of movement task, which has led to the finding being considered a law of motor control. One explanation for Hick's law, in simple terms, is that, when there are more S–R alternatives, the participant must process (i.e., think about) more information to be able to identify and produce the appropriate response. As humans can only process a limited amount of information in a given time, RT is slower when there is more information to be processed.

As with Fitts's law, the choice RT task described here might seem at first glance to be of limited relevance to movements made in sport and exercise. However, Hick's law helps explain performance in real sports, especially sports in which responding faster conveys a performance advantage. Consider a defensive team in football that knows the opponent's offense has two key running plays and two key passing plays and then observes the opponent's only ball carrier get injured so that running plays are no longer an option. At the line of scrimmage, the defense knows there are now only two possible play options, not four. In terms of Hick's law, the number of S–R alternatives has been halved, affording the defense a quicker RT (by 150 milliseconds) at the snap. Hick's law is also reflected in findings from studies of skilled athletes' preparation for upcoming competitions. For example, David Eccles and his colleagues presented evidence that skilled athletes gather information affording the identification of (and thus a reduction in uncertainty about) the types of stimuli that will be presented during a competition. An example of this process is when athletes and coaches in soccer or football watch game film of an upcoming opponent to identify patterns of play unique to that opponent or when kayakers and orienteers explore the river and forest, respectively, in which they will compete (under time pressure) to identify in advance the demands unique to these environments. According to Hick's law, these information-gathering activities, which reduce uncertainty about the types of stimuli that will be presented during a competition, lead to quicker RTs during that competition.

Conclusion

In conclusion, there are three well-established laws of movement learning and control: the law of practice, Fitts's law, and Hick's law. The law of practice describes the relationship between practice and learning; Fitts's law describes the relationship between movement speed and accuracy; and Hick's law describes the relationship between the time taken to prepare a movement response and the number of possible movement response alternatives. The relationships described by these laws apply to many different populations and types of movement in sport and exercise. The laws afford the identification of practice-related conditions that promote movement learning and predictions about how individuals will perform in situations requiring movement. As such, the laws are fundamental within the discipline of sport and exercise psychology (SEP).

David W. Eccles

See also Anticipation; Information Processing; Learning; Motor Control; Motor Learning; Practice; Skill Acquisition

Further Readings

Eccles, D. W., Ward, P., & Woodman, T. (2009). The role of competition-specific preparation in expert sport performance. *Psychology of Sport and Exercise, 10,* 96–107.

Ericsson, K. A., Krampe, R. Th., & Tesch-Römer, C. (1993). The role of deliberate practice in the acquisition of expert performance. *Psychological Review, 100,* 363–406.

Lee, T. D. (2011). *Motor control in everyday actions.* Champaign, IL: Human Kinetics.

Magill, R. A. (2007). *Motor learning and control: Concepts and applications.* New York: McGraw-Hill.

Schmidt, R. A., & Lee, T. D. (2011). *Motor control and learning: A behavioral emphasis* (5th ed.). Champaign, IL: Human Kinetics.

LEADERSHIP IN SPORT: MULTIDIMENSIONAL MODEL

An established model of leadership in sports is Packianathan Chelladurai's multidimensional model of leadership (MML). This model was the substance of a doctoral dissertation in management science. It represented a synthesis and reconciliation of the models of leadership found in the mainstream management literature. These preexisting models tended to focus more on either the leader, or the member, or the situation. However, as leadership is a concept that encompasses all three factors—the leader; the members; and the organizational context including goals, structures, and processes—it was reasonable to propose the model illustrated in Figure 1.

A unique feature of the model is that it includes three states of leader behaviors. *Required behavior* (Box 4) is the set of prescriptions and proscriptions of the situation in which leadership occurs. Required behavior is mostly defined by the situational characteristics (Box 1) that include the goals of the group, the type of task (e.g., individual vs. team, closed vs. open tasks), and the social and cultural context of the group. The nature of the group defined by gender, age, skill level, and such other factors would also partly define required behavior. *Preferred behavior* (Box 6) refers to the preferences of the followers for specific forms of behavior (such as training, social support, and feedback) from the leader. Members' preferences are a function of their individual difference characteristics (Box 3) such as personality (e.g., need for affiliation, tolerance for ambiguity, attitude toward authority) and their ability relative to the task at hand. Members are also aware of the situational requirements; thus, their preferences are influenced by those requirements. The *actual behavior* (Box 5, i.e., how the leader actually behaves) is largely based on leader characteristics (Box 2) in terms of personality, expertise, and experience. However, the leader would also be constrained to abide by the requirements of the situation (Box 4) and to accommodate member preferences (Box 6) as well.

Another significant feature of the MML is its *congruence hypothesis.* That is, the model specifies that the desired outcomes of individual and team performance, and member satisfaction will be realized if the three states of leader behavior are congruent with each other. Any misalignment among the three states of leader behavior would diminish performance and/or satisfaction. Further, if there is continued discrepancy between actual leader behavior and the other two states of leader behavior, the leader's position within the group would become untenable. The dynamic nature of leadership is highlighted in the model with backward arrows indicating feedback from attained

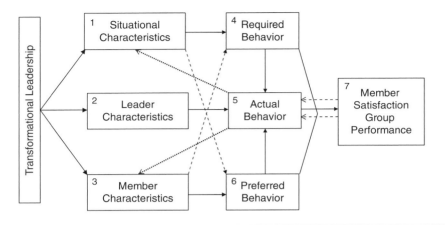

Figure 1 Multidimensional Model of Leadership

Source: Adapted from Chelladurai, P. (2007). Leadership in sports. In G. Tenenbaum & R. C. Eklund (Eds.), *Handbook of sport psychology* (p. 17). New York: Wiley. Used by permission.

performance and/or member satisfaction. That is, the leader may begin to exhibit more of task-oriented behaviors if she or he feels that the performance was below expectations. On the other hand, leader behaviors may begin to be more interpersonally oriented if it is felt that members were low on morale and/or satisfaction.

In 2007, Chelladurai made one significant modification to the model. It was the incorporation of the concept of transformational leadership into the multidimensional model. In his view, leadership exhibited by coaches is largely concerned with pursuit of excellence. In the process of pursuing excellence, the person is transformed from a relatively unaccomplished novice into an expert performer. Thus successful coaches do exhibit transformational leadership and, as such, incorporating the concept into the model was necessary as well as easy. In essence, the coach as the leader transforms member characteristics in terms of aspirations and attitudes and changes the situational requirements by articulating a new mission and convincing the members of the viability of the mission and their capacity to achieve that mission.

The idea (as shown in Figure 1) that transformational leadership influences leader characteristics (Box 2) would be most relevant where a coach has one or more assistant coaches. That is, the chief coach would attempt to transform the assistant coaches in the same way he or she would transform player characteristics. If there is only one coach, it would mean that the coach would change his or her own characteristics to fit the transformational mold and attempt to change the

situational characteristics as well as the characteristics of the members as indicated by the dotted arrows flowing from actual behavior (Box 5) to situational characteristics (Box 1) and to member characteristics (Box 3).

A theory is useful only to the extent that the variables of the study can be measured and the relationships among the variables can be verified. With this in mind, Chelladurai developed the Leadership Scale for Sports (LSS) to measure the three forms of leader behavior contained in the model. It is composed of 40 items to measure these five dimensions of leader behavior: *training and instruction* (13 items), *democratic behavior* (9 items), *autocratic behavior* (5 items), *social support* (8 items), and *positive feedback and rewarding behavior* (5 items). The response format is a 5-point scale ranging from (1) always; (2) often, about 75% of the time; (3) occasionally, about 50% of the time; (4) seldom, about 25% of the time; to (5) never. The scale has been used to measure athletes' preferences, their perceptions of their coaches' behavior, and coaches' perceptions of their own behavior pertaining to those five dimensions of behavior.

The psychometric properties of the LSS have been verified and supported in several studies. However, the subscale of *autocratic behavior* has been shown to be weak in almost all studies. One reason for such low internal consistency estimates is that the items in the subscale relate to three different forms of behavior—being aloof, being authoritative, and making autocratic decisions. Another conceptual issue that plagues the dimension of autocratic behavior is that whether a coach should be autocratic or democratic is dependent on the attributes of the problem in question. The items in this subscale do not capture the situational contingencies. The entry on "Decision-Making Styles in Coaching" (this volume) deals with contextual differences that indicate the degree of participation by team members in decision making.

There has been an attempt to improve the LSS by James J. Zhang and his colleagues. Their Revised LSS includes the five dimensions, the instructions, and the response format of the original LSS. It also includes a new dimension titled *situational consideration* behaviors. However, the Revised LSS has not been subjected to confirmatory analyses and the new dimension is subsumed by the original five dimensions. Therefore, parsimony would dictate the use of the original LSS.

Commentary

Both the MML and the LSS have been used and tested in several studies. Much of the research on the notion of congruence suggested in the model has been restricted to only two states of leader behavior—preferred behavior and perceived behavior used as a proxy for actual behavior. While the notion of congruence between these two states of leader behavior has been largely supported, it is disappointing that the congruence among all three states of leader behavior has not been tested adequately. Researchers could have omitted required behavior from consideration because of the difficulty of measuring required behavior. In his original research, Chelladurai employed the average of coaches' reporting of their own behavior as a surrogate of required behavior. Future research may consider asking expert coaches specifically about what should be the required behavior in a given situation defined by age, gender, ability level, goals of the program, and so on. The average of these responses may be used as required behavior in the relevant situation.

In developing the LSS, Chelladurai resorted to the leadership scales then popular in the mainstream management literature such as the Leadership Behavior Description Questionnaire (LBDQ). He collated more than 100 items from these scales and reworded them to suite the coaching context. However, he was forced to reduce the scale to 99 items because the computers available at his university at that time could not handle more than that number of items. He administered the initial questionnaire to members of the

university basketball teams in Canada and derived five dimensions of leader behavior through exploratory factor analysis. Subsequent research studies employing the more sophisticated confirmatory factor analysis has supported the robustness of the LSS. While these steps are acceptable, it is necessary to generate sport specific items, group them into meaningful categories, administer the questionnaire to different teams in different sports, and subject the data to confirmatory factor analyses. Furthermore, the LSS does not tap into the dimensions of transformational leadership, which has been recently incorporated into the MML. It is expected that future research will focus on refining the existing subscales and developing new subscales for transformational leadership.

Finally, it must be noted that although the MML was advanced in research related to leadership in athletics, the model itself is applicable to any context (e.g., business, industry, military) where leadership is a critical process. The model, after all, is a synthesis of other models from business and industry. Thus, reversing the process and applying the model to other contexts including business and industry is feasible. While the situational and member characteristics may vary from context to context, the concepts of required, preferred, and actual behavior are meaningful in any context. On a different note, Chelladurai included group performance and member satisfaction as the outcome variables. But other outcomes such as individual performance, individual growth, group cohesion, group solidarity, commitment, identification, and organizational citizenship can easily be accommodated in the model. Further, business outcomes such as profitability, market share, and return on investments can be used as outcome variables.

Packianathan Chelladurai

See also Autonomy-Supportive Coaching; Coach–Athlete Relations; Coaching Efficacy; Decision-Making Styles in Coaching; Group Characteristics; Leadership in Sport: Transactional and Transformational Learning; Leadership in Sport: Trait Perspectives; Team Building

Further Readings

Chelladurai, P. (1978). *A contingency model of leadership in athletics.* Unpublished doctoral dissertation, Department of Management Sciences, University of Waterloo, Waterloo, ON, Canada.

Chelladurai, P. (1993). Leadership. In R. N. Singer, M. Murphy, & K. Tennant (Eds.), *The handbook on research in sport psychology* (pp. 647–671). New York: Macmillan.

Chelladurai, P. (2007). Leadership in sports. In G. Tenenbaum & R. C. Eklund (Eds.). *Handbook of sport psychology* (3rd ed., pp. 113–135). Hoboken, NJ: Wiley.

Chelladurai, P., & Carron, A. V. (1978). *Leadership.* Ottawa: CAHPER, Sociology of Sport Monograph Series.

Chelladurai, P., & Riemer, H. (1998). Measurement of leadership in sports. In J. L. Duda (Ed.), *Advancements in sport and exercise psychology measurement* (pp. 227–253). Morgantown, WV: Fitness Information Technology.

Chelladurai, P., & Saleh, S. D. (1980). Dimensions of leader behavior in sports: Development of a leadership scale. *Journal of Sport Psychology, 2*(1), 34–45.

Zhang, J., Jensen, B. E., & Mann, B. L. (1997). Modification and revision of the Leadership Scale for Sport. *Journal of Sport Behavior, 20*(1), 105–121.

LEADERSHIP IN SPORT: SITUATIONAL AND CONTINGENCY APPROACHES

Shortly after World War II, Ralph Stogdill published a highly influential review paper in which he concluded that effective leadership is not derived through the expression of some set of personality traits but is invariably dependent on a range of situational factors that include the context in which leaders find themselves, as well as the alignment of various personal characteristics of the leader with the qualities, activities, and goals of those being led. In essence, Stogdill suggested that effective leadership occurs as a result of the interaction that takes place between a person and his or her environment.

Fiedler's Contingency Model

Over the next three decades (1950s to 1970s), a number of theoretical frameworks emerged that sought to examine the various situational characteristics upon which effective leadership is *contingent*. Perhaps the most widely studied situational or contingency model of leadership corresponds to Fred Fiedler's contingency model. Although the majority of research that tested this model was conducted within organizational units, it is

noteworthy that his foundational work in this area was conducted with high school basketball teams. According to Fiedler, leadership effectiveness is contingent upon both the leader's preferred style of interacting with others and the favorableness of the situation (also referred to as *situational control*). Fiedler suggested that leaders are typically either task oriented or relationship oriented, with task-oriented leaders primarily interested in maximizing goal or performance attainment among followers, whereas relationship-oriented leaders are primarily concerned with maximizing interpersonal connections with followers. Fiedler further theorized that the effectiveness of the leader's personal style (i.e., task- vs. relationship-oriented) is dependent on three situational dimensions that include the quality of leader–member relationships, the clarity and structure of the task and goals being pursued, as well as the extent to which the leader possesses formal authority and power. When each of these is maximized, the situation is described as being most favorable—or in other words the leader has the greatest amount of situational control.

The core tenet of Fiedler's model is that under conditions of high *and* low situational control (or favorableness), a task-oriented leader is preferable; however, under conditions of moderate situational control, a relationship-oriented leader is theorized to be most effective. Specifically, Fiedler contended that a more direct, task-oriented approach is beneficial when members have complete clarity in terms of what is expected and the leader has established authority as well as support (i.e., high-quality relationships) from those being led. Conversely, when teams or organizations are beset with instability and volatility (i.e., low situational control), Fiedler suggested that a highly structured and task-oriented approach would also be most appropriate to instill order out of chaos. However, within teams or organizations beset by moderate situational control (e.g., involving some goal or task uncertainty or diminished power available to the leader), Fiedler suggested that a leader who can adeptly manage the interpersonal relationships among group members would be most likely to evoke better individual performances, rather than a leader who takes a more authoritative task-driven approach.

Although meta-analytic evidence has provided some support for Fiedler's model within organizational settings, research in this area has also been the target of considerable debate and criticism on both conceptual and methodological grounds. One of the most vociferous concerns that has been leveled at work in this area corresponds to the assessment of leadership styles in these studies. Specifically, Fielder's contingency model was operationalized by measuring a leader's interpersonal style via an *indirect projective assessment.* Specifically, the least preferred coworker (LPC) scale involves the appraisal, by the focal leader, of *another person* (i.e., his or her LPC) to make an inference about whether the leader's interpersonal style is task- or relationship-oriented. In sum, the very nature of what a LPC score actually represents has been markedly questioned, and with it the validity of the model itself. In the context of sport, other than Fiedler's early work with youth basketball teams, only a few studies have directly sought to test the theoretical tenets of this model, and these have generally demonstrated inconclusive and mixed results. For example, in one study by Anne Marie Bird, members of winning (i.e., theorized to reflect high situational favorableness) Division II U.S. university volleyball teams perceived their coaches to be more task-oriented, and losing (i.e., low situational favorableness) teams perceived their coaches to be more socioemotional. However, the opposite effect was found for Division I volleyball players, where winning teams perceived their coaches to be more socioemotional, and losing teams perceived their coaches to be more task-oriented.

House's Path–Goal Theory

Another prominent situational and contingency model of leadership corresponds to Robert House's path–goal theory. However, unlike Fiedler's model, which focused on the effectiveness of personality factors that were contingent on the situation, House's model focused on the effectiveness of various leadership *behaviors* that were contingent on various situational constraints. Specifically, the extent to which leaders engage in four types of leadership behavior (directive path–goal clarifying behavior, supportive behavior, participative leader behavior, and achievement oriented behavior) was theorized to translate into effective leadership (as indicated by improved affective states, motivation, and performance among followers) but that these leadership behavior–subordinate outcomes were theorized to be dependent on various task-related situational constraints (e.g., clarity or ambiguity of task demands) as well as the attributes and characteristics of those being led (i.e., team member's preferences for independence). For example, path–goal clarifying behavior utilized by leaders was theorized to be particularly effective when followers experience role ambiguity but was expected to be a relatively redundant form of leadership behavior when followers are clear about their role responsibilities and task demands.

Chelladurai's Multidimensional Model of Leadership

Although research that directly sought to test the tenets of House's path–goal theory in sport settings is somewhat limited, early work by Packianathan Chelladurai and his colleagues found that different coaching behaviors are preferred in different sport contexts (e.g., closed vs. open sport) by athletes with different characteristics (e.g., males vs. females). Interestingly, Chelladurai built upon his initial tests of the path–goal model to develop his multidimensional model of leadership (MML). Specifically, the MML recognized that leadership effectiveness is contingent upon both the behaviors displayed by the leader *and* the preferences of the athletes being coached as well as the demands of the situation. Parenthetically, in addition to drawing from House's path–goal theory, Chelladurai also drew from elements of Fiedler's contingency model in developing his MML. Specifically, Chelladurai recognized that the behaviors utilized by coaches, and the effectiveness of these behaviors are, to some extent, shaped by the interaction of the coach's personal characteristics (e.g., personality traits) with the situational context in which the coach operates. In sum, the contingency and path–goal approaches developed by Fiedler and House, respectively, provided an important basis for Chelladurai's model, which to date has been one of the most extensively used models of leadership in sport.

Hersey and Blanchard's Situational Leadership Theory

The final contingency model described here corresponds to Paul Hersey and Ken Blanchard's situational leadership theory (also referred to as a *life cycle theory*). The core tenet of this theory is that the effectiveness of task- and relationship-oriented leadership behaviors is contingent upon the relative *maturity* levels of those being led.

According to Hersey and Blanchard, the extent to which task-oriented behaviors should be used decreases as the maturity of followers increase. Additionally, the degree to which relationship-oriented behaviors should be used forms an inverted U pattern, whereby at low and high maturity levels relationship-oriented behaviors should be used minimally, while at moderate levels of maturity they should be used more frequently. In workplace settings, empirical support for the life cycle theory has been mixed. In sport settings, the findings have been inconclusive at best and on a few occasions have been directly contrary to the theoretical postulates of this framework. For this reason, the life cycle theory has not generated much traction within the field of sport psychology (SP), although researchers and practitioners have generally recognized that coaches should adapt their coaching behaviors to the developmental levels (vis-à-vis maturity) of their athletes.

Conclusion

When taken together, the contingency approaches to leadership that have been developed over the past 60 years have provided an invaluable basis for recognizing that the utility of various leadership behaviors in sport is dependent, to some extent, on the situation in which leaders (i.e., coaches and captains) and followers find themselves (i.e., a *person x situation* interaction). Collectively, these frameworks have also played a major role in informing more recent (and sport-specific) models of leadership such as Chelladurai's MML.

Mark R. Beauchamp and Luc J. Martin

See also Leadership in Sport: Multidimensional Model; Leadership in Sport: Social Cognitive Approaches; Leadership in Sport: Trait Perspectives

Further Readings

Bird, A. M. (1977). Team structure and success as related to cohesiveness and leadership. *Journal of Social Psychology, 103,* 217–223. doi: 10.1080/00224545.1977.9713320

Blanchard, K. H., Zigarmi, D., & Nelson, R. B. (1993). *Situational Leadership* after 25 years: A retrospective. *Journal of Leadership & Organizational Studies, 1*(1), 21–36. doi: 10.1177/107179199300100104

Chelladura, P., & Saleh, S. D. (1978). Preferred leadership in sports. *Canadian Journal of Applied Sport Sciences, 3,* 85–92.

Fiedler, F. E., Hartman, W., & Rudin, S. A. (1952). *The relationship of interpersonal perception to effectiveness in basketball teams* (Technical Report No. 3). Urbana-Champaign, IL. Contract n60ri-07135 between University of Illinois and Office of Naval Research. Retrieved from http://www.archive.org/stream/relationshipofin03fied#page/n7/mode/2up

House, R. J. (1996). Path-goal theory of leadership: Lessons, legacy, and reformulated theory. *Leadership Quarterly, 7*(3), 323–352. doi: 10.1016/S1048–9843(96)90024-7

Klenke, K. (1993). Meta-analytic studies of leadership: Added insights or added paradoxes. *Current Psychology, 12*(4), 326–343. doi: 10.1007/BF02686813

Schriesheim, C. A., Tepper, B. J., & Tetrault, L. A. (1994). Least preferred co-worker score, situational control, and leadership effectiveness: A meta-analysis of contingency model performance predictions. *Journal of Applied Psychology, 4,* 561–573. doi: 10.1037/0021-9010.79.4.561

Stogdill, R. M. (1948). Personal factors associated with leadership: A survey of the literature. *Journal of Psychology, 25,* 35–71. doi: 10.1080/00223980.1948.9917362

LEADERSHIP IN SPORT: SOCIAL COGNITIVE APPROACHES

The core tenets of social cognitive theory (SCT) focus on the interrelationship among three sets of factors—namely personal, environmental, and behavioral. These factors are often described as being part of a reciprocal causal network whereby environmental, personal, and behavioral factors interact to determine a range of attitudinal and behavioral consequences. One of the key underpinning factors of the SCT approach is that it recognizes that human interactions do not occur in a vacuum; rather, they occur in an ever-changing environmental context, and this context influences the nature and outcomes of these interactions. For example, an identical set of interactions may produce one set of outcomes in a particular context (e.g., elite level sport) but different outcomes in another context (e.g., a youth physical education [PE] setting). Another key underpinning assumption of SCT is that humans are all different and that these differences will influence the nature and outcomes of their interactions with others. That is, an identical set of interactions will have a different impact depending on the personality of the individuals involved. For example, individuals high in self-esteem may respond differently to coach criticism than individuals low in self-esteem. SCT models of leadership that have been developed in the context of sport delineate the complex *social* and *cognitive* processes that influence coach behavior as well as the effectiveness of those behaviors on athlete and team outcomes. The major SCT models included in this entry are mediational model of leadership (MML), the coaching effectiveness model (CEM) of leadership, motivational model of the coach–athlete relationship (MMCAR), and coach-created motivational climate (CCMC).

Mediational Model of Leadership

The MML—developed by Ronald Smith, Frank Smoll, and their colleagues—delineates the complex interaction between person, environment, and behavior that typifies an SCT approach. The core of the model specifies that coach behaviors influence athlete perceptions and recall, which, in turn, influences athlete's evaluative reactions. One of the underlying principles of the MML is that the effects of coach behaviors is mediated through the *meaning* that athlete's give to their coaches' behaviors. That is, an athlete's appraisal of his or her coach's behaviors serves as the mechanism through which a coach influences that athlete's attitudes toward the coach and their sporting experience in general. For example, if an athlete perceives a coach to be supportive and helpful, he or she will likely have a positive attitude toward their coach and their sporting experience in general. These positive experiences will then likely lead to enhanced psychological well-being (PWB) (e.g., self-esteem), enhanced performance, and continued participation in their sport. Conversely, if an athlete views his or her coach as being overly critical and unsupportive, they are likely to form negative attitudes toward their coach and their sporting experience in general. This is likely to lead to a reduction in self-esteem, performance and reduced participation in their sport.

As a core tenet of this model, an understanding of the variables that can influence coach behaviors, athletes' perceptions and recall of these behaviors, and athlete evaluative reactions to these behaviors is critical. To this end, the MML identifies factors that are theorized to influence coach behaviors,

athlete perception and recall of coach behaviors, and also factors that are theorized to influence the athlete's evaluative reactions to coach behaviors. Coach behavior is hypothesized to be determined by three sets of factors including coach *individual difference variables, situational factors*, and *coach perceptions of athletes' attitudes*. For example, the MML hypothesizes that a coach's normative beliefs impact the way in which they behave. Coach normative beliefs refer to what the coach believes is his or her primary role. For example, one coach may believe that her primary role is to win, whilst another coach may believe her primary role is to promote personal growth and enjoyment. The MML hypothesizes that coaches with a normative belief of winning will display more punitive, authoritarian behaviors, and will be more regimented in their approach than those coaches who see their role as promoting athlete growth. The second broad factor that is theorized to impact coach behavior is situational factors. For example, current game status (i.e., winning, losing or tied) is theorized to impact coach behaviors such that coaches will tend to display more punitive behaviors when losing. The third broad factor that is proposed to influence coach behavior corresponds to coaches' perceptions of player attitudes. For example, a coach will likely behave differently toward an athlete who he believes has a contentious maladaptive attitude compared to an athlete who they believe has a positive attitude.

Athletes' perception and recall of coach behaviors are primarily determined by how coaches actually behave but also by a range of athlete individual difference variables and situational factors. For example, trait anxiety (TA) experienced by an athlete is an individual difference variable that reflects a dispositional tendency to selectively attend to threat-related information in the environment. Because of this attentional bias toward threatening stimuli it is likely that athletes with high TA will interpret a coach's behavior as being more threatening in nature (e.g., more punitive and less reinforcing behaviors) than those athletes with low TA. An example of a situational variable that might impact athlete perception and recall of coach behaviors is the pressure of the situation (e.g., practice vs. competition vs. championship finals). In highly pressured situations, athletes may become more aware of pressure-relevant cues in the environment, such as critical and controlling coach behaviors. As such, athletes are likely to report experiencing more of these types of behaviors in highly pressured situations.

Athletes' evaluative reactions of their perceptions and recall of coach behaviors are also proposed to be influenced by athlete individual difference variables and situational factors. For example, following on from the previous rationale regarding the influence of TA on perception and recall of coach behavior (i.e., perceive that her coach is displaying more threatening behaviors), TA is also theorized to impact evaluative reactions to these coach behaviors. That is, athletes with high TA perceive punitive coach behaviors to be more threatening than those with low TA. Thus, not only will TA influence the amount of punitive coach behavior that they perceive themselves as receiving but will also influence the magnitude of the effect of these behaviors.

Studies that have tested the tenets of the MML have found that coaches who display more reinforcement of desirable behaviors and effort combined with encouragement and technical instruction toward mistakes are liked by their athletes; the athletes have more fun, and athletes like their teammates more. Coaches' self-ratings of their own behavior tend to be uncorrelated with athletes' ratings of those same behaviors. However, athletes' ratings of their coaches' behavior are often correlated with expert observers' ratings of coach behaviors. Furthermore, supportive coach behaviors are generally associated with positive attitudes toward the coach, and punitive behaviors are generally related to negative attitudes toward the coach. Finally, team win–loss records have been found to be unrelated to athletes' liking of the coach. However, athletes' perceptions of their parents liking of the coach are related to win–loss records (athletes on winning teams perceived that their parents liked their coach more than athletes on losing teams).

The MML formed the basis for the development of a prominent coaching effectiveness training program by Smith and Smoll that was designed to enable coaches to relate more effectively to their athletes. This training program involves targeting (and modifying) coaches' behaviors in order to enhance the sport experience of their athletes. Five guidelines underpinning this coaching effectiveness training program are to (1) focus on effort and enjoyment rather than winning at all costs, (2) emphasize a positive approach to coaching, (3) establish norms around interpersonal helping behaviors, (4) involve athletes in decision making (DM), and (5) enhance self-awareness of coaches. This program has been shown to be effective in modifying coach behaviors, developing athlete self-esteem and enjoyment, liking of the coach and teammates, and reducing attrition rates in sport.

Coaching Effectiveness Model

The CEM, which was developed by Thelma S. Horn, is one of the most recent models of coaching that has emerged from a social cognitive perspective. The CEM, in some respects, can be considered an extension of the MML. Many of the predictions and pathways specified in the CEM are consistent with those specified in the MML. For example, both models highlight the importance of coach behaviors and athletes' evaluative reactions of these coach behaviors. However, the CEM also extended the MML by identifying and adding more explicit mediational pathways to the coaching process. These mediational pathways have been added to both the antecedents of coach behavior and the effects of coach behavior. For example, where the MML specifies that coach individual difference variables and situational factors can combine to impact coach behavior the CEM posits that the effects of these factors on coach behaviors is mediated by coaches' expectancies, values, beliefs, and goals. Furthermore, the CEM identifies that coach behavior directly impacting athlete performance has an indirect effect on athlete performance via athlete self-perceptions, beliefs, and attitudes. These in turn impact athlete motivation and performance.

The various linkages and relationships specified in the CEM are based on a wide range of theoretical models. For example, the link between coach expectations and coach behaviors is supported by principles of self-fulfilling prophecy theory. Achievement goal theory (AGT) is also used to provide a rationale for identifying factors that impact coach behaviors. Specifically, the CEM hypothesizes that coaches who have more of a task orientation display behaviors that are consistent with that task orientation and, for example, emphasize self-referent goals rather than goals that involve comparisons with others. Given that the core principles of the CEM are largely similar to the MML, the research that supports the main tenets of the MML also support the CEM.

Motivational Model of the Coach–Athlete Relationship

Genevieve Mageau and Robert J. Vallerand's MMCAR is premised upon self-determination theory (SDT) contentions. Similar to the other models discussed in this entry, the MMCAR specifies antecedents and consequences of coach behavior. The main difference of the MMCAR from the other models is that the MMCAR is almost exclusively grounded in SDT. In line with the principles of SDT, the MMCAR hypothesizes that the impact of coach behaviors on athlete motivation is mediated by the satisfaction of the three basic needs for *autonomy*, *relatedness* and *competence*. That is, the more coaches satisfy these three basic needs, the greater the athlete's self-determined motivation will be.

The MMCAR also identifies the coach's personal orientation (either autonomy supportive or controlling), coaching context, coach perception of athlete behavior, and motivation as determinants of coach behavior. For example, coaches' expectations of their athletes' ability are likely to influence the behavior that they display toward athletes. Specifically, according to the MMCAR, a coach who has low performance expectations of an athlete is likely to send messages of mistrust, emphasize mistakes, and ignore success in that athlete (i.e., exhibit behaviors that are likely to thwart need satisfaction). The MMCAR also identifies structure that a coach provides as being important in forming athlete perceptions of competence. Namely, structure in the form of specific instructions from the coach provides athletes with information by which to gauge their progress. Without sufficient feedback, athletes cannot experience progress, thus thwarting their need for competence. Lastly, coaches' involvement with the athlete (i.e., demonstrating care for the athlete's welfare) is theorized to make the athlete feel more related to the coach and thus satisfy their need for relatedness.

The MMCAR posits eight key indicators that are theorized to be consistent with the satisfaction of the three basic needs in athletes: provide a rationale for tasks, acknowledge athletes' feelings and perspectives, provide athletes with opportunities for initiative taking and independent work, provide

noncontrolling competence feedback, avoid overt control, avoid criticisms and controlling statements, avoid tangible rewards for interesting tasks, and prevent ego involvement in athletes. There is a large body of evidence that supports the core principle of the MMCAR that satisfaction of the basic needs for autonomy, relatedness, and competence is positively associated with the internalization of motivation. There is also research evidence that supports the notion that coaches who display an autonomy supportive style of leadership have positive effects on athletes, whereas coaches that display more controlling behaviors tend to have negative effects on their athletes.

Coach-Created Motivational Climate

Developed by Joan Duda and Isabel Balaguer, the CCMC approach to examining leadership in sport is grounded in the principles articulated in AGT. Consistent with the other models of leadership described in this entry the CCMC specifies antecedents of coach behavior (e.g., coach individual difference variables, situational characteristics, and coaches' perceptions of athletes' attitudes), and it also delineates the consequences of coach behavior via specific mediating mechanisms. However, the CCMC diverges from the other models in that all the effects of coach behavior are proposed to operate predominately through the creation of task-involving and ego-involving climates. Based on the work of John Nicholls, AGT posits that there are two fundamental higher-order goals—namely, task and ego goals. Task goals refer to goals that are primarily articulated around self-referent criteria and involve factors such as effort and improving skill level, whereas ego goals are primarily articulated around the demonstration of superior competence in relation to others. The CCMC model posits that coaches create climates that promote either task-involvement or ego-involvement, which in turn impact the types of goals that athletes set. The types of goals that athletes set (or the reference by which they evaluate their performance) have an impact on their own attitudes, motivation, and behavior.

A substantial body of research has generally supported the predictions of the CCMC. For example, task-oriented climates have been found to be related to a large number of positive outcomes, such as self-determined motivation, satisfaction, effort, enjoyment, persistence, team cohesion, collective efficacy (CE), and sportsmanship behavior among athletes. Furthermore, ego-oriented climates have been found to be related to maladaptive coping strategies, anxiety, worry, tension, and amoral sport behaviors.

Conclusion

The social cognitive approaches to leadership that have been developed within the field of sport psychology provide strong evidence that coaches play a significant role in shaping athletes' experiences. The models and theories of coach leadership that have emerged from the social cognitive perspective have identified in excess of 20 factors that are theorized to influence coach behaviors. These factors can be subsumed under the broad headings of coach individual difference variables, situational variables, and contextual variables. In excess of 15 coach behaviors have been identified with three different methodologies of measurement (observer rating, coach self-report, and athlete rating). The main findings to emerge from the social cognitive paradigm of sport leadership can be summarized as follows:

a. The coach plays a central role in influencing the athlete experience.

b. Athlete cognitive evaluations of coach behaviors are the primary mediator of the impact of coaches' behavior.

c. Coaches who provide their athletes with autonomy supportive environments provide positive reinforcement and structure, demonstrate care for their athletes, create task-oriented environments, and avoid controlling behaviors tend to engender positive outcomes in their athletes.

d. Coaches' individual differences, situation, and context play a major role in determining coach behavior.

e. Athletes' individual difference variables influence their perceptions and evaluations of their coaches' behaviors.

f. Athletes' individual difference variables moderate the effectiveness of coach behaviors.

g. Coaches' self-perceptions of their behaviors often appear to be incongruent with athlete perceptions and observer ratings of those same coach behaviors.

In sum, it is apparent that the social cognitive approach has been very influential in helping researchers and coaches understand the process of influence in a sport context. It is also apparent that the different models that have been proposed share similar features at a general level (e.g., they all specify antecedents of coach behavior and propose outcomes of coach behaviors) but differ substantively at a specific level (e.g., the specific antecedents of coach behavior that are identified, the specific variables involved in the coach behavior influence process, and the primary theoretical grounding employed). Finally, it appears that the coach has an incredibly difficult yet very important job in developing his or her athletes toward both optimal performance and PWB.

Calum Alexander Arthur

See also Achievement Goal Theory; Coach–Athlete Relations; Coaching Efficacy; Expectancy-Value Theory; Leadership in Sport: Trait Perspectives; Relational Efficacy Beliefs in Coach–Athlete Relations; Self-Determination Theory; Transformational and Transactional Leadership

Further Readings

Duda, J. L. (2001). Achievement goal research in sport: Pushing the boundaries and clarifying some misunderstandings. In G. C. Roberts (Ed.), *Advances in motivation in sport and exercise* (pp. 129–183). Champaign, IL: Human Kinetics.

Duda, J. L., & Balaguer, I. (2007). Coach-created motivational climate. In T. S. Horn (Ed.), *Advances in sport psychology* (3rd ed., pp. 239–267). Champaign, IL: Human Kinetics.

Chelladurai, P. (2007). Leadership in sports. In G. Tenenbaum & R. C. Eklund (Eds.), *Handbook of sport psychology* (3rd ed.). New York: Wiley.

Hardy, L., Jones, G., & Gould, D. (1996). *Understanding the psychological preparation for sport: Theory and practice of elite performance*. Chichester, UK: Wiley.

Horn, T. S. (2008). Coaching effectiveness in the sport domain. In T. S. Horn (Ed.), *Advances in sport psychology* (3rd ed., pp. 239–267). Champaign, IL: Human Kinetics.

Mageau, G. A., & Vallerand, R. J. (2003). The coach–athlete relationship: A motivational model. *Journal of Sport Sciences, 21,* 883–904.

Smith, R. E., & Smoll, F. L. (2007). Social cognitive approach to coaching behaviors. In S. Jowett & D. Lavallee (Eds.), *Social psychology in sport* (pp. 75–90). Champaign, IL: Human Kinetics.

Smoll, F. L., Smith, R. E., Barnett, N. P., & Everett, J. J. (1993). Enhancement of children's self-esteem through social support training for youth sport coaches. *Journal of Applied Psychology, 78,* 602–610.

Weinberg, R. J., & Gould, D. (2011). *Foundations of sport and exercise psychology* (5th ed.). Champaign, IL: Human Kinetics.

LEADERSHIP IN SPORT: TRAIT PERSPECTIVES

An enduring question within the field of sport and performance psychology concerns the origins of effective leadership (as displayed by both coaches and athletes) and, in particular, whether displays of leadership can be attributed to the emergence of any underlying set of personality traits. In the early 20th century, much research interest, especially within the field of organizational psychology, focused on the role of personality as a predictor of leadership. Following World War II, this interest receded considerably, largely in response to a prominent review paper by Ralph Stogdill. In this, he concluded that the development of leadership does not occur as a result of a set of personality traits but rather through the complex interactions that exist between leaders and followers, as well as the varied situations in which leaders find themselves. In short, he emphasized that situational factors are more salient than personality traits in determining leadership effectiveness and that although people might emerge as leaders in one context they may not in another.

From the 1960s through the 1980s (which coincided with the pronounced development of sport psychology as a recognizable field of study), a number of alternative paradigms to the trait leadership perspective gained prominence. These reflected a growing recognition of the role that social, situational, and self-regulatory processes play in the development of leadership. Indeed, during this time period, and as a reflection of research especially within the field of organizational psychology, interest in the study of personality traits in relation to leadership in sport began to wane. To a large extent, the diminished interest in trait approaches to leadership within sport can be traced to the highly variable and inconclusive nature of the research findings. For example, although some studies reported evidence that some personality traits were associated with improved ratings of leadership ability among athletes, very different patterns of findings were observed across many other replication investigations. It has been suggested that the failure to identify a clear pattern of associations between personality traits and leadership behaviors in sport was due, to a large extent, to the widespread use of conceptually limited and atheoretical approaches alongside deficiencies in measurement, which failed to explain how the extensive number of traits being measured might be related to the criterion variables of interest. As a prominent example of this, an instrument called the Athletic Motivation Inventory (AMI) was developed in the late 1960s, which was purported (by the authors of that instrument) to assess a range of personality traits associated with, and predictive of, athlete success. Specifically, the AMI was designed to assess traits that included "drive," "leadership," "responsibility," and "mental toughness." Following publication of the AMI, several scholars raised concerns with the use of this instrument (which was widely marketed for use in professional sports), highlighting that no published evidence for the reliability or predictive validity of measures derived from this instrument was ever provided.

Balanced against this backdrop has been a resurgence of interest in the study of personality traits and leadership in recent years, especially within the field of organizational psychology (interestingly, this interest has not been matched within SP). The impetus for this renewed focus can be ascribed to the general recognition of the five-factor model (FFM) of personality, which provided a unifying framework to organize the most salient dimensions of the personality construct. The five personality traits incorporated within the FFM include extraversion, neuroticism, conscientiousness, agreeableness, and openness to experience. In a prominent meta-analytic review by Timothy Judge and his colleagues, the personality traits subsumed within the FFM were not only implicated in the prediction of which people tended to emerge within leadership positions (i.e., leader emergence) but also predicted indicators of leadership effectiveness. Specifically, four out of the five traits (namely, extraversion, conscientiousness, neuroticism, and openness to experience) were found to be related to measures of both leader emergence and leader effectiveness, with extraversion demonstrating the strongest correlation with both criterion measures. When taken together, the five traits displayed noteworthy multiple correlations with both leader emergence ($R = .53$) and leader effectiveness ($R = .39$).

Unfortunately, only four studies included within that meta-analysis were conducted with athletes and coaches. As such, any inferences regarding the extent to which these effects might be evident in sport settings are limited. Nevertheless, it is entirely conceivable, for example, that those who "emerge" into positions of leadership within sport teams would be athletes who are more vocal and outgoing (i.e., score higher on extraversion). In short, it would be interesting to examine whether the same patterns of findings reported by Judge and his colleagues are also evident within the context of leadership in sport (e.g., team captains).

With the emergence of the FFM as a viable framework to understand leadership processes in sport, there is some recent evidence that the *concordance* of personality traits between coaches and their athletes is related to improved indicators of relationship quality. Specifically, in a study by Ben Jackson and his colleagues, when athletes were found to display a high degree of concordance (i.e., similarity) with their coaches in terms of extraversion and openness to experience this was found to be related to higher levels of commitment and relatedness among both coaches and athletes. Conversely, when athletes and coaches were found to be dissimilar on these personality traits, this was found to be related to lower levels of commitment and relatedness between both parties. In summary, and in spite of the recent dearth of research on trait leadership perspectives in sport, advances in personality science, including the widespread acceptance of the FFM, may have the potential to advance our understanding of leadership among athletes and coaches alike.

Mark R. Beauchamp and Luc J. Martin

See also Extraversion–Introversion; Leadership in Sport: Situational and Contingency Approaches; Leadership in Sport: Social Cognitive Approaches; Personality and Psychological Characteristics of Athletes; Personality Tests; Personality Traits and Exercise

Further Readings

Jackson, B., Dimmock, J. A., Gucciardi, D. F., & Grove, J. R. (2011). Personality traits and relationship perceptions in coach-athlete dyads: Do opposites really attract? *Psychology of Sport and Exercise, 12,* 222–230.

Judge, T. A., Bono, J. E., Illies, R., & Gerhardt, M. W. (2002). Personality and leadership: A qualitative and quantitative review. *Journal of Applied Psychology, 87,* 765–780.

Stogdill, R. M. (1948). Personal factors associated with leadership: A survey of the literature. *Journal of Psychology, 25,* 35–71.

Tutko, T. A., Lyon, L. P., & Ogilvie, B. C. (1969). *Athletic Motivation Inventory.* San Jose, CA: Institute for the Study of Athletic Motivation.

LEADERSHIP IN SPORT: TRANSACTIONAL AND TRANSFORMATIONAL

Over the past 25 years, there has been considerable interest in the application of the *transactional* and *transformational* leadership paradigm to understanding the effects of leadership behaviors in relation to various psychological (e.g., motivation, self-confidence) and behavioral (e.g., individual and team performance) outcomes among those being led. Originally conceived within political and organizational settings, the transactional and transformational leadership paradigm (also referred to as transformational leadership theory) has been studied across numerous domains of human achievement including (but not limited to) financial services, multinational project teams, military combat units, sport teams, and education. The basis for sustained academic inquiry can largely be traced to the seminal work of Bernard Bass, who differentiated between transactional and transformational leadership, as well as the subcomponents of those leadership dimensions. Broadly conceived, the essence of transactional leadership involves a series of exchanges (or transactions) between leader and follower, whereby leaders make use of rewards and reinforcement to foster compliance and encourage followers to meet previously agreed-upon standards. Transformational leadership, on the other hand, takes place when leaders go beyond their own self-interests and inspire, encourage, and stimulate others to exceed minimally expected standards.

Components of Transactional and Transformational Leadership

Transactional leadership is conceptualized as including both *management-by-exception* and *contingent reward* subcomponents. Management-by-exception includes both active and passive forms. Active management-by-exception involves actively monitoring the behaviors of those being led and taking corrective action when necessary. Passive management-by-exception involves waiting until problems become serious before intervening and reprimanding those being led. Contingent reward involves the clarification of expectations and providing rewards and recognition that is contingent on successful goal attainment.

In the context of sport, the active monitoring of athletes' competencies and actions and taking corrective action when necessary is seen as the foundation of "good coaching." Similarly, coaches providing praise and recognition when athletes perform well is seen as an important basis for bolstering their self-confidence and acts as an invaluable barometer, letting athletes know whether they are meeting their coaches' expectations.

From the perspective of transformational leadership theory, however, these transactional dimensions are theorized to be insufficient to maximize salient follower outcomes. This is not to suggest that these leadership behaviors are problematic. They are far from it. It is rather that the more active forms of transactional leadership (i.e., active-management by exception and contingent reward) provide a basis (or a bare minimum) for effective leadership, and in order to get the best out of those being led (i.e., exceed minimally expected standards), these transactional leadership behaviors need to be supplemented with transformational practices. Bass referred to this process as an *augmentation effect*, whereby the effects of transformational leadership build upon (and indeed supersede) the effects of transactional leadership.

Although a few different conceptual models have been advanced, it is generally recognized that transformational leadership is composed of four behavioral subcomponents. These include *idealized influence, inspirational motivation, intellectual stimulation,* and *individualized consideration.* Idealized influence involves—to use the old adage—"doing the right thing because it's the right thing to do." In essence, it involves acting as a role model, engendering the trust and respect of others, and articulating and acting on the leader's personally held value system. In sport settings, this might involve ensuring the coach practices what she preaches and following through on her words, even if it involves following the path of most (not

least) resistance. Inspirational motivation involves articulating a compelling vision of what is possible, setting high expectations of others, as well as displaying considerable optimism and enthusiasm about what others can accomplish. In sport, this might involve a coach conveying to his athletes, his philosophy for working effectively as a cohesive team, and also raising team members' expectations about what they can accomplish personally and collectively. Intellectual stimulation involves encouraging others to look at various challenges, assumptions, and problems from new and alternative perspectives and actively involving them in decision-making processes. From a coaching perspective, this might involve relinquishing some power and responsibility to one's athletes and having them become active agents in shaping adaptive team norms, strategizing, and developing group goals. Finally, individualized consideration involves paying attention to, and acting to satisfy, individuals' personal and psychological needs. In sport, this might involve coaches tailoring their training programs to align with each athlete's individual strengths and improve upon their weaknesses, ensuring that sufficient time is allocated to listening to their specific concerns or challenges.

Empirical Evidence From the Sport Domain

Although considerable research has been devoted to examining the transactional and transformational leadership paradigm in organizational settings, its application in the field of sport psychology (SP) is relatively recent. In one of the first studies to examine the external validity of the transformational leadership construct in the context of sport, Danielle Charbonneau and her colleagues investigated the extent to which perceptions of transformational leadership predicted motivation and sport performance among youth athletes. In this study, transformational leadership predicted elevated levels of athlete performance, and this relationship was mediated via elevated levels of intrinsic motivation.

Consistent with a core tenet of transformational leadership theory, research has also provided some support for the augmentation hypothesis specified earlier. Specifically, in the context of martial arts classes, displays of transactional leadership utilized by sensei (i.e., coaches) were found to be significantly related to three indicators of coaching effectiveness. These included measures of student satisfaction with the coach, self-report measures of "extra" effort, as well as student perceptions of coaching effectiveness. Most notably, however, the results of this study revealed that the effects of transactional leadership in relation to these three criterion measures were significantly augmented by the effects of transformational leadership in predicting higher levels of those same outcomes.

In addition to predicting enhanced individual-level outcomes, a growing number of studies have sought to identify the potential effects of transformational leadership behaviors in relation to group-level outcomes. Consistent with work conducted within occupational settings, elevated levels of transformational leadership have been found to be associated with improved task and social cohesion. In other work, conducted within the context of youth (ice-) hockey teams, when coaches were found to make use of transformational leadership behaviors, this was associated with a lower likelihood that athletes would engage in aggressive behavior. In this study, the relationship between transformational leadership and athlete aggression was mediated by team aggression levels. Taken together, this suggests that coaches have the ability to shape the culture and climate within a given team (in this case in relation to maladaptive or deleterious behaviors) and that this climate, in turn, can play a substantive role in shaping individual-level athlete outcomes.

One area of inquiry that has received considerable attention outside of the field of SP concerns the extent to which transformational leadership behaviors are shaped by heritable factors, early childhood experiences, or through intervention later in life. Some estimates, based on recent twin studies (involving comparisons of monozygotic and dizygotic twins), place the level of heritability in transformational leadership behaviors at just under 50%, which suggests that both nature *and* nurture play a substantive role in bringing about these behavioral characteristics. Although research has yet to examine the genetic bases of leadership behaviors among coaches and athlete leaders in sport, there is some evidence to suggest that the family environment can play an important role in developing transformational leadership behaviors among young athletes in sports. In a prominent study by Anthea Zacharatos and her colleagues, researchers examined the relationship between the leadership behaviors displayed by youth athletes and the leadership behaviors provided by their parents. In this work, parents' displays of transformational leadership were found to be associated with their adolescent children's displays of transformational leadership (based on self-ratings as well as ratings provided by their teammates and their coach). Furthermore, when adolescents made use of transformational leadership behaviors in the sport team context they were rated by both their teammates and coach as being more effective. This suggests that the home environment created by parents, and the manner in which parents interact with their children, can shape, to some extent, the development of transformational leadership among youth. In terms of the extent to which transformational leadership can be trained through intervention, this remains a question that has yet to be empirically tested within the context of sport. However, in organizational, military, and more recently within educational settings, a growing number of intervention studies have been conducted, which support both the viability and efficacy of transformational leadership training programs. In these studies, transformational leadership has been found to be amenable to change (i.e., trainable) and thus enhanced through intervention, resulting in improved cognitive (e.g., self-efficacy, self-determined motivation) and behavioral (e.g., achievement, performance) outcomes among those being led. In light of the moderate to large training effects derived within these studies, this would suggest that such intervention initiatives might have considerable value within the sporting domain.

Transformational Leadership and Physical Activity Engagement

Recently, researchers have begun to examine the transformational leadership behaviors utilized by teachers in relation to the behavioral engagement of students within physical education (PE) classes. While work in sport settings has primarily been concerned with the extent to which transformational leadership behaviors utilized by coaches might be related to performance-related outcomes among athletes, research in educational settings has primarily centered on the extent to which transformational leadership behaviors used by PE teachers might be related to health-enhancing cognitions and physical activity (PA) outcomes among adolescents. Recent studies indicate that when PE teachers make use of transformational leadership behaviors in their interactions with their students, their students tend to respond with improved self-efficacy beliefs, more self-determined motivation, and greater engagement in PE classes. Furthermore, there is evidence that when PE teachers consistently display transformational leadership behaviors in their interactions with their students this not only predicts effortful behaviors by adolescents within class time but, perhaps more importantly, also predicts greater engagement in PA behaviors during their leisure time. This finding points to substantive cross-domain effects, with PE teachers influencing adolescent behavioral engagement beyond the confines of the school.

Consistent with studies conducted within industrial and organizational settings, there is also evidence that transformational leadership behaviors used by PE teachers can be developed through short-term (1-day) training programs, resulting in elevated motivational responses among students. Transformational leadership training initiatives have typically taken a social-learning approach, whereby leaders are provided with exemplars of transformational leadership, opportunities to practice and receive feedback on their leadership behaviors, as well as make use of self-regulatory processes (e.g., goal setting) to maximize their sustained use of transformational leadership over time. In light of the omnipresence of professional development workshops for teachers, such training programs have the potential to maximize the quality of interactions between teachers and their students.

Conclusion

The transactional and transformational leadership paradigm has received a growing amount of empirical attention within both the sport performance literature and the field of educational psychology. Studies to date point to the predictive utility of the transformational leadership construct in relation to a range of adaptive athlete and student outcomes. Future work, however, is clearly warranted to test the effectiveness of interventions guided by transformational leadership theory, especially in sport settings in relation to enhancing coach behavior, as well as salient athlete–team outcomes (e.g., motivation, group cohesion, individual and team achievement).

Mark R. Beauchamp

See also Athlete Leadership; Cohesion; Team Building; Transformational Parenting

Further Readings

Bass, B. M. (1997). Does the transactional–transformational leadership paradigm transcend organizational and national boundaries? *American Psychologist, 52,* 130–139.

Beauchamp, M. R., & Morton, K. L. (2011). Transformational teaching and physical activity engagement among adolescents. *Exercise and Sport Sciences Reviews, 39*(3), 133–139.

Callow, N., Smith, M. J., Hardy, L., Arthur, C. A., & Hardy, J. (2009). Measurement of transformational leadership and its relationship with team cohesion and performance level. *Journal of Applied Sport Psychology, 21,* 395–412.

Charbonneau, D., Barling, J., & Kelloway, E. K. (2001). Transformational leadership and sports performance: The mediating role of intrinsic motivation. *Journal of Applied Social Psychology, 31,* 1521–1534.

Chaturvedi, S., Arvey, R. D., Zhang, Z., & Christoforou, P. T. (2011). Genetic underpinnings of transformational leadership: The mediating role of dispositional hope. *Journal of Leadership & Organizational Studies, 18*(4), 469–479.

Rowold, J. (2006). Transformational and transactional leadership in martial arts. *Journal of Applied Sport Psychology, 18,* 312–325.

Tucker, S., Turner, N. A., Barling, J., & McEvoy, M. (2010). Transformational leadership and children's aggression in team settings: A short-term longitudinal study. *The Leadership Quarterly, 21,* 389–399.

Zacharatos, A., Barling, J., & Kelloway, E. K. (2000). Development and effects of transformational leadership in adolescents. *The Leadership Quarterly, 11,* 211–226.

LEARNING

The ability to learn defines much that is unique about human behavior and underlies many aspects of sport and exercise psychology (SEP). Attempts to develop sweeping laws of learning have generally been unsuccessful, and it is unlikely that a universal theory of learning can be developed. Learning is often described as a process during which lasting changes occur in the potential that an individual has for a specific behavior. Such changes are a consequence of experience within a particular environment, rather than attributes of growth or development or temporary changes caused by fatigue, boredom, injury or even drugs or aging. Some authors define learning as a "biological device" that facilitates primarily adaptive changes that extend an individual's capability to survive.

This entry provides a much-condensed summary of learning as it has been understood over the past 120 years of study. Influential concepts and theories of learning are discussed in a relatively chronological sequence, and an effort is made to show how the theories culminate in recent approaches to learning in sport and exercise. Behaviorist theories regard learning to be an observable effect of the environment on an organism's behavior, whereas cognitive theories regard learning to be relatively permanent storage of knowledge as processes or representations in the brain. Constructivist theories consider learning to be the active construction of knowledge about the world. Jerome Bruner (1915–), for example, argued that learning is primarily driven by an active process of discovery about the meaning of information.

Learning by Association

A forerunner to any of these approaches, and probably the firstborn theory of learning, held that learning was a consequence of the formation of associations through experience. A person may feel pain on the first occasion that he or she goes running and thereafter associate exercise with pain as a consequence of learning the stimulus–response (S–R) relationship. Learning by association primarily is a function of conditioning. Ivan Pavlov (1849–1936) first demonstrated this as classical conditioning. By presenting food at the same time that he sounded a bell, Pavlov conditioned dogs to associate the idea of food with the sound of a bell. The dogs thereafter salivated when they heard a bell, regardless of whether food was present. Pavlov's work paved the way for behaviorism, as conceptualized by John Watson (1878–1959), who rejected subjective inferences about the influence of cognition on behavior in favor of objective measurement of external, overt actions. Watson argued that conditioning is the key mechanism that underlies learning in animals and humans. He argued that all are born *tabula rasa* (a blank slate), and the environment governs how each learns to behave. Watson (1930) famously claimed that the aim of psychology is "to predict, given the stimulus, what

reaction will take place; or, given the reaction, state what the situation or stimulus is that has caused the reaction" (p. 11).

Shaping to Learn

An important building block of behaviorism was provided by Edward Thorndike's (1874–1949) "Law of Effect," which states that behaviors are likely to be repeated if they are followed by favorable (e.g., pleasant) consequences but will eventually cease if they are followed by unfavorable (e.g., disagreeable) consequences. Thorndike showed that cats trying to reach a food outside a puzzle box eventually pressed a lever that gave them access to the food and that over trials they became faster at pressing the lever because of the favorable outcome associated with that response. In essence, the cats had learned from the consequences of their behaviors. Thorndike's work gave rise to operant (instrumental) conditioning, as demonstrated by B. F. Skinner (1904–1990). Skinner showed that behaviors could be modified by the type of consequence that followed a desired response. That is, a behavior would occur with greater frequency if it was reinforced and with less frequency if it was punished or even be extinguished if there was no consequence. Skinner also showed that behaviors could be gradually modified (shaped) by reinforcing iterations that approximated the desired response. Coaches often use shaping to modify an inappropriate technique in sport, or chaining to link appropriate responses together. A coach might use verbal praise to reinforce gradual increases in the height of the ball toss when a child serves at tennis, for example, and chaining might involve linking the ball toss to knee bend, followed by the swing of the tennis racquet, the snap of the wrist at contact, and finally the follow-through.

Many criticisms have been directed at behaviorism. For example, even when a behavior has been learned through conditioning, individuals, and animals, clearly can change the behavior if new information becomes available. Gestalt psychology abandoned the step-by-step S–R approach to learning in favor of an approach in which behaviors were seen to be driven by dynamic patterns of information available in the environment as a whole. But the great criticism of behaviorism, as embodied in Sigmund Freud's (1836–1939) psychodynamic approach, was that by considering only objective, observable behaviors, behaviorism ignored the influence of cognition, internal mental states of mind, on behavior.

Thinking to Learn

Cognitive approaches to learning differ from the behaviorist approach in that they define learning in terms of relatively permanent changes in organization and storage of information as a consequence of experience, rather than relatively permanent changes in behavior itself. Consequently, internal mental processes, such as information encoding and processing, perception and memory, and insight or intuition are seen to be key factors in learning, which mediate the relationship between a stimulus and a response.

Cognitive theories therefore try to account for the influence of internal thought processes on learning. Albert Bandura (1925–) proposed that internal psychological factors (the person), external observational factors (behavior), and the situation all interact to influence social-interpersonal forms of learning. *Social learning theory,* now called *social cognitive theory* (SCT), proposed that most learning occurred observationally, via modeling, and the tendency for a person to persist at it was governed by factors such as the person's sense of their own capability to carry out the required behavior effectively (i.e., self-efficacy).

Multistore models of memory that propose separate sensory, short-term, and long-term stores for information and multicomponent models of memory that explain how task-relevant information is temporarily stored and manipulated have provided a popular framework for examining the role of internal mental processes in learning. Evidence suggests that long-term memories (LTMs) present as rewired patterns of activation that require a process of consolidation to be laid down permanently, whereas short-term memories present as patterns of neural activation that are somehow prolonged by working-memory mechanisms such as subvocal rehearsal. Working memory facilitates a crucial component in most cognitive approaches to learning, which is verbal hypothesis testing about contingencies associated with actions, especially in terms of reasoning and problem solving. B. F. Skinner even delineated between rule-governed behavior and contingency-shaped behavior, because behaviorist approaches have difficulty accommodating the

tendency for humans to verbally mediate behavior. Skinner argued that behaviors that solve a problem can arise from direct shaping by contingencies (operant condition) or from rules that are hypothesized by the person solving the problem or from instructions provided by an agent with prior experience of the problem. In sport, a particular behavior may be shaped gradually by its consequences or by verbal rules that the athlete acquires by hypothesis testing or by instructions from a coach who has previously acquired the relevant information.

Conscious and Unconscious Awareness of Learning

An important distinction that arises from the cognitive approach to learning is between conscious and unconscious aspects of behavior, most recently approached within the context of implicit and explicit learning. Much of our interaction with the environment is implicit, resulting in accrual of knowledge without conscious awareness and sometimes without even intent to learn. Experimental studies of implicit learning began in the 1960s, when Arthur Reber used Markovian grammar chains to study the way in which participants learned knowledge underlying complex tasks. When participants memorized lists of exemplars (letter strings) created using the artificial grammars, they could distinguish between grammatically correct and incorrect exemplars that they had not seen previously, even though they were unable to consciously express knowledge of the grammatical rules that supported their decisions.

The double dissociation between performance of a task and the ability to express knowledge that guides performance of that task has been demonstrated using other paradigms. For example, in the serial reaction time task (SRTT), participants are required to rapidly depress keys that match positions indicated on a monitor. When the same sequence of positions (usually about 12–15) is repeated on trials, participants learn to anticipate each position in the sequence and thus respond by depressing the matching keys very rapidly. Few participants become consciously aware that they are responding to a specific sequence of key presses and fewer still can report the sequence, suggesting that the sequence may have been learned implicitly.

Implicit and Explicit Motor Learning

The conscious and unconscious dichotomy has been applied to learning in SEP in the context of implicit and explicit *motor* learning. Left to their own devices, humans display a pervasive tendency to acquire declarative knowledge explicitly when they learn motor skills. Usually, this knowledge is accrued by instructions from an agent (such as a teacher or coach) and conscious hypothesis testing during a trial-and-error process in which the learner makes attempts to move in a way that solves the motor problem. In particular, visual feedback about the outcome of each attempt is used to confirm or refute the hypotheses that are tested. Take, for example, a father and son at a golf driving range. The father may instruct his son to hold the golf club in a particular way. The son may use this grip but see that the ball travels to the left. Consequently, the son may try a different grip and watch closely to see if the ball travels in the desired direction. If the grip works, it is likely that the information will be stored as declarative knowledge for further use.

The ability to test hypotheses and store and manipulate information that can be used to make motor responses is made possible by the information-processing capabilities of working memory. Implicit motor learning tries to discourage hypothesis testing about motor responses or disrupt working memory storage of information that can be used for hypothesis testing, thereby limiting the amount of declarative knowledge that is accumulated during learning. For example, when motor learners carry out a secondary working memory task, such as tone counting or random letter generation, they tend to be unable to test hypotheses about the primary motor task that they are practicing. Consequently, they learn the primary motor task implicitly. Other methods devised in the context of SEP cause implicit motor learning by reducing the commission of errors during practice or providing reduced feedback about the outcomes of the movement. These methods prevent working memory involvement in learning by removing the necessity or the ability, respectively, to test hypotheses. If a performer does not make an error when executing a movement, there is little point in testing a hypothesis; if a performer does not become aware of the outcome of each movement, it is not possible to test the outcome of a hypothesis. Another method

that has been used to facilitate implicit motor learning entails presentation of a movement analogy (e.g., "kick like a dolphin"), which describes an appropriate technique by which to achieve the desired movement response, without the need to present explicit instructions. Analogy learning is only effective if the similar concept upon which it is based (a dolphin's tail movement) is understood by the learner. While it is unlikely that any form of human motor learning is purely implicit or explicit, implicit motor learning techniques appear to reduce conscious access to task-relevant knowledge and thus reduce potential destabilization of automatic movement by conscious thought processes.

Rich Masters

See also Adaptation; Feedback; Motor Learning; Movement; Practice; Skill Acquisition

Further Readings

Atkinson, R. C., & Shiffrin, R. M. (1968). Human memory: A proposed system and its control processes. In K. W. Spence & J. T. Spence (Eds.), *The psychology of learning and motivation: Advances in research and theory* (Vol. 2, pp. 89–195). New York: Academic Press.

Baddeley, A. D., & Hitch, G. J. (1974). Working memory. In G. A. Bower (Ed.), *Recent advances in learning and motivation* (Vol. 8, pp. 47–89). New York: Academic Press.

Bandura, A. (1986). *Social foundations of thought and action: A social cognitive theory.* Englewood Cliffs, NJ: Prentice Hall.

Bruner, J. (1960). *The process of education.* Cambridge, MA: Harvard University Press.

Masters, R. S. W., & Maxwell, J. (2008). The theory of reinvestment. *International Review of Sport and Exercise Psychology, 1,* 160–183.

Masters, R. S. W., & Poolton, J. M. (2012). Advances in implicit motor learning. In N. J. Hodges & A. M. Williams (Eds.), *Skill acquisition in sport: Research, theory and practice* (2nd ed., pp. 59–75). London: Routledge.

Pavlov, I. P. (1927). *Conditioned reflexes: An investigation of the physiological activity of the cerebral cortex* (G. V. Anrep, Trans. & Ed.). London: Oxford University Press.

Reber, A. S. (1967). Implicit learning of artificial grammars. *Journal of Verbal Learning and Verbal Behavior, 5,* 855–863.

Skinner, B. F. (1984). An operant analysis of problem solving. *The Behavioral and Brain Sciences, 7,* 583–613.

Thorndike, E. (1932). *The fundamentals of learning.* New York: AMS Press.

Watson, J. (1930). *Behaviorism.* New York: Norton.

LIMBIC SYSTEM

The limbic system is composed of a group of brain structures associated with various functions, most notably emotion, cognition, fear, and motivation. There is considerable variation in what structures researchers consider to constitute the limbic system, though the two primary structures of the system are consistently noted to be the amygdala and hippocampus. It should be acknowledged that the concept of the limbic system as the predominant view of the limbic system as the locus of emotional regulation of emotional regulation is considered by many to be flawed because it is overly simplistic. Some researchers in mainstream psychology have suggested that the concept of the limbic system be abandoned altogether. Nonetheless, the key structures of the limbic system (i.e., the hippocampus and amygdala) play important regulatory roles in behavior and may factor into some of the psychological effects seen with exercise. Both the amygdala and hippocampus have demonstrated important links with emotion, cognition, and the adaptation to stress.

The Limbic System and the Stress Response

Perhaps one of the main reasons that the limbic system is associated with the stress response and behavior is because of the direct links that it shares with the hypothalamic-pituitary-adrenal (HPA) axis. The HPA axis, hippocampus, and amygdala (along with the autonomic nervous system [ANS] and dorsal raphe nuclei) all respond to stressful stimuli. Furthermore, these areas also influence corticotropin-releasing hormone (CRH), serotonin, and other endocrine responses associated with stressful stimuli. The stress responses appear to be mediated through mineralocorticoid and glucocorticoid receptors in target organs as well as in the limbic system itself. In conjunction with serotonergic input from the dorsal raphe nuclei, the amygdala and hippocampus help integrate cognitive and behavioral responses associated with the HPA axis during exposure to stressors, including exercise. Neuroanatomic pathways between the hippocampus and hypothalamus provide for integration of metabolic, emotional, and cognitive information.

As further evidence of the link between the limbic system and the HPA axis, glucocorticoids have structural and functional impacts on the hippocampus. Marked impairment of cognition has been noted with chronic exposure to stress. Additionally, chronic stress induces direct changes in CRH and CRH gene expression in the hippocampus as well as a variety of morphological changes associated with cognitive impairments. It appears that exercise, along with other positive stimuli such as an enriched environment, can counteract these deleterious effects and promote neurogenesis. Optimal challenge or stimulation positively influences limbic system development. An inverse-U relationship appears to exist for the effects of stress on hippocampal function and structure. Stressors of a moderate intensity, such as exercise, effectively enhance hippocampal-related cognitive function. On the other hand, excessive or chronic stressors impair cognition and, as noted previously, produce negative changes in the hippocampus and related gene expression.

The hippocampus plays a central role in regulating cognitive and endocrine responses and adaptations to stressors, including exercise. Part of this regulatory role is derived from the inhibition that the hippocampus exerts over HPA axis activation. It is also important for terminating HPA axis activity following stressor exposure in order to promote systemic recovery. The hippocampus exerts negative feedback on the paraventricular nucleus under situations of high glucocorticoid secretion in order to decrease CRH secretion. Additionally, there is a counterregulatory influence by the glucocorticoids on hippocampal activity that results from acute stress. Under these conditions, the link between stress, the hippocampus, and the amygdala should also be recognized as stressors that impair the hippocampus yet enhance amygdala activation. This enhanced amygdala activation is particularly pronounced in the bed nucleus of the stria terminalis (BNST), which is a key projection site that has been associated with anxiety. Anxiety may manifest itself as such things as excessive worry and apprehension, physical tension, heightened cardiovascular tone, and, in animal models, freezing behaviors and decreased free-roaming.

Hippocampal Influences on Depression and Cognition

Dysfunction in the limbic system has been implicated in the development of depression and stress-related disorders. One of the mechanisms by which certain antidepressants appear to exert effects is through upregulation of neurotrophic factors, particularly brain-derived neurotrophic factor (BDNF), in the limbic structures. Further support for the link between the limbic system and depressive etiology is the fact that a number of morphological and metabolic changes occur in the hippocampus of individuals suffering from depression. It may partly be through this pathway that exercise exerts its effects on depression and anxiety. BDNF increases in the hippocampus in response to exercise and facilitates use-dependent neuronal growth. Despite the BDNF downregulation that is common during intense or prolonged stress, secretion is upregulated during exercise. Furthermore, there appear to be at least 33 exercise-regulated hippocampal genes, many of which are involved in growth factor and neurotrophic factor signaling and production. One growth factor in particular that is stimulated by exercise, VGF, appears to be involved in energy balance, synaptic plasticity, and has demonstrated antidepressant actions.

There is some evidence that brain uptake of insulin-like growth factor-1 (IGF-1) from endocrine or paracrine sources is necessary for exercise-induced hippocampal neurogenesis. Additionally, exercise helps halt the stress-induced efflux of glutamate from the hippocampus that can be detrimental to hippocampal structure and function. Activity-related increases in norepinephrine and serotonin may also have mediating roles in neurogenesis and cell proliferation, respectively.

The Amygdala: Emotion and Adaptation

The amygdala attributes emotional valence and arousal to external stimuli and integrates adaptive responses to stressors. The basolateral region of the amygdala integrates with the hippocampus to derive contextual information from stimuli. The centromedial area has projections to the lateral hypothalamus to help control blood pressure and projections to the BNST to regulate HPA activation. Because of these anatomical connections, amygdalar activation directly stimulates HPA axis responses and allows the limbic system to play a key role in regulating psychological and physiological adaptations to stressors, including exercise.

The amygdala plays a key role in emotional behaviors, fear conditioning, reward, and nociception. Much like the hippocampus, chronic stress can affect neuronal morphology and synaptic plasticity in the amygdala. This may be impacted significantly with exercise, though limited data currently exist to support this. The amygdalar CRH systems appear to be activated by stressors of a predominantly psychological nature, which may be related to cognitive interpretations of the nature of the exercise stimulus.

Shawn M. Arent

See also Brain; Cognitive Function; Emotional Responses; Mental Health; Stress Reactivity

Further Readings

Hand, G. A., Phillips, K. D., & Wilson, M. A. (2006). Central regulation of stress reactivity and physical activity. In E. O. Acevedo & P. Ekkekakis (Eds.), *Psychobiology of physical activity* (pp. 189–201). Champaign, IL: Human Kinetics.

LeDoux, J. E. (2000). Emotion circuits in the brain. *Annual Review of Neuroscience, 23,* 155–184.

Sapolsky, R. M. (2003). Stress and plasticity in the limbic system. *Neurochemical Research, 28,* 1735–1742.